Women's Sports Medicine and Rehabilitation

Edited by

Nadya Swedan, MD, FAAPMR

Consulting Medical Staff
North Shore University Hospital
Manhasset, New York

Courtesy Medical Staff
North Shore University Hospital
Glen Cove, New York

Medical Director
La Palestra Center for Preventative Medicine
New York, New York

Medical Director
The Physical Medicine and Rehabilitation Center
Orlin and Cohen Orthopedic Associates, LLP
Rockville Centre, New York

AN ASPEN PUBLICATION®
Aspen Publishers, Inc.
Gaithersburg, Maryland
2001

The author has made every effort to ensure the accuracy of the information herein. However, appropriate information sources should be consulted, especially for new or unfamiliar procedures. It is the responsibility of every practitioner to evaluate the appropriateness of a particular opinion in the context of actual clinical situations and with due considerations to new developments. The author, editors, and the publisher cannot be held responsible for any typographical or other errors found in this book.

Library of Congress Cataloging-in-Publication Data
Women's sports medicine and rehabilitation/edited by Nadya Swedan.
p. ; cm
Includes bibliographical references and index.
ISBN 0-8342-1731-7
1. Women athletes—Health and hygiene
2. Women athletes—Wounds and injuries.
3. Women athletes—Rehabilitation I. Swedan, Nadya.
[DNLM: 1. Athletic Injuries—rehabilitation. 2. Athletic Injuries—prevention and control.
3. Musculoskeletal Physiology. 4. Sex Factors. 5. Sports Medicine—methods. 6. Women.
QT 261 W872 2001]
RC1218.W65 W667 2001
617.1'027'082—dc21
00-050428

The front cover photograph is copyrighted by David Silverman and has been reprinted with permission.
The back cover photograph is copyrighted by Jane Wexler Photography and has been reprinted with permission.

About Aspen Publishers • For more than 40 years, Aspen has been a leading professional publisher in a variety of disciplines. Aspen's vast information resources are available in both print and electronic formats. We are committed to providing the highest quality information available in the most appropriate format for our customers. Visit Aspen's Internet site for more information resources, directories, articles, and a searchable version of Aspen's full catalog, including the most recent publications: **www.aspenpublishers.com**
Aspen Publishers, Inc. • The hallmark of quality in publishing
Member of the worldwide Wolters Kluwer group.

Editorial Services: Nora McElfish
Library of Congress Catalog Card Number: 00-050428
ISBN: 0-8342-1731-7

Printed in the United States of America

1 2 3 4 5

Dedication

To Mom, the first woman athlete I knew, and Dad, the first doctor. You always taught me to believe that, with hard work and persistence, all dreams can be achieved. I dedicate this book to you in return for the confidence you inspired as you encouraged and challenged me to be as athletic as my brother, financing one new sport after another. You never separated me from him in any activities and always provided me equal opportunity. I am so grateful for this because now as an adult I have the courage to try most anything; I am indebted to you for fostering this attitude and nurturing my abilities. Without these invaluable lessons and endless support, this book would have been neither completed nor complete.

Table of Contents

Contributors

Joseph T. Alleva, MD, FAAPMR
Instructor
Department of PM&R
Northwestern University Medical School
Medical Director
Outpatient Services
Evanston Northwestern Healthcare
Glenview, Illinois

Holly S. Andersen, MD, FACC
Assistant Professor of Medicine
Attending Cardiologist
The New York Presbyterian Hospital
Weill Cornell Medical Center
New York, New York

Michelle Andrews, MD, FAAOS
Orthopaedic Surgeon
Sports Medicine Specialist
Attending Physician
Cincinnati Sportsmedicine and Orthopaedic
    Center, Inc.
Cincinnati, Ohio

Marlisa Brown, MS, RD, CDE, CDN
Registered Dietitian
President
Total Wellness Inc.
Bay Shore, New York

Karen A. Carlberg, PhD, FACSM
Professor of Biology
Eastern Washington University
Cheney, Washington

**Gloria C. Cohen, MD, CCFP, FACSM, Dip Sport Med
(CASM)**
Sports Medicine and Family Practice Physician
Sarah Lawrence College
Health Services and Athletics
Bronxville, New York

Ellen Coven, MA
President
Fitwise Programs Inc.
Jericho, New York

Geoffrey Crowley, PT
Physical Therapist
Toowong Rehabilitation Centre
Toowong, Australia

Diane L. Dahm, MD, FAAOS
Orthopaedic Surgeon
Assistant Professor
Mayo Medical School
Consultant
Department of Orthopaedics
Mayo Clinic
Rochester, Minnesota

Carol Van Rossum De Costa, MD, MS, FAAPMR
Medical Director
Rehabilitation Medicine and Sports Services, PC
Brooklyn, New York
Assistant Attending
Mt. Sinai Services
Queens, New York
Team Physician
Medgar Evers College/N.Y. Sharks
Brooklyn/Long Island, New York

Kerry Gill DeLuca, MD, FAAPMR
Clinical Instructor
Brown University School of Medicine
Physiatrist
University Rehabilitation
East Providence, Rhode Island

Sheila A. Dugan, MD, PT, FAAPMR
Instructor
Harvard Medical School Department of PM&R
Director of Musculoskeletal Rehabilitation
Spaulding Rehabilitation Hospital
Boston, Massachusetts

Camille Duvall
Five-Time World Professional Water Skiing Champion
New York, New York

Mary Ann Everhart-McDonald, MS, MD, FAAPMR, FAAEM
Clinical Assistant Professor
Department of PM&R
Ohio State University
Attending Physician
Grant/Riverside Methodist Hospitals
Columbus, Ohio

Lorraine A. Fitzpatrick, MD
Professor of Internal Medicine
Director, Women's Health Fellowship
Mayo Clinic and Mayo Foundation
Rochester, Minnesota

Doreen Greenberg, PhD
Adjunct Professor
Richard Stockton College
Pomona, New Jersey

R. Norman Harden, MD
Director
Center for Pain Studies
Rehabilitation Institute of Chicago
Chicago, Illinois

Stacy A. Harris, MD, FAAPMR
Physiatrist
Annapolis, Maryland

Linnea S. Hauge, PhD
Assistant Professor
Educational Specialist
Department of General Surgery
Rush University
Chicago, Illinois

Sandra J. Hoffmann, MD, FACP, FACSM
Associate Professor, Medicine
Michigan State University
Kalamazoo, Michigan

Thomas H. Hudgins, MD, FAAPMR
Instructor
Department of PM&R
Northwestern University Medical School
Attending Physician
Evanston Northwestern Healthcare
Evanston, Illinois

Benjamin F. Johnson, EdD
Associate Professor
Department of Kinesiology
Georgia State University
Atlanta, Georgia

Karen Judy, MD, FAAP
Assistant Professor of Pediatrics
Rush Presbyterian St. Lukes Medical Center
Chicago, Illinois

Donna A. Lopiano, MS, PhD
Executive Director
Women's Sports Foundation
East Meadow, New York

Suzanne Meth, MS, ATC, CSCS
Athletic Trainer/Exercise Physiologist
La Palestra Center for Preventative Medicine
New York, New York

Carol A. Mushett, MEd, CTRS, CSW
Clinical Instructor
Department of Kinesiology
Georgia State University
Atlanta, Georgia

Alan Morris, DPM, FACFAOM
Attending Physician
North Shore University
Glen Cove, New York
Long Island Jewish Hospital
New Hyde Park, New York

Heidi Prather, DO, FAAPMR
Assistant Professor
Physical Medicine and Rehabilitation
Department of Orthopaedic Surgery
Washington University School of Medicine
St. Louis, Missouri

Kenneth J. Richter, DO
Medical Director of Rehabilitation Services
St. Joseph's Mercy Oakland Hospital
Pontiac, Michigan
Clinical Associate Professor
Michigan State University
East Lansing, Michigan

Nadya Swedan, MD, FAAPMR
Consulting Medical Staff
North Shore University Hospital
Manhasset, New York
Courtesy Medical Staff
North Shore University Hospital
Glen Cove, New York
Medical Director
La Palestra Center for Preventative Medicine
New York, New York
Medical Director
The Physical Medicine and Rehabilitation Center
Orlin and Cohen Orthopedic Associates, LLP
Rockville Centre, New York

Amie S. Ward, PhD
Assistant Professor of Clinical Neuroscience
Columbia University College of Physicians and Surgeons
New York, New York

Maxine Weyant, MD, CAQ, AAFP
Sports Medicine
Seattle Orthopedic and Fracture Clinic
Seattle, Washington

Foreword

Medical doctors (and others the public holds in high esteem and credibility) have a tremendous social responsibility to provide a balanced perspective on disease, illness, and injury. History demonstrates that they have failed to do so:

- In the late 1800s, when women were emancipated from the home by the bicycle, doctors wrote in respected medical journals of the dreaded disease "bicycle face." Imagining the pain of a female sitting astride a bicycle, they warned of a wrinkled face response and the permanence of such disfigurement. The effect of such warnings was to keep women away from this recreational sport.
- In the 1920s, after the first running of the women's 800 meters in the Olympic Games, an irresponsible journalist erroneously reported that all 11 runners had collapsed. In fact, nine ran, all nine finished, and one fell at the finish. Medical doctors followed with cautions about the lack of aerobic capabilities of women because of their smaller hearts, lungs, and circulatory capacities, and the event was dropped from the Olympic program. It was not until the 1950s that a women's running event more than 200 meters was reintroduced to the Games.
- Throughout the 1930s, medical doctors warned that high-stress sport would have a negative impact on a woman's reproductive system.
- In the 1980s and 1990s, medical doctors warned the public about eating disorders and the female athlete triad (eating disorders/osteoporosis/amenorrhea), which affected female athletes in the image sports of figure skating, gymnastics, and diving.
- In the 1990s, medical doctors suggested hormonal deficiencies and a woman's Q angle (angle between hip and knee) anatomical deficiency in support of the popular media (notably a major article in *Sports Illustrated*) heralding anterior cruciate injuries as the new scourge in women's sports.

The simple phenomenon of medical doctors giving their attention to these developments coupled with lack of balanced reporting in the media creates fear and has a deterrent effect on the participation of girls and women in sport. In all these situations the medical establishment made premature pronouncements.

It is so important for physicians and other health professionals to ask the right questions and consider all possible causative factors:

- What is the result of women not having access to the best coaches and not learning good mechanics in basic skills?
- What is the result of women not laying down a solid strength base early in their athletic careers, the result of not having the same access to weight rooms and strength coaches as their male counterparts?
- What is the result of less highly trained women at the high school level entering high-powered college programs, where they are immediately taxed at levels far beyond their physical strength and endurance levels? Is this producing fatigue over time that increases susceptibility to injury?

Similarly, physicians must ask whether gender bias exists in their profession that has an impact on how they consider the health status of women. Are the predominantly male medical and media professions too eager to reinforce the strength and dominance of men and dismiss the abilities of women in sport?

I travel all over the country as a public speaker. I love talking to high school boys because they reflect the male view before the veil of political correctness disguises their true feelings. When we begin these conversations, it is terribly important to them for me to acknowledge that males are better athletes than females. "Males jump higher, throw farther, run faster, dunk basketballs better, and are more interesting to watch than female athletes," they say, heads nodding in unison. They listen intently as I ask, "Who is the better athlete, Mike Tyson or Sugar Ray Leonard?" Initially struck silent by the question, they then respond with considerable chagrin, "That's not a fair question! Those are boxers in two different weight classes. They don't compete against each other. They are both great boxers." To which, I quietly respond, "Exactly." Why the need to have dominance acknowledged?

The point is an important one. Any examination of differences between the genders must (1) carry a strongly worded reminder that different does not mean "less than," (2) emphasize that the benefits of sports for women far outweigh any negatives, and (3) be grounded in sound hypotheses and research. This book is a fine example of such an effort.

WHY A BOOK ON WOMEN'S SPORTS MEDICINE?

Differences exist between the genders, experiential, social, psychological, and physiological, that must be considered when examining the female athlete. Female sport participation is a relatively recent phenomenon, such participation having been historically discouraged because of sex role stereotyping. Before 1970, a woman was allowed to be only a caretaker (wife, librarian, teacher, nurse, social worker), decorative object, or sex object. Today's standard is an active female who is permitted to use her body to compete, to demonstrate strength and endurance, and to pursue the same professions as her male counterpart.

Although she may not be as prepared as her male counterpart for elite level sport participation, as a result of not being allowed to develop the same strength base or to experience the same range of sports, this radical change is good for women's health. The sedentary life of our grandmothers and mothers that has led to one of every two women older than the age of 60 being osteoporotic is probably past, at least for those generations of women 40 and younger. Female participation in sports and fitness will continue to increase, led by the permissiveness of this stereotype and even influencing the activity habits of older women. Capitalism will reinforce the American woman's active lifestyle. This huge and lucrative market will be wooed by the sporting goods and apparel industry. So, the good news for physicians and other health professionals is that they will continue to see more girls and women playing sports and needing their services.

The bad news is that the primary contributing factors underlying female injuries in sports will not be going away any time soon. A dinosaur group is still making decisions about the employment of quality coaches for girls' teams, access to weight rooms, assignment of athletic trainers and promotions personnel, and the quality of athletic facilities provided to girls' teams. All these factors are related to injury prevention. Until these folks retire, women's sports in our schools and open amateur sports will experience a safe sport gender gap.

Girls continue to enter organized sport 2 years later than boys and with less experience and skill. Parents are still pushing their sons to be great athletes and telling their daughters that sport is when you can play with your friends and have fun. This "importance of skill" message must become consistent to both genders because the No. 1 reason children stay in sport is because it is fun. If you do not have skill, you do not have fun. It is simply no fun to strike out three times in a row. These cultural remnants of stereotyping girls will not go away overnight, and they will continue to have a detrimental impact on how quickly girls can overcome historical discrimination in sport.

These gender differences will be accentuated by non-gender-related factors. Boys and girls still have to contend with coaches continuing to hurt players because of the dominant philosophy that "more is better" and "no pain, no gain." We are in desperate need of a national system of coach training and certification. Not only will coaches continue their tendency to overtrain and overstress, they will do so without proper knowledge of biomechanics and basic exercise physiology. No change appears to be in sight regarding the continuation of a trend toward increased sports specialization, given the fact that college athletic scholarships and professional sport salaries are more visible and desirable as the "golden ring." Such single sport focus will continue to breed overuse injuries and must be condemned by physicians and other health professionals.

Fathers will continue to dominate as key influencers of female athletes (we are still 5–10 years away from the first generation of female athletes training their daughters), and girls will continue to be pushed as their fathers have pushed their brothers. Our children have an extraordinary need to please.

Maybe even more threatening is the fact that this and the next generation of young athletes will continue to seek ways of differentiating themselves and will explore ever more dangerous and complex extreme sports.

Both girls and boys will experience less developmental free play because of concerns for their safety. Organized play will simply not provide the balanced general, basic motor skill activity they need early in life. Children need both and they are not getting it. Few people realize that we have lost almost all our physical education programs. Only one state still requires mandatory physical education K–12 (Illinois).

We must also recognize that female athletes will continue to suffer from being forced into male model choices of sports. Over the last 20 years, schools have dropped women's field hockey and gymnastics because male athletic directors did not understand those sports or did not want to pay the salaries necessary to provide good coaches. Male coaches of male teams, who teach violence and aggression as the modus operandi of elite play, will coach girls and transmit this same message.

As the scholarship and professional sport stakes for female athletes become more apparent to both parents and their daughters, girls, like their male counterparts, will become increasingly susceptible to natural substance abuse. Fortunately, continued pressure to maintain slim and appealing bodies may deter female athletes from embracing steroids as a forbidden substance of choice—one instance in which the negative imperative to be beautiful may benefit women.

Another good news/bad news story will be that of older women entering the world of regular physical activity because of concern for their health and fear of debilitation. These women have little experience with rigorous physical activity and will need to progress gradually if their injury risk is to be reduced. Time will continue to limit women's participation in sports. If a woman chooses to add sport to her life, it will come at the expense of sleep. Her mate is not taking any responsibilities off her plate, and work has become almost mandatory for both men and women in our society.

The challenges are before us. A balanced perspective on injury and participation is essential. A strong emphasis and consistent message on the importance of exercise, fitness, and sports participation for girls are critical. Clear and specific instructions to parents and educators—in plain, unambiguous language—are essential. Knowledge about the differences between men and women and how those differences affect their sports participation, susceptibility to injury, and rehabilitation is critical. This is where this work begins.

Donna A. Lopiano, MS, PhD
Executive Director
Women's Sports Foundation
East Meadow, New York

Foreword

I was nervous and confident at the same time, not unusual for a summer Sunday morning for me. It was the finals, and my last regular season chance on the Water Skiing Pro Tour to wrap up a fourth consecutive year as World Pro Slalom Champion, take home some serious coin, and put the World Pro Overall title out of anyone else's reach (Figure F–1).

That was the time to rise to the occasion. I was slated to go head to head in the long distance jumping event with a woman I had been competing against all my life, Deena Mapple. I had beaten her a few times that season in jumping, which was her specialty. But, with a win in the jump event and a win in the slalom event, I would effectively put the title out of Deena's reach and would win my first World Pro Overall Title. The jumping event went well for me despite windy conditions, and I managed to eke out a win over Deena by just 2 feet. This set the stage for a slalom skiing showdown between Deena and me.

I felt ready to go after a win earlier in the day and, with the slight edge I held for the World Pro Overall title, I felt pretty positive. My training had paid off, and I was at my peak. With just three big events left, this event, the tour finals in Minneapolis, and the World Championships, where I was favored to win my second amateur world slalom title, I felt that day could be the start of something big.

The Oklahoma City site is a skier favorite. Many record performances have been recorded on this narrow lake with clean, clear water. The boat drivers were all in their grooves. Conditions and circumstances were ideal. But, as the men's events wore on, I could see and hear the flags and banners snapping in the dusty breeze; the wind started to pick up. On this particular site, wind speed must exceed 20 mph to mar the near ideal conditions, and it wasn't that windy yet.

My slalom draw pitted me against Deena in the first of the brackets. The winner would go on to take a shot at the Oklahoma City tour stop's slalom title. In water skiing's head-to-head slalom competition, two boats are used at the same time. One skier runs the slalom course, and as soon as the waves have cleared, the second competitor goes through the course at the same speed and rope length. We wished each other luck and leapt into the water. In the semifinal, skiers were required to start at the 28-off rope length, which reduced the normal 75-foot ski rope to 47 feet. Deena and I both completed these passes of six buoys easily. Next, we both shortened to 32-off, and we both made all six buoys yet again. The winds seemed to be picking up as I scanned the shoreline for flags that were beginning to snap in a wicked crosswind.

Deena started toward the course at 35-off rounding buoy one. With the rope only 40 feet long and the buoys nearly 38 feet out from the centerline of the slalom course, a skier only had 2 feet to spare to round the buoy. As she headed toward the second buoy, she started to get into trouble. With the wind blowing across the course, she had to ski directly into the wind, which created drag and reduced her velocity, causing a narrow turn. She was indeed very narrow into the second buoy and managed somehow to scramble around three, four, and five but had no chance to make the sixth and final buoy in the course. Her official score was 5 at 35-off.

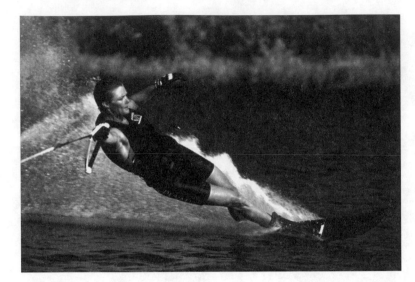

Figure F–1 Camille Duvall during Race Preparation.

All the women competitors on the tour could easily run this pass, so I knew that either the nerves had bitten her (not likely) or the conditions were rapidly deteriorating.

To win this bracket all I needed to do was get around any part of the sixth buoy. This would have positioned me for the slalom final and effectively put the Overall Tour title out of Deena's, or anyone else's, reach. I had the benefit of watching Deena's run, so I had a pretty good idea of how I needed to adjust to take to all six buoys at 35-off.

I signaled my driver to pull me out of the water. I visualized using all my power and an edge as sharp as a knife to ski against the wind so that I wouldn't suffer the same fate as Deena. I came into No. 1 and shot out of the buoy a little farther down course than I would have liked (Figure F–2). I leveraged against the red and white Mastercraft Boat with its 351 horsepower engine as hard as I could. As I approached the second wake, I heard the roar and felt the wall of wind slowing my progress out to the buoy. Buoy two was my good side turn, and even though I was narrow, I was able to at least stay in the game. I raced for the third buoy with the wind at my back and got pushed very far down course. I turned around three, and I knew that I had to hold my body position strong. As the rope snapped tight, I waited for the level 3 G-force and inertia to sling me to the far side of the course at 70 mph. Approaching the fourth buoy, I felt the wind pushing against me. I made an aggressive hard turn, but I was very far down course. I looked up and saw that I was not on the line to make it outside of the fifth buoy. Somehow I managed to get the tip of my ski around 5, and I realized at that moment, the sixth buoy was possible. I prayed that my 5'11" inch reach would do the trick. I again lowered my shoulder and leaned against the powerful speeding boat and felt myself rocket, in the space of about 45 feet, to 70 mph. I felt the

two wakes rush under my feet in quick succession like speed bumps. Now I had about a nanosecond to make my decision. I could play it conservatively and tie Deena, or I could throw my ski and body desperately out around the buoy. If I hit the buoy, I knew I was facing a hard slapping fall that would probably leave me sore and bruised. But I wasn't prepared for what happened next.

As I changed edge, I saw that the tip of my O'Brien ski was on a trajectory for a head-on collision with the buoy. I stretched out to the max, knowing that my right hip and elbow would start to skid along the water at any moment.

The tip of my ski hit the sixth buoy and bounced to the outside edge of the buoy, good for ¼ buoy! I didn't have time to think another thought; I was slammed to the water with the force of a tidal wave. I felt my right arm, which held the towrope snap backward, as if a speeding train had just hit it. My arm was now swinging wildly behind me, and I was a human torpedo diving a fathom underwater. My eyes were forced wide open, the sudden impact of the fall had folded my eyelids back. The water was so clear that I saw the neon orange buoy dancing in the water above me. As I struggled toward the surface, I realized I couldn't move my right arm. It simply felt like it wasn't connected to my body. My life vest popped me to the surface. I gasped for a breath because the intensity of the fall had compressed all the air from my lungs. But my main thought was to search down course to make sure that the boat time was good and I was given the ¼ of a buoy score.

The Mastercaft towboat quickly arced back toward me at the same time as the safety boat raced to me, and the safety swimmer jumped into the water beside me to make sure I was conscious. My driver, Jack Walker, who pulled me from the water more than once during falls in competition, asked,

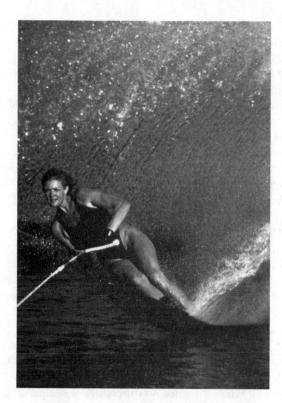

Figure F–2 Camille Duvall Fully Healed after Injury and Rehabilitation.

"Camilley, what happened to your eyes?" My lids were still folded upward, and as I reached up to try to roll them down an unbearable pain stabbed me in my right shoulder. I only wanted Jack to tell me what the official score was, that the time was good, and to get me out of the water. The official score came back 5 ¼ at 35-off, but the boat time was .001 slow! Which meant I had to take a re-ride or forfeit the win.

Competition rules allowed for a 3-minute injury break or more if the chief judge felt it was appropriate. I was definitely going to need more. The safety crew pulled me from the water on a stretcher and rushed me to the waiting ambulance. My brother, Sammy, and my friends crowded around to see if I was all right. I thought, "I don't want to go to the hospital, I just want to be checked and if nothing is broken take my re-ride." I could see the anxious faces of my brother and my friends peering through the door of the ambulance as the paramedics examined me. Diagnosis: slight concussion, no broken bones, but a possible dislocated shoulder. I was allowed to sit up and felt okay. But my shoulder was throbbing and felt very unstable in its socket.

The paramedics advised against returning to competition, but too much was at stake for me. I signed the release forms with my left hand (I'm right handed) and was let out of the ambulance. Then I managed, with the help of my brother and fellow competitors, to wiggle into my gear. The rules stated

I had to start my re-ride at the point the time went awry, that's the 35-off rope length. While I physically prepared, I mentally prepared; I justified the amount of pain I must endure to myself, "one pull out for the gate, one pull around each buoy. All told it would amount to only six pulls in pain. Was I ready to give up years of preparation and hard work for that? No way!"

I skied out of the water with one hand on the line, because I saved my strength for the slalom course. I pulled out for the gates and was shocked at the level of pain I felt. I started to reconsider my decision to ski, reasoning that maybe I did have a concussion or that I was crazy to do this. I edged through the gates and put my left arm out to turn the No. 1 buoy. My right hand came off the handle as usual but did not obey my commands. It was difficult to get my hand back onto the handle for the next "slingshot" pull. Somehow, I did it. I crossed over the wakes and changed my edge and started my reach for buoy two, which required me to reach out with my nearly useless right arm. I simply couldn't extend my arm to the side or even hold on to the handle. The catapult of my wake crossing and the force of the boat traveling at 34 mph in the opposite direction snatched the rope from my hand. No amount of willpower or mind game could will the handle in my hand. My body simply took over and said NO!

Fast forward home to Florida—the office of Dr. Michael Fulton, the US Water Ski Team doctor. Doc looked at my X-ray films and determined that, no I had not dislocated my shoulder, but as it had been extremely abducted, he placed me in a sling to be re-examined in 3 days. At that point, we pulled out all the stops with anti-inflammatory medication and electric stimulation, with the addition of the most aggressive rotator stabilization and strengthening plan my injury could take to get me to the point where I could ski at the World Championships in 3 weeks and defend my title. Of course, there was very little ski training to be done at this time. With the aggressive intervention of a cortisone shot coupled with steroidal anti-inflammatory dose pack, known as a "bute burst," at least I was on the mend, but my shoulder was still swollen and stiff. Dr. Fulton had exhausted every possible avenue for treatment at this point. During this time I was involved in a freak accident and was nearly electrocuted.

An electrical cord attached to our 500-gallon gas tank, used to refuel our training boat, had been accidentally damaged and managed to tumble into the lake at the edge of our gas dock. As I turned on the gas pump to help my brother refuel our boat, I grounded myself with 220 volts and could not let go of the gas pump. After what seemed like an eternity of being shocked to the point that every muscle in my body was cramping and I started to lose consciousness, I was inexplicably thrown away from the electricity source. I was rushed to a local emergency room and thoroughly tested.

Besides being tired and drained, my most serious injury was a subluxation of the biceps tendons to my left and only good arm! I went to US team training camp before the World Championships in England sore, unsure of myself, and with both arms dangling like a ragdoll's.

The freezing water temperatures of England helped to keep the swelling down in my right shoulder and with some adjustment to my style I could run competitive scores, but the pain was severe. Dr. Fulton and I made the decision to administer another cortisone shot, which of course would make the shoulder ache but dull some of the intense pain I was feeling. The entire team gathered round to watch the procedure and lend their support. In a stroke of luck, we managed to time the injection just right. The world preliminaries went well for me; I made the cut for slalom and jumping. Trick skiing was more difficult for me because it requires full range of motion of the shoulder, and mine was functional only to the front of the body under the stresses of skiing.

The World Championship finals dawned as a typical fall English day, temperatures hovering around 50 degrees and a slight foggy rain falling on Thorpe Park in London. With a team victory on my mind and defending my slalom title on the line, I was psyched even with the bad weather.

In the slalom event, I managed to put a seemingly winning score on the board only to have it bested by ½ a buoy on a belated re-ride by another competitor, which was requested after the event was officially over. It was an upsetting and unfair way to lose a gold medal in world competition, especially in light of my injury, but silver would have to do. In the jump event, I ended up with a bronze, a mere 24 inches behind the leaders. Talk about close! Ultimately, I pulled my share of the load for my teammates with my performances, earning team points for my individual medals: silver in slalom, a bronze in jumping, and a bronze in overall. The US Team's unbroken string of victories was secured before the men even took to the water.

Fast forward to the United States 6 weeks later. After intensive shoulder rehabilitation, we were not seeing significant improvement. Dr. Fulton ordered new tests. A bone scan revealed a broken humeral head! The humeral head of my right shoulder had been cracked like an egg in the fall in Oklahoma. The fracture had not been detected on conventional X-ray examination. It was amazing that I was even able to ski with what amounted to a break in the ball section of my humeral head.

Dr. Fulton referred me to Dr. Jim Andrews, founder and head of Alabama Sports Medicine, for a consultation. I found myself in Birmingham, Alabama, the next day and on the operating table that night! Judging from the photographs on the walls of pro athletes singing Dr. Andrews' praises, I knew I was in the best of hands. The state-of-the-art operating theater at Alabama Sports Medicine has seen the likes of Roger Clemens, Bo Jackson, and many other top-flight athletes.

After examining me and repeating the bone scan, Dr. Andrews planned to shave off the calcium deposit that had formed along the break, which was healing, and take off the rough edges of my torn rotator cuff. My husband watched the operation from behind the glass while Dr. Andrews chatted with him throughout the procedure. After he completed the main procedure, he used his scope to get an inside look at the rest of my shoulder and found a small bony hook at the end of the acromion. He promptly asked my husband if he thought I would want to have it removed to have a greater range of motion.

"I hate to play God with a World Champion, but I think we can make her even better than ever," said Andrews. "What do you think? I need your permission to do the additional procedure." Byron told him with a laugh, "If she wakes up and finds out you could have made her better than before and didn't do it, Dr. Andrews, then the only question will be which one of us she tries to kill first!"

Dr. Andrews is a big believer in perfecting your personal rehabilitation procedure before your operation; he knows the kind of dedication professional athletes have to their sport, and rehab is treated no differently at Alabama Sports Medicine. As tough as any coach, the staff push an athlete through range of motion and guide each exercise until all are perfect. I found out myself soon enough. In the morning, less than 12 hours after my operation, my husband came to visit me and I was not in my room. Thinking something had gone wrong, he rushed to the nurses' station for information. The nurse simply smiled and told him I was already in rehab! My husband found me sweating away in the rehab room with my hand in a pulley raising my arm over my head.

I was extremely fortunate to have the highest level of aggressive sports medicine care during the mid 80s, a time when typically that type of care was offered to male athletes only. I believe this was due to the lack of female professional athletes. If you weren't making your living in your sport, you received the least aggressive course of treatment. After all, who needs a perfect shoulder to drive the kids to hockey practice? I was treated with the newest techniques, and it made a huge difference in my life. I recovered from a potentially career-ending injury and went on to become World Pro Slalom Champion for a fifth time. And to this day, I stay in touch with and think fondly of Dr. Fulton and Dr. Andrews for believing in me and treating me as a serious, real athlete with a will to win.

After I retired from skiing in 1993 due to a collapsed vertebral artery, I tried my hand at sports broadcasting, another male-dominated profession. I do believe that my experiences hanging around the locker room with guys allowed me to come to the job with a different perspective than a woman who had not competed in sports. In fact, my first job outside of water skiing was at the X-games, which led to my hosting the outdoor ESPN adventure show *Men's Journal*. This show required athletic talent to interview rock climbers on third pitch of a multipitch rock climb at 1,500 feet, white-water raft the mighty Futalfu river in Chile, and bike trek 50 miles across the floor of Death Valley in June! Of course, my personal favorite is sideline reporting for the WNBA. Having been an athlete on that level, I have an idea of what players are going through. The past 2 years I've also spent acquiring my broadcasting certificate from New York University; this included a live television internship working with New York Knicks, Rangers, and Yankees. All of this required *some* dedication with the busy lives of my two young children, for whom I am an active hockey mom. I know I am a better mom with all this experience, and my kids appreciate my athleticism.

All in all, I'd say that the discipline of sports carries over into my everyday existence, from the values I try to instill in my children for sports, to the way I prep for sideline reporting for the WNBA, and even preparing myself for yoga class. I can't think of one negative aspect of being an athlete.

Camille Duvall
Five-Time World Professional Water Skiing Champion
New York, New York

Preface

Humans have always admired physical strength, speed, agility, and athletic prowess. Still, only recently has society openly nurtured and admired these qualities in women. Gender equality is still not fully established, and on the health and fitness front, a focus on women's sports medicine is still evolving. The multidimensional health benefits of athletic involvement cannot be substituted; however, associated medical and musculoskeletal impairments can occur. With the increasing involvement of women in all types of exercise activities, trends are being realized.

Our role as health care professionals is to identify and educate those susceptible to specific health and injury risks, including social, psychological, physiological, and musculoskeletal. These are unique to sports and individuals. In response to the demands of female athletes, education and medical and musculoskeletal research is becoming more gender specific. Historically, society has admired women involved in aesthetic sports, as girls idolized gymnast Nadia Comaneci, swimmer Donna de Varona, and figure skater Dorothy Hamill. With sleek, lithe physiques, they performed graceful, athletic, noncontact activities, with minimal and close-fitting dress. Unfortunately, these sports are those with the greatest rates of eating disorders, menstrual disorders, and even stress fractures. Often, strict diets and rigid overtraining are encouraged by coaches, judges, and parents. We now are aware of the measurable physiological and psychological morbidity and mortality that can be a consequence of such early discipline.

Fortunately, the publicity, popularity, and success of women's sports teams, including soccer and basketball, exemplify a healthier ideal for the desired female physique. The physical qualities of well-fed and trained muscular athleticism are now recognized as beautiful, and also give function to form. Gender-specific fitness and sports magazines now include *Sports Illustrated for Women*, *Golf for Women*, *Outdoor Magazine for Women*, *Muscle and Fitness for Women*, and *Skiing for Women*, exemplifying the acceptance of female athletes at all levels. Fashion models now include athletes such as Gabrielle Reece, world class beach volleyball player, Rebecca Lobo of the WNBA, and Anna Kournikova, pro tennis player. Young girls now have team sports idols and grow up playing multiple sports including soccer, softball, field hockey, and martial arts. It is refreshing to hear girls recite their school sports in lists of threes, one for each season.

The acceptance and encouragement of girls in all types of athletics have improved fitness and health of women overall. Still, in all athletics, acute and chronic injuries do occur. Appropriate diagnosis, treatment, rehabilitation, and prevention are the cornerstones to injury management. Knowledge of training and sports activities is essential to assisting athletes at all levels; personal involvement in athletics is ideal.

This book sums up all that is important to me. To be a well-rounded physician and athlete has been a lifelong and ongoing vision. From early years in the pool learning discipline, endurance, and team spirit; high school years playing varsity tennis and swimming; and collegiate years of varsity crew; to medical school years teaching aerobics and recent summer competing in triathlons, I have developed and maintained insight to all levels of athleticism. As a physiatrist I cherish the holistic aspects of health and wellness, and continuously exemplify and encourage balanced exercise and injury prevention. As a person I fill my leisure time with tennis, golf, skiing, running, biking, and swimming, and I delight in trying new sports.

It is my honor to be able to present this text. Most contributors are also women with personal involvement in athletics, providing the motivation to research and write this text with discipline, perseverance, heart, and soul. All are thrilled to contribute to the field of women's sports medicine, assisting health care professionals to optimally evaluate, treat, and rehabilitate women at all levels of athletic involvement. I can now smile proudly in reflecting back when I was told, by a prominent physician, that women could not be in sports medicine because they are not allowed in locker rooms.

This text may be read as a book, or used as a reference. It is designed to be practical and informative. Regardless, it is expected that it assists, enlightens, and challenges your knowledge of women's sports medicine, rehabilitation, health promotion, and injury prevention.

Acknowledgments

A contributed book such as this is a collaboration of immeasurable human talents and time, and I hope to offer some insight for the reader to appreciate all the invaluable assistance I have been fortunate to receive. To begin, this book would have never existed without the vision and expertise of Amy Martin of Aspen Publishers, Inc.; an athlete herself, she had the confidence in me and ability to make this book a reality. Also at Aspen, thanks to Mary Anne Langdon and Nora McElfish.

I am honored to have a foreword by Donna Lopiano, executive director of the Women's Sports Foundation (WSF), and recognized pioneer in developing equality in female athletics. I credit the WSF as an endless library of information and member list of women who cherish female athletes. They are at the forefront of research and development essential to women in sports. Also active in the WSF and women's sports, world champion water skier Camille Duvall is gratefully acknowledged for her foreword providing insight on injury in competition.

Thanks to Daniel Kron, founder of SportsForWomen.com, for sharing resources and introducing me to contributors. Thank you to U.S. Olympic Center Information Specialist Patricia Olkiewicz, and at Brown University, Sports Information Director Christopher Humm; both donated invaluable photographs. I am ever grateful to Pat Manocchia and Erik Stevens and the staff and members of La Palestra, a health and fitness center fostering a wealth of wisdom and experience.

Thank you to gracious models Shannon Malone DeScarfino, Jenifer Silverman, Carol Silver, and Colleen Lange. Thanks to Judy Donahue and Kofi Sekyi Amah for their generous offer of time and photography talents. Thank you to Ellen Schoniger for inspiring photos of her athletic daughter. Thank you to physical therapists Jennifer Russo and Maya Poinar for practical insight on rehabilitation.

My contributions would never have been as well researched without the help of Kate Zippert at North Shore University Manhasset's library. At The Physical Medicine and Rehabilitation Center, thanks to the staff and therapists who contributed time in their busy schedules. Special thanks to my assistant, Diane Hamsley.

I am blessed with the best in family, friends, and peers, without whom this would never have been achieved. Special thanks to Marla Bobowick; as my dearest friend and mentor, your wisdom, experience, and insight into book creation have been invaluable. Friends who supported me with additional medical insight and vision include Dr. Jake Elliott, Dr. John McIntyre, and especially Dr. Dan Brzusek, who identified the need for women to treat women, and encouraged and facilitated my first presentations on the female athlete. Thank you to my parents for their endless encouragement and support and to my brother for being the most challenging athletic companion while growing up. Thank you to Rob, for understanding my time restrictions, providing endless encouragement, and helping with crucial technological assistance.

I am grateful for the encouragement and support I have received endlessly since my residency at the Rehabilitation Institute of Chicago. Specifically, I thank Dr. Henry Betts, Dr. James Sliwa, Dr. James Kelly, Dr. John McGuire, and Dr. Elliot Roth, who fostered the academic physiatrist in me; Dr. Joel Press and Dr. Jeff Young taught me the best of musculoskeletal medicine. All set high standards that remain with me daily.

Finally, thank you to the contributors, without whose hard work, insight, and enthusiasm this book would have been impossible. Most importantly, I acknowledge the past and present contributions of girl and women athletes at all levels, working hard for health, fitness, self-respect, recognition, and equality.

Introduction
The Evolution of the Female Athlete

"The tragedy in life is not reaching your goal; it's not having a goal to reach."

Willye White, five-time Olympian and medalist, track and field

---

A textbook on women's sports medicine cannot be limited only to women who are active in "sports." Although the number of professional and elite women athletes competitive in organized athletics continues to grow, the field of sports medicine must accommodate both genders and new types of activities. Women are frequently involved in both aerobic and nonaerobic activities, which are not necessarily competitive sports but still require physical stamina, strength, and discipline. These "nonsports" athletic activities include walking, hiking, aerobics, dance, exercise classes, personal training, inline and ice skating, martial arts, yoga, and Pilates. All types of musculoskeletal repetitive activity with exertion not only enhance women's health and well-being, but also challenge it with acute and chronic injuries, eating disorders, and stress-related illnesses. Just as sports health differences between genders are both subtle and direct, research to date has been both detailed and limited. This book presents current insights, original and researched, on women in sports with guidelines toward developing the optimum sports health plan. The following historical reflection on the evolution of female athletes today will provide a foundation to the personality and cultural differences that are as important to health and well-being as the physiological and anatomical differences.

HISTORY OF THE FEMALE ATHLETE

Prior to the recent days of athleticism, middle- and upper-class women were cherished for pale skin, absence of musculature, and frailty. This was a social status symbol. They were identified as childbearers and wives, and it was society's, even medicine's, belief that strenuous activity challenged childbearing. The cultural ideals of fashion and motherhood strongly opposed physical activity. Women were discouraged from going outdoors and wore corsets that applied up to 21 pounds of pressure on their abdomen to narrow their waists.[1(p 264)] Toward the late Victorian era, women were gradually allowed to participate in "skirt sports," such as archery, croquet, bowling, tennis, golf, and bathing (swimming in a wooden box rolled into the water). All activities required full-body concealment, and exertion was not allowed. Still, this was the beginning of sport as socialization.

Unfortunately, the Victorian voice of physicians upheld society's misguided prohibitions, reflecting the conservative tone of medicine in general. Middle-class and upper-class women were regarded as frail creatures whose health centered around their uterus. Doctors visited women frequently in their homes and described menstruation as illness, during which time no physical activity should take place. Exercise was thought to compromise a woman's health and ability to bear children.[2(p 76)] These conservative medical recommendations persisted through the first half of the century. A highly publicized 1936 *Scientific American* article suggested that muscular development interferes with motherhood;[3] after World War II, the Amateur Athletic Union supported and publicized a study that concluded with a female doctor's quote that athletic competition during menstruation can hinder a woman from "being a normal mother."[1(p 270)] Dr. Spock, in his book on parenting and motherhood, also shifted the focus away from women as athletes.

Still, this was a time of paradox for women. Those who were not middle or upper class toiled in the fields, chopped wood, and built homes, performing more intense physical labor than many men. Slave women worked as hard as men, and, still, these women had children. For the middle-class and upper-class women, the "safety bicycle" of 1885 (with front and back wheel of even height) provided an initial step in allowing women more freedom and acceptance in physical activity.[4] The bicycle symbolized not only physical freedom, by providing a self-powered mode of transportation, but also psychological freedom, by allowing independence of transportation. To accommodate, bloomers became acceptable, beginning a new functional trend in fashion. Single sex educational settings provided environments and opportunities for athleticism. Banned not only from competing in, but often from spectating mens' sports, women developed their own events. The first all-female track meet was held in 1895 at Vassar,[5(p 4)] and other colleges soon followed.

Despite prevalent taboos on physical activity of middle-class and upper-class women, industry recognized the sociological and psychological benefits of exercise and sport. Women were encouraged to participate to promote unity and improve work relations.[6] In the late 1800s, sports activities were offered to employees in the cotton mills of Lowell, Massachusetts. Calisthenics were also introduced as 10-minute breaks during the day for National Cash Register Company employees in 1894. Dance and exercise classes were also sponsored and encouraged during lunch and in the evenings. In 1916 the Women's National Bowling Association was formed and soon included prize money.[6(p 110)] Those women in the workforce functioned as both mothers and wage earners; they were not excused for pregnancy or maternity leave.

A survey in 1921 revealed 36 of 51 companies offered women's teams, including tennis, bowling, basketball, volleyball, and hockey; a survey of companies in 1940 revealed that 35% of companies had bowling teams for women.[6(p 109)] Companies sponsored softball and basketball tournaments to promote public relations and loyalty. Company teams competed against one another, and games were well attended. Soon, corporations recruited athletes to increase their teams' success. Mildred "Babe" Didrikson, frequently recognized as the greatest woman athlete of the century, began her athletic career in 1930, when she was recruited for her basketball skills (for a secretarial job) by the Employers Casualty Insurance Co.[7(p 265)]

The 1920s through the end of World War II marked the "golden age of women's sports," because women were recognized for aesthetic athleticism. In 1919, women's fashion was once again revolutionized, when Suzanne Lenglen debuted at Wimbledon wearing a calf-length, arm-exposing dress[7(p 147)]; the public and athlete herself attributed this to allowing her to be more aggressive in her play. She became highly regarded for her fashion and femininity, wearing chiffon and winning with "dancelike" maneuvers on the court.

She is regarded as one of the first celebrity female athletes, transforming tennis into an enthusiastically spectated sport. In 1926, a 2-million-person ticker tape parade received Gertrude Ederle after she completed the English Channel swim nearly 2 hours faster than the five men who swam it before her.[7(p 82)] Fame was also familiar to Amelia Earhart, who, in 1928, was the first woman to fly solo across the Atlantic.[7(p 81)] As a teenager, Jackie Mitchell was the subject of controversial publicity when she struck out Lou Gehrig in a 1931 exhibition game.[8(p 43)] In 1945, the all-American girls professional baseball league's success peaked with 10 teams and close to 1 million fans.[8] These popularized figures represented to the public the strength and stamina women were capable of.

Just as mens' sports were the epitome of masculinity, women's sports glorified their femininity. In the 1930s, players participated in beauty contests during the Amateur Athletic Union's national championship. Beauty contests were often associated with many women's sporting events; companies used the combined tournaments for publicity and advertising. Corporate sponsors and team owners encouraged women athletes to wear attractive, body-revealing clothing to increase spectators at sporting events; shorter satin-trimmed shorts and tight shirts sparked public controversy, increasing attendance at the Dallas Cyclones basketball game from 150 to 5000 in the late 1920s.[6(p 114)] In 1949, the best-attended women's softball team was known to be "the most beautiful softball team in the world." Players were known to be selected for character, "feminine charm," and ability to play, in that order.[6(p 117)] Swimmer Esther Williams and skater Sonja Henie (Figure I–1) represented this glamorization, as they became movie stars.

The first Olympic events open to women were swimming and diving in 1912. With the persistence of Alice Milliat, founder of the Federation Sportive Feminie International, women gradually gained entrance into additional Olympic events; in 1928, the first women Olympic athletes competed in track and field events.[5(p 6)] Olympic participation set the stage for successful women athletes to flourish in other arenas as well. The great Babe Didrikson (Figure I–2) qualified for six 1932 Olympic events. Allowed to compete in only three, she won two gold medals and a silver medal. She then turned to basketball, baseball, and golf. She became an advocate for cancer survival treatment because she returned to her record-breaking professional golf career and won the US Open after surgical treatment for colon cancer.[7(p 265)] Representing Holland, Fannie Blankers-Koen, mother of two at age 30, won three gold medals in track and field events at the 1948 Olympics.[5(p 13)]

After World War II, American woman returned to their primary roles as wives and mothers. There was a resurgence of conservative ideals among society. However, African-American women did not face similar restrictions. Alice

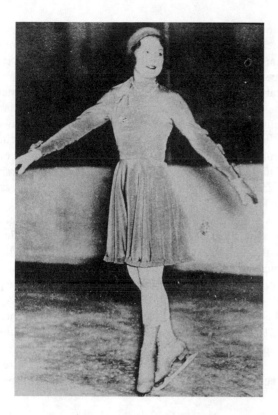

Figure I–1 Sonja Henie at the 1928 Winter Olympics.

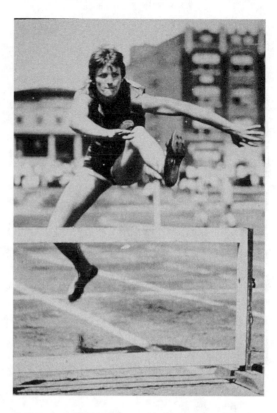

Figure I–2 Babe Didrikson at the 1932 Summer Olympics.

Coachman, the first black woman to win an Olympic gold medal, was also the only American woman to win a medal in the 1948 track and field events (Figure I–3). She went on to fight segregation in the South, along with discrimination against women. Although white colleges opposed track and field events for women, two black colleges—Tuskegee and Tennessee State—nurtured them.[5(p 15)] The 1950s and 1960s provided Olympic opportunity for women trained brilliantly at these colleges, including Wilma Rudolph, who overcame a childhood of illnesses and leg bracing (Figure I–4). Her drive and determination turned her into a multiple Olympic gold medallist in 1960 and world record holder in sprint distances.[7(p 209)]

As women developed strength and recognition at the collegiate and Olympic levels, they began to demand more equality and rights. In 1967, the Commission on Intercollegiate Athletics for Women (CIAW) was established to sanction and sponsor tournaments and championships. Over the next 5 years, as the needs of governance increased and the male-predominant National Collegiate Athletic Association threatened takeover, the CIAW handed the torch to the Association for Intercollegiate Athletics for Women (AIAW), a substructure of the National Association for Girls and Women in Sport (NAGWS).[9] Shortly thereafter, the most credited breakthrough for equality in women in sports, the education amendments of 1972, Title IX, was enacted, stating:

> No person in the United States shall, on the basis of sex, be excluded from participation in, be denied the benefits of, or be subjected to discrimination under any education program or activity receiving Federal financial assistance....[10(p 3)]

Full compliance was mandated by elementary schools in 1976 and high schools and colleges by 1978. Enforcement was lax, and Title IX was reinforced by the 1988 Civil Rights Restoration Act, although opposed by the National Collegiate Athletic Association (NCAA). Still, while equality in funding and competition increased, organizations specific to women's sports, including the AIAW, became integrated into the stronger male-dominated NCAA.[9] This led to a decrease in the number of female coaches and athletic administrators as women's sports organizations became integrated into male programs.

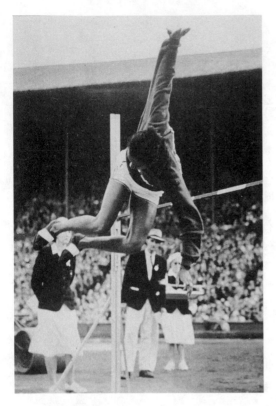

Figure I–3 Alice Coachman at the 1948 Summer Olympics.

BEYOND TITLE IX

Champion women athletes continued to make history by breaking down gender barriers with significant events, including "The Battle of the Sexes," when Billie Jean King defeated Bobby Riggs in a highly publicized tennis match in 1973. King went on to found the Women's Sports Foundation (WSF) with Donna DeVarona, the youngest member of a US Olympic team ever, world record-holding swimmer, and the first woman network sports broadcaster.[7(p 72)] Anita DeFrantz, Olympic rower, established a woman's voice in athletics, earning the Olympic Order Medal of Bronze for leading the opposition against the 1980 Moscow Olympic boycott. DeFrantz now runs the Amateur Athletic Foundation and serves on many athletic boards, including the International Olympic Committee,[7(p 71)] currently leading the movement to increase the percentage of women on the Olympic board. Wilma Rudolph established the Wilma Rudolph Foundation to motivate children through athletics.[7(p 209)] Julie Croteau is one of many women first in athletics, first to play on a collegiate men's varsity baseball team, recruited for a semi-professional team, and asked to coach a division 1 men's NCAA baseball team.[11(pp 19–20)]

The WSF, established in 1974 to provide monetary and political support to girls' and women's sports, has played a vital role in the growth of girls' and women's sports. A source and initiator of research, scholarships, organizations, education, advocacy, and publicity on girls and women in sports, the WSF also sponsors conferences and events that benefit the future of female athletes. The WSF also supports and reinforces gender equity in schools and athletic organizations and serves as a functional enforcement office of Title IX. As a source of athletic funding, sponsorships, and scholarships, it has played a vital role in the careers of many athletes.

The importance of funding cannot be underestimated—many elite athletes have experienced challenges of finance affecting training, opportunity, and health. Poorly funded athletes may have to work extensive hours, resulting in improper rest and training, or lack appropriate nutrition, equipment, coaching, and health care. The effects of increased funding and equality for women athletes are represented in the 27% increase of female participation in the 1996 summer Olympic games, "the games of the women."[12(p 593)]

It is evident that, armed with their physical strength and accomplishments, successful women athletes aspire to

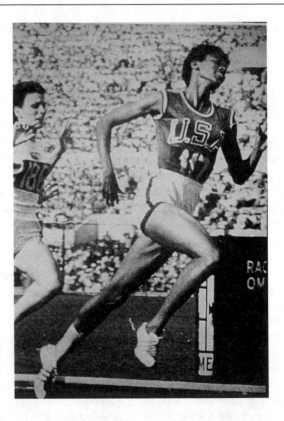

Figure I–4 Wilma Rudolph at the 1960 Summer Olympics.

groundbreaking achievements. Women athletes frequently develop into advocates for girl's and women's rights not just in sports, but for equality in all aspects of life. A history of women's victories can be made that rivals men. The 1999 world cup championship US women's soccer team also won the gold medal in the 1996 Olympics. The "magnificent seven" gold medal–winning US Olympic gymnastics team received instant celebrity status. The press and public embraced Kerri Strug as a hero after she displayed courageous grace, style, and brute determination and strength as she landed her Olympic championship vault with a severely sprained, fractured ankle. The United States profited in the glory of Title IX "babies" because three premier Olympic events for women—softball, soccer, and ice hockey—were dominated by championship US women as they all won the first-ever gold medals.

Culture and the media play an omnipotent role in the popularity of women as athletes. One cannot ignore the superstardom many female athletes have developed. In the 1980s, this was reserved for stars of the "glamour sports": gymnasts like Mary Lou Retton and Nadia Comaneci, ice skaters including Dorothy Hammill and Katarina Witt, and swimmer Tracy Caulkins. Now, the "glamour sports" are expanding to include team and aggressive sports; young girls now hang posters of soccer stars Mia Hamm and Julie Foudy, women's NBA players Sheryl Swoopes and Rebecca Lobo, and skier Picabo Street. Women's boxing has even been popularized with the success and grace of "Madame Butterfly," Laila Ali.

This recent exposure is crucial because it gives girls role models and idols to identify with; even fashion magazines are now filled not only with pages of sickly thin adolescent forms but also strong, muscular athletic heroes. The women's world cup soccer championship the summer of 1999 drew as many TV viewers as the men's National Basketball Association finals, spiraling the players into a frenzy of publicity and celebrity status. The winning US women's world cup soccer team, appealing to both sexes and all ages, has created a publicity explosion for women in sports. These athletes have maintained high standards as athletic heroes and role models in life. The inclusion of women in most military forces, the increasing number of scholastic and collegiate sporting events available to women, and the ever-growing number of women's Olympic and professional sports events reinforce the strength of the movement toward equity of women in sports.

PUSHING THE LIMITS

A study by Nattiv and colleagues[13] surveying college students in 1993–1994 found that athletes overall were more likely to engage in "risky" behavior, such as drinking alcohol and not wearing seatbelts. Although this likelihood is much greater in men than women overall, the female athletes profiled were found to engage in these behaviors and also were more likely to engage in physical fights and use smokeless tobacco. The frequency of symptoms of the female athlete triad (disordered eating, irregular or absent menses, and osteoporosis) was also higher.

The intensity of training and competition for female athletes and importance of performance and level of athletic achievement now are nearly equal to that of male athletes. Unfortunately, steroids and performance-enhancing drugs are increasing in frequency of abuse by female athletes. Recent statistics indicate that women and girls have doubled their use in the past decade. Ephedrine abuse and addiction are common in women who wish to reduce body fat and increase energy.[14]

It has been noted that the same driving personality traits that make a successful competitive athlete, including being goal-oriented, compulsive, and perfectionist,[12(p 596)] are similar to those associated with eating disorders.[15(p 304)] In addition, studies suggest that athletes with eating disorders began sports-specific training earlier than athletes with normal eating patterns.[16(p 449)] A new term has evolved, "anorexia athletica," appropriate as a description for the frequency of disordered eating among athletes.[16(p 449)] It is not only "athletes" who are vulnerable to these stressors. The overparticipant in fitness classes or excessive jogger often has body image, nutritional, stress injury, and overuse injury issues. The importance of body image at all ages and level of activity cannot be underemphasized.

Certain sports that require aestheticism and lithe bodies encourage drastic measures to lose weight, including laxative abuse, binging and purging, and bulimia. Self-mutilation has also been reported as athletes become obsessed with unrealistic and unhealthy ideals of physical perfection. Coaches pressure girls and women to become thinner so that they can "turn faster" as skaters, support their body easier as gymnasts, and be more streamlined as swimmers. These and other athletes are now being asked to pose in fashion and sex magazines and Internet sites. The money-making capacity of this attractive body image is also enticing to women of all ages. The complex issues that female athletes must face are endless; the cultural ideals of femininity and thinness in contrast to the muscular physique associated with athletic success can lead to identity conflict. The health risks associated with extreme aestheticism are becoming evident.

GENDER DIFFERENCES IN SPORT PERSONALITY

Most coaches agree on their use of gender-specific coaching techniques. As the coach in the movie *A League of Their Own* exclaimed, "there's no crying in baseball!" after critiquing a player, represents, women tend to take criticism to heart and respond better to positive reinforcement. It is a common perception that men generally are able to "leave their problems in the locker room," whereas women have difficulty compartmentalizing their emotions. Women respond better to communicative interaction; men like to be detached and use "pure muscle," because masculinity represents toughness, both verbally and physically.

Women tend to use their natural powers of socialization and negotiation on the playing field, which can place them at an advantage over strength and size. They are also known to be better listeners and are more compliant with coaches, therapists, and trainers. Author and professional basketball player Mariah Burton Nelson believes the increasing popularity of women as team players is a natural procession of socialization because women benefit from skills of friendship and communication. In addition, those who are successful athletes are natural leaders, have the self-confidence to take risks, take responsibility for mistakes, and ask for help.[17] Young girls gain friends and pride by being on teams, also developing a sense of identity.

The influence of athletic skill development at a younger age cannot be denied. Early reinforcement and practice of athletic skills, including balance, proprioception, speed, strength, and agility, prevent injuries later in life. Even today, girls are discouraged from physical play and encouraged to play with dolls or help with indoor housework, whereas boys play pick-up sports games and help with more physical house chores (carrying the garbage, raking, or mowing the lawn).

Women are known to perform sports with more finesse. In talking with a Women's National Basketball Association player who frequently spars with the Knicks, she states she uses the fact that she is a woman to "trash talk" the men, by making statements such as "you can't let a girl beat you!" She believes she also plays "smarter" by being more observant of other players' habits (ie, excessive dribbling), allowing her to outwit both men and younger, more aggressive women.

Women are known to be better climbers than men, are equally heralded as jockeys, and women cockswains (the driver and coach within the boat) in men's crews are common. Personality differences are also reflected in gender differences of skiing—women tend to assess the situation and negotiate a skillful way down the mountain, being more aware of other skiers.[18] They also want to ski "in control."

Overall, women, although less "aggressive" tend to be better at developing skills, negotiating play and course patterns, and tend to have more finesse. Less likely to play alone as girls, or exercise or play sports alone as women, they develop skills that allow them to be better "team players." Aggressiveness is not encouraged in many training programs in girl's and women's sports but is becoming more socially acceptable.

Public perception is that female and male athletic personalities are different. A 1997 study found that female athletes are perceived as goal oriented, organized, and rule governed; whereas men are perceived to be more aggressive, competitive, dominating, and controlling.[19] It is questioned whether these differences in perception are socialized or inherent to the gender differences. This contrast of what is expected and what is evolving contributes to the increasing popularity of women's sports as spectator sports—for example, the 1999 US Open Tennis tournament had more television viewers for women's than men's matches.

Rehabilitation of girls and women presents multifactorial gender differences. Personality differences prevail regardless of sex, but generally, women respond better to positive reinforcement, use socialization skills better, and positively respond to guided treatment sessions. Individualized programs designed with respect to strength, alignment, and muscle firing patterns are most successful. Some believe that women are more stoic with pain, perhaps residual from a history of women wearing tight corsets and small-fitting pointed shoes and giving birth. These established cultural ideals of sacrifice for the sake of fashion and maintaining an identity as a cheerful, uncomplaining, feminine woman continue today and overlap into athletic achievement ideals. In addition to restricting caloric intake, some girls avoid strength training for fear they will gain masculine physiques and callused hands. This leads to injuries and poor health.

All exercise requires forethought and training to prevent illness or injury. It is our job to provide the medical and health guidance that is important to overall well-being—preventive sports medicine is paramount. Encouraging early multidimensional athletic exposure is beneficial to future health. Treating female athletes with equal respect and opportunities as male athletes yet adapting to their gender differences can be challenging for some health care professionals. Sports medicine is only recently evolving to take female athletes as seriously as male athletes and support their quick return to play.

THE PRESENT

Today, girls have equal opportunity, recognition, and financial support to participate in sports. Statistics support the benefit of this, as those compiled by the WSF portrayed in a Nike athletic ad summarize:

> If you let me play
> I will like myself more
> I will have more self-confidence
> I will suffer less depression
> I will be 60 percent less likely to get breast cancer
> I will be more likely to leave a man who beats me
> I will be less likely to get pregnant before I want to

I will learn what it means to be strong
If you let me play sports[18(p 14)]

Studies assessing actual personality characteristics among women reveal the athletes to be "…more intrinsically motivated, assertive, achievement oriented, independent, and self-sufficient than nonathletic women.[15(p 301)] In addition, trends suggest that mood patterns of elite athletes reveal less tension, depression, and anger.[15(p 302)] Robert Sullivan, in a July 19, 1999, *Time* magazine writes about the women's world-cup winning soccer team: "Daughters of Title IX, they've never been told what they cannot do. They feel good about themselves. They feel free to make choices and to put their personalities—and other assets—on exhibit."[20] This is the essence of women's sports. Women get the same gratification out of athletic activity as men. The notion of masculine athleticism is being replaced by the term "athletically feminine."[18(p 29)] The athletic female personality and physique are now revered as a symbol of strength and perseverance.

New advances in gender-specific gear, equipment, and clothing are developing exponentially. Stores and online services that cater to women's fitness are becoming increasingly popular, and women's sections of sporting stores are expanding. Sports bras have evolved from the early compressive types to more shapely, comfortable versions. Womens' ski boots provide a narrower, more flexible heel and boot and are combined with individual binding placement and shorter, more flexible skis. Soccer cleats for women are built with narrower heels. Helmets and caps are made to accommodate ponytails. Backpacks are designed to fit a woman's generally smaller shoulders and wider hips. Bike seats are shaped to fit more comfortably, often with pressure relief in the midsection. Softball gloves are made for smaller hands. Shorter golf clubs, lighter bowling balls, and lighter windsurfing equipment are also regularly available. Even ACL braces are now being made specifically for female athletes.

Within sports, rule differences persist, including women's golf tee locations, smaller women's basketballs, and decreased number of sets in women's tennis. Unfortunately, earnings and winnings of competitive athletes still average less than half for women than men. In addition, the number of women coaches and leaders in athletic arenas are significantly lower than men, as well as their salaries.[21(p 292)] Women are challenging these differences.

Commercial sponsors now cater specifically to women, decreasing the frequency of male-dominated television commercials during sporting events. Well-respected athletic personalities such as Mia Hamm challenging Michael Jordan in a Gatorade ad are reminiscent of Jackie Mitchell pitching a 1931 exhibition game against Lou Gehrig, of Babe Didrikson Zaharias striking out Joe DiMaggio in a 1954 exhibition game, of Billie Jean King's defeat of Bobby Riggs in 1973 in the *Battle of the Sexes*, of Jean Balukas defeating Willie Mosconi in the billiards "CBS Challenge of the Sexes" in 1975, and, most recently, of the defeat of boxer Loi Chow by equally sized Margaret "Tiger" MacGregor in 1998.

There are still many firsts contributing to women's sports history. Recent women's successes surpassing that of men[22] include Susan Butcher as the first to be a three-time consecutive Iditarod winner and Teresa Edwards as the first four-time Olympic basketball team player. The first girl to qualify for the NFL pass, punt, and kick competition, Kendra Wecker, placed second in 1995. Lyn St. James, the only woman on the Indianapolis Racing League circuit, has set multiple speed records. Women athletes with disabilities are also setting new standards of play as Neroli Fairhall of New Zealand competed as a wheelchair athlete in archery, and Sonya Bell in 1997 became the first blind runner to compete at a high school track championship.

Sports medicine is beginning to recognize gender differences. The American College of Sports Medicine (ACSM) was one of the first organizations to identify gender-related sports issues. Women's Sports Medicine Centers, the first started several years ago in Manhattan, are being developed nationwide. The *Journal of Athletic Training*'s April–June, 1999, issue was entirely devoted to knee injuries in women. Nearly monthly, new research is published addressing patterns of musculoskeletal injuries and activity-related medical issues in women. More and more, research is investigating the differences between men and women in sports. More and more, medical care specialties and training are identifying the unique experiences and needs of female athletes.

Organizations such as WSF, ACSM, Women Sport International, Women's Initiative, Olympic Committee's Medical Commission, along with individual women's professional organizations are raising awareness of health risks. These and other organizations are instituting preventive strategies and research. In 1999, the National Institutes of Health sponsored a meeting to establish research in women's sports injuries. Educational programs for coaches and trainers, medical forums for health professionals, and awareness initiatives of athletes at all ages are expanding. Actions to decrease the frequency of health risks (notably, components of the female athlete triad) have included raising the age limit required for competition in elite tennis and gymnastics.[23(p 96)]

THE FUTURE

Over the past century marked by significant women, society has developed acceptance and recognition of female athletes at all levels. The revolution of athletic equality is just beginning. Each Olympics, more women's events are added. Each year, more women run marathons, participate in triathlons, play team sports, and lift more weights. Each month, studies are presented on female athletic injuries and their prevention. As girls begin sports at younger ages and are provided with an equal caliber of coaching and training, trends of injury and styles of play may become more similar among the sexes. The sports and health community will continue to become more aware of health and injury risks, prevention, and treatment. In addition, the amount of injuries will decrease as girls begin athletics at younger ages and women continue to use their forethought and finesse to prevent injuries. They will continue to flourish in their "athletic feminism" as prevalence of eating disorders, bone imbalances, and body image concerns decline. Women will continue to gain mental and physical strength and no longer feel vulnerable on city streets, corporate offices, training rooms, and playing fields. Newly empowered, girls and women will comfortably label themselves "athletes." With the assistance of publications like this, women athletes of all calibers will preserve the health benefits and defy the injury statistics. The reader is encouraged to use this information, challenge it, and develop further protocols and research to fill current voids.

REFERENCES

1. Lutter JM. History of women in sports: societal issues. *Clin Sports Med.* 1994;13:263–279.

2. Vertinsky P. Women, sport, and exercise in the 19th century. In: Costa DM, Guthrie SR. *Women and Sport: Interdisciplinary Perspectives.* Champaign, IL: Human Kinetics; 1994:63–82.

3. Howell R. *Her Story in Sport: A Historical Anthology of Women in Sports.* West Point, NY: Leisure Press; 1982.

4. Nelson MB. Introduction. In: Smith L, ed. *Nike Is a Goddess: The History of Women in Sports.* New York: Atlantic Monthly Press; 1998: ix–xix.

5. McElroy K. Track and field: somewhere to run. In: Smith L, ed. *Nike Is a Goddess: The History of Women in Sports.* New York: Atlantic Monthly Press; 1998:3–29.

6. Emery L. From Lowell Mills to the Halls of Fame: Industrial League Sport for Women. In: Costa DM, Guthrie SR. *Women and Sport: Interdisciplinary Perspectives.* Champaign, IL: Human Kinetics; 1994:107–121.

7. Layden J. *Women in Sports.* Santa Monica: General Publishing Group; 1997.

8. Nutt AE. Baseball and softball: swinging for the fences. In: Smith L, ed. *Nike Is a Goddess: The History of Women in Sports.* New York: Atlantic Monthly Press; 1998:33–54.

9. Hult JS. The story of women's athletics: manipulating a dream. In: Costa DM, Guthrie SR. *Women and Sport: Interdisciplinary Perspectives.* Champaign, IL: Human Kinetics; 1994:83–106.

10. Reith KM. *Playing Fair: A Guide to Title IX in High School & College Sports.* 2nd ed. Women's Sports Foundation; 1994.

11. Powe-Allred A, Powe M. *The Quiet Storm: A Celebration of Women in Sport.* Indianapolis: Masters Press; 1997.

12. Wiggins DL, Wiggins ME. The female athlete. *Clin Sports Med.* 1997;16: 593–611.

13. Nattiv A, Puffer JC, Green GA. Lifestyles and health risks of collegiate athletes: a multi-center study. *Clin J Med.* 1997;7:262–272.

14. Gruber AJ, Pope HG. Ephedrine abuse among 36 female weightlifters. *Am J Addict.* 1998;7:256–261.

15. Barnett NP, Wright P. Psychological considerations for women in sports. *Clin Sports Med.* 1994;13:297–313.

16. Beim G, Stone DA. Issues in the female athlete. *Orthop Clin North Am.* 1995;26:443–449.

17. Nelson MB. Learning what "team" really means. *Newsweek.* 1999; July 19:55.

18. Carbone C. *Women Ski.* 2nd ed. Boston: World Leisure Corporation; 1996.

19. Pedersen DM. Perceived traits of male and female athletes. *Percept Motor Skills.* 1997;85:547–550.

20. Sullivan R. Goodbye to heroin chic. Now it's sexy to be strong. *Time* 1999;July 19:62.

21. Lopiano DA. Equity in women's sports. *Clin Sports Med.* 1994;13: 281–296.

22. Women's Sports Foundation. National Girls and Women in Sports Day promotional materials. New York: The Foundation; 1999.

23. Schnirring L. What's new in treating active women. *Physician Sportsmedicine.* 1997;25:91–98.

Rehabilitation Concepts

Nadya Swedan

INTRODUCTION

A sports medicine text is incomplete without the inclusion of rehabilitation techniques and treatment. Currently, established principles of injury treatment, including surgery, are *not* gender specific. However, there are recommendations and impressions that can be derived from clinical experience and implied from the injury patterns and health risks identified in women. To begin rehabilitation treatment, proper injury assessment and prescription are essential. Early identification and treatment are key to efficient recovery from and further worsening of injury. The role of the health care provider, therapist, and coach should be individualized and specific for each individual, specific to activity, age, and gender.

PHASES OF THERAPY

Acute

Acute rehabilitation addresses pain and swelling while maintaining as much strength and range of motion as possible within the specified restrictions. During this time, the athlete may be splinted or immobilized, have range of motion or weight bearing precautions, and may be taking medication for pain or swelling. Activities including sports may be limited, and, unless suffering from a minor injury allowing continued play, the athlete is disabled from her regular activity and even handicapped with respect to her athletic society.

Recovery

Recovery, or restorative rehabilitation, begins when there are no further precautions; the goal is restoring strength to 75% to 80%[1(p 5)] and normal range of motion. The athlete should be primarily pain free and may return to modified training or activity, with respect to the sport.

Functional

Functional rehabilitation returns the athlete to play and normal activity. Because this puts maximum stress on the injury site, it is wise for the athlete to continue guided training and rehabilitation for 2–4 weeks to ensure complete recovery and prevent reinjury.

Prehabilitation

Prehabilitation may be recommended during preseason training or after the initial screening preparticipation physical. An athlete may have her own concerns for injury risk, with bothersome aches from the prior season or sustained during another sport or activity. This is the ideal setting for initiating a functional, sports-specific prehabilitation and injury prevention program.

GENDER-SPECIFIC THERAPY

Rehabilitation follows similar principles to coaching, because the therapist becomes the "coach" during rehabilitation "training." Coaches and therapists, in general, note personality differences in communicating with female and male athletes. As described in the Introduction, men tend to take criticism as a challenge, while women are more sensitive to negative cues. Overall, women respond better to positive reinforcement with communication and empathy. Both genders seem to feel more comfortable with therapists and health care providers of their own sex.

Women change physiologically and emotionally throughout the month; pain sensitivity and psychological well-being change with hormonal fluctuations of adolescence, menstrual cycles, and menopausal symptoms. Recent research has focused on strength and ligament laxity in relation to hormonal cycles and pregnancy. In puberty and adolescence, phases of growth affect growth plate integrity, flexibility, proprioception, coordination, and balance. Health care and rehabilitation providers must consider this and realize that day-to-day variations also occur secondary to nutrition, sleep, emotional well-being, and fatigue. Performance both in the gym and on the field is related to this delicate balance. As with all sports medicine techniques, therapy should always be individualized. Women should be given autonomy and choices during the course of their rehabilitation and credited with their motivation, insight into their own needs and emotions, and physical and mental flexibility.

Body image is an ongoing concern, particularly for active women who depend on peak physique to perform. Girls and women often describe a slight weight gain as making them feel unattractive, heavy, and slow; in contrast, men might describe weight gain as making them feel "stronger." Amount of exercise is an important component of a woman's body image along with caloric intake. Injury decreases activity and caloric expenditure; it is quite common for a woman to express concerns that she may gain weight because of reduced activity. This can add to feelings of discouragement and a sense of some loss of control because her main method of weight control becomes limited. Many athletes are exercise dependent and have fears of weight gain[2]; reactive depression and feelings of hopelessness can occur. Alternative exercises should be explored to fill the sense of loss and maintain fitness and weight. The athlete's social schedule is also likely to be affected. With respect to all the multidimensional possible consequences of injury, sports psychology counseling should be made available. (Refer to Chapter 22, Psychology and the Injured Female Athlete.)

Certain equipment and exercises may need modification to fit and adapt to a woman's physique, strength, alignment, and flexibility. Resistance should be assessed daily and begin at an appropriate level. Because most fitness and rehabilitation equipment, particularly strength machines, is designed for men, other exercise programs may need to be developed.

Although female athletes may come to a therapist and physician with less inherent intrinsic strength than men, they often have other attributes that may make them more effective and efficient responders to rehabilitation. In general, improved communication skills, greater flexibility, and balance and coordination skills commonly benefit the injured female athlete. Women are also more open to cross-training techniques, usually having trained in multiple environments to nurture their athleticism. In addition, because they are more likely to participate in alternative and complementary medicine techniques, as outlined in the latter part of this chapter, combining these with traditional methods of treatment should be considered.

THE KINETIC CHAIN

The "kinetic chain" is a term used more frequently to describe the anatomical and functional relationship of the distal to proximal joints to the pelvis and scapula to the spine. As described by W. Ben Kibler, "Individual body segments and joints, collectively called the *links*, must be moved in certain specific sequences to allow efficient accomplishment of the tasks."[3(p 16)] The kinetic chain is an excellent concept for both assessing and rehabilitating weakness and injury (Table P–1). In clinical pain and injury assessment, the advice "look above and below the pain or injury site" is useful. For example, the source of hip pain can be the lumbar spine, as a radiculopathy, or the knee as iliotibial band syndrome. In performing sports-specific tasks, this concept can be applied during training to increase speed, strength, technique, and prevent injuries.

It is clear that in assessing a woman in sports the kinetic chain is essential because many gender differences historically have been attributed to malalignment or, more appropriately, "unique alignment." To reinforce weakness, pain, or inflexibility proximally results in inefficient, compensating, and impaired distal movements. Velocity, proprioception, and strength all become subject to compensation; their normal coordination can become dysfunctional. With respect to the general belief that women rely on finesse, coordination, and skill more than men, a disrupted kinetic chain can become disabling to both elite and noncompetitive athletes. (Refer to Chapter 7, Clinical Biomechanics.)

Table P–1 Kinetic Chains of Sports Activities

Sporting Activity	Kinetic Chain
Baseball pitch	Ground → plant leg → hip and trunk → landing leg
	Ground → plant leg → hip and trunk → shoulder → elbow → wrist → hand
Running	Ground → plant leg → pelvis → landing leg
Freestyle swimming	Hand, wrist, and elbow → shoulder → hip and trunk → opposite shoulder → hand, wrist, and elbow
Soccer kick	Ground → plant leg → plant pelvis and trunk → kicking hip → knee → foot

NEUROLOGIC TECHNIQUES IN REHABILITATION

Proprioception, reaction time, and muscle firing all depend on the circular communication between muscle, peripheral nerves, and the central nervous system. Maintaining efficient functioning of sensorimotor pathways during injury and rehabilitation is beneficial to optimal recovery with minimal decrease in athletic ability and skill. Regular assessment and training of the nervous system can also facilitate quicker return of reaction time, balance, and technique after injury. Also, this enhances psychological well-being with immeasurable positive effects on healing. Neurologic fine-tuning and training does not necessarily mandate associated physical movement.

Mental imagery can take many forms. *Soothing imagery* is used to diminish pain by mentally escaping to a private, relaxing, pleasing, peaceful place. *Performance imagery* is widely used among professional athletes to enforce proper technique, winning plays, and flawless performance. *Healing imagery* requires an understanding of the physical injury so visual scenes of mending can occur.[4] Imagery includes not only visualization but also other sensory experiences including sounds, sensations, and smells. This is sometimes used with, or as adjunct to, relaxation therapy. Therapy should include both therapist and self-guided sessions. Imagery goals should be established and reevaluated periodically.

Goals of Rehabilitation Imagery

- Stimulate central nervous system
- Maintain technique
- Manage pain
- Facilitate relaxation
- Facilitate healing
- Improve concentration
- Restore sense of control
- Manage anxiety

Clinical Guideline

Proprioceptive neuromuscular facilitation (PNF) techniques utilize bilateral repetitive neuromuscular patterns to restore function and movement.[5] The techniques are directed at the body as a whole using concentric, eccentric, and static muscle contractions to promote functional movement through facilitation, inhibition, strengthening, and relaxation of muscle groups. The treatment patterns use motion in all three planes and are combined and modified by the therapist, depending on the condition and needs of each individual. The treatment should be intensive and encourage the athlete to push her limits without increasing pain or prolonged fatigue. This technique uses the benefit of neuronal cross firing of multiple pathways, allowing strength gains in one area by also training supporting, surrounding, and contralateral sites.[6] Diagonal, spiral patterns of movement are also used. During immobilization or relative rest, maximizing desired activities on the noninjured side is beneficial to restoring strength once movement can be returned.

Goals of PNF

- Decrease pain
- Increase range of motion
- Increase strength, coordination, and control of motion
- Develop a proper balance between motion and stability
- Increase endurance

Clinical Guideline

EMOTIONAL AND PSYCHOLOGICAL CONSIDERATIONS

Injury is an event resulting from a loss of control, either intrinsic or extrinsic. Injury results from an undesired, uncontrolled situation—secondary to play surface, position of landing, other players, or other conditions. Often, injury is caused by external events. The injured athlete is then thrust into the hands of medical providers who prescribe restrictions, treatment, rehabilitation, and sometimes surgery—more events an athlete feels unable to control.

The goal of sports health providers is for functional recovery, an objectively measurable achievement. Recovery, however, is very subjective, as athletes with similar injuries continue to have variable return to play times, in response to multiple factors. Psychobiology has as important an influence as biomechanical and physiological factors. The therapist, trainer, coach, and physician need to allow the athlete to feel in control. As described by Doyle, Gleeson, and Rees in "Psychobiology and the Athlete with Anterior Cruciate Ligament Injury,"[7] subjective sensations of functioning are not always related to objective functioning. This can be quite limiting in progress because an athlete may perform too little or too much both in and out of the rehabilitation setting. Unfortunately, none of the current measures of functional recovery (ie, Tegner and Lysholm scale, Cincinnati rating system) have reliably accounted for individual subjective recovery.

In assessing a woman's rehabilitation and recovery, time schedules can only be estimated predictions. There are both external and internal factors affecting rehabilitation success. Patient effort, cooperation, and verbal input are essential to the achievement of optimal recovery. Success can be maximized with mutual trust between athlete and clinician with consideration of her emotions and opinions. The physician, therapist, and trainer must treat each woman individually with respect to precautions and activities allowed at home. More compliant athletes should be given more freedom and control to perform activities outside the therapeutic or supervised environment.

External Influences of Rehabilitation Success

- Correct diagnosis
- Medical treatment (medications, precautions)
- Surgical treatment
- Immobilization
- Motivating rehabilitation environment
- Team support
- Coach support and contact
- Family and friend support
- Stability of physical environment
- Consistency of physician, therapist, trainer, and coaching goals
- Equipment
- Appropriate modalities
- Patient awareness of rehabilitation plan and goals

Clinical Guideline

Internal Influences of Rehabilitation Success

- Appropriate rest
- Nutrition and hydration
- Positive outlook
- Flexibility
- Strength
- Proprioception
- Soft tissue and bone healing
- Pain
- Perception of biomechanical healing
- Emotional profile
- Athlete's understanding of rehabilitation plan and goals
- Compliance
- Confidence in treatment plan and performance outcome

Clinical Guideline

OVERTRAINING

Beware the perfectionist, compulsive, competitive profile. The woman athlete who asks for more therapy and training sessions, performs home or gym exercises several times daily, continuously compares herself to others, or asks to frequently increase resistance and repetitions is likely to be overtraining. In these athletes, the importance of rest must be reinforced, and often scheduled; this includes sleep and relative rest from activity, particularly during rehabilitation from injury. This type of athlete may be quite common, particularly at the elite level, because a successful athlete is disciplined and determined. Ensure that her goals are realistic and obtainable within an adequate time frame.

Although recent literature has attempted to establish hormonal measures of overtraining, there have to date been no reliably measurable indicators establishing that an athlete is overtraining. The clinician must consider other signs of overtraining. A tireless schedule can be exhausting and inefficient, leading to anxiety, irritability, frustration, and impaired performance. Reviewing her social schedule—including work and home—in addition to her therapy and training schedules, and prioritizing what is most valuable to recovery, is as important to recovery and rehabilitation as actual training. The athlete who also works, has a family, or has other commitments in addition to athletics, may be overwhelmed with her responsibilities, and, if not balanced with rest and relaxing techniques, will have more difficulty recovering from injury.

Maintenance of general health is essential to musculoskeletal healing. Blood pressure and pulse should be monitored intermittently; weight is a more delicate issue. The athlete involved in rehabilitation should not focus on weight and accept that during decreased activity she may gain slightly but will likely return to her normal weight as she returns to her athletic activities. Nutritional counseling should be available to ensure balance if she is decreasing her caloric intake. Including a multivitamin with added iron and calcium is recommended if calories are restricted.

UNDERSTANDING REHABILITATION

To comprehensively include full treatment of athletic injury, the following section is a review of standard rehabilitation concepts used in therapeutic sports medicine.

Before beginning therapeutic exercise and treatment, medical and musculoskeletal histories must be reviewed by the therapist, and physician prescriptions for therapy should be specific with regard to precautions, specifically medical, range of motion, and weight bearing. In athletes with hypertension or hypotension, blood pressure should be monitored during evaluation and periodically throughout treatment. Medical and surgical precautions and presence of surgical hardware, open wounds, or infection should be clearly understood before initiating any modalities. Pain levels should be addressed at each session. Pain medication use, compliance with therapy and home program, and changes in function and activity should be periodically reviewed as a measure of progress.

Exercise Terminology

Resistance: the force or weight against which a movement is performed. This can be provided by gravity, elastic bands of various thickness and resistance, exercise, medicine and/or plyometric balls, free weights, and machines.

Repetitions: the number of motions performed for each exercise.

Isometric exercise: holding a position of muscle contraction without movement. This provides maximal muscle force and tension,[8(p 10)] although the lack of movement limits its functionality. This is highly used when there are range of motion precautions or when pain limits mobility.

Concentric exercise: resistance with the strongest muscle contraction movement (ie, arm curl is a concentric exercise for the biceps).

Eccentric exercise: resistance as a muscle unit lengthens (ie, slowly lowering the arm curl is an eccentric biceps exercise). This type of exercise is most likely to cause muscle soreness.

Isokinetic exercise: consistent resistance with both contracting and lengthening a muscle maintaining constant speed (ie, Cybex machine provides isokinetic exercise).

Plyometric exercise: uses bursts of forceful contractions with preload and stretch involving both eccentric and concentric movements[8(p 10)] (ie, throwing and catching a ball, squat-jumps) (Figures P–1 to P–3).

Closed-chain kinetic exercise: constant contact of the distal extremity with a constant reactive force (ie, squats, StairMaster, push-ups). This is safest in acute rehabilitation because exercises remain controlled and usually in one plane; plyometric or landing forces are restricted (Figure P–4).

Open-chain kinetic exercise: allowing the distal extremity to move away freely from the force (running, walking, biceps curls). This challenges the neuromuscular system as the plane of exercise becomes three dimensional (Figure P–5).

Modalities

Selecting appropriate treatment plans and modalities must be individualized with weekly assessment of improvement and pain ratings. Clinical experience enforces this because some patients feel certain modalities are "a waste of time" or may even be pain inducing. Others become dependent on modalities. Benefits and precautions of various modalities can be controversial among rehabilitation providers. In addition, current research is limited in its ability to measure objective benefits of many of the modalities commonly used[9]; therefore incorporating individual subjective measurements is crucial.

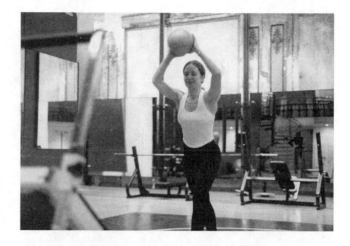

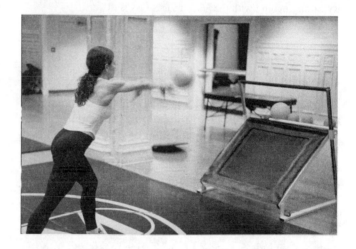

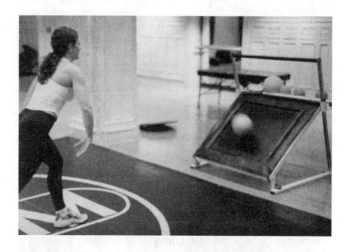

Figure P–1, P–2, P–3 Plyometric Upper Extremity Strengthening and Retraining Using Full Range of Motion, Proprioceptive Skills, and Resistance.

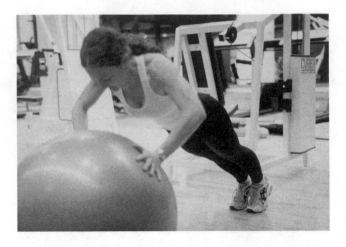

Figure P–4 Closed-Chain Scapula Stabilizing and Upper Extremity Strengthening with the Use of the Swiss Ball.

Cold Applications

Cryotherapy. Cryotherapy is likely the most common of patient and therapist used modalities, particularly in the sports medicine setting; application of cold results in both local and distal vasoconstriction.[10] Metabolism and inflammatory mediator release is decreased; pain threshold is increased.[11] Sensory and motor nerve conduction is slowed. Cryotherapy is used clinically to reduce pain, inflammation, and muscle spasms. Acutely, cold treatment decreases bleeding and hemorrhage and traumatic edema.[12] Conduction methods include ice and cold packs, ice massage (proposed to lower limb temperature quicker than ice bags),[13] and ice

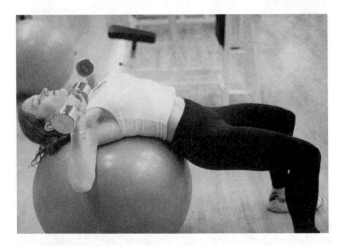

Figure P–5 Open-Chain Scapular Stabilizing and Upper Extremity Strengthening.

baths for extremities or large areas. Cryocuffs, providing both compression and cryotherapy, are effective in the acute injury and postsurgical setting.

Cryokinetics. Cryokinetics is the application of cold therapy in conjunction with stretching. In this way it reduces pain and decreases muscle spindle firing allowing stretching. Vapo-coolant sprays (ethyl chloride and fluoromethane) for spray and stretch techniques are often used, but some consider their use controversial because of proposed ozone layer damage.

Contraindications to cold therapy include hypersensitivity/urticaria reactions, Raynaud's phenomenon, paroxysmal cold hemoglobinurias, and conditions of decreased sensation or ischemia.

Heat and Ultrasound

Heat. Increasing local temperatures[10,14] results in vasodilation and muscle relaxation, increases cell permeability and capillary flow, increases tissue metabolism, decreases muscle spasms, increases nerve pain threshold, and allows extensibility of connective tissue and increased joint range of motion. Superficial heat, one of the most well-tolerated modalities, is frequently used in the form of silica gel hot packs, moist Thermophore packs, and paraffin treatments. Convective heat[10] includes fluidotherapy and radiant heat, which provides a weightless, noncontact, dry heat. Deep-heating modalities include ultrasound and microwave diathermy.

Precautions are required because of the vasodilatory effects of heat when treating areas of acute inflammation and in severe hypotension because heat can decrease blood pressure. Heat therapy must be used cautiously in pregnant women and patients with metabolic and cardiac decreased temperature sensitivity. Contraindications include patients with fever or those who have difficulty maintaining body temperature. Malignancies may metastasize because of increased blood flow.[15]

Ultrasound. High-frequency sound waves applied over a focal area[16] are proposed to result in heat-induced and vibration-induced separation of collagen fibers and increased membrane permeability. The deepest penetrating of the heating modalities, ultrasound heats to 2 inches below the surface, mostly at tissue interfaces, least in adipose tissue. Clinically, ultrasound is used to decrease scar tissue formation, decrease pain and swelling, and increase flexibility.[17] It is used to increase joint mobility and reduce scar tissue; the heating effect promotes blood flow, which can be effective in nonacute inflammation. It can also desensitize painful areas including neuromas and tight musculature. Ultrasound can be either pulsed, thought to cause less heating,[18] or continuous. Treatment lasts 5 to 10 minutes over a small area with frequencies ranging from .5 to 3 watts/cm. For effects of heating, doses of at least 1.5 W/cm are required.[16] Phonophoresis is the use of ultrasound for transdermal application of medications similar to iontophoresis (see following paragraphs).

Contraindications to ultrasound include treatment over sites of metallic implants or joint replacement; near pacemakers; over cavities including the eye or gravid uterus (causes cavitation of fluid); at sites of active bleeding, infection, malignancies; or over the carotid sinus or cervical ganglia. Ultrasound should not be used over bony prominences, over incompletely healed fractures, over growing endplates, or over acutely inflamed joints.[17]

Hydrotherapy

Hydrotherapy. The viscosity of water provides increased resistance with higher velocity movements, and the most resistance is offered in downward movements as the buoyancy of the body must be resisted. Hydrotherapy includes pool therapy, Hubbard tank, and whirlpool. Frequently used with athletes, pool therapy provides low resistance and buoyancy[10] to allow partial weight-bearing activities, reproducing those that are restricted during the rehabilitation process. This allows sport-specific activities and movement maintenance. Whirlpool treatments also relieve pain and muscle spasm. Hubbard tanks can be used to exercise in or to provide heating or cooling to larger body areas. Full body immersion should not exceed 102°; whirlpool temperatures should not exceed 113°.

Contrast Baths. Alternating warm and cold baths are often used for acute muscular or soft tissue injury. The affected limb is placed alternatingly in a warm bath for 100 to 110°F for 4 to 6 minutes followed by cold bath 55 to 65°F for 2 to 4 minutes for a total treatment time of 20 to 30 minutes.

Electrical Stimulation

Electrical Stimulation. Electrical currents stimulate nerve and muscle to result in decreasing pain, edema, and spasticity.[10,19,20] Soft tissue benefits of electrical stimulation include increased circulation, muscle stimulation and reeducation with prevention of atrophy, and decreased fibrosis. Low-voltage continuous direct current is also used to promote fracture healing and in settings of osteoporotic or stress fractures. Neuromuscular electrical stimulation is specifically used over motor points in coordination with isometric contraction to facilitate recruitment of motor units. Overall muscle strength has not been proven to increase; however, with selective stimulation of type II fibers, it is proposed that submaximal strength may be increased along with muscle firing force.[21]

Transcutaneous Electrical Stimulation (TENS). Electrical stimulation of afferent pain neurons relieve musculoskeletal pain and spasticity. A "TENS" device is a portable unit that patients can use at home for symptom relief. Frequency and intensity are varied to provide different types of analgesia.[22] *Conventional TENS* with high-frequency (50–100 Hz) low-intensity provides quick, short-acting gate-controlled synaptic pain inhibition and can be used continuously in some populations. *Low-frequency or acupuncture-like TENS* causes discomfort with or without muscle contractions with low-frequency, high-intensity stimulus producing beta-endorphin release. This provides delayed-onset but longer acting pain relief. *Burst-mode TENS* alternates high and low frequency with muscle contraction. *Hyperstimulation TENS* is high-frequency, high-intensity stimulation with quick and prolonged pain relief once the initial discomfort of probe initiated muscle stimulation is overcome. These techniques can be combined or alternated and are often used in settings of chronic pain.

Iontophoresis. In iontophoresis direct current transfers ionizable medications transdermally.[23] The medications, most commonly dexamethasone sodium phosphate (Decadron) either with or separately from lidocaine, are localized and slowly absorbed. Iontophoresis is most effective for focal soft tissue inflammation, including tendinitis, epicondylitis, and fasciitis. Other uses include treatment of neuromas, arthritis, and "shinsplints." Iontophoresis of acetic acid[23] has been used for treatment of calcific tendinitis, myositis ossificans, and plantar fasciitis.[24] Additional medications include salicylates and diclofenac.[25] In addition to precautions associated with each medication, burns are the greatest risk of use because resultant posttreatment pink skin can mask epithelial damage. Treatment time is usually 10 to 20 minutes and is not recommended on a daily basis.

Contraindications of electrical stimulation, TENS, and iontophoresis include anesthetic skin, cardiac pacemakers, and treatment during pregnancy, particularly during the first trimester. The carotid sinus should be avoided. Mucous membranes, eyes, and open skin areas should be avoided. In patients with epilepsy use near the head is not advised.

Spinal Traction

Spinal traction provides either continuous, sustained, or intermittent distractive force on the spinal segments to stretch and relax paraspinal muscles, ligaments, and capsules and open up vertebral and foraminal spaces.[26,27] Intradiscal pressure and pressure on nerve roots can be reduced. Traction can be very effective for treating symptoms of radiculopathy. Cervical traction, between 10 and 35 pounds, is always done in slight flexion; increasing the resistance and position of flexion targets lower cervical spine segments. Lumbar traction, between 65 and 200 pounds, can be done either prone or supine, unilaterally or bilaterally, with varying degrees of hip flexion. Before beginning mechanical traction, manual resistance should be applied to determine tolerance and optimum symptom-relieving position. A study in *Spine* in 1997[28] reported average lumbar lengthening of 6 mm and a reduction in lumbar curvature.

Absolute contraindications to traction include spinal infections, carcinomas, central nervous system signs or pressure alterations, osteoporosis, fracture, abdominal hernias, and aneurysm. Severity of rheumatoid arthritis (RA) must be established; cervical traction in RA is contraindicated. Relative contraindications include pregnancy, hyperlaxity, acute injury, inflammatory processes, anxiety, and cardiac or respiratory limitations.[26(pp 92–93)] *Adverse effects include pain, dizziness, orthostatic hypotension, nausea, and visual disturbances.*

Massage

Described as the world's oldest medical modality,[29] massage is the use of applied rhythmic pressure and stretching to soft tissues (see Table P–2). Local mechanical benefits include increasing venous return and loosening of adhesions; reflexive diffuse effects include increased circulation, relaxation, vasodilation, decreased pain, and enhanced well-being. Massage can be done manually (thought to be most effective because tissues can be assessed by the therapist during treatment) and with mechanical devices. Subjective benefits of massage include relaxation, decreased muscle soreness and tightness, improved sleep, and improved mood. Recent research suggests improved immunity,[30] prevention of delayed-onset muscle soreness,[31] and reduced anxiety and increased alertness.[32] Top Olympic trainers and professional athletes often rely on weekly massage to improve circulation and decrease soreness of stressed and intensely trained muscles.

Contraindications include infectious/contagious or open skin conditions, fever, varicosities, phlebitis, tumors, and thrombocytopenia.[33]

Biofeedback

Biofeedback is a means of monitoring and modifying physiological parameters such as heart rate, muscle tension, and sweat response by means of "psychophysiological self-regulation."[34(p 410)] The most widely used type of biofeedback is electromyographic monitoring of motor unit action potentials.[35] In the athletic training setting, electromyographic biofeedback can be used to teach muscle-firing patterns and maximize isolated muscle recruitment (see Table P–3). It can also be used for relaxation, pain management, decreased stress response, and improved musculature control at specific sites.

Table P–2 Types of Massage Therapy

Swedish	using stroking (effleurage), kneading (petrissage), friction, percussion (tapotement) and vibration
Acupressure	pressure points—also known as "Shiatsu"
Connective tissue	pulling strokes thought to stimulate a cutaneovisceral reflex; includes "rolfing"
Soft tissue mobilization	stretching and pulling strokes to increase flexibility
Myofascial release	addressing trigger points with stretch and light pressure
Mechanical	use of percussion, vibration, and suction devices
Hydromassage	water provides pressure and movement
Intermittent compression	used for edema

Alternative Therapy

The increasing popularity of alternative forms of therapy has been the focus of many medical studies. The division between conventional and alternative modalities is decreasing. The expansion of hospitals and health centers adding alternative and complementary medicine suites and the popularity of holistic and homeopathic treatments and practitioners reflect this trend. Medical research supports some of these methods; those particular to rehabilitation can be quite effective. Wainapel, Thomas, and Kahan surveyed an outpatient rehabilitation population in a study published in 1998[36] to evaluate the frequency of use of massage, chiropractic care, vitamin and mineral supplementation, and acupuncture. Of the subjects, 29.1% had used at least one of these treatments, with 53% reporting efficacy. Most treatments were sought for musculoskeletal pain.

Table P–3 Biofeedback Types and Measurement Parameters

Electromyographic (EMG)	muscle tension
Thermal	skin temperature
Electroencephalograph (EEG)	brain waves
Electrodermal response (EDR)	sweat glands
Perineometer	anal sphincter, pelvic floor
Plethysmography	blood pressure
Pressure, force, or position	force on external devices

Women have been noted to comprise up to two-thirds of the US population seeking alternative and complementary medical care with a particular bias for reproductive health care.[37] Other studies also support a greater percentage of women users.[36,38] Documented personality traits of consumers of alternative medicine include higher education, higher mind-body awareness, and greater sense of well-being.[39] An additional reason for use is patient desire for sense of autonomy.[40] The psychological benefits of alternative therapies include those associated with relaxation techniques and improved sense of well-being. Additional benefits include improved mood, decreased pain behavior, and increased activity levels. These factors provide a beneficial influence on physiological health and recovery from injury and are quite effective in women athletes with a holistic mindset.

Manipulation

Maneuvers to increase joint range of motion with mechanical or reflex relaxation can be done as both high-velocity thrust and slow nonthrust rhythmic or oscillation techniques.[10] In particular, craniosacral and spinal manipulation must be performed only by a skilled, licensed practitioner. If used, manipulation should only be in conjunction with other active modalities and exercise to maintain benefits. Long-term use is not indicated.

Contraindications include hematological, musculoskeletal, and neurological disease processes; malignancy; and fracture. Complications increase with high-velocity manipulations; high-velocity and rotational manipulation of the cervical spine are not advised because of the possibility of vertebrobasilar accidents. Other described adverse effects of spinal manipulation include progression of herniated discs and central nervous system effects including stroke.[41]

Acupuncture

Acupuncture involves the insertion of small-gauge solid needles into multiple acupuncture points, usually penetrating underlying muscle tissue. Effects are cumulative, and repeated sessions are required. Acupuncture is proposed to release opioid peptides[42] and is also acknowledged as a form of hyperstimulation analgesia. Indications include menstrual pain, depression, immune dysfunctions, stress, and insomnia.[10] Musculoskeletal disorders with positive responses to acupuncture include epicondylitis, fibromyalgia, and myofascial pain syndromes.[42]

Contraindications include anticoagulation and bloodborne and local infections. Complications are needle and technique related; vasovagal reactions can also occur.

Relaxation Techniques

The most popular of alternative therapy types, relaxation techniques can often be done without a practitioner. Commonly used relaxation techniques include meditation, yoga, biofeedback, massage, hypnosis, and imagery.

Energy Healing

Energy healing includes magnets, therapeutic touch, Reiki, and religious group spiritual healing.[38] Magnets are proposed to increase blood flow to painful areas. They are worn in self-adhesive patches, bracing, bandages, and are also available as shoe inserts, pillows, and cushions. A noninvasive, passive, pain-free modality with no reported ill effects to date, there are virtually no limits to the types of pain magnets are used for.

Holistic Healing

Holistic healing methods often integrate combinations of meditation, laying of hands, reflexology, crystals, scents, and holistic medications. Precautions should be used in regard to medications that are not approved by the Food and Drug Administration and often mysterious in their content. Patients should be monitored periodically to ensure that treatment is benign.[43] Communication encourages trust and can prevent avoidance of concordant conventional treatments if necessary.

CONCLUSION

Consistent with most medical treatments, although women comprise a greater population of health care consumers,[37] there has been little research on female-specific therapeutic techniques. It is anticipated that this will improve. A study on anterior cruciate ligament (ACL) rehabilitation[44] found women required an average of 6 more rehabilitation treatment sessions but achieved similar long-term and short-term results. The greater incidence of ACL tears in female athletes has focused medical and sports care on gender-specific injury prevention and rehabilitation. Protocols specific to women are being developed in response to demand.[45,46] Although research is still lacking, this text strives to expand gender-specific therapy to include all dimensions of sports rehabilitation. The future is promising as younger female athletes are being trained with greater amounts of conditioning, coaching, and medical care, and, as clinicians and researchers recognize and meet the demands unique to women's sports medicine.

REFERENCES

1. Herring SA, Kibler, BW. A framework for rehabilitation. In: Kibler WB, Herring SA, Press JA, Lee PA, eds. *Functional Rehabilitation of Sports and Musculoskeletal Injuries*. Gaithersburg, MD: Aspen Publishers; 1998:1–8.

2. Wilfley DE, Grilo CM, Brownell KD. Exercise and regulation of body weight. In: Shangold MM, Mirkin G. *Women and Exercise: Physiology and Sports Medicine*. 2nd ed. Philadelphia: FA Davis Company; 1994:27–54.

3. Kibler WB. Determining the extent of the functional deficit. In: Kibler WB, Herring SA, Press JA, Lee PA, eds. *Functional Rehabilitation of Sports and Musculoskeletal Injuries*. Gaithersburg, MD: Aspen Publishers; 1998:16–19.

4. Taylor J, Taylor S. *Psychological Approaches to Sports Injury Rehabilitation*. Gaithersburg, MD: Aspen Publishers; 1997:197–217.

5. Adler SA, Beckers D, Buck M. *PNF in Practice: An Illustrated Guide*. Berlin: Springer-Verlag; 1993.

6. Bell GW. Aquatic sports massage therapy. *Clin Sports Med*. 1999;18:427–435.

7. Doyle J, Gleeson NP, Rees D. Psychobiology and the athlete with anterior cruciate ligament (ACL) Injury. *Sports Med*. 1998;26(6):379–393.

8. Young JL, Press JA. In: Kibler WB, Herring SA, Press JA, Lee PA, eds. *Functional Rehabilitation of Sports and Musculoskeletal Injuries*. Gaithersburg, MD: Aspen Publishers; 1998:10–15.

9. Nordin M, Campello M. Physical therapy: exercises and the modalities: when, what and why? *Neurol Clin North Am*. 1999;17:75–89.

10. Tan JC. Physical modalities. In: Tan JC, ed. *Practical Manual of Physical Medicine and Rehabilitation*. St. Louis, MO: Mosby; 1998:133–155.

11. Swenson C, Sward L, Karlsson J. Cryotherapy in sports medicine. *Scand J Med Sci Sports*. 1996;6(4):193–200.

12. Fond D. Cryotherapy. In: Hecox B, Mahreteab TA, Weisberg J. *Physical Agents: A Comprehensive Text for Physical Therapists*. Norwalk, CT: Appleton & Lange; 1994:193–202.

13. Zemke JE, Andersen JC, Guion WK, McMillan J, et al. Intramuscular temperature responses in the human leg to two forms of cryotherapy: massage and ice bag. *J Orthop Sports Phys Ther*. 1998;27(4):301–307.

14. Hecox B. Clinical effects of thermal modalities. In: Hecox B, Mahreteab TA, Weisberg J. *Physical Agents: A Comprehensive Text for Physical Therapists*. Norwalk, CT: Appleton & Lange; 1994:115–124.

15. Sicard-Rosenbaum L, Danoff JV, Guthrie JA, Eckhaus MA. Effects of energy-matched pulsed and continuous ultrasound on tumor growth in mice. *Phys Ther*. 1998;78:271–277.

16. Hayes KW. Ultrasound. In: Hayes KW. *Manual for Physical Agents*. 5th ed. Upper Saddle River, NJ: Prentice Hall Health; 2000:43–55.

17. Sweitzer RW. Ultrasound. In: Hecox B, Mahreteab TA, Weisberg J. *Physical Agents: A Comprehensive Text for Physical Therapists*. Norwalk, CT: Appleton & Lange; 1994:163–192.

18. Young S. Ultrasound therapy. In: Kitchen S, Bazin S, eds. *Clayton's Electrotherapy*. 10th ed. Philadelphia: WB Saunders; 1996:243–267.

19. Snyder-Mackler L. Electrical stimulation for tissue repair. In: Robinson AJ, Snyder-Mackler L. *Clinical Electrophysiology*. 2nd ed. Baltimore: Williams & Wilkins; 1995:313–332.

20. Mehreteah TA. Clinical uses of electrical stimulation. In: Hecox B, Mahreteab TA, Weisberg J. *Physical Agents: A Comprehensive Text for Physical Therapists*. Norwalk, CT: Appleton & Lange; 1994:283–293.

21. Mysiw WJ, Jackson RD. Electrical stimulation. In: Braddom RL. *Physical Medicine and Rehabilitation*. Philadelphia: WB Saunders; 1996.

22. Foley RA. Transcutaneous electrical nerve stimulation. In: Hayes KW. *Manual for Physical Agents*. 5th ed. Upper Saddle River, NJ: Prentice Hall Health; 2000:121–147.

23. Ciccone CD. Iontophoresis. In: Robinson AJ, Snyder-Mackler L. *Clinical Electrophysiology*. 2nd ed. Baltimore: Williams & Wilkins; 1995:335–358.

24. Japour CJ, Vohra R, Vohra PK, Garfunkel L, Chin, N. Management of heel pain syndrome with acetic acid iontophorosis. *J Am Podiatr Med Assoc*. 1999;89(5):251–257.

25. Demirtas RN, Oner C. The treatment of lateral epicondylitis by iontophoresis of sodium salicylate and sodium diclofenac. *Clin Rehabil*. 1998;12(1):23–29.

26. Wilding J. Mechanical spinal traction. In: Hayes KW. *Manual for Physical Agents*. 5th ed. Upper Saddle River, NJ: Prentice Hall Health; 2000:91–102.

27. Weisberg J. Spinal traction (distraction). In: Hecox B, Mahreteab TA, Weisberg J. *Physical Agents: A Comprehensive Text for Physical Therapists*. Norwalk, CT: Appleton & Lange; 1994:397–417.

28. Janke AW, Kerdow TA, Griffiths HJ, et al. The biomechanics of gravity-dependent traction of the lumbar spine. *Spine*. 1997;22(3):253–260.

29. Yates J. *A Physician's Guide to Therapeutic Massage: Its Physiological Effect and Their Application to Treatment*. Vancouver, BC: Massage Therapists Association of British Columbia; 1990.

30. Ironson G, Field T, Scafidi F, et al. Massage therapy is associated with enhancement of the immune system's cytotoxic capacity. *Int J Neurosci*. 1996;84:205–218.

31. Ernst E. Does post-exercise massage treatment reduce delayed onset muscle soreness? A systematic review. *Br J Sports Med*. 1998;32(3):212–214.

32. Field T, Ironson G, Scafidi F, et al. Massage therapy reduces anxiety and enhances EEG pattern of alertness and math computations. *Int J Neurosci*. 1997;86:197–205.

33. Field T. Massage therapy. In: Jonas WB, Levin JS. *Essentials of Complimentary and Alternative Medicine*. Philadelphia: Lippincott-Raven, Publishers; 1999:383–391.

34. Green JA, Shellenberger R. Biofeedback therapy. In: Jonas WB, Levin JS. *Essentials of Complimentary and Alternative Medicine*. Philadelphia: Lippincott-Raven, Publishers; 1999:410–425.

35. Poe WJ, Sander AP. Electromyographic feedback. In: Hayes KW. *Manual for Physical Agents*. 5th ed. Upper Saddle River, NJ: Prentice Hall Health; 2000:189–199.

36. Wainapel SF, Thomas AD, Kahan BS. Use of alternative therapies by rehabilitation outpatients. *Arch Phys Med Rehabil*. 1998;79:1003–1005.

37. Beal MW. Women's use of complementary and alternative therapies in reproductive health care. *J Nurse Midwifery*. 1998;43:224–234.

38. Eisenberg DM, Davis RB, Ettner SL, et al. Trends in alternative medicine use in the United States, 1990–1997: Results of a follow-up national survey. *JAMA*. 1998;280:1569–1575.

39. Owens JE, Taylor AG, Degood D. Complementary and alternative medicine and psychologic factors: toward an individual differences model of complementary and alternative medicine use and outcomes. *J Altern Complement Med*. 1999;5:529–541.

40. Astin JA. Why patients use alternative medicine: results of a national study. *JAMA*. 1998;279:1548–1553.

41. Ernst E. Adverse effects of spinal manipulation. In: Jonas WB, Levin JS. *Essentials of Complimentary and Alternative Medicine*. Philadelphia: Lippincott-Raven Publishers; 1999:176–179.

42. National Institutes of Health. Acupuncture. *NIH Consensus Statement*. 1997;15:1–3.

43. Eisenberg DM. Advising patients who seek alternative medical therapies. *Ann Intern Med*. 1997;127:61–69.

44. Barber-Westin SD, Noyes FR, Andrews M. A rigorous comparison between the sexes of results and complications after anterior cruciate ligament reconstruction. *Am J Sports Med*. 1997;25:514–526.

45. Wilk KE, Arrigo C, Andrews JR, Clancy WG. Rehabilitation after anterior cruciate ligament reconstruction in the female athlete. *J Athletic Training*. 1999;34:177–193.

46. Cook G, Burton L, Fields K. Reactive neuromuscular training for the anterior cruciate ligament-deficient knee: a case report. *J Athletic Training*. 1999;34:194–201.

PART I

Musculoskeletal Considerations

CHAPTER 1

Gender Differences in Muscle Morphology

Suzanne Meth

INTRODUCTION

There are a number of ways to compare gender differences in strength and an even greater number of reasons why differences exists at all. It is obvious that men and women respond differently to similar weight training programs, but actually they both have the same capacity to build strength when related to total muscle mass.[1,2] Recently, more research has been focusing on strength training in women to understand how anatomical or physiological differences affect performance. When comparing all the cells of a male and a female, the only physical differences lie in the reproductive system.[3] One cannot differentiate the gender origin of a tissue when compared on a laboratory table.[3]

ANATOMY

Anatomical Gender Differences—Women vs Men[1,4]

- 3–4 inches shorter
- 25–30 pounds lighter
- 10–15 pounds (8%–10%) more body fat
- 40–45 less pounds of fat-free weight (bone, muscle, organs)
- Less muscle mass supported by narrower shoulders
- Shorter extremities

Clinical Guideline

All these factors combined (see Clinical Guideline above) give men a mechanical advantage over women which en-

ables them to handle more weight and generate more power.[5] In addition, men who have larger shoulder girdles may also have a higher center of gravity, which can increase the ability to develop upper body strength. Women generally have wider pelvises, which will then lower the center of gravity and decrease the potential to gain upper body mass. A wider pelvis may also lead to an increased Q angle which can negatively affect optimal patterns of muscle firing in lower extremities.[5–7] The major anatomical strength differences occur between men and women in stature and muscle fiber size. These structural differences are only a matter of degrees but are enough of a mechanical limitation for women who are trying to gain maximal strength.[1,5]

PHYSIOLOGY

Physiological characteristics of skeletal muscle in both men and women do not differ significantly.[4,8] The most important hormones for muscle fiber and strength development are the androgenic hormones testosterone and androstenedione.[1] These hormones are anabolic and contribute to muscle hypertrophy and decreasing body fat percent. Resting testosterone concentrations can vary considerably, but the average woman has between $\frac{1}{2}$ and $\frac{1}{10}$ the blood level that a man has.[4,9,10] Some women have higher than average testosterone levels and therefore may have greater potentials for strength and power development.[1,10] Most studies show that women do not demonstrate significant exercise-induced increases in testosterone after different types of heavy resistance exercise.[1,10] A decreased amount of androstenedione can limit muscle development in both men and women, but it appears that the absolute androstenedione response is similar in both genders. Women also have higher quantities of estrogen, a hormone that can interfere with potentials for muscle growth by increasing body fat stores.[9] These factors together help us understand why women often do not make muscle size gains that are comparable to those of men.[2]

MENSTRUAL CYCLE

Research that explores how the menstrual cycle affects strength training and muscle development is limited.[5,10] Although there seem to be some hormonal and other differences, it is generally accepted that the menstrual cycle has no significant deleterious effects on training.[2,6,11] In 1997, Fleck and Kraemer[4] found that women had higher resting growth hormone levels during the early follicular phase of their menstrual cycle (the days immediately after menstruation) compared with growth hormone levels in men. This hormone will affect skeletal muscle growth in response to resistance training, and levels may be affected by type and amount of resistance used and rest period durations.[4,10] One study found that women who were not taking oral contraceptives significantly (11%) increased their quadriceps and handgrip strength during the middle of their menstrual cycle (ovulation) compared with their luteal and follicular phases.[12] More research is needed to examine the effects of the menstrual cycle on strength and power performance.

MUSCLE

The amount and location of muscle tissue strongly affect potentials for gaining strength, as do the muscle fiber type and the quantity of muscle fibers that one is born with.[5] It is difficult to study the exact changes in human muscle tissue after resistance training, because most assessments are merely estimations reached by studying percent body fat and limb circumference changes.[3] To date, there are an equal number of studies showing that women have either less than or the same number of muscle fibers as men, so it is difficult to conclude whether the actual number of muscle fibers differs significantly between genders.[4] Men appear more muscular simply because their individual muscle fibers are larger than those in women, but the quantity of fibers does not appear to significantly differ.[3,5]

Most studies have not found any major gender differences in type I (slow-twitch) and type II (fast-twitch) muscle fiber distributions.[1,3,5,13] When comparing fiber area, men appear to have larger slow and fast twitch muscle fibers than women.[3] Studies show that fast-twitch fibers are larger than slow-twitch fibers in trained men and women and untrained men, but they are of similar size in untrained women, because they do not have developed fast-twitch muscle fibers.[3] Athletes of both genders participating in the same sport (ie, male and female powerlifters or male and female sprint-

ers) seem to have similar muscle fiber compositions, but two studies have shown that men may have a greater fast-twitch/slow-twitch fiber area ratio.[2,5] Staron et al[14] demonstrated that all the muscle fiber types (types I, IIA, IIAB, and IIB) can hypertrophy similarly in both sexes, assuming that the exercise stimulus and intensity are sufficient. In summary, differences in strength gains between men and women seem not to be affected by muscle fiber type or adaptation but rather by cross-sectional area and muscle fiber number.[6]

Unit for unit, female muscle tissue does not differ from a male in potentials for force development.[13]

Clinical Guideline

STRENGTH

Strength is defined as the maximal force that can be exerted by a muscle or group of muscles and as a quantitative measure can be looked at in two different ways.[14] Absolute strength is simply the amount of weight that one can lift (ie, 30 kg) and is usually how we speak of our individual strength. Relative strength relates this 30 kg to an individual's muscle mass (ie, 50 kg of lean muscle mass can lift 30 kg). Men appear to demonstrate larger *absolute* increases in strength and degree of muscle hypertrophy than women when both undergo identical weight training regimens.[5,13] Over time, women and men make the same *relative* gains in muscular hypertrophy after a resistance training program.[3,8] Studies have shown that in some exercises (squat, bench press, leg press, isometric knee extension), women actually achieved greater relative gains.[5] One study, in which men and women trained their elbow flexor muscles (biceps) for 20 weeks, demonstrated that the women actually showed greater relative strength increases than the men, even though muscle size increased similarly among the genders.[15] Because muscle cross-sectional area (muscle fiber size multiplied by the number of muscle fibers) is directly related to the ability to produce force, individuals who have larger muscles are able to lift more weight.[4,10] When comparing strength to lean body mass (body weight without fat) or cross-sectional area, women are about equal to men and are just as capable of developing strength relative to total muscle mass.[1,4]

The ability of a muscle to produce force is independent of gender: A 15-cm^2 cross-sectional area of an elbow flexor muscle can produce about 19 kg of force for both men and women.[16]

Clinical Guideline

The average woman can produce about two-thirds of the force of the average man, but muscular strength differences between genders depend on which muscle groups are compared.[1,5,9,10] Absolute gender differences are less in lower body muscles; leg strength as it relates to units of lean body weight can actually be slightly greater in women than in men.[4,9] This is in part because both sexes use their legs to perform similar activities (walking, stair climbing).[8,9] It has also been proposed that women may tend to avoid upper body strengthening activities more because of sociocultural reasons.[6,8] A simple explanation for upper body strength differentials between the sexes may be that women have a lower proportion of their total lean body mass in their upper body.[4] This may warrant additional upper extremity strength training(ie, add one or two sets to an existing exercise or add one or two different exercises) if a female athlete is preparing for competition that relies heavily on upper body strength or power.[4] This is not to say that the program should significantly differ from a man's, but that a larger portion of the total training volume could emphasize the upper body musculature.[4]

There appear to be no significant gender differences in adaptations to resistance training, except for the amounts of muscle hypertrophy.[5,8] An average woman responds to weight training with a slight increase in muscle girth and a decrease in intramuscular and subcutaneous fat stores, with little change in limb circumference.[5] Lean body mass will increase as muscle tissue grows, but no significant corresponding change in weight will occur unless dietary intake decreases. The increased vascularity often observed in highly muscular men usually will occur only in highly trained women who also possess a low level of subcutaneous fat.[3,8]

Muscle physiologists often perform research using bodybuilders as study subjects in order to see extreme changes in muscle histology. A study that compared female bodybuilders to untrained men found that the women possessed less strength in their upper bodies, but no significant differences were found in lower body strength.[5] Relatively speaking (taking body weight into account), there was no significant difference in strength for either the upper or the lower body.[5,13] Another study on elite male and female bodybuilders demonstrated that muscle cross-sectional area was two times greater in male bodybuilders than in female bodybuilders, but when expressed relative to lean body mass or per centimeter body height, the difference was reduced to 35%.[16] Yet another study on nationally ranked male and female bodybuilders actually found no difference in muscle fiber cross-sectional area.[5] Male and female bodybuilders do not seem to differ in force production relative to lean muscle mass, but with so few data comparing muscle fiber size between genders, it is difficult to draw any conclusions. We can see from observing female bodybuilders that it is indeed possible to make large gains in muscle mass, although the most probable explanation (excluding steroid use) is that of genetic endowment.[3,8] Female bodybuilders usually have less than normal levels of subcutaneous fat, dehydrate themselves, and "pump up" immediately before a bodybuilding routine, which will increase muscle blood flow to engorge the muscle, thereby increasing its size.[3,8] Their training regimens may also focus on the body parts that need to be brought up to the standard size of the other muscles in their physique.

Women gain relative strength at the same rate as (or faster than) men when performing identical resistance training programs.[2,3,4,13] One reason may be that women begin weight-training regimens at lower resistances than men.[3] Research suggests that if given similar training protocols, gender differences in strength gains are due mostly to differences in percent muscle mass.[8] Because women have less absolute upper body muscle mass than men, when you eliminate body fat and compare strength to lean body mass, men still dominate in upper body strength, but lower body gender differences disappear.[8] It has also been speculated, but not scientifically supported, that broader hips and an increased Q angle (hip-knee angle) may give women an advantage in squatting exercises.[8] Notice that many successful male and female powerlifters tend to have shorter than average legs.

Training Recommendations

No evidence exists to suggest that women should strength train any differently than men.[1,3,5,13,14,17] Assuming equal nutrition, the rate and degree of improvement in strength should be equal between genders.[13] Significant gains in muscle strength and endurance can be achieved by use of a training program 3 to 4 days a week.[8] Any changes in muscle mass or muscle fiber characteristics are minimal once anyone of either gender has reached a high degree of muscularity and competitiveness.[18]

Strength Training Recommendations

- The training program should incorporate four to five exercises that use major muscle groups in both the lower and upper body.[7]
- Your program should be periodized by altering your exercise choices, rest periods, and quantity of sets, repetitions, and intensity.
- Higher repetitions (12–15) are used for endurance training, whereas maximal strength gains can be achieved using lower repetitions (5–8).[7]
- Multijoint, multiplanar, functional free weight exercises should be used to optimize neuromuscular coordination, movement patterns, balance, and speed during power training.[1,3]

- For the lower body, free weight exercises should be incorporated that emphasize foot-based (closed chain) exercises, such as stepping, lunges (forward and diagonal), and squats.[1,3]
- Upper body exercises should include functional activities: push-ups, bench and incline presses, pull-downs and pull-ups, rowing, and shoulder raises.[1]
- Back extensions and abdominal work are necessary for core stabilization and strength and for preventing lower back injuries.
- Advanced exercises such as plyometrics, power cleans, hang cleans, push presses, snatches, and clean and jerks should be performed with proper technique after a solid base of strength has been established.[1]

Clinical Guideline

FLEXIBILITY

Research shows that women are generally more flexible than men.[19,20] Evidence for this difference appears in anatomical and physiological attributes. Depending on the type of pelvis they inherit, women with broader and shallower pelvises may have a greater range of motion in the hips.[19,20] One study that looked at hundreds of subjects tested during adolescence and again 18 years later showed that men had less flexibility than women only in their hamstring muscles.[21] Women also have greater elbow extension because of a shorter upper arc in the olecranon process than men.[19] Of course, the effects of the types of exercise that women are socially conditioned to perform may also have an effect on gender differences in flexibility.[19]

REFERENCES

1. Ebben WP, Jensen RL. Strength training for women; debunking myths that block opportunity. *Phys Sports Med.* 1998;26:86–97.
2. Lewis DA, Kamon E, Hodgson JL. Physiological differences between genders; implications for sports conditioning. *Sports Med.* 1986;3:357–369.
3. Wells CL. *Women, Sport, and Performance—A Physiological Perspective.* 2nd ed. Champaign, IL: Human Kinetics; 1991.
4. Fleck SJ, Kraemer WJ. *Designing Resistance Training Programs.* 2nd ed. Champaign, IL: Human Kinetics; 1997.
5. Holloway JB, Baechle TR. Strength training for female athletes; a review of selected aspects. *Sports Med.* 1990;9:216–228.
6. Sanborn CF, Jankowski CM. Gender-specific physiology. In: Agostini R. *Medical and Orthopedic Issues of Active and Athletic Women.* Philadelphia: Hanley & Belfus, Inc; 1994:23–28.
7. Sanborn CF, Jankowski CM. Physiologic considerations for women in sport. *Clin Sports Med.* 1994;13:315–327.
8. Costa DM, Guthrie SR. *Women and Sport—Interdisciplinary Perspectives.* Champaign, IL: Human Kinetics; 1994.
9. Fox EL, Bowers RW, Foss ML. *The Physiological Basis for Exercise and Sport.* 2nd ed. Dubuque, IA: Brown and Benchmark Publishers; 1989.
10. Baechle TR, ed. *Essentials of Strength Training and Conditioning. National Strength and Conditioning Association.* Champaign, IL: Human Kinetics; 1994.
11. Miskec CM, Potteiger JA, Nau KL, Zebas CJ. Do varying environmental and menstrual cycle conditions affect aerobic power output in female athletes? *J Str Cond Res.* 1997;11:219–223.
12. Sarwar R, Niclos BB, Rutherford OM. Changes in muscle strength, relaxation rate and fatiguability during the human menstrual cycle. *J Appl Physiol.* 1996;493:267–272.
13. Cureton KJ, Collins MA, Hill DW, McElhannon FM Jr. Muscle hypertrophy in men and women. *Med Sci Sports Exer.* 1988;20:338–344.
14. Staron RS, Malicky ES, Leonardi MJ, Falkel JE, Hagerman FC, Dudley GA. Muscle hypertrophy and fast fiber type conversions in heavy resistance-trained women. *Eur J App Phys Occup Physiol.* 1990;60:71–79.
15. O'Hagan FT, Sale DG, MacDougall JD, Garner SH. Response to resistance training in young women and men. *Int J Sports Med.* 1995;16:314–321.
16. Alway SE, Grumbt WH, Gonyea WJ, Stray-Gundersen J. Contrasts in muscle and myofibers of elite male and female bodybuilders. *J Appl Physiol.* 1989;67:24–31.
17. Campos JL. *Comparison of strength development of adult males and females undergoing dynamic weight training.* Iowa; Graduate College of the University of Iowa; 1980. Thesis.
18. Alway SE, Grumbt WH, Stray-Gundersen J, Gonyea WJ. Effects of resistance training on elbow flexors of highly competitive bodybuilders. *J Appl Physiol.* 1992;72:1512–1521.
19. Atter MJ. *Science of Flexibility.* 2nd ed. Champaign, IL: Human Kinetics; 1996.
20. Cyphers M. Flexibility. In: *Personal Trainer Manual—The Resource for Fitness Instructors.* San Diego, CA: American Council on Exercise; 1991:275–292.
21. Barnekow-Berkvist M, Hedberg G, Janlert U, Jansson E. Development of muscular endurance and strength from adolescence to adulthood and level of physical capacity in men and women at the age of 24 years. *Scand J Med Sci Sports.* 1996;3:145–155.

BIBLIOGRAPHY

1. Ikai M, Fukunago T. Calculation of muscle strength per unit cross sectional area of human muscle by means of ultrasonic measurement. *Int Z Angew Physiol.* 1968;26:26–32.
2. Laubach L. Comparative strength of men and women: a review of the literature. *Aviat Space Environ Med.* 1976;47:534–542.

CHAPTER 2

The Shoulder and Upper Extremities

Diane L. Dahm

INCIDENCE OF INJURY

Sports in which upper extremity injuries are seen frequently include gymnastics, swimming, volleyball, tennis, racquetball, and golf. Overuse injuries of the upper extremities are common in these sports. Traumatic injuries to the upper extremity are frequently seen in sports such as alpine skiing, snowboarding, and rollerblading. In general, similar injury rates are seen in men's and women's sports with comparable rules.[1]

Certain injuries have been reported to occur with higher frequency in women. Aagaard[2] has reported a higher incidence of serious shoulder injuries in female volleyball players despite a similar overall incidence of injury in men and women. Shoulder pain secondary to impingement has been reported to be more common in female than in male swimmers.[3,4]

Injuries More Common in Women

- Serious shoulder injuries in volleyball
- Shoulder pain caused by impingement in swimmers
- Stress injuries to the distal radial physis in gymnasts
- Wrist and elbow injuries in golfers
- Thoracic outlet syndrome
- Stress fractures caused by osteoporosis

Clinical Guideline

Similarly, thoracic outlet syndrome is three times more common in women than in men.[5] In young adolescent gymnasts, wrist pain caused by stress fractures of the distal radial physis is more commonly seen in women.[6] Fractures occurring as a result of decreased bone mineral density are also of particular concern in the female athlete. In the sport of golf, injury patterns also seem to differ by gender. Although male professional and amateur golfers most frequently report lower back injuries, among female professional golfers, injuries to the left wrist are most frequently reported, and among female amateur golfers, injuries to the elbow are most frequently reported.[7]

Although sports participation in general exposes the female athlete to risk of upper extremity injury, participation in sports involving the use of the upper extremities may also serve to prevent neck and shoulder symptoms in girls. Neimi[8] studied 718 high school students and found a significantly greater incidence of neck and shoulder symptoms in girls compared with boys of the same age. Girls involved in sports requiring dynamic use of the upper extremities complained of significantly fewer neck and shoulder symptoms than those participating in activities or hobbies involving static postures of the upper limbs.

GENDER DIFFERENCES IN ANATOMY AND KINESIOLOGY

On average, women have approximately two-thirds the absolute strength and power output of men, with a proportionately greater difference in absolute upper body strength.[9] This is likely due to a combination of factors, including decreased average height, arm length, shoulder-to-hip width, muscle fiber, and total cross-sectional area in women versus men. Despite a common perception that women have an increased "carrying angle" of the forearm that could theoretically make acquisition of throwing skills more difficult, Beall[10] found no significant difference in the carrying angle between men and women of various ages. However, a woman's relatively shorter arms, narrower shoulders, and decreased lean muscle mass likely result in decreased mechanical advantage for force production in the upper extremities. It is important to note that when strength is expressed per unit of muscle cross-sectional area, men and women have the same potential for force production.[11] Similarly, muscle strength and hypertrophy responses are similar for men and women when measured from a pretraining baseline.[11]

The role of hormonal differences relative to strength training, ligamentous laxity, and susceptibility to injury is still being researched. Decreased fine motor skills have been reported by Posthuma et al[12] in women with premenstrual symptoms, perhaps contributing to increased risk of injury in this particular group of women. Most such research has focused on athletic injuries to the lower extremity and, in particular, the anterior cruciate ligament. On the basis of a scarcity of current research, no firm conclusions can be drawn regarding the influence of hormonal fluctuations on upper extremity injuries in female athletes.

SPECIFIC INJURIES: DIAGNOSIS AND MANAGEMENT

Shoulder

The shoulder joint allows for extreme mobility of the upper extremity. It is made up of the humeral head, which articulates with the glenoid, a rather shallow bony socket that is deepened by a fibrocartilaginous rim known as the glenoid labrum. The highly mobile shoulder joint is stabilized by the joint capsule and associated glenohumeral ligaments and the surrounding rotator cuff musculature (Figure 2–1). The rotator cuff consists of the subscapularis, supraspinatus, infraspinatus, and teres minor muscles (Figure 2–2). The scapular stabilizing muscles—the trapezius, rhomboids, latissimus dorsi, and serratus anterior—are important in proper positioning of the scapula and thus also contribute to stability of the shoulder joint.

Impingement Syndrome/Instability

Shoulder pain in female athletes may occur for several different reasons. Relatively poor upper body strength, shorter upper extremities, improper technique, generalized laxity, and overuse may be contributing factors. Primary impingement, secondary impingement, and laxity with recurrent subluxation will be discussed.

Primary impingement syndrome and associated rotator cuff tendon pathological conditions have been well described by Neer.[13] This is typically seen in the more mature overhead

athlete or swimmer. Associated factors include a downsloping acromion, os acromiale, and undersurface acromioclavicular joint spurring, as well as dysvascular changes and tendon degeneration, which may occur in the aging athlete's shoulder. These factors may result in encroachment on the subacromial space and microtrauma with eventual tearing of the rotator cuff.[13,14]

Instability may also be a cause of secondary impingement-like symptoms, particularly in younger athletes.[15] Repetitive overhead activities, with the arm in abduction and external rotation, stress the anterior capsule and in the setting of glenohumeral laxity may cause secondary fatigue and rotator cuff strain. Similarly, impingement of the undersurface of the rotator cuff on the posterior superior glenoid labrum has been described in overhead athletes and may be exacerbated by subtle instability.[16]

Glenohumeral laxity with recurrent subluxation or dislocation may cause pain and apprehension in certain positions, depending on the primary direction of instability, which may be anterior, posterior, inferior, or multidirectional. For example, a volleyball player with anterior instability may feel apprehension with the arm in an abducted, externally rotated position during the initial phase of a serve or spike. Likewise, the same player with posterior instability might complain of apprehension with the arm in an adducted and internally rotated position during follow-through after spiking the ball.

History and physical examination are of utmost importance. The most common complaint in both primary and secondary impingement will be increased pain with overhead activities or activities performed with the arm outstretched. Pain is often poorly localized but may be anterior, posterior, or superior. Athletes may complain of pain while throwing, pitching a softball, serving or spiking a volleyball, performing swimming strokes such as freestyle or butterfly, or weight training using the bench or military press. A lack of endurance in these activities is also a common complaint. There is often no history of traumatic injury. In primary impingement syndrome, night pain is common, as are complaints of inability to sleep on the side of the affected shoulder. The classically described impingement signs in forward elevation and abduction and internal rotation are typically positive (Figure 2–3).[13,17] Weakness of the rotator cuff is often present.

With secondary impingement, pain is often present only during the offending activity, for example, during the cocking and early acceleration phases of throwing. Jobe et al[15] have described a "relocation test" in which the involved shoulder is abducted to 90° and externally rotated (Figure 2–4). An anterior force on the humeral head will cause pain in the athlete with mild instability and secondary impingement. This is thought to be due to impingement of the undersurface of the supraspinatus on the glenoid rim. Posterior

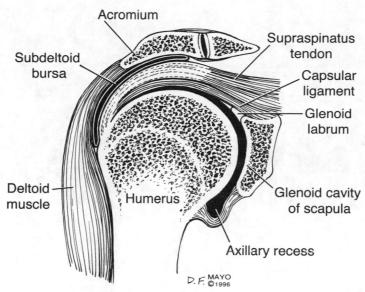

Figure 2–1 Coronal Section through Joint.

pressure on the humeral head restores the space between the glenoid and rotator cuff, thus relieving the pain and constituting a positive test.

Athletes with recurrent instability typically exhibit a positive apprehension test. This is similar to the previously described relocation test, in that for anterior instability the test is also performed with the arm abducted to 90° and externally rotated with anterior stress applied to the humeral head. This maneuver will typically cause apprehension and a sense that the shoulder may subluxate or dislocate rather than pain (Figure 2–5). A posterior apprehension test is performed with the arm abducted and internally rotated and

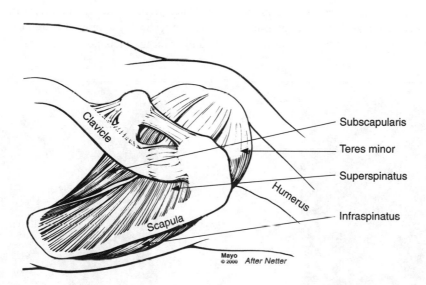

Figure 2–2 Muscles of Rotator Cuff.

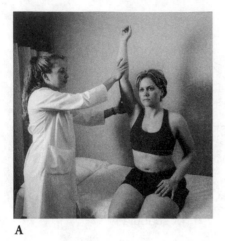

A

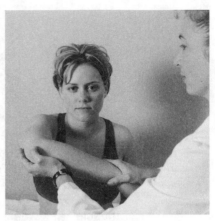

B

Figure 2–3 Impingement Signs.

results in apprehension when posterior stress is applied to the humeral head. The involved shoulder should always be compared with the uninvolved side, and increased anterior, posterior, and inferior glenohumeral translation should be documented. A sulcus sign may be demonstrated by applying downward pressure on the arm with the arm at the side and suggests inferior laxity, which is often seen in the setting of multidirectional instability. Patients should be examined for signs of generalized ligamentous laxity, such as elbow, metacarpophalangeal, and knee hyperextension, and the ability to approximate the thumbs to the forearms.

Diagnostic studies include x-ray studies, magnetic resonance imaging (MRI), and examination under anesthesia. X-ray studies may be helpful in the older athlete to look for degenerative arthritis or spur formation and in the setting of traumatic instability to visualize a Hill-Sachs impression fracture or bony Bankart lesion. MRI may be helpful to

visualize a glenoid labral tear or rotator cuff tear. Examination under anesthesia may be necessary to define the presence and direction of instability.

The mainstay of treatment for all the preceding conditions is conservative management. This includes relative rest from the offending activity and anti-inflammatory measures that may include a short course of nonsteroidal anti-inflammatory agents (NSAIDs), ice, and occasionally a subacromial corticosteroid injection. A stretching program with emphasis on the posterior capsule is initiated. Exercises for pain-free strengthening of the rotator cuff and dynamic scapular stabilizers are important, with the goals of improving scapulothoracic rhythm and improving strength and endurance. Proprioceptive training is also important, particularly in the setting of shoulder instability. Sport-specific training techniques should be emphasized, as well as cross-training for maintenance of generalized conditioning during

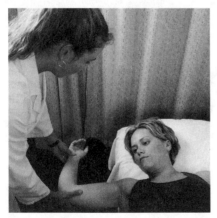

Figure 2–4 Relocation Test.

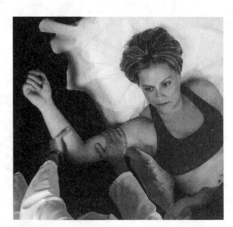

Figure 2–5 Apprehension Test.

the rehabilitative period. Proper technique and form should be emphasized, and abnormal muscular substitution patterns should be recognized and corrected. This program is continued for at least 6 months, after which surgical management may be considered if symptoms continue. Pure subacromial impingement may be treated with a subacromial decompression with resection of a prominent beaked acromion, subacromial spur, or hypertrophic bursa. For athletes with anterior instability and secondary impingement, treatment may include an anterior capsulolabral repair, often combined with debridement or repair of any concomitant rotator cuff pathosis. For pure anterior instability, surgical repair of labral pathology and associated capsular laxity is undertaken. Athletes with generalized ligamentous laxity and multidirectional instability may require a more extensive capsular shift procedure.[18] Habitual voluntary shoulder dislocation has been found to be more common in women. It is important to recognize this phenomenon, because such patients should be treated nonoperatively in most cases (Figure 2–6).[19]

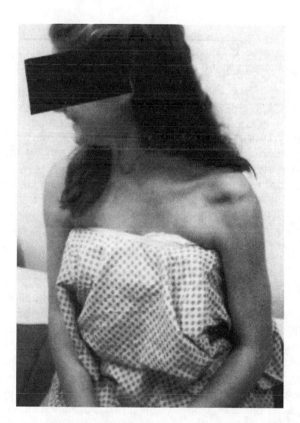

Figure 2–6 Voluntary Instability. This adolescent patient is subluxing her humerus inferiorly through asymmetric muscle contraction.

Shoulder Impingement and Instability

Primary impingement	Night pain, classic "impingement test" positive, subacromial spur formation
Secondary impingement	Pain primarily with activity (ie, throwing), relocation test positive, secondary rotator cuff inflammation
Instability	Apprehension greater than pain, increased glenohumeral translation, may be multidirectional

Clinical Guideline

Voluntary Instability

It is important to recognize the habitual voluntary dislocator. This patient readily demonstrates an ability to dislocate the shoulder by abnormal muscle-firing patterns. This phenomenon is more common in women and is sometimes associated with psychiatric disturbance. These patients are generally poor surgical candidates and are best treated with rehabilitation.

Clinical Guideline

Suprascapular Nerve Entrapment

Suprascapular nerve entrapment is a recognized cause of shoulder pain in the overhead athlete and is frequently observed in volleyball players.[20] Injury to the suprascapular nerve may occur with compression at the spinoglenoid notch by a ganglion cyst[21] or by direct compression or traction of the infraspinatus branch of the suprascapular nerve between the lateral border of the scapular spine and medial margin of the rotator cuff during extremes of shoulder motion or with significant eccentric contraction of the infraspinatus muscle (Figure 2–7).[20,22] Patients may complain of pain at the posterior aspect of the shoulder or cosmetic abnormality caused by atrophy of the infraspinatus muscle. It has been estimated that 20% of high-level volleyball players show clinically evident atrophy of the infraspinatus muscle.[20] Electromyographic examination typically reveals denervation of the infraspinatus muscle without involvement of the supraspinatus muscle. MRI may demonstrate atrophy of the infraspinatus muscle and may show a space-occupying mass such as a ganglion cyst at the level of the spinoglenoid notch and occasionally a superior labral lesion that can lead to ganglion cyst formation.[23] Management depends on the proposed cause of the suprascapular nerve injury. Conservative management consists of relative rest from the

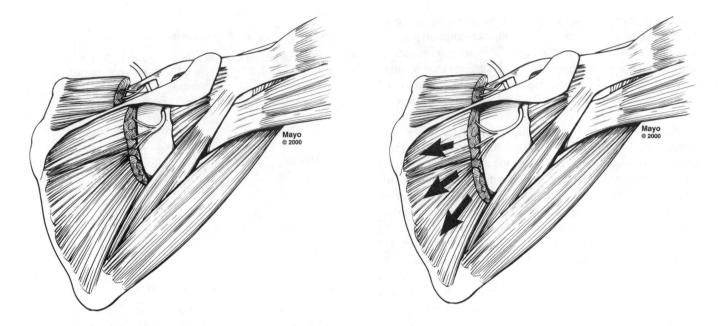

Figure 2–7 Mechanism of Suprascapular Nerve Impingement at the Base of the Scapular Spine Caused by Contraction of the Infraspinatus Muscle.

offending activity, which in volleyball typically involves performance of a "floating service" or volleyball spike, as well as attempted strengthening of the external rotators to reestablish muscle balance and function. Surgical treatment is indicated with failure of conservative management. Direct compression of the infraspinatus branch of the suprascapular nerve between the lateral border of the scapular spine and medial margin of the rotator cuff has been treated with spinoglenoid notchplasty with satisfactory results.[22] Compression by a ganglion cyst is treated with ganglion excision and treatment of any concomitant pathological condition such as a superior labral lesion.

Twenty percent of high-level volleyball players show clinically evident infraspinatus muscle atrophy, thought to be caused by chronic suprascapular nerve injury.

Clinical Guideline

Thoracic Outlet Syndrome

Thoracic outlet syndrome is a relatively uncommon cause of referred pain to the shoulder in athletes; however, it is seen three times more commonly in women than in men.[5] It is sometimes seen in athletes with long, thin necks, especially dancers.[4] It has also been described in aquatic athletes.[24] It is thought to be caused by compression of the nerves and

vessels to the upper extremity as they course between the scalene muscles, over the first rib, and into the axilla. Etiologic factors include poor suspension of the shoulder girdle, tension on the scalene muscles, or anatomical abnormalities such as a cervical rib or an anomalous scalene muscle insertion. Relatively weak shoulder girdle muscles or excessively large breasts may predispose an athlete to thoracic outlet syndrome.[4,5] Swimmers in particular are known for their poor posture and forward position of the shoulders, which may lead to downward pressure of the clavicle on the first rib.[24]

The athlete typically complains of pain and paresthesias that radiate from the neck and shoulder to the medial aspect of the forearm and hand. Symptoms are exacerbated with overhead activity. The swimmer may complain of inability to keep the fingers together and control movement of the hand during the pull-through phase of the swimming stroke. Likewise the water polo player may have difficulty grasping and throwing the ball.[24] Several tests on physical examination have been described that may suggest the diagnosis (Figure 2–8). Wright's test is performed by abducting and externally rotating the arm at the shoulder while palpating the wrist pulses. Reproduction of symptoms or a change in radial pulse suggests the diagnosis. Adson's maneuver is performed by pulling down on the patient's arm during deep inhalation with the head turned away from the affected side. Again, obliteration or diminution of the radial pulse supports the diagnosis of thoracic outlet syndrome. Bracing the shoulder in a military position or direct pressure on the shoulder may exacerbate symptoms. The overhead exercise test consists of repetitive finger flexion and extension with the arm in an overhead position and typically reproduces symptoms within 30 seconds.[5] A complete shoulder and cervical spine examination should be performed to rule out primary shoulder pain or instability or cervical nerve root impingement as a cause for the patient's symptoms. Radiographs of the cervical spine and an apical lordotic chest x-ray film should be obtained to rule out cervical spine disorders or evidence of a cervical rib.

Treatment includes anti-inflammatory medications and rest from the offending activity. Stretching and control of spasm in the cervical muscles, including the scalene, pectoralis major and minor, trapezius, levator scapula, and sternocleidomastoid, are beneficial. This is followed by strengthening of the scapular stabilizing muscles, including the trapezius, rhomboids, and levator scapula. Postural training is important, as is adequate support for large breasts.[4] Rarely, after failure of conservative management, surgical treatment is performed. This may include scalenotomy, scalenectomy, and/or first rib resection.

Predisposing Factors for Thoracic Outlet Syndrome

- Female gender (3:1 predominance)
- Long, thin neck
- Weak shoulder girdle musculature
- Large breasts

Clinical Guideline

Stress Fracture

Stress fractures about the shoulder girdle are uncommon. Still, the diagnosis should be considered in any female athlete involved in an upper-limb–dominant activity who has insidious onset of pain and bony tenderness. The postmenopausal athlete and the young amenorrheic female athlete may be at particular risk for stress fractures because of lower bone density.[25] Rib stress fractures may be seen in female rowers and golfers and are thought to be due to repetitive stresses applied to the posterolateral rib cage by the serratus anterior, rhomboids, trapezius, and external oblique muscles.[26,27] In rowers these fractures are most often associated with long-distance training and heavy load per stroke.[27] The athlete will complain of posterolateral chest pain aggravated by rowing or with trunk rotation during the golf swing. Coughing or deep breathing may also cause pain. The affected ribs will be tender to palpation. Treatment consists of a period of rest from the offending activity, cross-training to maintain

conditioning, and local modalities for pain relief. A rib belt may increase support for the rib cage and provide additional pain relief. Pain-free strengthening of the serratus anterior, rhomboids, and trapezius muscles should be emphasized after acute symptoms have subsided and the ribs are no longer tender. In rowing, it has been proposed that using a truncated arm pull-through technique and a decreased layback position at the end of the stroke combined with equipment changes to decrease length of the lever arm may yield a decreased risk of rib stress fractures.[27]

Stress fractures of the humeral shaft have been described in adolescent male baseball pitchers and tennis players.[28] They are thought to be due to a high level of repetitive stress placed on immature bone, possibly aggravated by a period of rapid growth. As more young female athletes participate in such activities, the incidence of such fractures may increase. It is a common misconception that, compared with overhead pitching, the underhand motion performed in windmill softball pitching creates less stress on the arm, resulting in fewer injuries. In reality, it has been shown that high forces and torques are experienced at the shoulder and elbow during the delivery phase of the windmill softball pitch with peak compressive forces equal to 70% to 98% of body weight.[29] Thus, the upper extremity in softball pitchers may be at risk for repetitive stress injury. The presentation of stress fractures of the humeral shaft is similar to that of fractures in other areas, with insidious onset of pain and tenderness, often with an acute increase in pain with completion of the fracture. Diagnosis is confirmed by x-ray examination; however, occasionally a bone scan or MRI is needed, particularly in the early symptomatic period. The mainstay of treatment is rest from the offending activity, pain-relieving modalities, and gradual resumption of pain-free activity.

The Elbow

The elbow links the shoulder to the hand and allows for motion in flexion, extension, pronation, and supination. The lateral epicondyle, medial epicondyle, and olecranon are easily palpated bony landmarks (Figure 2–9). The lateral epicondyle serves as the origin of the supinator-extensor muscle group, and the more prominent medial epicondyle serves as the origin for the flexor-pronator muscle group. The medial or ulnar collateral ligament provides a constraint to valgus instability of the elbow, whereas the lateral ligamentous complex provides lateral and posterolateral stability. Lateral epicondylitis is the most commonly seen problem about the elbow in athletes.[30] This syndrome occurs equally in male and female athletes. In a study of more than 500 tennis players, it was found that women past the age of 40 had an increased risk of lateral epicondylitis developing, particularly when participating in greater than 2 hours of

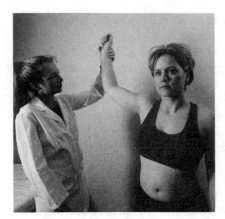 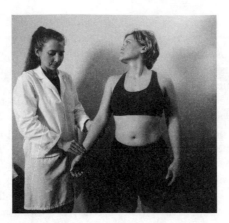 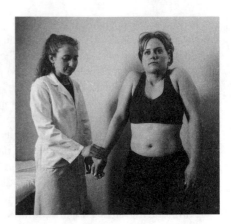

Figure 2–8 Test for Thoracic Outlet Syndrome. A, Wright's test; B, Adson's maneuver; C, military shrug.

racquet time per week.[31] Other sports requiring repetitive forearm motion such as volleyball, golf, and other racquet sports have been implicated in the development of lateral epicondylitis.

Lateral epicondylitis likely begins as an injury to the origin of the extensor carpi radialis brevis with subsequent local tissue degeneration.[32] The presence of associated local tissue inflammation is debatable. Athletes will have pain in the lateral epicondylar area, which is typically insidious in onset. Examination will reveal tenderness just distal and anterior to the lateral epicondyle (Figure 2–10). Resisted wrist and finger extension with the elbow in full extension will cause pain. Treatment includes relative rest from the offending activity and pain-relieving modalities such as ice and NSAIDs. A forearm support band placed just distal to the elbow may help relieve discomfort by decreasing stress at the wrist extensor origin. Stretching of the wrist extensors followed by pain-free strengthening is also performed. Occasionally, a corticosteroid injection may provide symptomatic relief.

The use of proper technique and equipment should be emphasized. In tennis or other racquet sports proper grip and racquet size are important and should be appropriate for a player's palm size. Decreasing string tension may also help in dispersion of forces placed on the forearm extensors. The use of lighter racquets, low-vibration materials, and playing on softer surfaces may also prevent recurrence.[33] Surgical management is considered if symptoms persist beyond 1 year and most commonly consists of excising the pathological portion of the extensor carpi radialis brevis tendon origin and repairing the residual defect.[32]

Medial epicondylitis refers to an overuse syndrome of the flexor pronator mass. It has been reported to occur with increased frequency in men, but is also seen in women.[33] The athlete will complain of chronic medial elbow pain, which is increased with activities involving wrist flexion and pronation such as tennis, golf, or bowling. Examination will reveal tenderness to palpation just anterior to the medial epicondyle and pain with resisted flexion and forearm pronation. Grip strength may be decreased. Treatment is similar to that for lateral epicondylitis, beginning with rest, pain-relieving modalities, stretching, and pain-free strengthening with gradual return to exercise through technique modification or retraining. Specific technique modifications include avoiding hitting the ball late with the head of the racquet behind the elbow on contact.[34] Equipment modifications similar to those noted previously in the prevention of lateral epicondylitis may be used. Surgical management is considered with the failure of conservative treatment and includes debridement of the abnormal tissue at the common flexor origin.

Valgus Extension Overload

An increased valgus angle or carrying angle of the elbow combined with relative ligamentous laxity in lower upper body strength may predispose an athlete to traction injuries to the medial elbow structures and compressive injuries to the posterior and lateral structures termed "valgus extension overload."[35] This syndrome is most commonly seen in baseball pitchers but may also occur in field sports, such as javelin or shotput, or gymnastics where the gymnast uses her elbow as a weight-bearing post. Valgus extension overload can result in medial sided elbow pain because of ulnar collateral ligament sprains, strains of the flexor pronator muscles arising from the medial epicondyle, or tension on the medial epicondylar physis in the skeletally immature athlete. Ulnar nerve symptoms may also be present. Valgus overload can also result in impingement of the olecranon process to the medial wall of the olecranon fossa with formation of posterior and posteromedial osteophytes, which may cause pain and limitation of extension on physical examina-

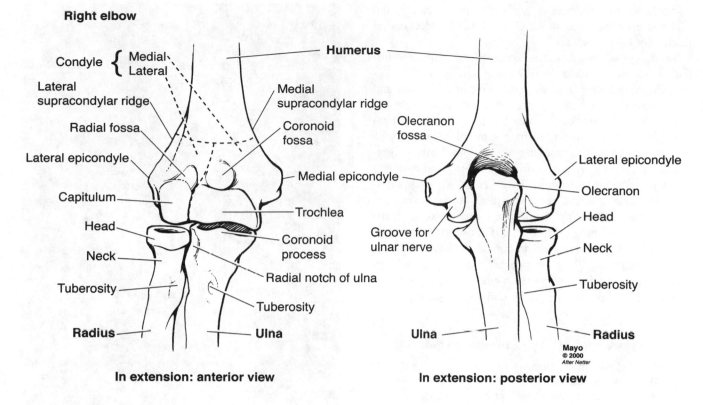

Right elbow

In extension: anterior view

In extension: posterior view

Figure 2–9 Bones of Elbow.

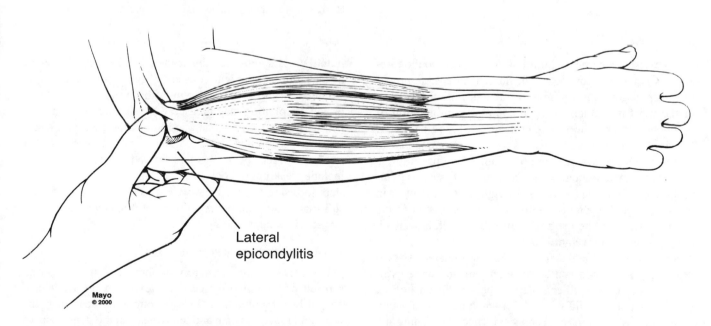

Lateral epicondylitis

Figure 2–10 Physical Examination Demonstrating Tenderness over the Common Extensor Origin Often Localized to the Extensor Carpi Radiolis Brevis.

tion.[35] In addition, valgus overload can result in compression of the radiocapitellar joint, which can lead to osteochondral fracture of the capitellum.[36]

Treatment of valgus extension overload syndrome initially involves rest from the offending activity, use of pain-relieving modalities, and strengthening of the elbow and wrist flexors and extensors, strengthening primarily of the flexor pronator muscles that assist with dynamic stabilization of the elbow. Sporting technique modifications may be needed. In gymnastics "locking of the elbow" in a weight-bearing position should be avoided. Pitching and throwing mechanics should be examined with particular attention to the entire kinetic chain, because injuries to the lower back and shoulder can result in increased stress placed on the elbow during pitching or throwing. If conservative management fails, surgical treatment to correct the specific pathological condition may be considered. This may include arthroscopic debridement of posteromedial osteophytes and/or reconstruction of a deficient ulnar collateral ligament.

Consequences of Valgus Extension Overload

- Ulnar collateral ligament sprain
- Flexor/pronator strain
- Medial epicondylar epiphyseal injury (in the skeletally immature athlete)
- Ulnar nerve symptoms
- Radiocapitellar osteochondral fractures

Clinical Guideline

The Wrist

The wrist is a complex joint linking the hand to the forearm, which allows for motion in flexion, extension, pronation, supination, and radial and ulnar deviation. Stability of the wrist is maintained by a complex configuration of ligaments linking the bones both dorsally and palmarly. Injuries to the hand and wrist are the most common types sustained during athletic competition.[37] Overuse injuries to the wrist are common, particularly in sports such as gymnastics, which use the wrist as a weight-bearing joint or in the sports requiring repetitive flexion and extension of the wrist such as fast pitch softball, volleyball, golf, basketball, racquet sports, and weightlifting.

Stress injury to the distal radial physis (radial stress syndrome) is a common source of wrist pain in young gymnasts.[38] The athlete will complain of pain in the area of the distal radial physis and will exhibit tenderness to palpation in this area. X-ray films may show evidence of widening and indistinctness of the epiphyseal plate with fragmentation and cystic changes in the metaphysis (Figure 2–11). Chronic

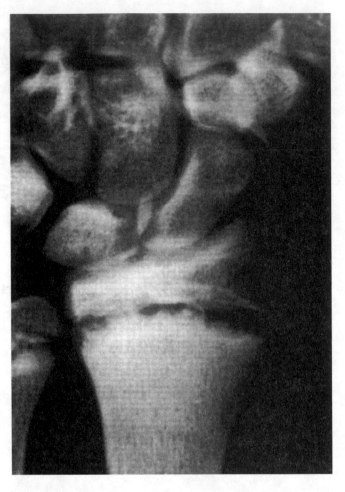

Figure 2–11 Physeal Stress Reaction. Widening of physis, cystic changes on metaphyseal side, and indistinct margins.

---

radial stress syndrome may lead to a widened, shortened distal radius. Treatment consists of rest and avoidance of weight-bearing activities through the wrist joint. A short period of splinting may be useful. Gradual return to activities with appropriate technique modifications is necessary. Improvement in upper body strength and technique is also important. Predisposing factors for radial stress syndrome include weak upper body strength, "jamming the wrist" for stability using a fixed hand-wrist position, the use of very soft mats, and multiple repetitions of maneuvers involving single arm weight bearing.[38]

Wrist Impingement Syndrome

Dorsal wrist pain caused by impingement may occur as a result of repetitive forced dorsiflexion of the wrist in a weight-bearing situation. This is commonly seen in gymnasts and is seen as pain and tenderness on the dorsal aspect of the wrist, often with associated synovitis or swelling of the dorsal wrist.[39] Treatment consists of initial rest along with NSAIDs and pain-relieving modalities followed by strengthening of the muscles about the wrist. Protection of the wrist from hyperextension either by taping or technique modifications is warranted.

Tenosynovitis of the Hand and Wrist

Tenosynovitis of the hand and wrist occurs commonly in golf and other sports involving repetitive use of the hand and wrist. During the golf swing using the left thumb of a right-handed golfer if hyperabducted may predispose to the development of de Quervain's syndrome in which there is pain and swelling involving the tendons within the first dorsal wrist compartment (Figure 2–12).[40] The woman's smaller hand may predispose her to this syndrome developing, particularly with use of ill-fitting gloves with too large of a grip. De Quervain's syndrome is thought to be more common in women during the postpartum period. Treatment consists of rest, splinting, NSAIDs, ice, and occasionally a corticosteroid injection into the tendon sheath. With failure of conservative management, surgical release of the tendon sheath may be considered.

Carpal Tunnel Syndrome

Carpal tunnel syndrome has been reported in athletes requiring wrist flexion with a tight grip, including cyclists and weightlifters. It is seen more frequently in women.[41] Symptoms include paresthesias in the distribution of the median nerve that result from compression of the nerve as it passes through the wrist. Common complaints include pain at night and while driving and pain after participating

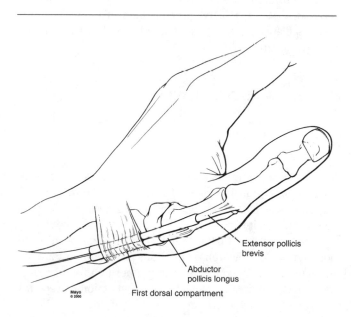

Figure 2–12 Anatomy of the First Dorsal Compartment.

in the offending sport. Treatment consists of rest, splinting, and NSAIDs. Corticosteroid injection is often performed to decrease local inflammation in the carpal canal. Surgical release of the carpal tunnel is performed for severe or recalcitrant cases.

CONCLUSION

In general, the nature and frequency of upper extremity injuries that occur in women's sports are similar to those seen in men's sports. However, certain upper extremity injuries have been reported to occur with greater frequency in women. A woman's relatively shorter arms, narrower shoulders, and decreased lean muscle mass may result in decreased mechanical advantage for force production in the upper extremity. In addition, hormonal differences between men and women may have an impact on strength training, ligamentous laxity, and susceptibility to injury. More research is required before firm conclusions can be drawn in this area. An upper body strength and conditioning program along with sports-specific training and technique modifications may reduce the risk of injury and contribute to enhanced recovery from injury in the female athlete.

CASE HISTORY 1

The patient is a 45-year-old female martial artist with no history of trauma. She complained of pain in the shoulder with any attempt at use of the arm in an outstretched or overhead manner. Her examination was remarkable for positive impingement signs, both in forward flexion and abduction with internal rotation. She had pain with manual muscle testing of the supraspinatus. There was no evidence of glenohumeral instability on examination. X-ray films were unremarkable. MRI showed inflammation within the substance of the supraspinatus tendon consistent with classic subacromial impingement and rotator cuff tendinitis (Figure 2–13). She was treated with a period of relative rest followed by pain-free stretching exercises, NSAIDs, and a subacromial corticosteroid injection. She was able to progress to rotator cuff strengthening within a period of 4 weeks and returned to her sport at 8 weeks.

CASE HISTORY 2

This patient is a 26-year-old female basketball player who injured her shoulder while rebounding. She suffered a forced abduction and external rotation injury and felt the shoulder partially "slide out." She complained of persistent pain, particularly with attempted rebounding and shot blocking despite an appropriate rehabilitation program. She also complained of a painful click in the shoulder with certain overhead motions. Her examination was remarkable for full

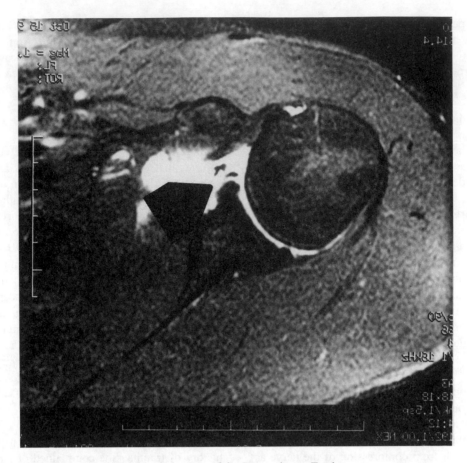

Figure 2–13 MRI Showing Inflammation within the Substance of the Supraspinatus Tendon.

range of motion of the shoulder with positive apprehension and relocation maneuvers. Classic impingement signs were negative. Plane x-ray films were unremarkable; MRI showed an anterosuperior labral tear (Figure 2–14). She was treated with arthroscopic labral repair followed by a rehabilitation program that emphasized strengthening of the rotator cuff and scapular stabilizers. She returned to basketball 6 months postoperatively.

CASE STUDY: SHOULDER INSTABILITY IN A RUGBY PLAYER

Geoffrey Crowley

Miss K, a state representative rugby union player, was identified in preseason screening as having multidirectional instability in both glenohumeral joints, with the left being worse than the right. She was told by a team doctor that her left side was so lax that she was certain to dislocate the shoulder soon. She was referred to physiotherapy for a preventive exercise program.

She was identified as having inadequate control of the scapula during movements of the upper limb, as well as rotator cuff weakness. Scapulothoracic control was seen as the first priority. During elevation, the scapula needs to be a stable base from which the rotator cuff can act to control glenohumeral translation.[42,43] Exercises for the rotator cuff muscles were performed with such resistance that scapula control was maintained.

Initially, setting of the scapula in a neutral position (a position of no elevation/depression, protraction/retraction, or rotation) was taught as the starting position for all movement. This requires an isometric co-contraction of *serratus anterior*, *upper trapezius*, and *lower trapezius*.

From the neutral scapula position, glenohumeral external and internal rotation in 0° abduction/flexion was begun to

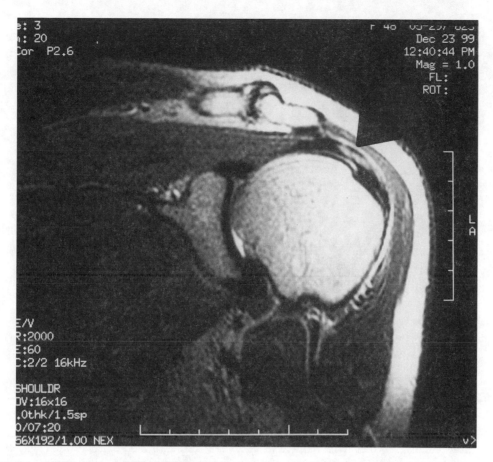

Figure 2–14 MRI Showing an Anterosuperior Lateral Tear.

activate the rotator cuff. Specific attention was paid to maintaining a stationary scapula while moving the arm (Figure 2–15).

The patient was instructed to perform this exercise with self-monitoring by watching scapula movement in a mirror and palpating the medial border of her scapula (Figure 2–16). Sets of 10 repetitions were repeated until fatigue (as indicated by loss of scapula control) occurred.

This exercise was mastered quickly (by the second treatment session) and progressed by using elastic tubing to add resistance to the rotation movement. Miss K could maintain a neutral scapula only with the lightest grade of elastic; therefore this grade was chosen. Heavier grades of tubing resulted in excessive scapula retraction/protraction when the exercise was performed. Closed kinetic chain exercises for *serratus anterior* facilitation were also prescribed, done initially in a wall push-up position, with attention to scapula control without excessive *upper trapezius*, *levator scapulae*, or *rhomboideus* activity. This closed kinetic chain position enhances the stabilizer action of the rotator cuff.[42]

The next progression was unloaded glenohumeral rotation at 45° of abduction. Again a stable scapula was attained before resistance was added. Unloaded abduction to 30° and flexion to 90° (stationary scapula) were added. The *serratus anterior* exercise was progressed into hands-and-knees. This was continued until the end of the second week of treatment.

More unstable positions of the glenohumeral joint were used as further progressions (ie, approaching 90° abduction) with internal and external rotation, again only adding resistance when unresisted scapula control was satisfactory. Similar exercises were added in prone and supine (eccentric control) positions.

The player took 4 weeks to achieve scapulothoracic and rotator cuff control to this level. At this point she was prescribed exercises for hypertrophy of the large prime mover muscles of the shoulder such as *deltoid*, *pectoralis major*, *biceps*, *triceps*, *trapezius*, and *latissimus dorsi*. One rationale behind training for hypertrophy is that in a contact sport, muscle bulk absorbs impact forces. Although these muscles

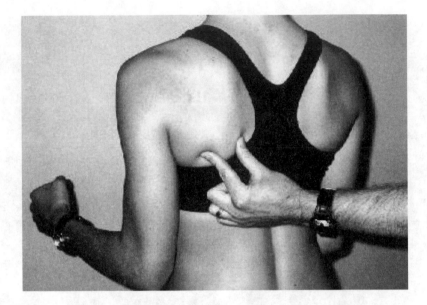

Figure 2–15 Internal and External Rotation at the Glenohumeral Joint Maintaining Scapula Stability.

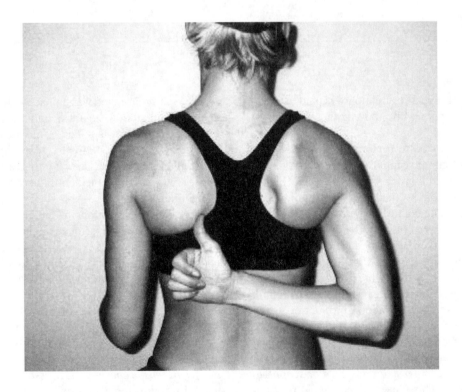

Figure 2–16 Self-Monitoring of Scapula Control with Glenohumeral Rotation.

do not directly stabilize the shoulder joint, they make dislocation less likely by acting as shock absorbers. Well-fitted shoulder pads also seem to reduce the incidence of dislocation (anecdotal evidence only!).

At the time of publication, Miss K had completed a full season of rugby union at club and representative level and had suffered no further problems.

REFERENCES

1. Arendt EA. Orthopedic issues for active and athletic women. *Clin Sports Med.* 1994;13(2):485.
2. Aagaard H, Jorgensen U. Injuries in elite volleyball. *Scand J Med Sci Sports.* 1996;6(4):228–232.
3. Kennedy JC, Hawkins R, Chrisoff WB. Orthopedic manifestations of swimming. *Am J Sports Med.* 1978;6:309–322.
4. Teitz CC. The upper extremities. In: *The Female Athlete. American Academy of Orthopedic Surgeons Monograph series.* AAOS, 1997.
5. Leffert RD. Thoracic outlet syndrome. *J AAOS.* 1994;2:317–325.
6. DiFiori JP, Puffer JC, Mandelbaum BR, et al. Factors associated with wrist pain in the young gymnast. *Am J Sports Med.* 1996;24:9–14.
7. McCarroll JR. The frequency of golf injuries. *Clin Sports Med.* 1996; 15(1):1–7.
8. Neimi S, Lafoska S, Kemila A, et al. Neck and shoulder symptoms and leisure time activities in high school students. *J Orthop Sports Phys Ther.* 1996;24(1):25–29.
9. Holloway JB. Individual differences and their implications for resistance training. In: Baechle TR, ed. *Essentials of Strength and Conditioning.* National Strength and Conditioning Association; 1994:152.
10. Beall RK. The carrying angle of the elbow. *Clin Orthop.* 1976;119: 194–196.
11. Holloway JB, Baechle TR. Strength training for female athletes: A review of selected aspects. *Sports Med.* 1990;9(4):216–228.
12. Posthuma BW, Bass MJ, Bull SB, et al. Detecting changes in functional ability in women with premenstrual syndrome. *Am J Obstet Gynecol.* 1987;156(2):275–278.
13. Neer CS II. Impingement lesions. *Clin Orthop.* 1983;173:70–77.
14. Flatow EL, Soslowsky LJ, Ticker JB, et al. Excursion of the rotator cuff under the acromion. *Am J Sports Med.* 1994;22:779–788.
15. Jobe FW, Kvitne RS, Giangarra CE. Shoulder pain in the overhead or throwing athlete. The relationship of anterior instability and rotator cuff impingement. *Orthop Rev.* 1989;18:963–975.
16. Walch J, Bioleau P, Noel E, et al. Impingement of the deep surface of the supraspinatus tendon on the posterior superior glenoid rim. An arthroscopic study. *J Shoulder Elbow Surg.* 1992;1:238–245.
17. Hawkins RJ, Kennedy JC. Impingement syndromes in athletes. *Am J Sports Med.* 1980;8:151–158.
18. Bigliani LU, Pollock RG, Owens JM, et al. The inferior capsular shift procedure for multidirectional instability of the shoulder. *Orthop Trans.* 1993;17:576.
19. Rowe CR, Pierce DS, Clark JG. Voluntary dislocation of the shoulder. A preliminary report on a clinical electromyographic and psychiatric study of 26 patients. *J Bone Joint Surg Am.* 1973;55:445–460.
20. Ferretti A, Carli A, Fontana M. Injury of the suprascapular nerve at the spinoglenoid notch. The natural history of infraspinatus atrophy in volleyball players. *Am J Sports Med.* 1998;26(6):759–763.
21. Ganzhorn RW, Hocker JT, Horowitz M, Switzer HE. Suprascapular nerve entrapment. *J Bone Joint Surg Am.* 1981;63:492–494.
22. Sandow MJ, Ilic J. Suprascapular nerve rotator cuff compression syndrome in volleyball players. *J Shoulder Elbow Surg.* 1998;7(5): 516–521.
23. Wang DH, Koehler SM. Isolated infraspinatus atrophy in a collegiate volleyball player. *Clin J Sports Med.* 1996;6(4):255–258.
24. Richardson A. Thoracic outlet syndrome in aquatic athletes. *Clin Sports Med.* 1999;18(2):361–378.
25. Holden DL, Jackson DW. Stress fractures of the rib in female rowers. *Am J Sports Med.* 1985;13:342–348.
26. Myburgh KH, Hutchins J, Fataar AB, et al. Low bone density is an etiologic factor for stress fractures in athletes. *Ann Intern Med.* 1990; 113:754–759.
27. Karlson KA. Rib stress fractures in lead rowers. A case series and proposed mechanism. *Am J Sports Med.* 1998;26(4):516–519.
28. Brukner P. Stress fractures of the upper limb. *Sports Med.* 1998;26(6): 415–424.
29. Barrentine SW, Fleisig JS, Whiteside JA, et al. Biomechanics of windmill softball pitching with implications about injury mechanics at the shoulder and elbow. *J Orthop Sports Phys Ther.* 1998;28(6):405–415.
30. Rettig AC, Pattel DV. Epidemiology of elbow, forearm, and wrist injuries in the athlete. *Clin Sports Med, The Athletic Elbow and Wrist.* 1995;14(2):289.
31. Gruchow HW. An epidemiologic study of tennis elbow, incidence, recurrence and effectiveness of prevention strategies. *Am J Sports Med.* 1979;7:234–238.
32. Nirschl RP. Elbow tendinosis/tennis elbow. *Clin Sports Med.* 1992; 11:851–870.
33. Plancher KD, Halbrecht J, Louric GM. Medial and lateral epicondylitis in the athlete. *Clin Sports Med.* 1996;15(2):283–305.
34. Ilfeld SW. Can stroke modification relieve tennis elbow? *Clin Orthop.* 1992;276:182–186.
35. Johnston J, Plancher K, Hawkins R. Elbow injuries to the throwing athlete in the athletic elbow and wrist, Part 2. *Clin Sports Med.* 1996;15(2):307–328.
36. Field LD, Altcheck DW. Elbow injuries. *Clin Sports Med.* 1995;14:59.
37. McCue FC, Ploska P, Alley RM. Athletic injuries to the hand and wrist. In: Johnson RJ, Lombardo J, eds. *Current Reviews in Sports Medicine.* Philadelphia: Current Medicine; 1994:42–51.
38. Carek P, Fumich R. Stress fracture of the distal radius. *Physician Sports Med.* 1992;20(5):115–118.
39. Griffin L. Upper extremity injuries. In: Pearl A, ed. *The Athletic Female.* Champaign, IL: Human Kinetics; 1991:235–250.
40. Murray PM, Cooncy WP. Golf-induced injuries of the wrist. *Clin Sports Med.* 1996;15(1):85–109.
41. Steyers C, Schelkun T. Practical management of carpal tunnel syndrome. *Physician Sports Med.* 1995;23(1):83–87.
42. Kibler WB. Shoulder rehabilitation: Principles and practice. *Med Sci Sports Exercise.* 1998;30(suppl):S40–S50.
43. Mottram SL. Dynamic stability of the scapula. *Manual Therapy.* 1997;2(3):123–131.

BIBLIOGRAPHY

1. Hakkinen K, Pakarinen A, Kyrolainen H, et al. Neuromuscular adaptations and serum hormones in females during prolonged power training. *Int J Sports Med.* 1990;11(2):91–98.

2. Sanborn CF, Jankowski CM. Physiologic considerations for women in sport. *Clin Sports Med.* 1994;13(2):315–325.

3. Wojtys EM, Huston LJ, Lendenfeld TN, et al. Association between the menstrual cycle and anterior cruciate ligament injuries in female athletes. *Am J Sports Med.* 1998;26(5):614–619.

4. Wreje U, Kristinsson P, Aberg H, et al. Serum levels of relaxin during the menstrual cycle and oral contraceptive use. *Gynecol Obstet Invest.* 1995;39:197–200.

CHAPTER 3

The Spine

Joseph T. Alleva and Thomas H. Hudgins

INTRODUCTION

Posterior element pain (spondylolysis/spondylolisthesis, and lumbar facet syndrome) account for 70% of the injuries involving the low back in the athletic population.[1] Discogenic pain, including herniated nucleus pulposus (HNP), annular tear, and degenerative disc disease, accounts for 25% of injuries in the lumbar spine in this same population.[1] A few studies have tried to identify factors that may predispose the athlete to these conditions, notably anthropometric and hormonal differences between the sexes. A study of female soccer players failed to reveal an association of low back pain with menstrual cycle or with the use of oral contraceptive medications.[2] Ultimately, although women athletes have a higher incidence of overuse and lumbar spine injuries,[3] and contact sports such as field hockey and soccer may have a higher incidence of low back pain in women compared with men,[4] the male and female athletes are essentially predisposed to the same conditions that result in low back pain.[5] This chapter will discuss the anatomy of the lumbar spine and the history, physical examination, diagnosis, and management of common conditions that affect the lumbar spine in the female athlete. These include spondylolysis/spondylolisthesis, facet syndrome, radiculopathy caused by HNP, and degenerative disc disease.

ANATOMY

The lumbar spine is made of five vertebral bodies. Each vertebral body contains corresponding anterior, middle, and posterior elements (Figure 3–1). The anterior element is composed of the vertebral body, which is largely responsible for sustaining all compressive forces, including gravity and muscle contraction. The middle element or the pedicle attaches the anterior and posterior elements and is responsible for forming a canal. It is thought to function as a transmitter of forces. The posterior elements are composed of the zygapophyseal (facet) joints (which are diarthrodial joints between the vertebral bodies), spinous process, and transverse process. These processes, along with mamillary and accessory processes, provide areas of muscle attachment and act as levers to create complex lumbar motions.

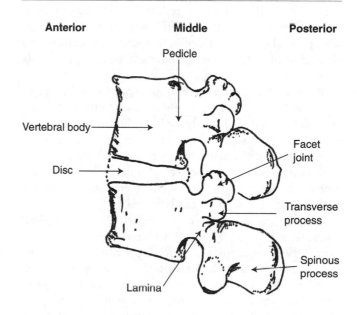

Figure 3–1 Illustration of the Vertebra, Columns, and Spaces.

The facet joints function to prevent excessive anterior translation and excessive rotation. They are composed of not only a cartilage interface but also a surrounding capsule and intervening meniscoid and synovial membrane. They receive nerve supply from the medial branch of the dorsal rami. The innervation of a particular facet joint is fairly complex in that it will receive nerve supply from the medial branch at that level and the level above. An example would be the L4–5 facet joint receiving medial branch innervation from L4 and L3.

The sacrum is composed of five fused vertebrae; it articulates with the pelvis and gives rise to four pairs of nerve roots. The pelvis itself is made up two innominates, which articulate anteriorly with the symphysis and posteriorly with the sacrum. The sacroiliac joint is also diarthrodial, receiving vast nerve supply from L3 to S2. It has limited range of motion.

The intervertebral disc is critical in spine anatomy. Although its main function is absorption, it also plays a vital role in lumbar stability. It provides separation from one vertebral body to another, thus allowing free passage of the spinal nerve roots. The disc is composed of two components, the annulus fibrosis and the nucleus pulposus. It forms one of the three joints in the three-joint complex, the other two of which are the concordant facet joints. The annulus fibrosis is an array of concentric laminae of collagen fibers. They are arranged in alternating approximate 65° angles. The inner fibers attach to the endplates, whereas the outer fibers are heavily innervated and serve a ligamentous role. The nucleus pulposus is a matrix of proteoglycans that binds water. It also contains phospholipase A, which has a major role in inflammation when the disc is disrupted. The innervation of the intervertebral disc is derived from the rami communicantes anterolaterally, the ventral rami posterolaterally, and the sinuvertebral nerves posteriorly. Histochemical studies have demonstrated that only the outer third of the annulus fibrosis contains nerve fibers.

At each intervertebral level of the spinal cord, a pair of nerve roots arises; they further divide into ventral and dorsal rami. The ventral rami supply the lower limbs, and the dorsal rami supply the back. The dorsal root ganglia sit in the most lateral aspect of the neural foramen and thus are spared in most nerve root pathological conditions. The spinal cord ends at approximately L1–L2, forming the conus. From that point on it gives rise to the cauda equina.

The muscles of the lumbar spine are elaborate in their orientation and mechanisms of action. As a whole they are termed the "erector spinae," which are multisegmental muscles. They consist of the iliocostalis and longissimus and function concentrically in extension and eccentrically to control flexion. Somewhat deeper to this include the multifidi muscles. These fill a similar role as the preceding muscles, but because of their insertion onto the transverse process, they also function toward controlling rotational activities. Just deeper to that layer of muscle are unisegmented muscles, the interspinalis and intertransversii. The quadratus lumborum attaches to the iliac crest and the twelfth transverse process and the twelfth rib. It functions eccentrically and concentrically to stabilize the spine in lateral bending. The abdominal muscles, which include the rectus abdominus, the internal and external obliques, and the transversus abdominus, form a cylinder around the trunk, connecting anteriorly with the linea alba and posteriorly with the thoracolumbar fascia. These muscles will also become critical when discussing lumbar stabilization techniques.[6,7]

SPONDYLOLYSIS/SPONDYLOLISTHESIS

Seventy percent of low back pain in the athlete can be attributed to the posterior elements of the spine.[1] This includes the pars interarticularis and the lumbar zygapophyseal (facet) joints. The pars interarticularis is the portion of the neural arch between the superior and inferior articular process. A defect/crack in this arch is known as spondylolysis.[8] Spondylolysis is derived from the Greek words "spondylos" meaning "spine" and "lysis" meaning "lytic lesion." Bilateral spondylolysis may lead to spondylolisthesis ("lysthesis" Greek derivation: "slippage"). Spondylolisthesis may also be seen with a unilateral defect and an elongated pars interarticularis.

The incidence of spondylolysis in the general population is 5% to 6%, most often seen in children ages 5 to 10 years old but rarely symptomatic.[9] A pars defect is an uncommon cause of back pain in patients older than 40 years old.[10(p 831)] The young population is at risk because the vertebral body grows faster than the posterior elements, contributing to a more lordotic posture and higher forces on the posterior elements. In addition, the pars interarticularis has not reached maximum strength, and the disc is less resistant to shear.[11] The stress on the posterior elements with bipedal motion contributes to spondylolysis. No cases have been demonstrated in newborns or nonambulatory cerebral palsy patients.[12]

The athletic population is more prone to spondylolysis and more likely to be symptomatic from this defect.[11] Anatomical studies have shown that shear forces are greater on the pars with extension of the lumbar spine and that repetitive flexion/extension will cause impingement on the pars from the cephalad vertebra, resulting in microfractures.[11] Gymnasts, figure skaters, swimmers who frequently butterfly kick, and divers are most prone to this injury. The incidence in female gymnasts ages 6 to 24 years old was found to be four times greater than in the general female population.[13,14] Figure skaters also have spondylolysis because of the repetitive lumbar flexion/extension during jumps. In addition, the presence of spina bifida occulta and a hyperlordotic posture has been associated with spondylolysis. The pars defect is at L5 in 60% of persons, L4 in 15% to 30%, and L3 in 2%.[10]

Although these abnormalities may result in low back pain, their presence does not necessarily result in symptomatic low back pain. Much controversy exists as to whether spondylolysis is a congenital or acquired defect. Wiltse has classified five types of spondylolysis: dysplastic, isthmic, degenerative, traumatic, and pathological. The dysplastic type represents a congenital deficiency. The isthmic is pertinent to the athletic population and can be further divided as a fatigue fracture, an elongated but intact pars, and an acute fracture.[9] The symptomatic spondylolysis in the athlete is typically an acquired overuse injury, resulting in a stress fracture of the pars interarticularis.[9] Overuse injuries are the result of repetitive micro-trauma overwhelming the tissue's ability to heal itself, leading initially to local inflammation.[15] In essence, the defect is an acquired lesion in patients with a hereditary predisposition and participating in high-risk athletic endeavors such as gymnastics.[10]

Clinical Presentation

The patient with symptomatic spondylolysis will complain of low back pain that may radiate into the buttock and posterior thigh. The pain will be exacerbated by lumbar extension; for example, a gymnast or diver will have pain during or after a back flip. However, although initially the discomfort may only be present with sports-specific activities, eventually the discomfort may be present during activities of daily living.[16] The patient may point to the belt line as the focal location of the discomfort.[17] The examination reveals a hyperlordotic posture with relative tightness of the hamstrings. This is thought to be tight in an attempt to stabilize the painful segment. A Phalen-Dickson sign may be present, whereby the patient demonstrates a knee-flexed, hip-flexed gait pattern.[12] The most significant finding on examination will be pain provocation with one-legged lumbar extensions on the ipsilateral side (Figure 3–2). A "step-off" may be palpated in the prone position at L4/L5 or L5/S1 segment in cases of spondylolisthesis.[12] In addition, a normal neurological examination is present. If present, radicular symptoms may indicate a high-grade slip (greater than 50%).

The differential diagnosis of posterior element pain includes lumbar strain/sprain, lumbar facet syndrome, and sacroiliac joint dysfunction. Women in their reproductive years may experience low back pain related to endometriosis (presence of endometrial glands and stroma outside the uterine cavity). The prevalence of endometriosis-related back pain approaches 10%.[18] Other gynecologically related back pain can occur as a result of fibroids, dysmenorrhea, pelvic inflammatory disease, and uterine prolapse. (Refer to Chapter 11, The Pregnant Athlete, for information on pregnancy and postpartum-related back pain.)

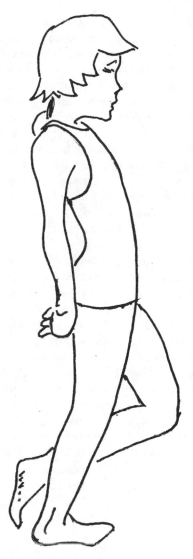

Figure 3–2 Pain Provocation with One-Legged Lumbar Extension Standing on the Ipsilateral Side of Spondylolysis/Spondylolisthesis.

Symptoms of Spondylolysis

- Localized "belt line" low back pain
- May radiate to buttock
- Relative tightness of hamstring
- Pain with extension activities

Clinical Guideline

Diagnosis

The clinical diagnosis may be confirmed by an oblique view x-ray film. The examiner should look for a defect in the neck of the "Scotty dog." A lateral view film examines for the presence of spondylolisthesis. This is graded 1 to 4, depending on the degree of displacement. Grade 1 represents 1% to 25% displacement compared with the cephalad vertebrae; grade 2, 26% to 50%; grade 3, 51% to 75%; grade 4, 76% to 100%. However, an x-ray film often will not demonstrate a pars defect. In cases in which the physician has a high index of clinical suspicion, but a negative x-ray, a single photon emission computed tomographic (SPECT) bone scintigraphy can help identify stress reactions of the pars not seen on x-ray examination.[19] The SPECT scan also distinguishes an acute active healing process from a chronic healed lesion.[20] A reverse/gantry angle computed tomography (CT) scan has also been shown to be a sensitive test to confirm the diagnosis of spondylolysis.[11] The CT scan is also helpful in distinguishing other causes of a positive bone scan such as osteoid osteoma. A magnetic resonance imaging (MRI) scan may also be used to make an early diagnosis[21] but is typically reserved for cases with radicular symptoms where disc pathology is suspected. If present, the pars lesion can be staged according to the radiographic studies: stage I stress reaction reveals a positive SPECT scan with a negative x-ray film, stage II "early spondylolysis" will show a fracture on CT scan with a negative x-ray film, stage III will show "progressive spondylolysis," and stage IV "terminal spondylolysis" will show a defect on oblique view x-ray films.[21] This staging will be helpful with prognosis and directing treatment. Therefore, if x-ray films are negative but the practitioner is highly suspicious of a pars lesion, it is recommended that further diagnostic tests such as a SPECT scan be obtained.

Treatment

Treatment focuses on promoting a lumbar flexion position and may or may not include the use of immobilization to promote healing of an acute injury. Ciullo[17] states that most of these lesions heal without medical attention. A reasonable approach for the symptomatic athlete is to restrict the inciting activity and implement a therapy routine that emphasizes lumbar flexion. This would consist of strengthening the deep abdominal muscles (internal oblique and transverse abdominus) and lumbar multifidi, maintaining intra-abdominal pressure and tension on the lumbar vertebra though the thoracolumbar fascia. This provides a "stiffening" effect on the lumbar spine.[22] Pelvic tilt exercises also promote strengthening of the abdominal muscles and flexibility of the lumbar paraspinal muscles. Flexibility of the hamstrings to reduce the excessive lordosis is also emphasized. Some authors advocate the use of a thoracolumbar orthosis such as a modified Boston brace to limit lumbar extension to promote healing of the lesion and reduce symptoms. With this approach, the brace is worn 23 hours a day and taken off only for hygiene and flexion exercises. Activities may continue while wearing the brace. This is continued for 3 to 6 months, and then the patient is gradually weaned from the brace during the day and then finally during sports-specific activities. Fifty-two of 67 patients with a documented pars lesion returned to full activity without symptoms with this approach. Six of the 67 patients required surgical intervention.[16] The average time to return to competition without symptoms was 7.3 months in 37 athletes with spondylolysis in another study. The symptom resolution correlated with bone scan resolution.[13,14] It is beyond the scope of this chapter to discuss surgical options, but indications for surgery may include spondylolisthesis progression, greater than 50% slip in skeletally immature athletes, persistent deformity and abnormal gait, and neurological deficits.[9]

In our opinion, a reasonable approach is to initially avoid any inciting factors and implement a flexion-bias physical therapy program. Once a comprehensive rehabilitation program has been completed and resolution of symptoms is attained, the athlete may gradually return to play. If symptoms occur with activities of daily living or persist despite physical therapy, a modified thoracolumbosacral orthosis to prevent lumbar extension should be worn 23 hours/day until symptoms improve. This may take 3 to 6 months, but activities may continue while the patient is wearing the brace. After 3 to 6 months, with decreasing symptoms and documentation of healing on bone scan, the brace can gradually be weaned over a 3-month time period.

Treatment of Spondylolysis

- Activity restriction exercises
- Bracing for refractory cases
- Relative rest from painful activity
- Lumbar stabilization with flexion bias
- Hamstring and dorsal muscle stretching

Clinical Guideline

LUMBAR FACET SYNDROME

As discussed previously, 70% of low back pain in the athletic population can be attributed to the posterior elements.[1] Posterior element pain is a nonspecific term that includes the pars interarticularis, spinous ligaments, and the zygapophyseal joint (facet joints). The lumbar facet joint is a true synovial joint with hyaline cartilage, a synovial membrane, and a fibrous capsule.[22] The joint is innervated by the medial branch of the dorsal rami at the level of the joint and one level above. The orientation of the lumbar facets prevents excessive rotation, lateral bending, and extension while facilitating lumbar flexion.[23] In theory, excessive lumbar extension stretches the joint capsule, irritating the nociceptive fibers of the medial branch. In addition, articular changes of the facet joint may occur similar to other synovial joints contributing to pain associated with this syndrome. Less likely, a fatigue fracture of the facet may result in localized low back pain. One published case study describes a 36-year-old female ballerina with chronic localized low back pain and a stress fracture of the inferior articular process of the L4 facet joint on CT scan. This diagnosis was confirmed by surgical exploration and relieved by debridement and removal of the non-union fracture.[24] Although the athlete may be first seen after an acute event with symptoms consistent with lumbar facet syndrome, this disorder is more likely the result of chronic microtrauma.[25] Osteopenia or osteoporosis can also contribute to spinal stress fractures.

Clinical Presentation

Facet syndrome is seen as a localized discomfort in the low back with occasional referral pattern into the buttock and posterior thigh rarely past the knee. This discomfort is exacerbated by lumbar extension. There is no pathognomonic sign on physical examination that rules in or rules out the diagnosis. Although unreliable, tenderness to palpation in the prone position may implicate a segment. Essentially, lumbar facet pain is a diagnosis of exclusion. There is no radiographic test to confirm the diagnosis, and abnormalities found on radiographic studies do not correlate with symptoms.[25] However, a series of two injections may be used for both therapeutic and diagnostic information. The differential diagnosis of posterior element pain includes facet syndrome, spondylolisthesis/spondylolysis, and central disc herniation. In addition, lumbar radiculopathy, discogenic pain, insufficiency fracture of the vertebral body and/or sacrum, myofascial pain, and sacroiliac joint pain should be included in the differential diagnosis of low back pain in the female athlete. The female athlete may also experience gynecological-related pain.

Rehabilitation

Conservative treatment of lumbar facet syndrome is similar to the approach taken with other causes of posterior element pain. The acute phase involves education, relative rest, and modalities to promote tolerance of a physical therapy program. The exercises prescribed should be individualized to the patient's biomechanical abnormalities. Similar to the treatment of spondylolysis/spondylolisthesis, an emphasis is placed on reducing the lumbar lordosis that increases stress and compressive load on the posterior elements, including the facet joints. This may be accomplished by strengthening the abdominal and gluteus maximus muscles and promoting

flexibility of the hip flexors, lumbar paraspinal muscles, and thoracolumbar fascia. Posterior pelvic tilt exercises are taught and should be performed in a variety of positions, including bent knee standing, straight leg standing, and sitting.[22]

If no clinical improvement is seen after 4 weeks of physical therapy, a diagnostic series of injections may be warranted. The injections are given directly into the facet joint or at the site of the medial branch of the dorsal rami at the level of the joint and one level above (see Figure 3–3). The first injection uses a short-acting anesthetic such as lidocaine to establish whether this results in reduction of symptoms. The second injection uses an anesthetic with a longer half-life such as bupivacaine to reduce the false-positive rate associated with a response to the initial injection.[23] Efficacy of long-term relief with use of anesthetic and corticosteroids with these injections has not been established. However, once the diagnosis has been explored with dual anesthetic injections, a neurotomy of the medial branch with radiofrequency ablation may be warranted.

LUMBAR RADICULOPATHY

Classically, lumbar radiculopathy is terminology that relates to the herniated nucleus pulposus (HNP). Literally taken, radiculopathy means a diseased nerve root. Injury to a nerve root stemming from disc pathosis is more complex than just mechanical deformation. It is for this reason that most radiculopathies resulting from a herniated disc do not require surgical intervention. Most patients with lumbar radiculopathy can be treated successfully without surgery; only 5% to 10% go on to require surgery.[26] Surgery for a herniated disc is performed 1.5 to 3 times more often in men than in women. However, lumbar radiculopathy appears to be equally distributed among the sexes.[27]

The nerve root is more susceptible to injury relative to its peripheral counterpart. Neuroanatomically, it lacks a well-developed epineurium, perineurium, and blood supply. From a vascular standpoint, animal studies have shown that pressure on the blood supply to the nerve is capable of producing anoxia and release of substance P.[28,29]

It has long been established that inflammation plays a large role in radicular pain. Substances such as phospholipase A are found in large contents within the nucleus pulposus itself. When released, these then can create an inflammatory cascade.[30,31] This self-perpetuating event then leads to increased levels of other inflammogens such as prostaglandins and leukotrienes, which may stimulate nociceptor receptors and or sensitize neurons to mechanical stimulation. Chemical mediators of pain such as vasoactive intestinal peptide, interleukins, nitrous oxide, and change in pH are being actively investigated as modulators of pain in radiculopathy.[32]

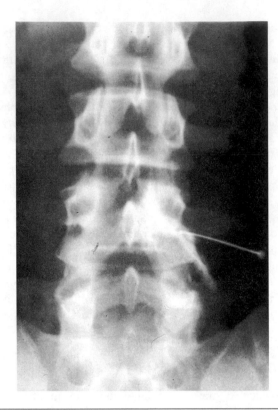

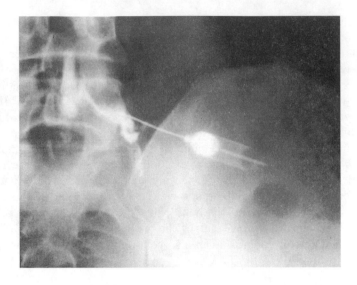

Figure 3–3 Transforaminal Injection.

Pathophysiology of Lumbar Radiculopathy

- Mechanical
- Inflammatory/chemical
- Vascular

Clinical Guideline

Clinical Presentation

Lumbar radiculopathy has a classic presentation. The level and type of disc herniations will dictate the symptoms. It is typically aggravated by flexion maneuvers and twisting maneuvers. It may also be aggravated by Valsalva maneuvers. Ninety to 95% of herniations involving the lumbar spine take place at L4–5 or L5–S1.[33] Discs also vary in their location within the neural foramina. The posterolateral disc, for example, will typically impinge the nerve root below that particular level. For example, an L4–5 posterolateral disc will typically result in an L5 radiculopathy. A far lateral disc, on the other hand, will typically involve the nerve above.[34] Central disc herniations are rather unpredictable in that they can irritate the nerve above, below, unilateral/bilateral, or present as discogenic pain.[35] See Table 3–1 for assistance in examination.

Patients will typically complain of low back pain and radicular symptoms along that particular dermatome. The physical examination includes an evaluation of strength, sensation, muscle stretch reflexes, and dural tension signs. The straight leg test is a dural tension sign that creates pain in the thigh and calf of the affected leg when lifted in the supine position. This was also described to have taken place below 70°.[36] Butler describes a host of sensitizing techniques for dural tension signs that are used for both diagnostic and therapeutic purposes. These maneuvers include assessment of the patient seated and supine while adding tibial, peroneal, and femoral biases in an attempt to localize le-

---

Table 3–1 Examination of Nerve Root Level

Dermatome	Root Level	MSR	Myotome
Upper thigh and groin	L1		HF/KE
Mid anterior thigh	L2	Patella	HF/KE
Medial femoral condyle	L3	Patella	HF/KE
Medial malleolus	L4	Patella	HF/KE
Dorsum of foot	L5	Hamstring	EHL
Lateral heel	S1	Achilles	PF
Popliteal fossa	S2	Achilles	PF

MSR, muscle stretch reflex; KF, knee flexion; KE, knee extension; EHL, extensor hallucis longus; PF, plantar flexion.

sions.[37] The crossed straight leg raise is positive when lifting the contralateral or asymptomatic leg produces posterior pain in the symptomatic leg and low back. This is thought to represent a large or sequestered disc.[38]

A lumbar shift, in which posture reveals translation of the pelvic girdle and shoulder girdle in opposite directions similar to a scoliotic appearance, will be apparent on physical examination. This almost always indicates disc pathosis and when present not only aids in diagnosis but also treatment and prognosis.[18,39]

Again, clinical presentation of a classic radiculopathy as a result of a herniated disc is fairly straightforward. However, piriformis syndrome, plexopathy, congenital stenosis, spondylolisthesis, and sacroiliac dysfunction are among those to be considered in the differential diagnosis.

Poor Prognostic Indicators of Lumbar Radiculopathy

- Positive crossed straight leg raise
- Persistent lumbar shift
- Declining neurological status

Clinical Guideline

Diagnostic Tests

Lumbar radiculopathy resulting from a herniated disc is largely a clinical diagnosis. However, in those situations in which the subjective complaints do not match the objective findings, further workup may be warranted. Testing is also warranted in patients who are declining clinically. In those cases, MRI is superior to CT scan for disc pathosis. Nomenclature one should be familiar with includes annular tear, bulge, protrusion, extrusion, and fragmentation/sequestration. Bulge is not a disc herniation; rather it is a symmetrical extension of the annulus beyond the margin of the vertebral endplates. Protrusion, which is a form of a herniated disc, represents focal contour abnormality of the outer annulus displaced by the nuclear material that is contained by the outer annulus. Extrusion, a more severe form of a herniated disc, represents penetration of the nuclear material through the outer annulus. It is further labeled transligamentous if it goes beyond the posterior longitudinal ligament. Finally, fragmentation or sequestration represents material separated from its disc origin.[40]

Myelography in conjunction with CT is typically used when diagnostic evidence (ie, an MRI) does not correlate with patient signs and symptoms. It is also helpful in distinguishing bone from disc pathosis if it is not clearly defined by the MRI. Finally, a patient can be evaluated functionally with myelography in flexion, extension, or lateral bending. This is an advantage over other diagnostic imaging in that it allows one to assess for segmental instability. However, this is an invasive test, and it does not accurately assess the lumbosacral junction and far lateral recess pathological conditions.[41] The natural history of disc herniations has been studied fairly extensively in the radiology literature. Numerous studies support spontaneous reduction in the size of nonsurgically managed disc protrusions and extrusions. This would certainly support conservatively approaching such a problem. In fact, a positive correlation exists between the degree of disc herniation and the subsequent regression. Plainly stated, larger discs tend to show a more significant resolution.[42,43]

Electrodiagnostic testing, more specifically electromyography (EMG)/nerve conduction studies, is another tool used to aid in diagnosis of radiculopathy. This is an extension of the physical examination that provides physiological information about muscle and nerve. With regard to radiculopathy, nerve conduction studies serve to rule out other processes such as plexopathy, compressive neuropathies, and peripheral neuropathies. It may be positive in severe radiculopathies. The H-reflex is a special type of conduction study that measures the afferent and efferent conduction of mainly the S1 root. It is the electrophysiological analog of the Achilles reflex. It is therefore helpful in diagnosing S1 radiculopathy when the Achilles reflex is present. EMG is the most valuable portion of the electrodiagnostic examination. However, abnormal findings such as decreased recruitment take 10 to 14 days after injury to manifest on the examination, and spontaneous activity (an indication of denervation) does not occur until 14 to 21 days after injury. Therefore, although the EMG test helps localize the root involved, prognosticate recovery, and elicit information regarding chronicity,[44] for optimal results one should wait 2 to 3 weeks after the injury before pursuing this study.

DISCOGENIC PAIN

Discogenic pain is thought to come about as a result of a tear in the annulus. It is therefore nonradicular. Because the outer fibers of the annulus fibrosis have nociceptive fibers and the intervertebral disc functions toward lumbar stability, the mechanism of pain can be inferred.[45,46] The inner two-thirds of the disc is aneural (Figure 3–4). Irritation of the outer annular nociceptive fibers probably occurs both mechanically and chemically. The former occurs as a result of direct trauma to that region and by the inevitable microinstability that ensues.[47–49] Chemical irritation of the annular nociceptors occurs in the presence of certain inflammogens. Inflammogens such as phospholipase A_2, cytokines, and bradykinins are known to exist and are subsequently released with disrupted discs.[30,50,51] Classification of these annular tears is typically made radiographically. The Dallas Discogram Scale (modified) essentially spans from grade 0 to grade 5, which represents normal to full-thickness tear with extra-annular leakage.[52] The Yu classification catego-

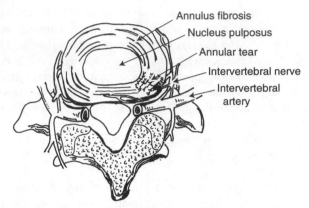

Figure 3–4 Cross-section of Vertebra and Intervertebral Disc with Annular Tear. Note the inner two-thirds of the disc is aneural.

rizes tears as either concentric, transverse, or radial. Radial tears probably receive the most attention.[53]

Clinical Presentation

The clinical presentation of discogenic (nonradicular)-type pain can vary. Typically lumbar pain is the prevailing symptom. Referral patterns commonly occur to the buttock, posterolateral thigh, and/or groin. Pain may be episodic or incapacitating and unilateral or bilateral. Aggravating factors include prolonged static postures, transitions from sitting to standing, and Valsalva maneuvers, especially coughing. Patients often report improvement of symptoms with lying supine with the hips and knees flexed at 90°.[54, 55] Discogenic pain can occur as a result of sports involving axial loading, such as weightlifting and rowing, and sports involving repetitive flexion coupled with twisting, including golf, tennis, softball, and gymnastics. In addition, equestrians are prone to discogenic pain given the repetitive compression of the lumbar spine. The differential diagnosis for discogenic pain includes injuries to the posterior elements (ie, facet, pars interarticularis), sacroiliac joints, and/or surrounding soft tissues. Again, gynecological factors must always be considered.

Just as description of this clinical entity can be vague, the physical examination is often nonspecific. In our experience, decreased lumbar range of motion with pain in extremes of flexion and extension is common. A negative neurological examination, presence of a lumbar shift, and positive spring test (see clinical guideline) are suggestive. Although expected to be negative, neural adverse dural tension signs may reproduce the discogenic pain. Tenderness is typically elicited in the surrounding soft tissue.

Spring Test

With the patient prone, the examiner places the palm of the hand over the spinous processes of the site of pain and

suspected site of the pathological condition. Posterior-to-anterior forces are applied at each level individually. A positive test is one in which less "spring" or movement is present at a particular level with corresponding symptom reproduction.[18]

Clinical Guideline

Diagnostic Testing

The "gold standard" for annular tears and subsequent discogenic pain is CT discography. However, the usefulness of discography remains controversial given its provocative nature.[56,57] The goal of discography is to assess whether radio-opaque dye is maintained in the nucleus by an intact annulus; if not, to what degree and to what pattern does it extravasate into the annulus. In addition, degree of symptom reproduction is observed to establish a specific site of pain. The test is most typically reserved for those who have persistent lower back pain with negative noninvasive diagnostic testing. Typically the patients have exhausted conservative measures and are likely to undergo more aggressive management. A subject of debate is the existence of a noninvasive study to establish similar diagnostic information. The "high intensity zones" observed in a disc on T2-weighted MRI images have drawn considerable attention (Figure 3–5). This bright spot sometimes found on the posterior margin of the annulus is thought to represent migrated nuclear material and/or contained inflammation.[58] In patients with symptomatic lower back pain, the high-intensity zone was found to correlate highly (>85% incidence) with positive discography.[54,58] There are studies that show less impressive correlation and the presence of a high-intensity zone in

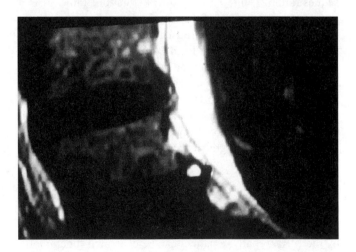

Figure 3–5 High-Intensity Zone; the Bright Spot Is Thought To Represent Migrated Nuclear Material and/or Contained Inflammation.

asymptomatic patients.[59–61] Clearly, MRI is not in a position to replace CT discography at this point.

Rehabilitation

The definitive nonsurgical treatment of acute discogenic lower back pain, be it radicular or nonradicular, is subject to some controversy. There is a wide array of approaches without general consensus. The goal of this section is to outline common approaches with the caveat that the ideal prescription is customized to a patient's physical examination. Numerous research shows that 95% of disc-related problems do not go on to surgery.[62] Studies show that conservatively treated herniated discs are comparable to surgically treated herniated discs.[63,64]

Generally, the acute phase of treatment is geared toward controlling pain. This can be typically achieved with a short period of relative rest (48 to 72 hours).[65] This may be coupled with the judicious use of modalities such as ice and electrical stimulation. Traction can be helpful. Medications usually include anti-inflammatories (nonsteroidal or steroid) with or without narcotic medications in an overall attempt to get the athlete to participate in a rehabilitation program.[66]

Spine stabilization exercises, also called dynamic stabilization, are probably the regimen that has received the most attention. The exercises attempt to provide back support, reduce microtrauma/pain, and allow healing within a "neutral spine position." This neutral spine position varies from patient to patient. It typically represents the position of the pelvis and spine where pain is minimal. It also represents a zone of functional stability for axial loading. Stabilization is thought to take place with an interaction between the thoracolumbar fascia, abdominal muscles (rectus, obliques, transversus), paraspinous musculature (polysegmental and unisegmental), and the gluteus musculature.[67,68] Assessing this in the office can be quickly achieved by evaluating pelvic tilt and pelvic clock maneuvers, whereby the patient demonstrates weakness in any direction of pelvic mobility and support.

Muscle Groups Providing Spinal Stabilization

- Thoracolumbar fascia
- Abdominal muscles
- Paraspinal muscles
- Gluteal muscles
- Hip and pelvic muscles

Clinical Guideline

Areas of relative weakness, for example, spine stabilizers, are typically opposed by areas of relative tightness (reflexive inhibition). Flexibility and strength of hip flexors, piriformis, and hamstrings should be carefully evaluated and addressed in rehabilitation to achieve optimal stabilization.[69] The modified Thomas test is a valuable screen used for the detection of hip flexor and knee extensor tightness. Figure 3–6 demonstrates more advanced spinal stabilization exercises, as the use of the Swiss Ball challenges balance and proprioception of the trunk in relation to the upper and lower extremities. For beginning stabilization, these exercises can be performed on a mat without the ball.

The McKenzie approach essentially divides back pain patients into three categories: postural, dysfunctional, and derangement syndromes. Derangement is the most relevant to this section. Basically, it represents internal displacement (ie, an HNP) leading to pain and loss of function, as well as possible deformity. The complex set of maneuvers attempts to identify postures and ranges of motion that "centralize" and/or reduce pain. It commonly involves lumbar extension, but it is a misconception to believe that it is solely an extension-based program. Patients whose radicular pain does not respond are thought to carry a poor prognosis.[70]

The usefulness of manual medicine in the treatment in discogenic pain is a subject of much controversy as well. The Agency for Healthcare Policy and Research guidelines recently supported its limited use in nonspecific back pain.[71] There have also been some recent reputable journal articles comparing both chiropractic treatment and osteopathic treatment techniques to physical therapy.[72,73] These authors believe that nervous tissue restrictions, soft tissue restrictions, and/or joint restrictions often accompany these painful states and should be assessed during the physical examination.[74,75] When used in conjunction with standard approaches, manual medicine techniques can customize a treatment approach toward a particular athlete, reducing pain and assisting in restoration of function. Tissue texture assessment, adverse neurological dynamic tension signs, sacroiliac motion testing, and dynamic assessment of transverse process symmetry can be quickly assessed during the routine physical examination.

Intuitively, cardiovascular fitness is essential to all fields of athletics and therefore should be part of every rehabilitation program. However, the role of exercise, more specifically, conditioning exercises, is not clearly defined with disc pathosis. Regarding nonspecific low back pain, studies are divided as to the specific preventive role of cardiovascular fitness.[76,77]

Return to play criteria are based on multiple factors. Resolution of lower back pain and radicular symptoms at rest and during the particular sport activity is of prime importance. Before returning to sports, neurological signs such as weakness or lack of sensation must be static, improved, or resolved. Furthermore, they should not impede performance or predispose to other injuries. Because of this, the final step in a rehabilitation program should include sports-specific evaluation and training. With disc pathological conditions,

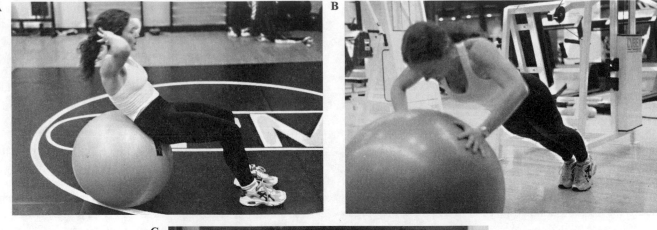

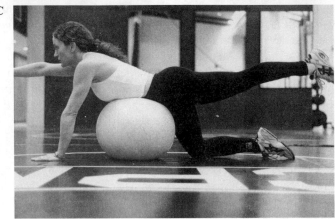

Figure 3–6 Spine Stabilization Exercises Using a Swiss Ball. A, flexion; B, neutral; C, extension, demonstrate more advanced spinal stabilization exercises, because the use of the swiss ball challenges balance and proprioception of the trunk in relation to the upper and lower extremities. For beginning stabilization, these exercises can be performed on a mat.

creating exercises that are functional can be most challenging. They should be both sports specific and complementary to the program described previously. Assessing for faulty mechanics and technique, particularly with sports involving lifting, lumbar rotation, and/or flexion, is essential.[5,78]

Injection techniques, such as epidurals and intradiscal steroid injections, have been poorly studied in discogenic pain. The surgical procedure of choice is lumbar fusion. Intradiscal electrothermal (IDET) therapy is a new minimally invasive procedure for discogenic pain. All studies thus far are encouraging but unpublished and uncontrolled.[79,80] This procedure functions by essentially navigating a catheter tip intradiscally, which contains a thermoresistive coil that delivers a targeted thermal treatment. The proposed goal of this treatment is to denervate the outer annular fibers so they become less pain sensitive and to remodel protein in the area of the annular defect. The success rates vary, depending on the study read but range from 50% to 80%. Today, no long-term studies have been completed.

Epidural steroid injection for lumbosacral radiculopathy had its first recorded use in the 1950s, and despite the minimal number of controlled trials since then, there have been more than 40 articles describing the experience of more than 4000 patients. Only four of those articles revealed unfavorable and/or no response to the procedure.[81] Rationale for use includes addressing the inflammatory cascade associated with compressive and/or chemical radiculopathy.[82] The use of fluoroscopy is recommended to prevent the documented 30% to 40% miss rate of blind epidural injections.[83,84]

CONCLUSION

Both the female and the male athlete is susceptible to similar syndromes that affect the lumbosacral spine. Certainly, different athletic endeavors stress certain segments of the lumbar spine. More studies are needed to examine specific sporting activities and the stresses absorbed by the lumbar spine in the female athlete. Comprehensive multispecialty evaluation is sometimes necessary. Early diagnosis and treatment are judicious in preventing chronic and more significant sources of back pain.

REFERENCES

1. Saal JA. Rehabilitation of sports-related lumbar spine injuries. *Phys Med Rehabil.* 1987;4:613–638.

2. Brynhildsen J, Akstrand J, Jeppson A, Tropp H. Previous injuries and persisting symptoms in female soccer players. *Int J Sports Med.* 1990;11:489–492.

3. Keene JS, Albert MJ, Springer SL, Drummond DS, Clancy WG. Back injuries in college athletes. *J Spinal Disord.* 1989;2:190–195.

4. Engstrom S, Johansson C. Soccer injuries among elite female soccer players. *Am J Sports Med.* 1991;19:372–375.

5. Brukner P, Kahn K. *Clinical Sports Medicine.* New York: McGraw-Hill; 1993.

6. Bogduk N. The lumbar disc and low back pain. *Neurosurg Clin North Am.* 1991;2:791–806.

7. White AA, Panjabi NM. *Clinical Biomechanics of the Spine.* Philadelphia: JB Lippincott; 1990.

8. Dietrich M, Kurowski P. The importance of mechanical factors in the etiology of spondylolysis. A model analysis of loads and stresses in human lumbar spine. *Spine.* 1985;10:532–542.

9. Stinson JT. Spondylolysis and spondylolisthesis in the athlete. *Clin Sports Med.* 1993;12:517–527.

10. Sinaki M, Mokri B. Low back pain and disorders of the lumbar spine. In: Braddom RL. *Physical Medicine and Rehabilitation.* Philadelphia: WB Saunders Company; 1996:813–850.

11. Congeni J, McCulloch J, Swanson K. Lumbar spondylolysis, a study of natural progression in athletes. *Am J Sports Med.* 1997;25:248–253.

12. Smith JA, Hu SS. Management of spondylolysis and spondylolisthesis in the pediatric and adolescent population. *Orthop Clin North Am.* 1999;30:487–497.

13. Jackson GW, Wiltse LL, Cirincione RJ. Spondylolysis in the female gymnast. *Clin Orthop Rel Res.* 1976;117:68–73.

14. Jackson DW, Wiltse LL, Dingeman RD, Hayes M. Stress reactions involving the pars interarticularis. *Am J Sports Med.* 1981;9:304–312.

15. Nadler SF, Wu KD, Galski T, Feinberg JH. Low back pain in college athletes. *Spine.* 1998;23:828–833.

16. Steiner ME, Micheli LJ. Treatment of symptomatic spondylolysis and spondylolisthesis with a modified Boston brace. *Spine.* 1985;10:937–943.

17. Ciullo JV, Jackson DW. Pars interarticularis stress reaction, spondylolysis, and spondylolisthesis in gymnasts. *Clin Sports Med.* 1985;4:95–111.

18. Geraci M, Alleva J. *Physical Examination of the Spine and Its Functional Kinetic Chain: The Low Back Pain Handbook.* Philadelphia: Hanley & Belfus; 1997:49–70.

19. Bellah RD, Summerville DA, Treves ST, Micheli LJ. Low back pain in adolescent athletes: detection of stress injury to the pars interarticularis with SPECT. *Radiology.* 1991;180:509–512.

20. Kanstrup IL. Bone scintigraphy in sports medicine: a review. *Scand J Med Sci Sports.* 1987;7:322–330.

21. Ralston S, Deir M. Suspecting lumbar spondylolysis in adolescent low back pain. *Clin Pediatr.* 1998;37:287–293.

22. O'Sullivan PB, Phyty G, Twomey LT, Allison GT. Evaluation of specific stabilizing exercise in the treatment of chronic low back pain with radiologic diagnosis of spondylolysis or spondylolisthesis. *Spine.* 1997;22:2959–2967.

23. Dreyer SJ, Dreyfuss PH. Low back pain in the zygapophyseal (facet) joints. *Arch Phys Med Rehabil.* 1996;77:290–300.

24. Deusinger RH. Biomechanical application for clinical application in athletes with low back pain. *Clin Sports Med.* 1989;8:703–715.

25. Fehallandt AF, Micheli LJ. Lumbar facet stress fracture in the ballet dancer. *Spine.* 1993;18:2537–2539.

26. Frymoyer J. Back pain and sciatica. *N Engl J Med.* 1988;318(5):291–300.

27. Heliovaara M, Knekt P. Incidence and risk factors of herniated lumbar intervertebral discs or sciatica leading to hospitalization. *J Chron Dis.* 1987;40:251–285.

28. Olmarker K, Holm S. Experimental nerve root compression: a model of acute, graded compression of the porcine cauda equina and analysis of neuro and vascular anatomy. *Spine.* 1999;16:61–69.

29. Conefijord M, Olmarker K. Neuropeptide changes in compressed spinal roots. *Spine.* 1995;20:670–673.

30. Saal J, Franson Z. High levels of inflammatory phopholipase-A2 activity in lumbar disc herniations. *Spine.* 1990;15:674–678.

31. Saal J. The role of inflammation in lumbar pain. *Phys Med Rehabil.* 1994;20:191–199.

32. Gordon S, Weinstein J. A review of basic science issues in low back pain. *Phys Med Rehabil Clin North Am.* 1998;9:323–343.

33. Bogduk, N. The causes of low back pain. *Med J Aust.* 1992;156:151–153.

34. Reid D. *Injuries and Conditions of the Neck and Spine. Sports Injury, Assessment and Rehabilitation.* New York: Churchill-Livingstone; 1992:739–839.

35. Hudgins TH, Alleva JT. Central vs. posterolateral disc herniations: differentiation by history and physical. Presented at the International Injection Society, 7th Annual Scientific Meeting, August 1999.

36. Hoppinfeld S. *Physical Exam of the Spine and Extremities: Physical Exam of the Lumbar Spine.* New York: Appleton-Century-Crofts; 1976:237–265.

37. Butler D. *Mobilization of the Nervous System.* New York: Churchill Livingstone; 1991:139–146.

38. Hudgins W. The crossed straight leg test. *N Engl J Med.* 1977;297:1127.

39. Donelson R, Silva G. Centralization phenomenon: its usefulness in evaluating and treating referred pain. *Spine.* 1990;15(3):211–213.

40. Herzog R. *MRI of the Spine in the Adult Spine: Principles and Practice.* Vol 1. New York: Raven Press; 1991:457–510.

41. April C. *Myelography in the Adult Spine: Principles and Practice.* Vol. 2. Philadelphia: Lippincott-Raven Press; 1997:443–467.

42. Bozzao A, Gallucci M. Lumbar disc herniation: MRI imaging of natural history of patients treated without surgery. *Radiology.* 1992;185:135–141.

43. Saal JA, Saal JS. The natural history of lumbar intervertebral disc extrusion treated nonoperatively. *Spine.* 1990:15;683–687.

44. Press J, Young J. *Electrodiagnostic Medicine, The Low Back Pain Handbook.* Philadelphia: Hanley & Belfus Inc; 1997:213–227.

45. Bogduk N, Tyran W. The innervation of the human intervertebral discs. *J Anat.* 1981;132:39–56.

46. Coppes M, Marani E. Innervation of painful lumbar discs. *Spine.* 1997;22:2342–2349.

47. Moneta G, Videman T. Reported pain during lumbar discography as a function of annular ruptures and disc degeneration a reanalysis of 833 discograms. *Spine.* 1994;1917:1968–1974.

48. Young J, Press J. The disc at risk in athletes: perspectives on operative and nonoperative care. *Med Sci Sports Exercise.* 1997;29:222–232.

49. Kotilanen E, Valtonen S. Clinical instability of the lumbar spine with microdiscectomy. *Acta Neurochir.* 1993;125(14):120–126.

50. Gronbald M, Virri J. A controlled immunohistochemical study of inflammatory cells in disc herniation tissue. *Spine.* 1994;19:2744–2751.

51. Willburger R, Wittenburg R. Prostaglandin release from lumbar disc and facet joint tissue. *Spine.* 1994;19:2068–2070.

52. Sachs B, Vanharanta H. Dallas discogram description: a new classification of CT discography in low back disorders. *Spine.* 1987;12:287–294.

53. Yu S, Haughton V. Comparison of MR and discography in detecting radial tears of the annulus; a postmortem study. *Am J Neuroradiol.* 1989;10:1077–1081.

54. Schellas K, Pollei S. Lumbar disc high intensity zones correlations with MRI and discography. *Spine.* 1996;21(1):79–86.

55. Liss H, Liss D. *History and Past Medical History. The Low Back Pain Handbook.* Philadelphia: Hanley & Belfus; 1997:31–49.

56. Nachemson A. Lumbar discography where are we today? *Spine.* 1989;14:555–557.

57. Maezawa S, Muro T. Pain provocation of lumbar discography as analysed by computed tomography/discography. *Spine.* 1992;17:1309–1315.

58. April C, Bogduk N. High intensity zone: a diagnostic sign of painful lumbar disc on magnetic resonance imaging. *Br J Radiol.* 1992;65(773):361–369.

59. Ito M, Kristine I. Predictive signs of discogenic lumbar pain on MRI with discography correlation. *Spine.* 1998;23(11):1251–1260.

60. Jensen M, Brandt-Zawadski M. MRI of the lumbar spine in people without low back pain. *N Engl J Med.* 1994;331:69–73.

61. Buirski G, Silberstein M. The symptomatic lumbar disc in patients with lower back pain: MRI appearances in both symptomatic and controlled population. *Spine.* 1993;18:1808–1811.

62. Dawson E, Johannes B. The surgical treatment of lower back pain. *Phys Med Rehabil Clin North Am.* 1998;19:489–497.

63. Saal J, Saal J. Nonoperative treatment of herniated lumbar vertebral discs with radiculopathy. *Spine.* 1989;14(4):431–437.

64. Weber H. Lumbar disc herniation: a controlled prospective study, ten years of observation. *Spine.* 1983;8:131–140.

65. Deyo R, Diehl A. How many days of bedrest for acute low back pain, a randomized trial. *N Engl J Med.* 1986;315:1064–1070.

66. Saag K, Cowdery J. Nonsteroidal antiinflammatory drugs balancing benefit and risks. *Spine.* 1994;19:1530–1534.

67. Kaul M, Herring S. Rehabilitation of the lumbar spine injuries in sports. *Phys Med Rehabil Clin North Am.* 1994;5:173–176.

68. Young J, Press J. The disc at risk in athletes: perspectives on operative and nonoperative care. *Med Sci Sports Exercise.* 1997;29:S222–S232.

69. Jull G, Janda V. Muscle and motor control in lower back pain: assessment and management: physical therapy of the lower back. *Clin Phys Ther.* 1987:253–278.

70. Donnelson R, Silva G. Centralization phenomena: its usefulness in evaluating and treating referred pain. *Spine.* 1990;15(3):2111–213.

71. Acute lower back problems in adults; assessment and treatment provided by the US Department of Health and Human Services. Washington, DC: The Agency of Healthcare Policy and Research, No. 14, December 1994.

72. Cherkin D, Deyo R. A comparison of physical therapy, chiropractic manipulation, and provision of an educational booklet for the treatment of patients with low back pain. *N Engl J Med.* 1998;339(15):1021–1029.

73. Andersson G, Lucente T. Comparison of osteopathic spinal manipulation with standard care for patients with low back pain. *N Engl J Med.* 1999;341(19):1426–1431.

74. Greenman P. *Concepts of Vertebral Motion Dysfunction. Principles of Manual Medicine.* Baltimore: Williams & Wilkins; 1985.

75. Butler D. *Mobilization of the Nervous System.* Edinburgh: Churchill Livingstone; 1991.

76. Battie M, Bigos S. A prospective study of the role cardiovascular fitness in industrial back pain complaints. *Spine.* 1989;14:141–147.

77. Cady LD, Bischoff DP. Program for improving health and physical fitness of firefighters. *J Occup Med.* 1979;21:269–272.

78. Reid, DC. *Sports Injury Assessment and Rehabilitation.* New York: Churchill Livingstone;1992:739–837.

79. Derby R, Bjorn E. Intradiscal electrothermal coagulation by catheter. IATS 11th Annual Meeting in San Antonio, Texas. May 1998.

80. Saal J. Percutaneous treatment lumbar disc derangement with a navigable intradiscal thermal catheter: a pilot study. NASS/APS 1st joint meeting, Charleston, SC. April 1998.

81. Bogduck N, Christophidis N. Epidural steroids in the management of back pain and sciatica of spinal origin. Position of the working party on epidural use of steroids in the management of back pain, National Health and Medical Research Council, Canberra, Australia, 1983.

82. Weinstein S, Herring S. Contemporary concepts in spine care; epidural steroid injections. *Spine.* 1995;20(16):1842–1848.

83. White A, Derby R. Epidural injections for the diagnosis and treatment of lower back pain. *Spine.* 1980;5:78–86.

84. Mehta M, Salmon N. Extradural block, confirmation of injection site by x-ray monitoring. *Anesthesia.* 1985;40:1009–1012.

CHAPTER 4

Pelvis and Hip Injuries in the Female Athlete

Heidi Prather

More women and girls are choosing to participate in sports and exercise. With this increase in participation, health care providers and exercise specialists will learn more about the management of sports- or exercise-specific injuries in women. In the past, sports medicine literature has often omitted discussions of pelvic injuries. This omission is likely related to a lack of research related to exercise and sports injuries specific to the pelvis. An overlap of problems involving the lumbar spine, hip, and pelvis exists as well. As a result, the health care provider needs to pull information from various sources, including primary care, orthopaedics, urology, physical medicine and rehabilitation, and obstetrics and gynecology. The female pelvis changes with aging. These changes occur as a result of hormonal changes, pregnancy, childbirth, and menopause. To provide comprehensive management of pelvic and hip problems in women, the health care provider must take into account these changes and adapt the therapeutic approach accordingly. Ultimately, a better understanding of specific anatomical, physiological, and biomechanical differences between men and women with regard to specific exercise or sport will decrease the number of "sidelined" female exercisers and athletes.

ANATOMY AND BIOMECHANICS

A good understanding of the anatomy and biomechanics of the hip and pelvis is essential in devising a comprehensive treatment program after an injury. Further awareness of the physiological changes that occur during the female life cycle is important.

The bony pelvis includes three bones that articulate at three joints. The ilium articulates with the sacrum at the sacroiliac joint. The lumbar spine articulates with the sacrum anteriorly by way of the lumbar disc and posteriorly by way of the L5–S1 facets. The lower extremity extends from the pelvis, including the femur articulating with the acetabulum at the hip joint. In general, the shape of the bony pelvis of the woman is broader than that of the man. The combination of greater femoral neck anteversion and shorter lower extremity limb length leads to a lower center of gravity for women compared with men.[1] This alignment suggests different adaptive or firing patterns in women versus men but not necessarily increased risk for injury.[2]

The sacroiliac joint (SIJ) meets the definition of a synovial joint, synarthrosis, and amphiarthrosis. The joint is "L"- or "C"-shaped with two lever arms that meet at the second sacral level where it interlocks (Figure 4–1). The sacral side is lined by thick hyaline cartilage, and the ilial side is lined with fibrocartilage. There are intraindividual and interindividual differences in the shape of the joint. The anterior fibrous capsule is well formed, but the posterior capsule is thinner and may have multiple plications. Accessory articulations may occur in up to 35% of the population. These are thought to occur as a result of degenerative changes over time.[3] Ligaments affecting stability of the joint include the intraarticular, periarticular, and accessory ligaments. The interosseous ligaments are the strongest ligaments supporting the joint and resist motion. The thin anterior ligaments pass between the psoas major and the obturator internus and provide a sling for the ilium and sacrum. The posterior ligament has three layers progressing from deep to superficial. The most superficial layer becomes continuous with the sacrotuberous and sacrospinous ligaments. As an accessory ligament, the sacrotuberous ligament

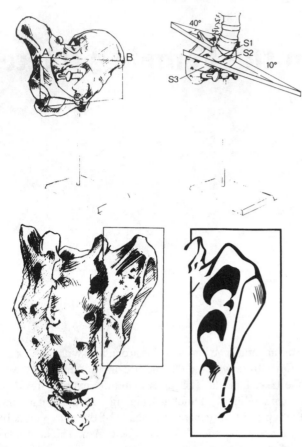

Figure 4–1 Interlocking of the Sacrum and the Ilium Occurs at the Second Sacral Level.

influences the joint through load and tension forces from the lower extremity and pelvis (Figure 4–2). The iliolumbar ligament also affects the joint by preventing anterior translation and rotation of L5. Vleeming et al[4,5] best describe the subtle motion changes that occur at the SIJ as a "self-locking mechanism." Stability of the interlocking mechanism is related to form and force closure. Form closure refers to joint surfaces that congruently fit together and require no extra forces to maintain stability. Force closure refers to a joint requiring outside force provided by muscles and ligaments to withstand load. If opposing forces do not have the appropriate form and/or force closure, the joint is less stable and more subject to shear force. The form closure in women is less congruent because of a wider pelvis and decreased joint space surface area compared with men. Force closure in women is susceptible to hormonal changes that occur during pregnancy. Increased joint laxity occurs related to elevated levels of relaxin and estrogen. These hormones return to baseline in the weeks and months postpartum but less predictably in women who breastfeed. Muscle groups operating at a biomechanical disadvantage during pregnancy and postpartum because of increasing abdominal girth, changes

in load transfer, and deconditioning may also alter force closure.

Self-locking Mechanism of SIJ

- Form closure—congruent fit of joint surfaces provides stability
- Force closure—muscles and ligaments provide forces to allow loads

Clinical Guideline

The thoracolumbar fascia is also important in load transfer from the lower extremity through the pelvis, lumbar spine, and abdominal muscles. The superficial lamina of the fascia facilitates transmission of forces from the lower extremity to the contralateral latissimus dorsi. These forces cross at the level of the pelvis and thereby may be a potential area of breakdown (Figure 4–3).[6] Muscles at the hip, pelvis, and lumbar spine provide indirect motion at the SIJ. Abdominal muscles affect motion at the ilium, pubis, and lumbar spine. The psoas connects the thoracolumbar fascia with the lower extremity and thereby may restrict lumbopelvic rhythm. Altered lower extremity and pelvic mechanics can then alter pelvic floor function, leading to secondary pain and potential incontinence. In particular, the obturator internus may be susceptible to overload (Figure 4–4). This muscle is a primary hip external rotator and abductor. If the gluteus medius is inhibited, the obturator internus is recruited as a hip abductor and may not be strong enough to respond to the load demand or repetition. As a result, an overuse syndrome may develop. Pain in the groin and pelvic floor may be the primary symptom. Other pelvic floor muscles such as the levator ani group must transfer load forces directly and indirectly across the SIJ and pubic symphysis. Although no literature to date describes the pelvic floor biomechanics in relationship to the female athlete, one should be suspect of dysfunction in athletes with unresolved hip, groin, and pelvic pain. Ligaments, fascia, and muscles supply force closure necessary for the SIJ to maintain stability. Gender differences in flexibility and range of motion that may affect performance have been well documented. Reports indicate that women have greater range of motion and flexibility.[7] This further suggests that relative imbalances in muscle length and strength may place the female athlete at risk for SIJ dysfunction.

Muscles Indirectly Affecting SIJ Motion

- Psoas
- Rectus abdominus

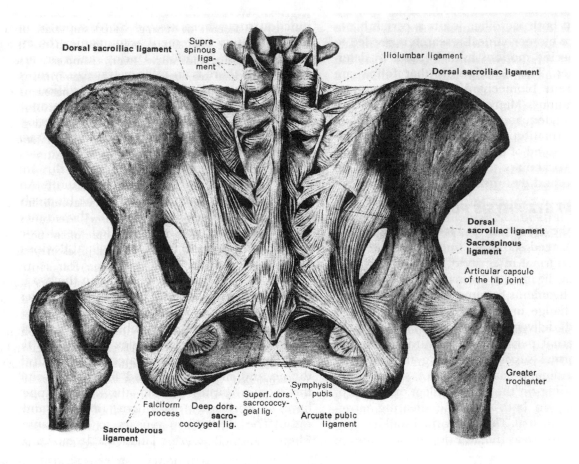

Figure 4–2 Ligaments of the Sacroiliac Joint with Direct and Indirect Affect on Joint Stability.

- Obturator internus
- Levator ani
- Thoracolumbar fascia
- Gluteal
- Hamstrings
- Latissimus dorsi
- Quadratus lumborum
- Erector spinae

Clinical Guideline

The innervation of the joint is from multiple root levels of the lumbosacral pelvis. The posterior joint receives innervation from L3–S3, whereas the anterior joint receives innervation from L2–S2. The primary innervation is thought to be from the S1 root level.[8] Because of the various levels of innervation, sacroiliac joint pain may have a variety of locations of pain. Similar to its primary level of innervation, SIJ pain often presents with S1 distribution symptoms in the form of pain and or numbness.

Joints Affecting SIJ Motion

- Lumbosacral spine segments
- Ilium
- Pubic symphysis
- Hip

Clinical Guideline

The biomechanics regarding the SIJ are complex. Most research has looked at one or two components of force and movement. Motion at the SIJ occurs indirectly (Figure 4–5). Body weight and postural changes may create or inhibit motion at the SIJ. Muscle groups surrounding the joint also cause indirect motion. These include gluteal muscles, hamstring muscles, hip external rotators, psoas, abdominal muscles, latissimus dorsi, quadratus lumborum, and erector spinae. Myofascial changes associated with these muscle groups will also alter mechanics. The SIJ forms the base of support for the spine. The joint receives and transmits

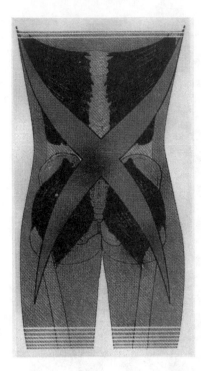

Figure 4–3 Force Transmission Occurs across Fascial Planes Directly Connecting the Upper Extremity with the Hip and Pelvis and Vice Versa. The sacroiliac joint is part of the base between the upper and lower extremities.

forces from the trunk, lower, and upper extremities. Forces absorbed through the SIJ allow changes in body weight transmission to occur while providing stability. SIJ motion is affected by motion at the spine, ilium, pubic symphysis, and hip. Studies have shown various ranges of motion, but most agree that approximately 4° of rotation and 1.6 mm of translation occurs.[9] The amount of joint motion decreases with age. Women have degenerative changes develop that restrict motion at age 50, whereas men have them develop around age 40. It is not clear that change in motion at one joint is the source of pain at that joint. Acquired hypermobility or hypomobility results in altered load transmission that may lead to muscle and other joint dysfunction resulting from adaptations. Women have relative changes develop in motion on the basis of hormonal fluctuations as well. During pregnancy, estrogen and relaxin play a key role in promoting increased ligamentous laxity. If the secondary stabilizers (musculature of the hip, spine, and pelvis) do not provide the stability needed, the joint may enter a relatively hypermobile state. Estrogen level changes continue in the postpartum period. This is also the time when the supporting musculature is developing new adaptive patterns as a result of the pregnancy and delivery. Again, these circumstances may place the female athlete at greater risk for injury. With

aging, degenerative changes direct the joint into a relative hypomobile state. Often, motion lost at the SIJ is attempted to be regained at another joint. Examples include the hip, lumbosacral segments, and pubic symphysis. So although changes in motion at the SIJ may not cause direct injury to the joint, they place peripheral joints at risk for altered adaptive patterns. Changes in adaptive patterns and mechanics may make these joints more susceptible to injury.

PAIN AND INJURY

Injuries or pain syndromes that develop in the hip and pelvis can be seen in a wide array of symptoms. Again, the risk factors for such injuries are often sport rather than gender specific. However, some injuries in women may be indicators of more serious systemic problems. An example is recurrent stress fractures in women with poor bone mineral density. For comprehensive care to be initiated, the health care provider must be aware of these scenarios. The following outlines hip and pelvic injuries that athletes and exercisers may encounter. These injuries occur in both men and women. Specifics regarding the female athlete will be included.

Bony Injuries

Weight-bearing exercise is protective because it helps build bone mass. However, excessive activity increases the risk of stress fracture. Determining what is excessive is specific to the individual's circumstances. Women participating in endurance-type exercise or sports are at increased risk for these fractures. Bony injuries involving the hip and pelvis may occur because of overuse and/or trauma. The hip joint accounts for 17% of all athletic injuries, most of which are overuse injuries.[10] Stress fractures may occur at various sites, including the ilium, lesser trochanter, femoral neck, pubis, and sacrum. Early diagnosis is important to prevent further injury or complete fracture. Recurrent stress fractures may be a sign of an underlying systemic problem. The health care provider needs to investigate reasons other than exercise or sports participation for repeated injury. The adolescent or young adult athlete should be questioned regarding other symptoms of the female triad. The older female athlete or exerciser should be ruled out for osteopenia or osteoporosis. Early intervention will decrease the risk of repeated injury.

Bony Pathology Causing Hip and Pelvic Pain

- Stress fractures
- Avulsion injuries
- Hip dislocation
- Acetabular labral tear

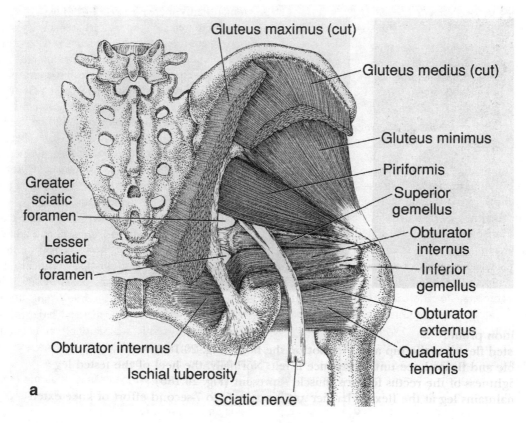

Figure 4–4 Obturator Internus Performs Its Function Primarily at the Hip. However, muscle imbalance and inhibition can lead to pelvic floor pain.

- Avascular necrosis
- Osteoarthritis
- Osteitis pubis

Clinical Guideline

Other bony injuries to the hip and pelvis are often sustained as a result of high impact or trauma. These include avulsion injuries, hip dislocation, and acetabular labrum tears. Avulsion injuries occur at the attachment of a tendon or ligament to bone. They occur as a result of a strong and rapid muscle contraction and are seen most commonly in adolescents participating in sports. The most common sites for avulsion injuries include the anterior superior and inferior iliac spines, lesser trochanter of the femur, ischial tuberosity, and iliac crest. Clinically, avulsion injuries are seen with tenderness at the site of muscle origin and demonstrate weakness of the isolated muscle. Similar in presentation to avulsion injuries is apophysitis. The latter is an inflammation at the tendon-periosteal junction but with no avulsion of bone. In contrast, apophysitis results from an overuse injury. Radiographs can differentiate the two injuries, because a fracture will be identified in avulsion injuries.

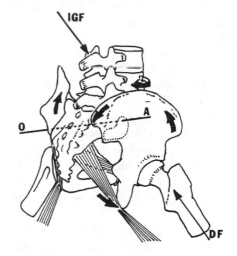

Figure 4–5 Motion at the SIJ Occurs Indirectly Related to Combinations of Motions Directly Occurring at the L5–S1 Junction, Ilium, Pubic Symphysis, and Hip. With heel strike shown on the right lower extremity, the deceleration force (DF) increases self-bracing to support the transfer of weight that is increased by the inertial-gravitational force (IGF). With counterrotation, the spine undergoes segmental deceleration. The sacrum moves on a force-dependent oblique axis (OA).

Common Sites of Avulsion Injuries

- Anterior superior iliac spine
- Anterior inferior iliac spine
- Lesser trochanter of femur
- Ischial tuberosity
- Iliac crest

Clinical Guideline

Hip dislocation is an uncommon sports injury. It often occurs during a high-impact trauma with the hip flexed and abducted while the knee is flexed. A posterior direction of dislocation is most common in sports injuries, resulting in the dislocated hip being seen in an internally rotated, adducted, and flexed position. Reduction of the dislocated hip should be attempted after a computed tomography (CT) scan has been completed to rule out acetabular fracture. Displaced acetabular fractures require open reduction and internal fixation.

Acetabular labrum tears often result from trauma or repetitive twisting injury. Presenting symptoms include a catching and giveaway sensation in the anterior hip and groin. Pain may occur with pivoting or transitional movements as when arising from a chair. Clicking may be noted when the hip is passively extended, internally rotated, and adducted.[11] Once x-ray studies have been completed and show no fracture, a magnetic resonance imaging (MRI) arthrogram has become accurate in identifying labral tears. Laparoscopic hip procedures now provide a minimally invasive definitive treatment.

Avascular necrosis of the femoral head again is uncommon in specific sporting or exercise events but may occur as the result of repetitive trauma. Those at increased risk include having a history of alcohol use/abuse and corticosteroid use. It most commonly occurs in men between 30 and 70 years of age. Clinical presentation includes sudden onset of hip and/or groin pain and change in gait pattern. Again, early diagnosis is important in improving long-term outcome. Radiographs may not show the early changes of vascular necrosis, and an MRI should be obtained in suspected cases.

Osteoarthritis is the most common hip disorder in the general population. The cause is multifactorial, including familial, obesity, and history of hip injury or disease. Men and women are equally prone to hip pathology. Recent studies outline concern for the development of an increased risk of hip osteoarthritis in women who participate in sports and exercise. Lane and colleagues[12] compared self-reported activity levels and hip x-ray films and pain in elderly women. Women who exercised more than four times per week had a marginally increased risk of hip osteoarthritis. Vingard et al[13] compared self-reported sports activities in women who underwent total hip replacement for osteoarthritis with controls without hip problems. Those with high sports exposure were 2.3 times more likely to have hip osteoarthritis develop, leading to total hip replacement. Both of these studies are retrospective and rely on the subject to recall activity level over a lifetime. Caution should be used in counseling women to abstain from physical activity because of the risk of osteoarthritis. Although activity may increase the risk of osteoarthritis, better skill training and prehabilitation for women in the future may show a plateau in the incidence of activity associated osteoarthritis.

Hip osteoarthritis in general may not be caused by a specific sports injury. Many exercisers and athletes must overcome the limitations of the osteoarthritis in order to participate. Managing an exerciser with hip pain related to osteoarthritis encompasses possibly altering the type of activity or weight bearing while trying to restore muscle, fascial, and capsular "mechanical balance." Prevention of impairing soft tissue adaptations such as a hip flexion contracture is essential in keeping the exerciser with hip osteoarthritis on the playing field.

Osteitis pubis is a syndrome involving bony change that often occurs as a result of an overuse injury. Pubic symphysitis and recurrent groin injuries may, in fact, be precursors to the degenerative changes described as osteitis pubis. Exercisers or athletes participating in repetitive kicking, pivoting, and running are at risk for this injury. Nonathletic risks also include previous bladder or prostate surgery or pelvic floor trauma. Symptoms at presentation include groin, anterior hip, and lower abdominal pain. The exerciser may have a recurrent or long history of "groin pulls." Antalgic gait and pain on palpation of the pubic symphysis that increases with resisted hip motion are often noted on physical examination. X-ray films may show sclerotic changes but oftentimes are normal. A bone scan may show asymmetric uptake at the pubic symphysis. MRI is helpful in delineating stress fracture from stress reaction. Arriving at the diagnoses of osteitis pubis takes coordination of history and physical examination, because adjunct testing is limited.

Sites of Stress Fractures

- Ilium
- Lesser trochanter
- Femoral neck
- Pubis
- Sacrum

Clinical Guideline

Soft Tissue, Nerve, and Muscle Injuries

Tendinitis, muscle strains, and muscle imbalances are common types of injuries in exercisers and athletes. Muscle and tendon dysfunctions can lead to friction and, at specific sites, cause bursitis. Several theories have been given regarding the concept of muscle imbalance. These are listed in Exhibit 4–1.[14] Therefore, trauma or injury is not the only way muscle imbalances develop. Jull and Janda[15] have studied muscle imbalance and adaptations in children and adolescents. They found a 21% incidence of short muscles in 115 school-aged children. Follow-ups at ages 12 and 16 showed that muscle tightness increased and then plateaued. These muscle imbalances did not correct without intervention. Muscles involving the hip and pelvis that are prone to tightness include the iliopsoas, rectus femoris, tensor fascia lata, short adductors, hamstrings, quadratus lumborum, and piriformis. Strains and muscle tears often occur in muscles that are prone to tightness. Tendinitis often occurs in weak, inhibited muscle groups. Examples at the hip and pelvis include the gluteus medius, gluteus maximus, abdominals, and quadriceps.[16] Identifying muscles functioning in a shortened position or that are inhibited is key to devising a rehabilitation or prehabilitation program.

Exhibit 4–1 Theoretical Causes of Muscle Imbalances

1. Postural adaptation to gravity
2. Neuroreflexive caused by joint blockage
3. Central nervous system malregulation (impaired programming)
4. Response to painful stimuli
5. Response to physical demands
6. Lack of variety of movement patterns
7. Psychological influences
8. Histochemical differences

Common Sites of Bursitis

- Greater trochanter
- Iliopsoas at ischial pectineal line
- Ischiogluteal
- Origin of obturator internus

Clinical Guideline

Bursitis can also accompany a primary muscle or tendon dysfunction. A bursa becomes fluid filled as a result of inflammation that develops because of friction. This friction occurs because a tendon is not able to glide efficiently across a region. This inefficiency may be because of bony protrusions or primary muscle or tendon injury. Common sites for bursitis involving the hip and pelvis include iliopsoas at the ischial pectineal line, greater trochanter of the hip, ischiogluteal area, and origin of the obturator internus. Determining the primary mechanism of injury will facilitate a treatment program and prevent reinjury.

Identifying the mechanism of injury in the history coupled with a comprehensive physical examination leads to a specific diagnosis. The health care provider must have a good understanding of muscle balance and function. Subtle imbalances of agonist and antagonist muscle groups are often not found on a standard physical examination. Muscle weakness sometimes cannot be identified unless the muscle is fatigued. Poor endurance in a quadriceps may be brought out with single-leg squats. Hamstring weakness may be detected with repeated wall squats or bridging from a supine position. Examining individual muscle length is also key in forming a specific rehabilitation prescription. If a tight iliopsoas goes unnoticed, a strengthening program for the hamstrings may be fraught with problems. A tight iliopsoas often leads to an anterior pelvic tilt. An increase in anterior pelvic tilt then leads to the hamstrings firing in a lengthened position. Strengthening the hamstrings in a lengthened position may lead to submaximal strength benefit, and overload may cause subsequent hamstring injury.

Observing quality of motion is also important. Examining lumbopelvic rhythm is an example of observing quality of motion. With forward flexion, the lumbar spine should move initially followed by the pelvis and hips. Initiation of motion from the pelvis or hip indicates a breakdown in muscle function. This may be a result of lumbar spine dysfunction or muscle imbalance at the hip and pelvis. Measuring fingertip distance from the floor at end range forward flexion is not as useful as determining the quality of motion demonstrated to achieve the position.

Recurrent muscle and tendon injuries must be carefully reviewed to avoid missing an underlying bony or systemic problem. If, indeed, the injury is recurrent to the soft tissue, the health care provider must investigate the mechanism of injury, training patterns, environmental factors, and equipment to ensure complete resolution. Specifying the precise muscle, tendon, or soft tissue involved in an injury leads to a specific treatment program and preventive maintenance program.

Several specific muscle imbalance syndromes occur at the hip and pelvis. Again, these are more sport or activity specific. They may be seen with a wide range of symptoms, including pain in the buttocks, groin, lumbar spine, and knee.

Piriformis syndrome may be seen with a variety of complaints. These include back and/or buttocks pain and lower extremity pain and/or numbness. The true syndrome by definition includes electrophysiological changes along the

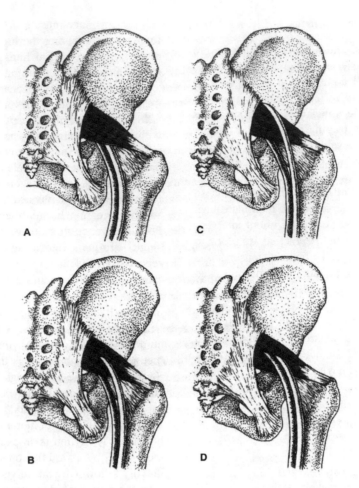

Figure 4–6 Four Variations of the Relationship of the Sciatic Nerve and the Piriformis Muscle. A, the most common route (85%) where all of the nerve fibers pass anterior to the piriformis; B, peroneal nerve fibers pass through the muscle and the tibial nerve fibers pass anterior to the muscle; C, peroneal nerve fibers pass up and over the muscle posteriorly and the tibial nerve fibers pass anterior to the muscle; D, tibial and peroneal fibers pass directly through the muscle.

distribution of the sciatic nerve as a result of compression by the piriformis. The sciatic nerve travels through the sciatic notch and passes anterior to the piriformis 85% of the time (Figure 4–6). Variations to this relationship exist. In 10% of the population, the sciatic nerve divides before passing through the gluteal region. The common peroneal portion passes through the piriformis, and the tibial portion passes anterior to the piriformis. In 2% to 3% of cadavers the peroneal portion loops superior and posterior to the piriformis, and the tibial portion travels anterior to the muscle. Another variation found in less than 1% of the cadavers is an undivided nerve that passes through the piriformis. Regardless of its position, the sciatic nerve is vulnerable to compression or irritation at the site of the piriformis.

The piriformis facilitates different motions at the hip on the basis of the position of the hip. In hip extension, the piriformis is an external rotator of the hip. In 60° of hip flexion the piriformis is an abductor. With the hip positioned at 90° of flexion, the piriformis internally rotates the hip.[17]

Because the muscle performs different motions in different hip positions, the examiner must include different positions to fully examine the muscle (Figure 4–7). Again, an imbalance in muscle length and strength may create a dysfunction resulting in pain.

Clinically, there are a number of patients who complain of a symptom complex related to piriformis dysfunction without electrophysiological changes on electromyography. This may be a result of inherent muscle weakness or show that neurogenic compression is only intermittent. Yet piriformis irritability and dysfunction may still occur even though electrodiagnostic testing does not fulfill the criteria for piriformis syndrome. Even if this does not meet the definition of piriformis syndrome, the area needs to be treated to prevent further regional breakdown in mechanics. A painful piriformis by history and on physical examination may be part of a symptom complex of another regional diagnosis. Examples include L5–S4 radiculopathy, intrinsic hip pathology, and sacroiliac joint dysfunction. These need to

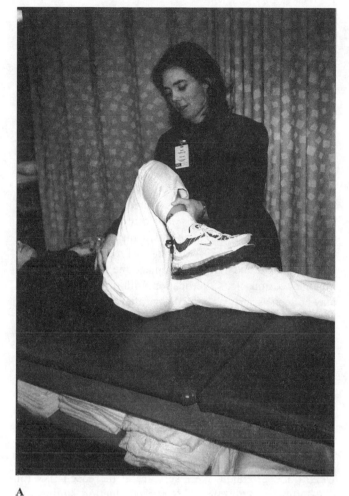

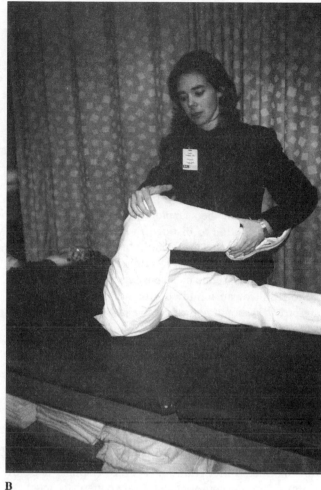

A   B

Figure 4-7 Piriformis Performs Different Functions Dependent on the Degree of Hip Flexion. Flexibility testing should be completed with the hip flexed greater than 90° and internal rotation, A, as well as less than 90° of hip flexion with external rotation, B.

be further investigated so as not to incompletely treat the athlete or exerciser. Activities that require one-legged activity or stance such as bowling or skating may place the athlete at risk for pain associated with the piriformis muscle. Shifting from one extremity to the other like running and using the stairstepper may also increase the risk for breakdown in mechanics.

Clinical Guideline: Piriformis Muscle Function

Position	Function
Hip extension	External rotation
60° flexion	Abduction
90° flexion	Internal rotation

Clinical Guideline

The exerciser may complain of low back, buttocks, and lower extremity pain and/or numbness. Lower extremity symptoms may not pass far beyond the gluteal fold or may involve the foot. On examination, pain with palpation of the muscle may be noted and further exacerbated with stretch or with resisted activation. The examiner must be careful to stretch and activate the muscle according to the function it performs in different hip positions. Specific positioning for testing relative muscle strength and length is essential to formulate a specific rehabilitation plan. Positioning may also bring out symptoms other than pain such as numbness or tingling, which should also be noted. Further internal palpation by rectal examination can help clarify the clinical diagnosis in questionable cases. Muscle stretch reflexes may be reduced, as well as sensory deficits, in the tibial and/or peroneal distribution.

Snapping hip syndrome is another common symptom complex that afflicts exercisers and athletes. A snapping or clicking sensation during activity may be associated with pain. The cause of the click is site specific. The most common cause is the hip suction phenomenon. Other intra-articular causes that should be carefully ruled out include subluxation, acetabular labral tear, loose body, and osteochondromatosis. Other common tendon causes include the iliopsoas snapping over the iliopectineal eminence and the iliotibial band moving over the greater trochanter. Exercisers or athletes with pubic symphysis instability may complain of clicking in the groin region. The instability may be related to trauma such as that experienced with childbirth or generalized ligamentous laxity. Determining the site of the clicking is important but can be difficult. The examiner should palpate the area of the snapping during active and passive hip range of motion to distinguish the structure.[18] Again, regional muscle imbalance should be considered once the source of snapping has been determined. The iliotibial band may tighten because the muscle is serving as a hip abductor as the result of an inhibited gluteus medius. The health care provider should not expect the snapping hip syndrome to remain resolved solely with iliotibial band stretching. Gluteus medius strengthening in the appropriate hip position will allow the iliotibial band to remain in its new lengthened position.

Other sources of pain and dysfunction include muscle imbalances causing relative overuse syndromes. Jull and Janda have described a muscle imbalance syndrome at the hip and pelvis as the pelvic crossed syndrome. This includes a muscle imbalance pattern of tight hip flexors and hamstrings with inhibited glutei and lumbar erector spinae muscles. Quality of muscle activation and firing patterns is noted. An example includes noting the succession of muscle firing in hip extension from the prone position. The order of firing involves the ipsilateral hamstring, gluteus maximus, contralateral lumbosacral paraspinals, contralateral thoracolumbar paraspinals, and finally the ipsilateral thoracolumbar paraspinals. Commonly, the gluteus maximus is weak and fires late in the sequence, which may then allow breakdown somewhere proximal or distal such as the lumbar spine or hip.[15]

Sahrmann[19] also describes a series of muscle imbalances at the hip called hip impingement syndromes. Anteromedial impingement is seen with groin pain with hip flexion and posterior pain with weight bearing. On physical examination there is anteromedial displacement of the greater trochanter with knee to chest. With hip extension, hamstring activity is dominant over gluteus maximus. Tightness may be found in the tensor fascia latae. Anterolateral impingement is seen with hip pain with weight bearing, which is relieved with external rotation of the lower extremity in stance. As a result, hip external rotators and hamstrings are tight. Proximal impingement syndrome is diagnosed in individuals with complaints of deep hip pain and pain on palpation lateral

to the tensor fascia lata. Pain may also be described in the inner thigh region. The exerciser may complain of early morning stiffness or discomfort that increases with activity. Decreased range of motion is found in a capsular pattern, including decreased hip flexion and internal rotation. Tightness is found in the iliopsoas, rectus femoris, and tensor fascia lata. Osteoarthritis is often found in association with this hip impingement syndrome.

Muscle contusions should be identified early in the athlete so as to rule out underlying bony injuries. A contusion usually develops as a result of a direct blow or trauma. A hip pointer occurs as a result of a blow to the anterior iliac crest. A tear to the muscle aponeurosis or avulsion of the apophysis should be excluded. Myositis ossificans may also develop as a result of muscle trauma. The athlete may have hardening of the hematoma and decreasing range of motion. Osteoblasts form within the hematoma to replace the fibroblasts in the traumatized muscle. Calcification within the muscle belly may be seen as early as 7 to 10 days after the injury on x-ray. The individual usually complains with concentric muscle contraction or passive stretch. Heterotopic bone growth may be evident between 2 and 3 weeks after the trauma. Bone scan may be positive before changes are found on x-ray.

Neurogenic pain should be considered in the differential for pelvic and hip pain. Meralgia paresthetica is one common nerve entrapment at the hip. The lateral femoral cutaneous nerve is entrapped in the pelvis as it crosses the groin medial to the anterosuperior iliac spine. Fibrous tunnels may exist that the nerve or branches may cross through. The overweight and pregnant exercisers are at increased risk for developing an entrapment. Nerve conduction studies are helpful in confirming the diagnosis. Reducing equipment or clothing restrictions at the hip and groin can be helpful in reducing symptoms.

Sacroiliac Joint Dysfunction

The SIJ is a controversial instigator of pain and dysfunction. Reasons for controversy include that the joint is narrow with only a few degrees of motion. The joint degenerates with aging and loses further motion.[9] The biomechanics regarding the joint are complex and are still in the process of being evaluated by researchers. There are no specific standards for evaluation of SIJ dysfunction. It is often a diagnosis of exclusion. Imaging of the joint commonly reveals changes associated with aging but does not distinguish asymptomatic from symptomatic individuals. For women, SIJ pain and dysfunction may be underdiagnosed because of coexisting gynecological problems or because of pelvic changes that occur during and after pregnancy that may be attributed to "having a baby."

The prevalence of SIJ pain is unknown. Bernard et al[20] reported that of 1293 patients with low back pain, SIJ dysfunction was thought to be the pain source in 22.5% on the basis of history and physical examination. Another study showed that 58% of those with SIJ dysfunction by history and physical examination had a history of trauma.[3] Sports and training equipment that require repetitive unidirectional pelvic shear and torsional forces may be important risk factors for SIJ dysfunction (Figure 4–8). These sports include skating, gymnastics, golfing, and bowling. Athletes can put asymmetrical shear forces through the SIJ when using a stairstepper, elliptical trainer, or workouts including step aerobics.

SIJ dysfunction may present in various patterns. However, athletes commonly complain of pain in the low back or buttock near the posterior superior iliac spine. Pain may radiate down the posterior leg or anterior into the groin. Pain may be exacerbated with repetitive overload activity, transitional movements, and unsupported sitting. There are no specific examination techniques or diagnostic tests that consistently or accurately identify SIJ pain. The examiner must have a clear understanding of biomechanics and process through a differential diagnosis, because SIJ dysfunction is often determined by exclusion. The physical examination should include the usual gait analysis, neurological, postural, joint range of motion, flexibility, and strength evaluation. Provocative testing such as Gaenslen's or Patrick's test may help direct the diagnosis, but a negative test does not exclude SIJ dysfunction.

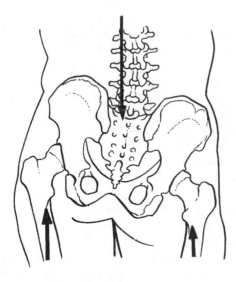

Figure 4–8 Activities Requiring Repetitive Unidirectional Pelvic Shear and Torsional Forces May Place the Athlete at Risk for SIJ Dysfunction. The arrows depict vertical converging forces from above (trunk force) and from below (ground force).

Differential Diagnosis of SIJ Pain

- Inflammation
- Instability
- Osteitis condensans
- Pelvic inflammatory disease
- Tumors
- Pregnancy
- Lumbar causes
- Infection
- Fracture

Clinical Guideline

The differential diagnosis of SIJ pain is all encompassing. Inflammation of the SIJ may occur as a result of metabolic changes, arthritis, trauma, or infection. Primary tumors of the SIJ are rare. Iatrogenic instability may result from graft harvesting. Osteitis condensans, increased density on the ilial side of the inferior SIJ, occurs in 2.2% of the multiparous female population and is usually self-limiting. Sacroiliitis may develop as a part of pelvic inflammatory disease. Changes that occur during pregnancy as described previously must be considered. Pain may be referred from other sites of dysfunction, including lumbar radiculopathy, lumbar facet joint pain, lumbar central or lateral recess stenosis, lumbar discogenic pain, hip disease, and Maigne's syndrome. Obtaining x-ray films of the SIJ is important to rule out infection, metabolic changes, fracture, or tumor. CT, MRI, bone scan, or single photon emission computed tomography provides more detailed information regarding the joint. Rarely will imaging clearly define SIJ dysfunction. The health care provider organizes information from the history, performs a physical examination that includes noting subtle changes in flexibility and strength, and rules out neurogenic causes. A diagnostic fluoroscopically guided SIJ injection can be helpful in confirming the diagnosis.

Pelvic Floor Dysfunction

Pelvic floor pain and dysfunction can cause considerable pain and impairment for the female exerciser and athlete. Unfortunately, sports literature rarely focuses on such problems and is often left as a "female problem." The pelvic floor is a group of muscles that must act in coordination with their surrounding joints, including the lumbar spine, SIJ, hip joint, and pubic symphysis. In addition, the pelvic floor must function in coordination with visceral structures. These include the bladder, vagina, uterus, ovaries, and colon. The muscles of the pelvic floor may respond adaptively to a primary visceral problem. An example includes an increase muscle tone that may occur in the levator ani on the ipsilateral side of an ovarian cyst. The athlete may have primary complaints of pelvic pain with urination, defecation, intercourse, and around the time of menstruation. Primary hormonal and visceral problems should be ruled out.

"Labels" Used for Pelvic Floor Dysfunction

- Myofascial pain syndrome
- Tension myalgia
- Hypertonis
- Muscle dyssynergia

Clinical Guideline

Adaptive patterns in the pelvic floor can also develop as a result of a primary joint injury. A hip with osteoarthritic changes and loss of range of motion may refer pain to the groin and pelvic floor. Muscle guarding may occur, causing increased tone within the pelvic floor. Increased muscle tone within the pelvic floor may lead to pain and dyssynergic problems. Primary muscle imbalances can also refer or cause subsequent pelvic floor muscle imbalance. An athlete with piriformis syndrome with an inhibited gluteus medius may develop obturator internus pain noted in the pelvic floor. The obturator internus acts as a secondary hip abductor. Overload may occur because of the inhibited gluteus medius with resultant obturator internus pain. Pelvic floor myofascial pain in female exercisers and athletes is often associated with asymmetrical tautness in the sacrotuberous ligament and the surrounding muscles and fascia. Because much overlap exists in hip, back, and pelvic injuries and dysfunction, the biomechanics of the pelvic floor should be addressed just as they are addressed for an external pelvic dysfunction.

Tension myalgia is another label often given to general pelvic floor pain. Diagnoses also included under this label include piriformis syndrome, levator ani syndrome, coccydynia, and vaginismus. Dysfunctions involving increased muscle tone of the musculoskeletal and urogynecological systems are often referred to as levator ani syndrome. Increased pelvic floor muscle tone may also be contributing components for individuals with low back pain, chronic pelvic pain with negative laparoscopy, endometriosis, interstitial cystitis, urethral syndrome, and sphincter dyssynergia. Women with these dysfunctions may complain of pain in the general region of the vagina, rectum, lower abdominal quadrants, and posterior pelvis. Other areas of discomfort can include the coccyx, pubic symphysis, and posterior thigh. Women may report functional limitations because of pain. These include dyspareunia, sexual dysfunction, and difficulty with voiding and constipation. Urinary frequency and urgency may also be present.

Increased muscle tone in the pelvic floor may occur for several reasons: direct trauma to the pelvis as with fractures or joint injuries involving the hip, ilium, and sacrum; abnormal use or adaptive muscle imbalance syndromes can contribute to increased pelvic floor muscle tone; and myofascial pain syndromes may occur primarily or secondary to trauma or muscle imbalance. Travell and Simons[21] have identified specific pelvic floor muscles that may cause symptoms. Trigger points within these muscle groups can refer pain. These muscles are listed in Exhibit 4–2. A history of sexual abuse, anxiety, depression, and general lifestyle stress can cause muscle tension.[22] Concomitant evaluation of psychosocial factors is imperative to evaluate and treat the pain syndrome comprehensively.

Evaluations for pelvic floor dysfunctions involving hypertonus include a manual pelvic floor, musculoskeletal, neurological, and posture evaluation. The internal and external pelvic floor examination identifies the specific location of the pain. The musculoskeletal and neurological examinations of the hip, pelvis, and lumbar spine help identify primary or secondary causes for pelvic floor pain. Surface electromyography (EMG) biofeedback evaluation performed with internal and external electrodes is helpful in determining baseline resting muscle activity. Tone changes that occur with position changes, exercise, or functional activities can also be identified.

When infection and other serious medical or skeletal causes have been ruled out, hypertonic pelvic floor muscle pain should be managed by addressing psychological, neurochemical, and mechanical factors. Physical therapy can address specific muscle imbalances with appropriate flexibility and strengthening exercises. Various techniques such as myofascial release, muscle energy, joint mobilization, and posture education can be incorporated. Surface EMG biofeedback is helpful in identifying the muscles with increased tone and facilitates relaxation techniques used to reduce tone. Modalities such as heat and cold may facilitate pain management and relaxation. When indicated, medications addressing neurogenic pain, sleep dysfunction, anxiety, and depression should be used concomitantly with physical therapy. Pelvic floor muscle dyssynergia is another cause of pelvic floor pain. Muscles must fire at the appropriate place, time, and intensity. If muscles are unable to coordinate contraction and relaxation, dysfunctions in micturition and defecation may occur. This complex of symptoms is referred to as pelvic floor dyssynergia. Several causes for pelvic floor dyssynergia exist. Pudendal nerve injury can result in sensory and motor deficits inhibiting appropriate muscle functioning. Improper technique during exercise that causes a bearing down on the pelvic floor rather than lifting of the pelvic floor can facilitate dyssynergia. Other neurological diseases or injury and inability to isolate pelvic floor muscle contraction from abdominal or gluteal muscle contractions can lead to muscle incoordination and dyssynergia.[23]

Pelvic floor biofeedback is especially helpful in the treatment of pain syndromes related to dyssynergia. Biofeed-

Exhibit 4–2 Trigger Points in Pelvic Floor Muscles

Muscles Susceptible To Trigger Point Formation Resulting in Pelvic Pain	*Muscles Susceptible To Trigger Point Formation Resulting in Iliosacral Pain*
Coccygeus	Coccygeus
Levator ani	Levator ani
Obturator internus	Gluteus medius
Adductor magnus	Quadratus lumborum
Piriformis	Gluteus maximus
Oblique abdominals	Multifidi
	Rectus abdominus
	Soleus

back facilitates coordination of muscle contractions at rest and during activities of daily living. Physical therapy must also focus on retraining pelvic floor muscle activity with proper breathing. This is especially important for the athlete performing high-resistance exercise such as weightlifting, rowing, and bicycling. Activities of daily living involving child care should also be evaluated. During the months after childbirth, lifting and carrying the child may facilitate a dyssynergic syndrome. Controlling contraction of the pelvic floor during exhalation facilitates the pelvic and respiratory diaphragms to act in synergy. A physical therapist can help facilitate training the pelvic floor to contract before lifting, laughing, or coughing. Medications for neurogenic causes may be indicated. Care must be taken to avoid medications that may adversely affect bladder function.

Another pelvic floor dysfunction that adversely affects female athletes is urinary stress incontinence. One survey[24] revealed 28% of a group of 144 elite nulliparous female athletes reported stress urinary incontinence during exercise or sports participation. Of the sports studied, gymnasts and tennis players reported a higher incidence of urine loss. The cause for incontinence in athletes is thought to be multifactorial. Contributing factors include inadequate abdominal pressure transmission, pelvic floor muscle fatigue, and changes in collagen or connective tissue.

High-impact sports requiring jumping and landing may place participants at greater risk for incontinence because of the sudden increase in intra-abdominal pressure. The pelvic floor muscles must be able to contract with enough speed and force to withstand repetitive deceleration of the visceral structures within the abdomen onto the pelvic floor. The levator ani in particular must have sufficient endurance and strength to support the pelvic organs in humans because of the upright posture.[25] The chronic pressure of gravity on the pelvic floor is rapidly increased with coughing, sneezing, running, and jumping. Despite ongoing investigations, the question remains as to whether athletes have stronger pelvic muscles or connective tissue because of long-term increases in intra-abdominal muscles. Nygaard[26] surveyed previous

female Olympic swimmers, gymnasts, and track and field participants from 1960 through 1976. The survey focused on the prevalence of urinary incontinence. The athletes were between 42 and 47 years of age at the time of the survey. No differences were found between athletes participating in high-impact or low-impact sports. Of the 104 responders, 8% and 10% of each group, respectively, reported daily or weekly incontinence. Therefore, a significant number of the athletes were reporting incontinence later in life regardless of the type of impact sport. With further investigations, the risk associated with exercise and sports may be found to be activity specific rather than associated with exercise in general.

Stress incontinence also occurs in nulliparous women without obvious risk factors associated with activity. Bo et al[27] found that nulliparous women with stress incontinence had a reduction in tissue collagen concentration compared with controls. Another study by Al-Rawi and colleagues[28] showed connective tissue differences in controls and women with genital prolapse. Sixty percent of the group with prolapse had joint hypermobility compared with 18% of those without prolapse. Collagen architecture or collagen with aging changes may place women at risk for incontinence. This may cumulate with the stress of high-impact activities during sports or exercise-producing stress incontinence.

The female athlete or exerciser who has given birth may have other contributing factors to the development of incontinence. Several studies[29–32] have shown significant denervation in pelvic floor muscles in women who have given birth vaginally. Denervation with subsequent muscle weakness requires adaptations in muscle function and tone to make up for the loss. Such adaptations may put the woman at risk not only for incontinence but also for myofascial pain syndromes as well.

Urinary incontinence in the nonelite athlete and general exerciser also occurs. Often this dysfunction goes underreported or unreported. Health care providers need to be made aware of such problems so they may be better addressed. In addition to the risk factors identified earlier, the athlete who is amenorrheic or having irregular menstrual cycles may have low estrogen levels. This can also contribute to the development of incontinence. The importance of completing a directed detailed history cannot be overemphasized. Women may need to be asked if they experience incontinence. Health care providers should not leave it to women to report the problem.

Proposed Etiology of Stress Incontinence

- Reduced tissue collagen
- Hypermobility
- Stress of high-impact activities
- Denervation in pelvic floor muscles

Clinical Guideline

Once stress incontinence during exercise has been identified, a thorough evaluation should ensue. Evaluation of other medical problems and medications that may predispose the woman to incontinence is necessary. A voiding diary is helpful in determining the individual's voiding and drinking patterns. This can also record the types of beverages consumed and number of incontinence episodes. The urine should be evaluated for infection with a urine dipstick test. Bladder catheterization should be completed within 5 minutes of voiding to measure a postvoid residual. A normal postvoid residual helps to rule out a voiding dysfunction. Assessing S2–S4 sensation by means of pinprick, pressure, and vibration along the vulva, perineum, and inner thighs is important to detect or rule out a subclinical neuropathic process or injury.

A general speculum examination by the primary care physician or gynecologist should be completed to rule out other medical reasons for urinary dysfunction. Palpation of the pelvic floor is important to assess muscle tone, strength, and coordination. The individual pelvic floor muscles should be palpated and their tone compared from side to side. Muscle strength of the pelvic floor musculature should be evaluated. Several grading systems describe muscle strength from absent to strong. These are listed in Exhibit 4–3. The examiner must observe for the individual's ability to contract the pelvic floor muscles without using accessory muscles and without bearing down. This muscle examination helps to determine whether the woman will be a good candidate for pelvic floor exercises. A specific prescription can then be written indicating if too much or too little muscle tone, strength, or coordination is a problem. If the woman reports urgency, frequency, or dysuria in the absence of infection, referral for urethrocystoscopy may be indicated. Other indications for referral include women with a history of smoking or those who are found to have microscopic hematuria. Full

urodynamic testing is indicated when conservative treatment fails, voiding dysfunction is found, or if a history of pelvic surgery or radiation therapy exists.

Treatment for urinary stress incontinence is tailored to the individual and her lifestyle. Lifestyle measures, support devices, and specific pelvic floor exercises are helpful in managing women whose incontinence occurs primarily during sports and exercise.

Voiding before exercise can be suggested if the exerciser with incontinence is not already doing so. Eliminating coffee and caffeine 2 to 3 hours before exercise can prevent diuresis, thereby decreasing bladder filling. Some women may have already severely reduced their fluid intake before exercise in attempts to decrease their incontinence. These women should be counseled on the need for proper hydration to prevent severe complications that may arise with dehydration.[33] Several types of intravaginal support devices are available and can be worn during exercise to help eliminate incontinence. Intravaginal pessaries and tampons have been found to be effective in up to 83% and 57% of users, respectively. Successful reduction in incontinence was correlated with the severity of the incontinence.[34] The Introl bladder-neck-support prosthesis is similar to a pessary but has projections that fit under the urethra to support it. This prosthesis was found to be 83% effective in one clinical trial.[35] All these devices help to prevent incontinence by supporting the bladder neck and urethra. However, their effectiveness is not universal.

Several barrier devices can be useful in controlling incontinence during exercise. These are placed on the external urethral meatus and are secured in place by adhesive material or suction. Barrier devices work by obstructing the external urethral meatus. They can be somewhat cumbersome in that they must be removed to void.

Management of Stress Incontinence

- Decrease caffeine intake
- Decrease fluid intake
- Intravaginal devices
- Biofeedback
- Physical therapy
- Muscle retraining and re-education
- Barrier devices
- Electrical stimulation
- Strengthening exercises

Clinical Guideline

Education in pelvic floor muscle relaxation, coordination, and strengthening is vital for the treatment of urinary stress incontinence in women who have been ruled out for overflow incontinence or other voiding dysfunction. Instructing

Exhibit 4–3 Pelvic Floor Muscle Strength Grading

Grading Scale	**Grading Scale**
0—none	0—no contraction
1—flicker	1—flicker, only with the muscle stretched
2—weak	2—a weak squeeze, two second hold
3—moderate	3—a fair squeeze, definite "lift"
4—good	4—a good squeeze, good hold with "lift," repeatable
5—strong	5—a strong squeeze, good lift, repeatable
Measure length of contraction up to 10 seconds	
Record number of repetitions up to 10	
Record number of fast 1-second contractions	

the patient in relaxation techniques to counteract increased pelvic floor muscle tone can easily be started during the internal palpatory pelvic examination. Adding biofeedback can be especially helpful. This technique of making the patient aware of physiological changes as a response to a voluntary action assists in controlling muscle tone. Simply the examiner commenting on the strength of a muscle contraction during the pelvic examination can accomplish biofeedback. More sophisticated forms include external perineal and intravaginal monitors that allow the patient to visualize the magnitude of her contraction or relaxation effort on a monitor. This equipment requires specific education in its use and can be expensive. Many companies offer rental programs to support an individual's temporary needs.

Facilitating muscle coordination is also important in the treatment of incontinence. The patient must be educated in the sequence of muscle contraction and relaxation with activities of daily living, voiding, and defecation. An example is the importance of contracting the pelvic floor muscles without performing a Valsalva maneuver. The latter increases intra-abdominal pressure, thereby increasing the amount of force required by the pelvic floor muscles to contract.

Contraction exercises are often used to increase tone and strengthen the pelvic floor muscles. Health care providers should be careful in their recommendations for strengthening exercises in the setting of incontinence. Stress urinary incontinence is not always associated with weak pelvic floor musculature. Often, dysfunction in muscle tone and coordination can be determined. If these are not first addressed, the patient may waste time attempting to strengthen muscles that are either not weak or have not been reset to their appropriate physiological length to accomplish strengthening. When weakness has been determined to be a part of the dysfunction, patients should be instructed in the proper technique during the palpatory physical examination. Close follow-up is needed to ensure follow through and problem solving. Devising a strengthening program should also be individualized to the patient's needs. A program might include a series of 5-second contractions followed by 10 seconds of relaxation performed for 10 minutes per day. The program may be upgraded by increasing duration and intensity as the patient's accomplishments progress. When satisfactory strength has been achieved, a maintenance program should be created to deter future recurrences. Vaginal cones may be used to facilitate vaginal strengthening. The patient can use a set of cones of various weights. Starting with the lightest cone, the patient holds it in the vagina for approximately 20 minutes one to two times per day. As the muscles become stronger, the cone is changed to a heavier weight.

Electrical stimulation is another technique that can be used in the treatment of stress urinary incontinence. This is a device that is inserted into the vagina and delivers a current. The current's amplitude and frequency are adjusted to the patient's comfort and sensitivity. The current produces an involuntary contraction of the pelvic floor muscles. This may be useful in assisting in the retraining and strengthening of these muscles. Several studies have shown this adjunct treatment device to be effective.[36,37]

Although urinary stress incontinence involves visceral structures, primary or secondary musculoskeletal dysfunctions are often identified. These need to be fully evaluated and treatment specified to the type of muscle imbalance, coordination, or tone problem. Incontinence has many social implications. Accurate and early diagnosis in the female athlete can prevent a progressive problem that might deter the woman from participating in exercise or sports.

REHABILITATION

A rehabilitation program for the exerciser and athlete must focus its outcome goal beyond resolution of symptoms. An appropriate program will focus on muscle and joint physiological restoration. Ultimately, this should prevent reinjury and future muscle imbalance. Pelvic pain and dysfunction rehabilitation includes restoration of lumbar spine, hip, and pelvis mechanics. Success in treatment relies on a specific and accurate diagnosis. The rehabilitation model that incorporates the injury cycle and negative feedback described by Kibler et al[38] and Herring[39] will be followed. Exhibits 4–3 to 4–5 outline the different stages of rehabilitation.

Bony Injuries

Acute Phase (1–3 days)

Bony injuries excluding fractures will be discussed here. During the acute phase of recovery, the *clinical symptom complex* and *tissue injury complex* are addressed with measures to decrease weight bearing and edema. Weight bearing on the lower extremity should be as tolerated. Crutches may be necessary in the initial stage. Ice and anti-inflammatory medications will facilitate control of swelling and pain. Isometric muscle contractions around the involved joint will provide compression to the joint and decrease the deleterious effects of immobilization. The exerciser or athlete can advance to the recovery phase of healing once pain and swelling are controlled, near normal range of motion is achieved, and strengthening is tolerated. Weight bearing is advanced as pain allows.

Recovery Phase (3 days–8 weeks)

The *tissue overload complex* and *functional biomechanical deficit complex* are further addressed during this phase. Flexibility of the capsule and muscles surrounding the hip is important. Particular attention should be given to the iliopsoas and hip adductors, because muscle tightness here can lead to tightening down of the capsule. Once full weight bearing is achieved, lower extremity balance and proprioceptive training can be accomplished. Trunk stabilization and closed kinetic chain strengthening exercises for the lower

extremity are added. Advancement to the maintenance phase takes place when the athlete or exerciser is pain free with impact activities, bony healing is complete, range of motion and flexibility are restored, and strength has returned to 75% of baseline. Appropriate radiographic imaging is required to ensure bone healing.

Maintenance Phase

The functional *biomechanical deficit complex* and *subclinical adaptation complex* are addressed. Sports and exercise-specific activities are advanced. Power and endurance strengthening are tailored to the individual's goals. Review of training schedule and techniques is important during this phase. Further ergonomics and equipment (shoes, orthotics, etc) should be completed. Trial of return to activity under the supervision of a physical therapist is especially helpful in problem solving. The exerciser or athlete can return to play if she remains pain free with full range of motion, has normal strength and balance, and demonstrates good mechanics while performing the activity. Again appropriate radiographic imaging should be completed as indicated to follow the progression of bony healing.

Sacroiliac and Pelvic Dysfunctions

Acute Phase (1–3 days)

Acute injury is often associated with a fall or marked increase in intensity, frequency, or duration of a specific activity. More commonly this dysfunction is progressive with fluctuations in symptoms. The woman may experience symptoms only during sports or exercise participation. In the

---

Exhibit 4–4 Acute Stage of Rehabilitation

Focus of treatment
    Clinical symptom complex
    Tissue injury complex

Tools
    Rest and/or immobilization
    Physical modalities
    Medications
    Manual therapy
    Initial exercise
    Surgery

Criteria for advancement
    Pain control
    Adequate tissue healing
    Near normal range of motion
    Tolerance for strengthening

Exhibit 4–5 Recovery Stage of Rehabilitation

Focus of treatment
    Tissue overload complex
    Functional biomechanical deficit complex

Tools
    Manual therapy
    Flexibility
    Proprioceptive, neuromuscular control training
    Specific, progressive exercise

Criteria for return to play
    No pain
    Complete tissue healing
    Essentially pain-free range of motion
    Good flexibility
    75–80% or greater strength, as compared with uninjured side, and good strength balance

acute setting anti-inflammatorics and icing arc helpful. Relative rest after an acute injury assists with pain management. This includes no running or excessive walking, because these activities often provoke SIJ pain. Identifying the activity that may aggravate symptoms is important, especially in those with a progressive onset of symptoms. In general, avoiding activities that require one-legged stance like bowling, skating, running, and stairstepper is helpful in alleviating symptoms. Correcting asymmetries in muscle length should start as soon as possible. This should be accomplished within the limits of pain. Muscle energy techniques are particularly helpful, because they require patient activation of muscle groups, and therefore pain tolerance is easily monitored. Special care should be taken with early treatment of the pregnant athlete or exerciser. Because of the usual hypermobility associated with pregnancy, stretching or mobilization that is too aggressive can further aggravate her symptoms.

Recovery Phase (3 days–8 weeks)

Once pain has been controlled and the injured area has been rested, correction of the *functional biomechanical deficit* and *tissue overload complex* becomes the rehabilitation focus. Balancing lower extremity muscle length and strength is important, because they have both a direct and indirect effect on the ilium and sacrum. Muscle length must first be restored. The iliopsoas commonly is found to be activating in a shortened position. This shortened position leads to an anteriorly rotated ilium. Hamstring strengthening cannot be accomplished until the iliopsoas is stretched. An anterior pelvic tilt forces the hamstring to work in a lengthened position. The hamstring is a key muscle to provide stability to the sacroiliac joint because of its direct and fascial connections to the sacrotuberous ligament. Other muscles commonly found to be working in a shortened position include the rectus femoris, tensor fascia lata, adductors, quadratus lumborum, latissimus dorsi,[16] and obturator internus. Achieving appropriate muscle flexibility may require several weeks of stretching two to three times per day. Once appropriate muscle flexibility has been achieved, strengthening of muscles that are inhibited by the biomechanical deficit can be completed. Neuromuscular re-education and facilitation techniques are helpful with this process. Closed kinetic chain strengthening should be attempted first and is incorporated into the lumbopelvic stabilization exercises. Muscles commonly found to be weak include the gluteus medius, gluteus maximus, lower abdominals, and hamstrings.

Belts can be used to provide compression and thereby proprioceptive feedback to the gluteal muscles. Sacroiliac joint belts are especially helpful in patients with hypermobility or significant muscle weakness. Care must be taken to ensure that the patient is able to apply the belt appropriately.

Other equipment such as orthotics and shoe modification must also be assessed. A shoe lift to correct a functional leg length discrepancy can be helpful in the acute setting to manage pain with weight bearing or ambulating. Further use of the shoe lift should be approached with caution, because the functional leg length discrepancy should be corrected with muscle rebalancing. An inappropriate shoe lift can promote a *subclinical adaptation complex*. Of course, anatomical leg length discrepancies should be determined as early in treatment as possible so the appropriate modifications can be completed. SIJ injections can be used as an adjunct to a physical therapy program if the athlete reaches a plateau or the program cannot be advanced because of pain provocation. The injections can also be used diagnostically, specifically if done under fluoroscopic guidance. Maigne et al[40] reported 18.5% of 54 patients diagnosed with SIJ pain responded to double SIJ block under fluoroscopic guidance. This study did not control for other treatments given and therefore accurately reports only what an injection alone can improve.

Progression to the maintenance phase of treatment includes absence of pain and inflammation, absence of functional joint and myofascial dysfunction, and return of approximately 75% of strength and flexibility as judged per the patient's preinjury baseline. Normal activities of daily living, especially walking, should not provoke symptoms.

Maintenance Phase

During this phase of rehabilitation the focus turns to correcting the *biomechanical deficits* and the *functional adaptation complex* (Exhibit 4–6). Recognizing the adaptations that have occurred in response to the injury is essential to prevent further injury on return to sport. A common example includes the role of the gluteus maximus to stabilize the pelvis posteriorly by means of attachments at the ilium and sacrotuberous ligament. If the sacroiliac joint dysfunction involves an anteriorly rotated ilium, correction of the inflexibility of the iliopsoas alone will be insufficient. If the gluteus maximus contractions are too weak to stabilize posteriorly, then stretch will be placed on the iliolumbar ligament as well. This in turn will lead to lower lumbar segmental restrictions that must be addressed during the treatment process. The piriformis muscle length should be assessed with the hip flexed greater and less than 90°. Stretching applied with the hip in either or both directions is necessary. Continued inflexibility of this muscle is often thought to be part of the source of recurrent pain. Although maintaining individual muscle flexibility and strength is important, retraining of multiple muscle groups to fire in coordination is focused on during this phase in rehabilitation. This can be facilitated with lumbopelvic stabilization, advance proprioceptive re-education, plyometrics, and exercise or sport-specific activities. Education regarding proper ergonomics

Exhibit 4–6 Functional Stage Rehabilitation

Focus of treatment
   Functional biomechanical deficit complex
   Subclinical adaptation complex

Tools
   Power and endurance exercise
   Sports-specific functional progression
   Technique/skills instruction

Criteria for return to play
   No pain
   Full pain-free range of motion/normal flexibility
   Normal strength and strength balance
   Good general fitness
   Normal sports mechanics
   Demonstration of sport-specific skills

---

in activities of daily living and work environment should be included. Careful attention to training techniques must also be incorporated into the program. Mechanics are reviewed with return to exercise activity to rule out breakdown in the stabilization that has just been completed. Return to sport or exercise routine should resume when a pain-free state without medications is achieved. Proper muscle balance in flexibility and strength should remain a part of the maintenance program. Careful monitoring during initial return can prevent reinjury.

SIJ hypermobility unresponsive to the preceding outlined program is a difficult problem. SIJ arthrodesis is proposed for instability. Long-term outcome studies thus far have not been completed, and it is unknown what happens to surrounding articulations with the lumbar spine, contralateral SIJ, and hip. Prolotherapy has been proposed as an invasive but less permanent option in such cases. This treatment is supported by the theory that stimulation of fibrosis by needling a ligament followed by infusion of sclerosing agent will stabilize ligamentous laxity. No prospective, controlled studies exist to date on the specific use of prolotherapy and SIJ dysfunction.

Muscle Strains Involving the Groin

Acute Phase (1–3 days)

Muscles most often involved in groin injury include the adductor longus at the proximal musculotendinous junction, tendon to osseus insertion onto the inferior pubic tubercle, or muscle belly. During the acute stage, ice and relative rest are important. The athlete or exerciser should avoid repeated hip abduction or resisted hip adduction. If pain is significant with weight bearing, crutches may be necessary to facilitate pain control. Stretching during this stage should be limited to a pain-free range. Modalities such as ice and electrical stimulation may be used as adjuncts to pain management. Anti-inflammatory medications can also help relieve edema and facilitate pain management.

Recovery Phase (3 days–6 weeks)

Again during this phase, the focus of rehabilitation turns to correcting the biomechanical deficits and tissue overload complex. Modalities and medications may be continued during the first few weeks for adequate pain management. Active range of motion is advanced in the pain-free range. Myofascial release and muscle energy techniques may further promote increased range of motion. The patient should be independent in self-stretching, pelvic tilts, and concentric contraction of the antagonistic hip abductors. Four to 6 weeks of superficial heat and ultrasound may further expedite muscle stretching. Strengthening is added during this phase. Initially this should be limited to multilevel isometrics within a pain-free range.

Proprioceptive re-education can be added with balance retraining. Care should be taken to monitor the position of the pubic symphysis during this phase. Muscle shortening or instability may be recognized by difference in pubic symphysis heights and rotation on palpation. Again muscle energy techniques can be useful in correcting this dysfunction. The patient can become independent in self-correction. Retraining proper sequence of firing of hip abductors is important. Balance must be achieved between the contraction of usually weak lower abdominal muscles and tight hip adductors. The latter address the functional adaptation complex. The patient advances to the maintenance phase when pain and inflammation are controlled. Range of motion should be pain free and symmetric on side-to-side comparison. There should be no limitation in activities of daily living, including walking, and no recurrent pubic symphysis dysfunction.

Maintenance Phase

During this phase, the *functional biomechanical deficit* continues to be addressed through stretching and strengthening of the adductor muscle group. Attention to the *tissue overload complex* is begun with avoidance of excessive strain and inflammation to the lateral hip and pelvic structures. In particular, avoidance of tensor fascia lata overuse is enforced and continued stabilization concentrating on coordinated lower abdominal contraction with the adductor group. Resistance can be added to the stabilization program and graduated to weights. Before weight training for hip abduction is initiated, proper sequence of muscle contraction should be noted. If not, the tensor fascia lata will continue to be strengthened, and the adductors will continue to be inhibited. In addition to advancing walking and running, kicking mechanics should be reviewed as well.

INJURY PREVENTION OR PREHABILITATION

The more the world of health care learns about sports and exercise-specific injuries in women and girls, the more we will know about developing prevention or, even better, prehabilitation programs. Experts are recognizing that women may be more susceptible than men to some injuries because of differences in training and skill. Girls are learning sport-specific skills at earlier ages. Time will tell whether more or different injuries unique to women will become more prevalent.

With regard to the hip and pelvis, prevention of injury should focus on the assurance of proper joint mechanics and balanced muscle flexibility and strength. This balance is an evolving process with aging, especially for women. As adolescents, some girls may tend to be prone to joint hypermobility and laxity, which places them at increased risk for injury. During the early adult years, trauma to the pelvic floor as a result of childbirth can place the woman at increase risk for pelvic floor pain, pelvic pain, and urinary incontinence. Some of these dysfunctions may be subtle and become clinically relevant when the woman returns to exercise or sport. With middle age, hormonal changes may facilitate soft tissue atrophy and soften bones, placing the woman at increased risk for overuse injuries. Surgeries involving the pelvis such as hysterectomies and bladder suspensions place the woman at risk for pelvic floor pain dysfunctions. Degenerative changes begin and may limit joint motion with subsequent loss in muscle flexibility. Again, some of these changes may cause symptoms only when the woman increases or changes her activity level. Adapting training and exercise prescriptions to the individual is important. Taking into account where she is in the life cycle of aging and hormonal changes is vital.

REFERENCES

1. Sady SP, Freedson PS. Body composition and structural compositions of female and male athletes. *Clin Sports Med.* 1984;3:755–777.

2. Ciullo JV. Lower extremity injuries. In: *The Athletic Female; American Orthopaedic Society for Sports Medicine.* Champaign, IL: Human Kinetics; 1993:267–298.

3. Bernard TN, Cassidy JD. The sacroiliac joint syndrome: Pathophysiology, diagnosis, and management. In: Frymoyer JW, ed. *The Adult Spine: Principles and Practice.* New York: Raven Press; 1991:2107–2130.

4. Vleeming A, Stoeckart R, Volkers ACW, Snijders CJ. Relation between form and function on the sacroiliac joint, part I. *Spine.* 1990;15:133–135.

5. Vleeming A, Stoeckart R, Volkers ACW, Snijders CJ. Relation between form and function on the sacroiliac joint, part II. *Spine.* 1990;15:133–135.

6. Vleeming A, Pool-Goudzwaard AL, Stoeckart R, VanWingerden J, Snijders CJ. The posterior layer of the thoracolumbar fascia. *Spine.* 1995;20:753–758.

7. Kibler WB, Chandler TJ, Uhl T, Maddux RE. A musculoskeletal approach to the preparticipation physical examination. *Am J Sports Med.* 1989;17:525–531.

8. Greenman PE. Clinical aspects of sacroiliac function during walking. *J Man Med.* 1990;5:125–130.

9. Vleeming A, VanWindergan JP, Dijkstra PF. Mobility of the sacroiliac joint in the elderly: A kinematic and radiology study. *Clin Biomech.* 1991;6:161–168.

10. Lloyd-Smith R, Clement DB, McKenzie DC, et al. A survey of overuse and traumatic hip and pelvis injuries in the athlete. *Phys Sport Med.* 1985;13:131–141.

11. Sim F, Scott S. Injuries of the pelvis and hip in athletes: Anatomy and function. In: Nichols JA, ed. *The Lower Extremity and Spine in Sports Medicine.* St. Louis, MO: Mosby;1986:1119–1169.

12. Lane NE, Hochberg MC, Pressman A, Scott JC, Nevitt MC. Recreational physical activity and the risk of osteoarthritis of the hip in elderly women. *J Rheumatol.* 1999;26:849–854.

13. Vingard E, Alfredsson L, Malchau H. Osteoarthritis of the hip in women and its relationship to physical load from sports activities. *Am J Sports Med.* 1998;26:78–82.

14. Bookout MR, Greenman PE, eds. In: *Exercise prescription as an adjunct to manual medicine syllabus.* Continuing Medical Education Course, Michigan State University College of Osteopathic Medicine, September 30–October 2, 1994.

15. Jull GA, Janda V. Muscles and motor control in low back pain: Assessment and management. In: Twomey LT, Taylor JR, eds. *Physical Therapy of the Low Back: Clinics in Physical Therapy.* New York: Churchill Livingstone; 1987:253–278.

16. Geraci MC. Rehabilitation of the hip and pelvis. In: Kibler WB, Herring SA, Press JM, eds. *Functional Rehabilitation of Sports and Musculoskeletal Medicine.* Gaithersburg, MD: Aspen Publishers, 1998:216–243.

17. Kapandji IA. *The Physiology of the Joints: Volume 2: The Lower Extremity.* Edinburgh, UK: Churchill Livingstone; 1970.

18. Fagerson TL. Diseases and disorders of the hip. In: Fagerson TL, ed. *The Hip Handbook.* Woburn, MA: Butterworth-Heinemann; 1998:39–95.

19. Sahrmann SA. A program for identification and correction of muscular and mechanical imbalance: Principles and methods. *Clin Manage.* 1983;3:23–28.

20. Bernard TN, Kirkaldy-Willis WH. Recognizing specific characteristics of nonspecific low back pain. *Orthopedics.* 1987;217:266–280.

21. Travell J, Simons D. *Myofascial Pain and Dysfunction: The Trigger Point Manual. Vol 2. The Lower Extremities.* Baltimore: Williams & Wilkins; 1992.

22. Walker E, Katon W, Harrop-Griffiths J, Holm L, Russo R, Hickok LR. Relationship of chronic pelvic pain to psychiatric diagnoses and childhood sexual abuse. *Am J Psychiatry.* 1988;145:75–80.

23. Wallace K. Female pelvic floor functions, dysfunctions, and behavioral approaches to treatment. *Clin Sports Med.* 1994;13:459–481.

24. Nygaard IE, Thompson FL, Svengalis SL, Albright JP. Urinary incontinence in elite nulliparous athletes. *Obstet Gynecol.* 1994;84:183–187.

25. Delancey JO. Structural support of the urethra as it relates to stress urinary incontinence: The hammock hypothesis. *Am J Obstet Gynecol.* 1994;170(6):1713–1720.

26. Nygaard IE. Does prolonged high-impact activity contribute to later urinary incontinence? A retrospective cohort study of female Olympians. *Obstet Gynecol.* 1997;90(5):718–722.

27. Bo K, Maehlum S, Oseid S, Larsen S. Prevalence of stress urinary incontinence among physically active and sedentary female students. *Scand J Sports Sci.* 1989;11:113–116.

28. Al-Rawi ZS, Al-Rawi ZT. Joint hypermobility in women with genital prolapse. *Lancet.* 1982;I:1439–1441.

29. Snooks SJ, Badenoch DF, Tiptaft RC, et al. Perineal nerve damage in genuine stress urinary incontinence: An electrophysiological study. *Br J Urol.* 1985;57(4):422–426.

30. Skoner MM, Thompson WD, Caron VA. Factors associated with risk of stress urinary incontinence in women. *Nurs Res.* 1994;43(5):301–306.

31. Allen RE, Hosker GL, Smith AR, et al. Pelvic floor damage and childbirth: A neurophysiological study. *Br J Obstet Gynaecol.* 1990;97(9):770–779.

32. Foldspang A, Mommsen S, Lam GW, et al. Parity as a correlate of adult female urinary incontinence prevalence. *J Epidemiol Community Health.* 1992;46(6):595–600.

33. Sherman RA, Davis GD, Wong MF. Behavioral treatment of exercise-induced urinary incontinence among female soldiers. *Milit Med.* 1997;162(10):690–694.

34. Nygaard I. Prevention of exercise incontinence with mechanical devices. *J Reprod Med.* 1995;40(2):89–94.

35. Haken J, Benness C, Cardozo L, et al. A randomised trial of vaginal cones and pelvic floor exercises in the management of genuine stress incontinence, abstracted. *Neurourol Urodynam.* 1991;10(5):393–394.

36. Sand PK, Richardson DA, Staskin DR, et al. Pelvic floor electrical stimulation in the treatment of genuine stress incontinence: A multicenter, placebo-controlled trial. *Am J Obstet Gynecol.* 1995;173(1):72–79.

37. Meyer S, Dhenin T, Schmidt N, et al. Subjective and objective effects of intravaginal electrical myostimulation and biofeedback in patients with genuine stress incontinence. *Br J Urol.* 1992;69(6):584–588.

38. Kibler WB, Chandler TJ, Pace BK. Principles of rehabilitation after chronic injuries. *Clin Sports Med.* 1992;11:668–669.

39. Herring SA. Rehabilitation of muscle injuries. *Med Sci Sports Exerc.* 1990;22:455.

40. Maigne JY, Aivaliklis A, Pfefer F. Results of sacroiliac joint double block and value of sacroiliac pain provocation tests in 54 patients with low back pain. *Spine.* 1996;21:1889–1892.

CHAPTER 5

The Knee

Michelle Andrews

INTRODUCTION

Knee injuries are a frequent and often devastating injury to female athletes.[1] The mechanism of injury can be an acute traumatic event or repetitive trauma caused by overuse. The injury may cause lost playing time or may decrease the athlete's ability to play at the top of her game. Studies have focused on the incidence of knee injuries in the female athlete and have given more insight into the rate of knee injuries,[2–16] various mechanisms of injury to the knee,[17–26] and outcomes of various treatments of knee injuries.[27,28] This chapter is designed to help identify common knee problems of the female athlete, to present current data pertinent in making the correct diagnosis, to review the available treatment options of those injuries, and to improve the ultimate outcome.

PAIN AND INJURY

Knee injuries may be classified as acute injuries related to a specific traumatic event (ie, ligament or tendon disruptions, meniscus tears, fractures, or dislocations) or as overuse types of injury such as tendinitis or synovitis. The athlete's conscious pain response to the injury is related to the neurosensory signals that are generated locally in the knee and received through the neural pathways to the higher central nervous system.

The author gratefully acknowledges the assistance of Julie Sanker.

Receptors and Chemical Stimuli

The knee has been found to have several types of receptors, including mechanoreceptors that respond to tension, pressure, traction or stretching, and free nerve endings.[29–31] Chemical mediators that stimulate these various receptors include bradykinin, histamine, and prostaglandin F_2. The interaction between the stimulation of these receptors and the activation of the neurosensory pathway with the ultimate conscious perception play a role in both the athlete's response to the injury and the rehabilitation process after injury and treatment.[32] Understanding and incorporating this information will improve treatment and rehabilitation of knee injuries in the female athlete.

The work of Dye et al.[33] involving the human knee attempts to map out the conscious neurosensory perception of the intra-articular components. The study found that the anterior synovium, fat pad, and joint capsule were subjectively graded with accurate localization as severely painful. The cruciate ligaments insertion sites and the capsular margin of the meniscus were also severely painful but poorly localized, and the least sensitive sites were the patellar articular cartilage, inner rim of the meniscus, and the midportion of the anterior cruciate ligament (ACL) (see Figure 5–1).

Input from the knee mechanoreceptors also plays a role in the events after injury.[34] Knee fluid aspiration (see Figure 5–2) will help to decrease chemical and mechanical irritants that stimulate the nociceptors in the knee. Control of pain with modalities such as cryotherapy or the use of nonsteroidal anti-inflammatory medication to decrease prostaglandin production allows the athlete to maximize rehabilitation and return to sporting activities. Balance and proprioception

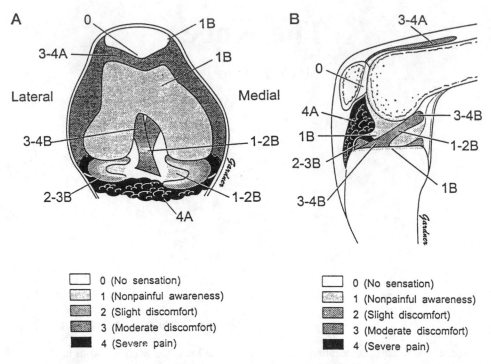

Figure 5–1 Neurosensory Mapping of the Internal Structures of the Knee. Coronal (A) and sagittal (B) schematic representations of the conscious neurosensory finding of the intra-articular structures of the knee. The right knee is illustrated. A, accurate spatial localization; B, poorly localized sensation.

skills are addressed in the later phases of the rehabilitation process. Proprioception is the cumulative neurological input to the central nervous system from all mechanoreceptors. In sports, proprioception gives the athlete joint position feedback and contributes to dynamic stability and protection.

GENDER DIFFERENCES IN ANATOMY

Anatomical gender differences as related to the female athlete include shorter legs; lower centers of gravity; smaller frames; wider pelvises; more flexibility; less well-developed musculature; greater percentage of fat per body weight; narrower femoral notch at the knee, increased genu valgum (knock-kneed), and increased tibial torsion. These gender differences represent average values. Significant variation of these values exists within each sex—that is to say, as much individual variation is seen within each sex as between the sexes.[35-38]

ANTERIOR KNEE PAIN

Anterior knee pain is a common problem in female athletes.[39,40] The cause of the pain is often related to the exten-

sor mechanism and the surrounding soft tissues. The patellofemoral joint may be involved, including chondromalacia of the patella or femoral trochlea. Other causes may be a painful and inflamed medial plica, bipartite patella, quadriceps tendinitis, prepatellar bursitis, patellar tendinitis, or malalignment problems, including subluxation of the patella or traumatic dislocations. Microfailure of the articular cartilage can stimulate cytokine production. With any of these problems synovitis and fat pad inflammation can occur. The differential diagnosis for anterior knee pain is listed in the Clinical Guidelines.

To help sort out the cause of the female athlete's knee pain, a detailed history and physical examination are crucial. In addition, appropriate diagnostic testing, including certain x-ray views, magnetic resonance imaging (MRI), computed tomography (CT), bone scans, and laboratory analysis of blood and aspirated knee joint fluid, allows the clinician to arrive at the correct diagnosis on the basis of anatomical structures.

Anterior Knee Pain Differential Diagnosis

- Patellofemoral chondromalacia

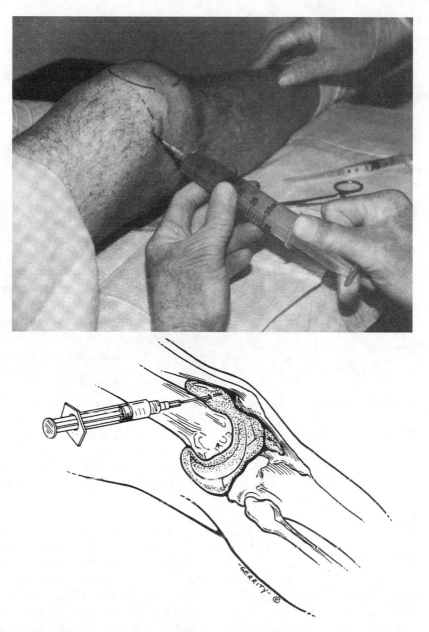

Figure 5–2 Knee Aspiration. A lateral approach into the distended suprapatella bursa is used for aspiration of the knee joint. Note the markings on the knee to indicate the point of needle entry. A skin pencil or wax crayon is often used, although pressing the needle hub against the skin produces a satisfactory temporary mark.

- Quadriceps tendinitis
- Prepatellar bursitis
- Synovitis
- Fat pad inflammation
- Plica inflammation
- Patellar tendinitis
- Loose bodies
- Meniscus tears
- Ligament injuries
- Patellar subluxation

- Patellar dislocation
- Patellar fractures
- Bipartite patella
- Osgood-Schlatter disease
- Larsen-Johansson disease
- Inflammatory arthritis
- Infection

Clinical Guideline

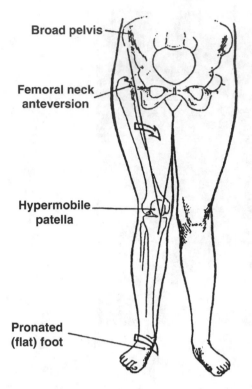

Broad pelvis

Femoral neck anteversion

Hypermobile patella

Pronated (flat) foot

Figure 5–3 Female Lower Extremity Alignment. Miserable alignment syndrome: femoral neck anteversion, hip varus, knee valgus, and external placement of tibial tubercle with pronation of the heel.

History and Physical Examination

Common complaints that female athletes with knee pain give include the sensation of creaking and grinding. This sensation may be due to roughness of the articular cartilage surfaces of the patellofemoral joint. Anterior knee pain going up and down stairs or inclines may be due to the shear forces at the patellofemoral joint. The "movie sign" or the inability to sit for prolonged periods of time is commonly mentioned by the female athlete with patellofemoral problems. If the symptoms of knee pain persist, quadriceps weakness may develop, and the sensation of knee instability may result.

Anterior Knee Pain: Common Complaints

- Creaking, grinding, popping
  Caused by chondromalacia or symptomatic plica
- Tightness
  Caused by swelling, inflammation, or an effusion

- Giving out
  Caused by quadriceps weakness
- Movie theater sign
  Inability to sit for a prolonged time

Clinical Guideline

Evaluation of the patellofemoral joint on physical examination requires a systematic anatomical approach. The physical examination may reveal an effusion or boggy synovitis. Palpation of the knee allows the examiner to anatomically delineate the structures that are painful, such as the inferior pole of the patella, the patellar tendon, the insertion of the patellar tendon on the tibial tubercle, the fat pads, the medial or lateral retinaculum, and the quadriceps tendon. Crepitus is noted through the arc of motion. The range of knee motion and patellar tracking through the range of motion must also be evaluated. Muscle weakness with particular attention to the vastus medialis obliquus (VMO) should be evaluated, as well as any tightness involving the quadriceps muscles, the hamstrings, and the iliotibial band.

Lower Limb Alignment

The lower extremity alignment of the female athlete may contribute to the occurrence of patellofemoral problems (see Figure 5–3). Female anatomy of the lower limb may result in an increased valgus force at the knee because of a broader pelvis, femoral neck anteversion, hip varus, knee valgus, external tibial torsion, and heel pronation.

Joint Laxity

Ligamentous laxity can play a part in women with anterior knee pain. Ligament laxity or loose jointedness is evaluated on physical examination at various joints and may be documented by hyperextension at the knees, elbows, and metacarpophalangeal (MCP) joints. The "thumb to wrist" sign supports the diagnosis of ligament laxity in the female athlete as does an increased sulcus sign at the shoulder and pes planus (flat foot) at the foot.

The Q Angle

Bony anatomy, including the size and shape of the patella and the femoral trochlea, the soft tissue structures (such as the muscles, tendons, and retinaculum), and knee joint position contribute to the patella's position. The resultant forces at the knee along with relative muscle weakness in the vastus medialis muscle can increase lateral pressures at the patella resulting in anterior knee pain and articular surface wear (see Figure 5–4). The Q Angle is routinely used to evaluate anatomical alignment of the lower extremity in regard to the patella. The Q Angle is measured from the anterior superior iliac spine to the center of the patella to the tibial tubercle (see Figure 5–5). In women, a Q Angle greater than 15° is considered abnormal. A high Q Angle produces a valgus force on the patella and can predispose the athlete to lateral patella subluxation or dislocation.[41]

Patellar Mobility

Further evaluation of the patella should include the mobility of the patella in superior and inferior directions and medial and lateral directions. Passive patellar tilt or the turn-up test (see Figure 5–6) evaluates tightness of the lateral structures of the patella.[42] Tightness of the lateral retinaculum may cause patellar tilting or contribute to excessive lateral compressive forces. Manual pressure on the patella by the examiner, the "patellar compression test," may elicit pain. Apprehension may be tested by gently pushing the female athlete's patella laterally. A positive test gives the examiner information about possible patellar instability.

RADIOLOGICAL EXAMINATION OF THE PATELLOFEMORAL JOINT

Standard radiographs to evaluate the patellofemoral joint consist of anteroposterior (AP), lateral, and axial views.[43] The AP view provides information as to the size, shape, and position of the patella in relationship to the femur. Patella

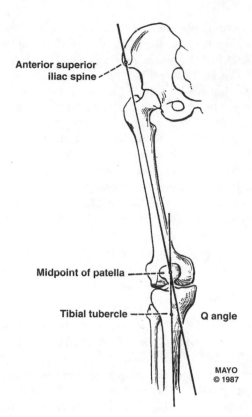

Figure 5–5 The Q-Angle (or Quadriceps Angle), Formed by Extension of Lines Drawn from the Center of the Patella Proximally to the Anterosuperior Iliac Spine and Distally to the Tibial Tubercle, Denotes Alignment of the Knee. Excessive Q angle predisposes the athlete to lateral patellar subluxation or dislocation.

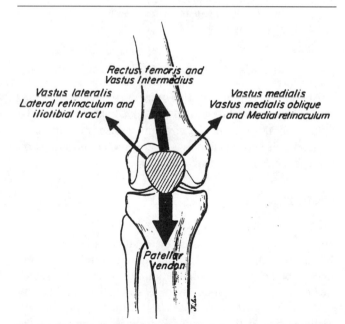

Figure 5–4 Patella Forces and Constraints on the Patella during Function. *Source*: F.H. Fu and M.J. Seel et al., Patellofemoral Biomechanics in *The Patellofemoral Joint*, J.M. Fox and W. Del Pizzo, eds., pp. 49–62. Reproduced with permission of The McGraw-Hill Companies.

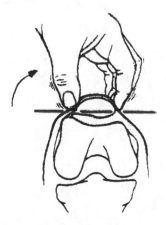

Figure 5–6 The Turn-Up Test. The examiner places a thumb on the lateral patella edge and fingers on the medial aspect of the patella to stabilize the patella. Then the lateral patella is lifted or tilted up. This tests the lateral retinaculum. *Source*: R.D. Ferkel, Lateral Retinacular Release, J.M. Fox and W. Del Pizzo, eds., *The Patellofemoral Joint*, (c) 1993, pp. 309–323. Reproduced with permission of The McGraw–Hill Companies.

fractures and bipartite patella may be noted on this view. The axial view with the knee flexed 30° to 45° can document tilt or subluxation of the patella in relationship to the femoral trochlea. The lateral view can be used to determine the relative patellar height (see Figure 5–7) and is useful to document patella alta or patella infera. Enlargement, fragmentation, sclerosis, and separation of the tibial tubercle on the lateral view may be found in mature athletes who had Osgood-Schlatter's disease in adolescence.

CT and MRI have also been used to evaluate the patellofemoral joint at various flexion angles and may provide further information to help the clinician in functional diagnosis and treatment of the female athlete with knee pain.

VARIOUS DISORDERS OF THE PATELLOFEMORAL JOINT

Jumper's Knee

"Jumper's knee"[41] is an overuse injury involving the extensor mechanism of the knee. The location of inflammation can be at the quadriceps tendon insertion at the superior patellar region, the patellar tendon insertion at the inferior pole of the patella, or at the patellar tendon insertion at the tibial tubercle (see Figure 5–8). This type of injury is commonly found in jumping sports such as volleyball and basketball. Symptoms have been classified and are presented in the Clinical Guidelines.[45]

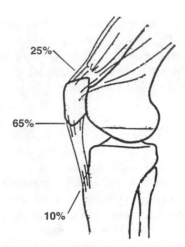

Figure 5–8 Location of Pain in Jumper's Knee.

Classification of Jumper's Knee According to Symptoms (after Blazina et al. 1973, as modified by Roels et al. 1978)

Stage	Symptom
1	Pain after practice or after a game.
2	Pain at the beginning of activity, which disappears after warm-up and reappears after completion of activity.
3	Pain remains during and after activity, and the patient is unable to participate in sports.
4	Complete rupture of the patellar tendon.

Clinical Guideline

The gross and microscopic pathological anatomy of tendinitis has been well described by Puddu et al.[46] and may be a pure tendinitis that involves inflammation of the peritenon, peritendinitis with tendinosis (inflammation or degeneration of the tendon), or pure tendinosis.

Medial Plica Syndrome

Medial patellar plica syndrome is another cause of anterior knee pain. Normally, the synovial plica originates on the superomedial wall of the knee joint and transverses the anterior compartment medially and inserts into the anteromedial fat pad. The plical tissue is soft, pliant, and highly elastic, enabling it to pass back and forth over the femoral condyles in knee flexion and extension.[47,48] With injury, the plica can become thickened and fibrous. The pathological plical band along the medial aspect of the knee can cause pain and is often palpated on knee examination (see Figure 5–9). With knee flexion and extension, the thickened plica can cause clicking and pain. The thickened plica may rub

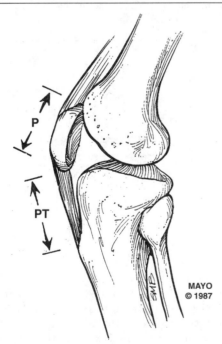

Figure 5–7 The Insall Ratio for Determining Relative Patellar Height. In normal knees, the height of the patella (P) should equal the height of the patellar tendon (PT).

across the medial femoral condyle and produce chondromalacia in the area of contact. Fat pad inflammation may be related (see Figure 5–10).

Chondromalacia Patella

Chondromalacia, or softening, fissuring, and fibrillation of the articular cartilage, may be the result of patellar malalignment and excessive shear forces or direct patellofemoral trauma. Chondral breakdown products are irritating and may cause an effusion and pain. Treatment algorithms for anterior knee pain address this issue with cryotherapy (see Figure 5–11), nonsteroidal anti-inflammatory medication, and physical therapy. Most successful protocols consist of quadriceps strengthening (see Figure 5–12). Straight-leg raises safely improve quadriceps function, and closed chain exercises can be used to avoid shear forces through a particular range of motion (ROM). Electrical muscle stimulation of the quadriceps in various positions (30°, 60°, and 90°) may also be beneficial. Exercises utilizing Thera-Band are helpful and convenient.

Anterior Knee Pain—Nonsurgical Treatment

- Medication
  NSAIDs
  Corticosteroids
- Activity modification
  Rest
  Avoid painful activity
- Physical therapy
  Strengthening
  Stretching and flexibility
  Patellar mobilization
- Modalities
  Heat
  Ice
  Electrical stimulation
  Iontophoresis
  Phonophoresis
- Intra-articular injections
  Corticosteroids
  Hyaluronate
- Repositioning methods
  Knee braces and neoprene sleeves
  Shoe orthotics
  McConnell taping

Clinical Guideline

A key component to any rehabilitation program is stretching tight structures around the knee. Patellar mobilization is also addressed by exercises to stretch the lateral retinaculum. Stretching the hamstrings (see Figure 5–13), iliotibial band

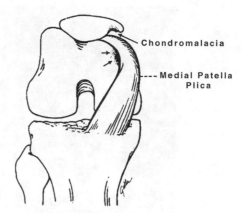

Figure 5–9 Medial Plica with Chondromalacia. *Source*: D. Patel and C.T. Laurencin et al., Synovial Folds–plicae, in *The Patellofemoral Joint*, J.M. Fox and W. Del Pizzo, eds., pp. 193–198. Reproduced with permission of The McGraw–Hill Companies.

(ITB) (see Figure 5–14), quadriceps, and gastrocnemius-soleus improves flexibility and function.

Taping and bracing (see Figure 5–15) have been used in the conservative treatment of anterior knee pain. Taping is based on the premise that the tape can provide enough traction on the patella to change the patellar position and thereby lead to significant changes in joint pressure.[49] Taping and bracing may improve acute symptoms, decreasing the irritation of the synovium by unloading those regions.[50] Shoe wear modification and inserts or orthotics to control foot pronation have also been used in the successful treatment of anterior knee pain.[51]

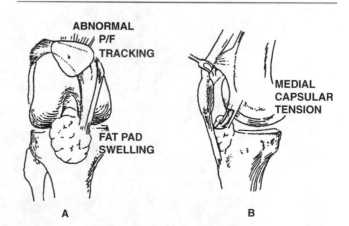

Figure 5–10 Triad Injury Combining Patellofemoral Friction (PF) and Subsequent Cartilage Debris with Fat Pad Hypertrophy (and Related Patellar Tendinitis) along with Medial Capsular Traction, or Plica Syndrome (Largely Caused by VMO Atrophy).

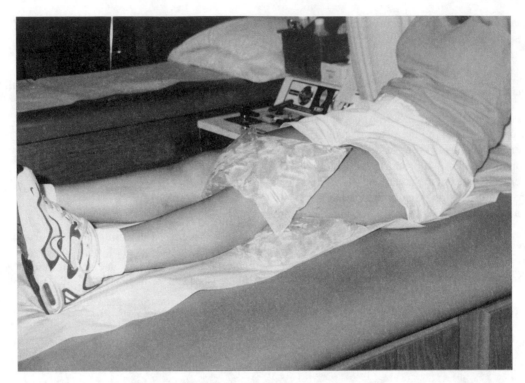

Figure 5–11 Cryotherapy. The use of ice to control swelling and pain after an acute knee injury.

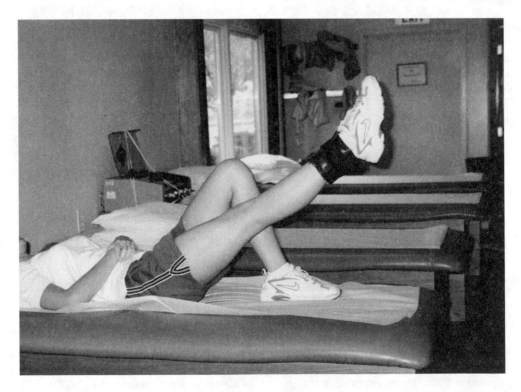

Figure 5–12 Straight-Leg Raises To Improve Isometric Quadriceps Strength.

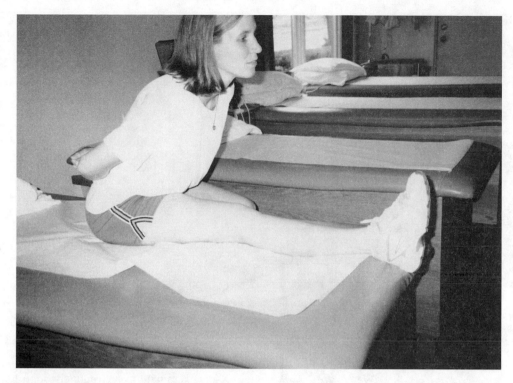

Figure 5–13 Hamstring Stretches.

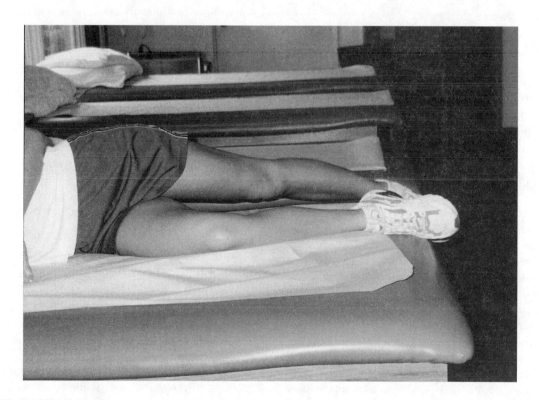

Figure 5–14 Iliotibial Band Stretches.

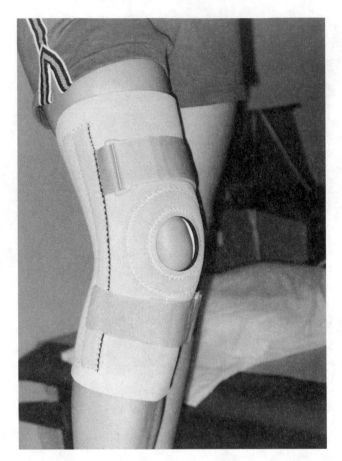

Figure 5–15 Patella Brace.

The outcome of patellofemoral pain syndrome has been shown to be related to the extension strength of the affected knee. Natri et al.[52] showed that restoration of good quadriceps strength and function in the affected extremity is important to good recovery for the patient.

Patellar Instability

Patellar instability may result in subluxation or dislocation of the patella. The female athlete may experience an acute lateral patellar dislocation during sports. The patellar dislocation can occur by a direct blow or may be due to quadriceps contracture with an externally rotated tibia. Associated dysplasia of the patella or the femoral trochlea may predispose the athlete to this type of injury.[53] The athlete commonly reports that her knee "went out of place." A large hemarthrosis and decreased range of motion of the knee can be present with tenderness along the medial retinaculum, and possibly a defect that may be palpated. Lateral retinacular tenderness is also common. If the patella spontaneously reduces, the diagnosis is somewhat more difficult to make correctly.

Consideration in Evaluating Acute Lateral Patellar Dislocations

1. Mechanism
   A. Direct blow
   B. Quads contracture
2. Predisposition
   A. Associated dysplasia
   B. No dysplasia
3. Osteochondral fracture
   A. Yes
   B. No
4. Severity
   A. Attenuation of medial capsule
   B. Rupture of medial capsule
   C. Avulsion fracture of medial capsule

Clinical Guideline

Source: J.L. Halbrecht and D.W. Jackson, Acute Dislocation of the Patella, J.M. Fox and W. Del Pizzo, eds. *The Patellofemoral Joint*, (c) 1993, pp. 123–134. Reproduced with permission of The McGraw–Hill Companies.

X-ray examinations are routinely done and may reveal an osteochondral fragment. Treatment of acute patellar dislocations depends on the presence of an osteochondral fracture and loose fragment (see Figure 5–16).[53] If no fragment exists, initial conservative treatment includes immobilization followed by an active exercise program.

Rehabilitation Goals

- Decrease inflammation
- Restore range of motion
- Regain muscular strength
- Regain muscular endurance
- Regain muscular power
- Regain muscular flexibility
- Maintain or improve cardiovascular fitness
- Develop proprioceptive awareness
- Develop proprioceptive agility
- Perfect functional skills, including sports-specific skills

Clinical Guideline

Source: L.Y. Griffin, Rehabilitation of the Knee Extensor Mechanism, J.M. Fox and W. Del Pizzo, eds., *The Patellofemoral Joint*, (c) 1993, pp. 279–290. Reproduced with permission of The McGraw-Hill Companies.

Initially, the rehabilitation goal is to decrease inflammation in the knee, decrease pain, restore range of motion (ROM), regain muscular strength and endurance, and improve flexibility. During rehabilitation, maintaining the athlete's cardiovascular fitness is important to her well-being and ultimate return to play. In the final stages, the development of proprioceptive awareness and agility skills with

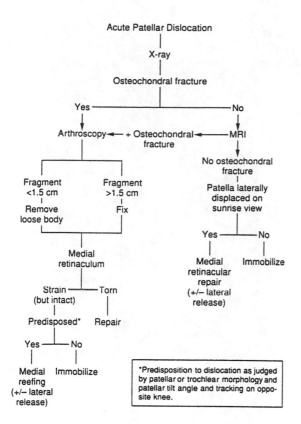

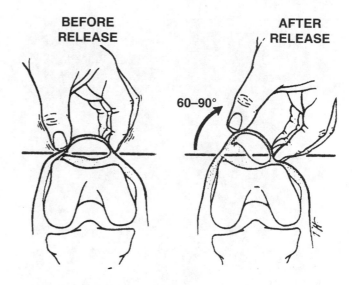

Figure 5–17 The Turn-Up Test. After surgical release, passive patellar after surgical tilt is done to achieve a goal of 60° to 90° tilt. *Source*: R.D. Ferkel, Lateral Retinacular Release, J.M. Fox and W. Del Pizzo, eds., *The Patellofemoral Joint*, (c) 1993, pp. 309–323. Reproduced with permission from The McGraw-Hill Companies.

Figure 5–16 Decision Tree for Acute Patellar Dislocation. *Source*: J.L. Halbrecht and D.W. Jackson, Acute Dislocation of the Patella, J.M. Fox and W. Del Pizzo, eds. *The Patellofemoral Joint*, (c) 1993, pp. 123–134. Reproduced with permission of The McGraw-Hill Companies.

the use of sports-specific skills and functional activities allow the athlete to return to her sport and prevent reinjury. Many rehabilitation protocols of patellofemoral problems are available.[54-56] Refer to the Patellofemoral Rehabilitation and Strengthening Program in Chapter 9, The Young Female Athlete.

Initially, conservative treatment regimens for anterior knee problems in the female athlete are recommended. Surgical treatment options are used if the athlete continues to have symptoms despite compliance of an aggressive rehabilitation program. Surgical treatment options include arthroscopic surgery to debride inflamed fat pads and synovium, excise pathological plica, and smooth articular cartilage roughness (chondroplasty). Multiple surgical options exist with the goal to improve patellar alignment, including lateral release of tight lateral retinacular structures (see Figure 5–17), medial reefing, and/or distal realignment procedures such as a medial tibial tubercle transfer. Tibial tubercle elevation and patellectomy are considered salvage operations for patellofemoral arthrosis and are rarely used in athletes. Each operation has been successful in treating anterior knee pain, but neither is without failures and complications.

Anterior Knee Pain—Surgical Treatment

- Arthroscopic debridement
  Synovectomy
  Chondroplasty
  Excision of inflamed plica
- Proximal realignment
  Lateral retinacular release
  Medial plication
- Distal realignment
  Media tibial tubercle transfer
- Tibial tubercle elevation
- Patellectomy
- Total knee replacement

Clinical Guideline

Iliotibial Band Tendinitis

Iliotibial band tendinitis (ITB) is an overuse injury affecting the lateral aspect of the knee. The ITB rubs over the lateral femoral condyle during knee flexion and extension (see Figure 5–18).[57] The ITB then becomes inflamed, causing pain and occasional swelling in this area. The athlete is often a runner, and she usually complains of gradual worsening of the lateral knee pain initially during running and eventually with walking.

The physical examination reveals pain with palpation along the lateral aspect of the knee. The tenderness may be elicited anywhere along the course of the ITB from the

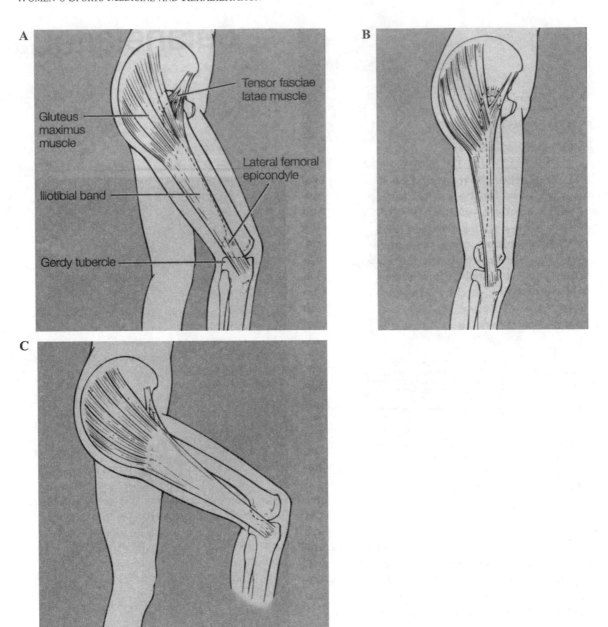

Figure 5–18 ITB Tendinitis. With the knee in approximately 30° of flexion (A), the iliotibial band lies over the lateral femoral epicondyle. With the knee between 30° and full extension (B), the iliotibial band is anterior to the lateral femoral epicondyle and assists in extension. With knee motion greater than 30° (C), the iliotibial band is posterior to the lateral femoral epicondyle and assists in flexion. *Source*: J.G. Aronen et al.: Practical, Conservative Management of Iliotibial Band Syndrome, *The Physician and Sportsmedicine*, Vol. 21, No. 6, Fig. 1 only, p. 60, (c) 1993. Reproduced with permission of The McGraw-Hill Companies.

lateral femoral epicondylar region superior to the lateral joint line to the insertion of the ITB at Gerdy's tubercle. Tightness of the tensor fasciae latae contributes to a positive Ober test. The Ober test places the athlete on her side with the affected extremity toward the ceiling. The examiner lifts the affected leg with a flexed knee and slowly brings it posterior and toward the examination table. Tightness of the ITB is shown when the knee does not touch the table or remains higher than the unaffected side (see Chapter 9).

Treatment includes cryotherapy, nonsteroidal anti-inflammatory medication, and ITB stretching exercises. Occasionally, iontophoresis or phonophoresis may be used, as well as a local corticosteroid injection. Training programs should be evaluated with particular attention to alternating running direction on a ramped track or sloped pavement. Avoiding hills and shortening the runner's stride may decrease her symptoms. Shoes may reveal an uneven wear pattern such as excessive pronation. Foot orthotics may be beneficial in this situation. Correction of a limb length discrepancy is also helpful.

LIGAMENT INJURIES

Anterior Cruciate Ligament Injuries

Knee ligament injuries in the female athlete have recently received considerable attention from the general public and the scientific community.[2,5,14,58] The increased rate of anterior cruciate ligament (ACL) injuries—particularly noncontact—in female athletes compared with male athletes in sports requiring jumping, turning, and twisting (ie, soccer, basketball, gymnastics) is well documented (see Figure 5–19).[3,6–11,13,15,18,19] The attention is well deserved in that these injuries tend to be functionally limiting and often require surgical treatment.

Female/Male Ratio of ACL Injuries

Studies: 1995 NCAA[7]   4:1
1993 Basketball[19]   8:1
1994 Soccer[11]   6:1
1990 U.S. Olympic Trials[58] 4:1
1999 H.S. Basketball[15]   4:1

Clinical Guideline

Factors Involved in ACL Injuries

Why female athletes have an increased rate of ACL injuries is an often asked question. The exact cause of this phenomenon is unclear, although many hypotheses abound.[4,20,59] Contributing factors that have been suggested for increased rates of ACL injuries in female athletes include anatomical differences such as lower extremity alignment,[60] femoral notch size and shape,[25,61] ACL strength, lower extremity muscle strength and imbalance,[16,24,62] ligamentous laxity[16,23,63,64] with resultant knee hyperextension,[65] tibial rotation and hormonal influences.[21,26] Extrinsic factors include training and conditioning issues with differences in inherited and acquired skills, proprioception and neuromuscular activation patterns,[64] order of hamstring muscle firing,[23] and the player's experience and the style of play.[19] Equipment factors such as shoe-floor interface have also been suggested as a factor in the increased rate of ACL injuries in female athletes.

Hypothesis ACL Injuries

- Anatomic differences
  Lower extremity alignment
  Notch size and shape
  ACL strength
  Muscle strength
  Ligamentous laxity
  Knee hyperextension and rotation
  Hormonal influences
- Coaching and conditioning
  Inherited and acquired skills
  Conditioning
  Motivation
  Coordination
  Proprioception (position sense and balance)
  Neuromuscular activation patterns
  Order of firing
  Experience
  Style of play
- Equipment
  Shoe-floor interface

Clinical Guideline

The ACL is the primary knee restraint to anterior tibial translation. In addition to serving a mechanical role, the ACL also has a sensory role in knee position sense (proprioception) detected by mechanoreceptors[30,31] located in the ligament. Without a functioning ACL, the female athlete will often experience a "trick knee," which gives out with jumping, turning, and twisting motions. These episodes of instability can cause further knee injuries, including other ligament injuries, meniscus tears, and injury to the articular cartilage of the knee.

History and Physical Examination

The injured athlete usually is initially seen in the office complaining that the knee gave out or shifted. She will often describe a twisting or hyperextension, noncontact, deceleration type of injury. There may have been a pop or ripping sensation. The female athlete experiences immediate severe knee pain with the inability to continue to play. Often, a large bloody effusion occurs over 24 hours with decreased ROM resulting from the pain and swelling.

History ACL

- Noncontact injury
  Planted foot
  Turning
  Twisting
  Deceleration
  Hyperextension
  Landing
- Sounds
  Pop
  Tearing
  Ripping

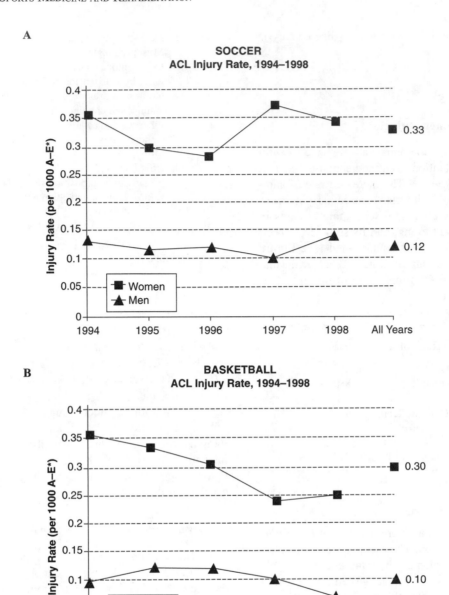

Figure 5–19 NCAA ACL Injury Rate in Soccer Players (A), and in Basketball Players (B) 1994–1998. *A–E = athletic exposures.

- Swelling
  Large intra-articular effusion
  Within 24 hours
- Instability
  Giving way
- Pain
- Inability to continue play

Clinical Guideline

A thorough knee examination provides critical information to arrive at an accurate diagnosis. The Lachman test is an extremely sensitive test to evaluate the ACL (see Figure 5–20). In the supine position the affected knee is placed at 30° of flexion. With the athlete relaxed, the examiner stabilizes the femur with one hand and applies an anterior force to the proximal tibia with the other hand. During the Lachman test, increased anterior tibial translation and quality of the end point are compared with the noninjured knee.

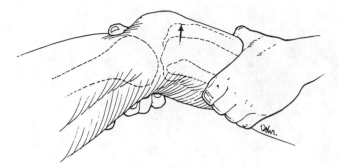

Figure 5–20 ACL Examination. The Lachman test for ACL injury.

Other special tests have been described to evaluate the ACL, including the anterior drawer, pivot shift, and reverse pivot shift.

KT-1000

The KT-1000 instrumented knee arthrometer (MEDmetric, San Diego, CA) allows for objective information on the amount of AP tibial translation. Studies[66-70] have shown reliable and reproducible results in detecting increased anterior tibial translation in an ACL-deficient knee by use of established examination techniques. The quality of the end point is also helpful in evaluating the female athlete's ACL-deficient knee (see Figure 5–21).

Differential Diagnosis

The differential diagnosis of ACL injuries includes meniscus tears, patellar subluxation or dislocation, osteochondral loose bodies, femoral osteochondritis dissecans, and patellar and tibial plateau fractures. Other ligament injuries may also occur.

ACL Injury Differential Diagnosis

- Meniscus tears
- Patellar subluxation
- Patellar dislocation
- Patellar fractures
- Femoral OCD lesions
- Osteochondral loose bodies
- Tibial plateau fractures
Other ligament injuries

Clinical Guideline

Radiological Examination

Routine x-ray examinations including AP, lateral, and axial views, allow for additional information when evaluat-

ing the female athlete's injured knee. Segond fractures[71] (a small fleck of bone at the lateral joint line, superior and anterior to the fibular head) and osteochondritis dissecans may be found. Further information may be obtained with MRI, a highly sensitive test in evaluating the integrity of the ACL (see Figure 5–22). Other concomitant injuries may be demonstrated.

Treatment of ACL Injuries

The treatment of the female athlete with an ACL injury must be individualized. Factors to consider include the age of the athlete, the type and level of activity, the degree of instability, the presence or absence of other lesions involving the knee, and the ability of the athlete to comply with the rehabilitation program.[72,73] The goal of any treatment program in an ACL-deficient knee is to prevent recurrent injuries and further damage to the knee (ie, meniscus tears, articular cartilage damage). Initially, physical therapy to regain knee range of motion and improve strength combined with modalities to control swelling and prevent muscle atrophy is used. Nonsurgical treatment of ACL injuries involves activity modification plus rehabilitation and functional bracing. Maximizing hamstring (an ACL agonist) strength and proprioceptive skills are identified as goals that optimize the outcome of ACL rehabilitation in female athletes.

Treatment ACL Injuries

- Nonsurgical
   Acute—to control pain, swelling, prevent muscle
    atrophy
   Medication—NSAIDs
   Physical therapy—PREs, ROM
   Modalities—ice, electrical stimulation
   Physical therapy—proprioception, strength,
    conditioning
   Brace—functional ACL brace
- Surgical
   Technique
    Open vs arthroscopic
    Intra-articular vs extra-articular
    One vs two incisions
    Graft selection—autograft vs allograft
     Bone—patellar tendon—bone
     Hamstrings
     Quadriceps
     Achilles tendon
   Notchplasty
   Isometry
   Fixation—interference screw, posts, bioabsorbable,
    etc.

Clinical Guideline

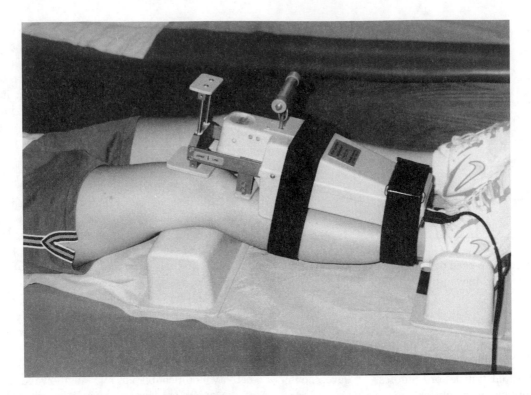

Figure 5–21 KT-1000 Evaluates Amount of Anterior Tibial Translation.

Surgical treatment[74] of ACL injuries (see Figures 5–23 and 5–24) has benefited from improved surgical techniques and equipment, along with fine-tuned postoperative reha- bilitation resulting in excellent outcomes.[27] Several techni- cal factors, including use of arthroscopic instrumentation, notchplasty, isometric tunnel placement, graft selection (see

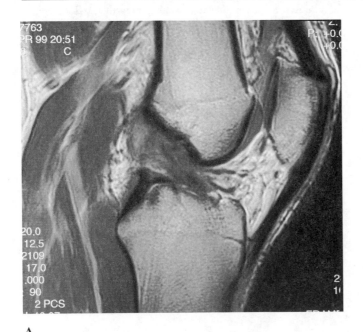

A

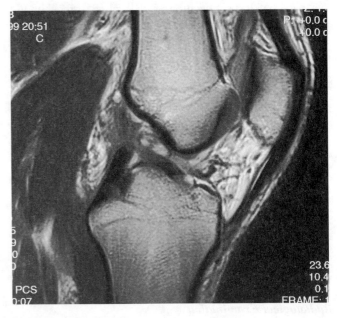

B

Figure 5–22 MRI Evaluation of ACL. A, T1 and B, T2-weighted MRIs of an acute ACL injury.

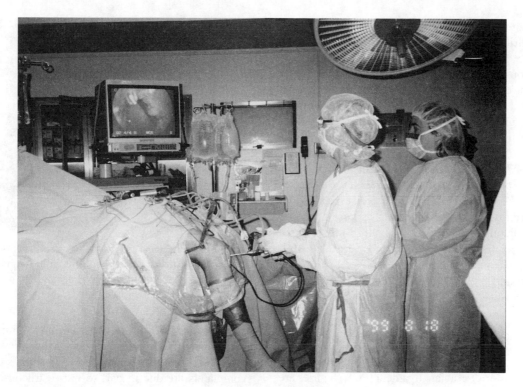

Figure 5–23 ACL Reconstruction. Intraoperative picture of arthroscopic ACL reconstruction.

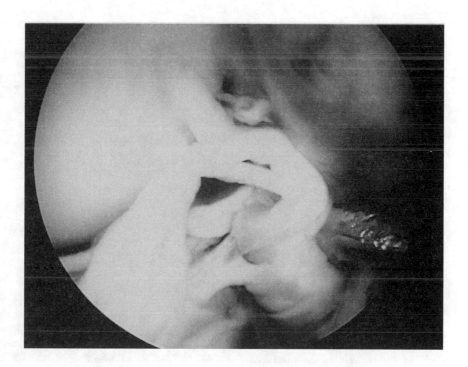

Figure 5–24 Acute ACL Tear. Intraoperative arthroscopic picture of an acute ACL tear.

Figure 5–25) and preparation, graft tension, and graft fixation, have contributed to successful outcomes in ACL surgery (see Figure 5–26).

Rehabilitation after ACL reconstruction plays an essential role in returning the female athlete back to her sport. Several postsurgical ACL reconstruction rehabilitation protocols are available.[75] In general, goals of rehabilitation after ACL reconstruction include controlling pain and swelling and achieving full knee extension immediately postoperatively (see Figure 5–27). Attention to the extensor mechanism is important and is addressed by quadriceps isometric exercises (see Figure 5–28), active assisted ROM exercises (see Figure 5–29), and electrical muscle stimulation as necessary (see Figure 5–30). Patellar mobilization is addressed early in the rehabilitation process. Focus is also on restoring full knee flexion and muscle strength. Exercises to improve proprioception and balance (see Figures 5–31 and 5–32) are essential and used in conjunction with sports-specific exercises.

Posterior Cruciate Ligament Injury

Fortunately, posterior cruciate ligament (PCL) injuries are not common athletic injuries. When this injury does occur, it is often the result of a fall directly on the knee or sliding into a base. PCL injuries may also occur in knee hyperflexion or hyperextension. The PCL is the main restraint of posterior tibial translation. The female athlete may not experience gross instability and may not have considerable pain or an

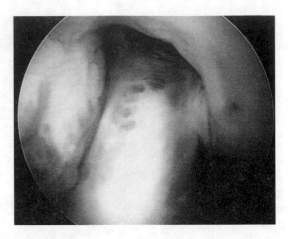

Figure 5–26 Reconstructed ACL. Intraoperative arthroscopic picture of bone-patellar tendon-bone autograft 3 months after reconstruction shows good vascularity of the graft.

effusion. Instability is not a common complaint even in the chronic PCL-deficient knee. More likely, the female athlete will have patellofemoral and medial side pain. These complaints are due in part to these structures (patella and medial meniscus) being secondary restraints to posterior tibial translation.

History and Physical Examination

A thorough physical examination can reveal an injury to the PCL. Most commonly, the posterior drawer test reveals

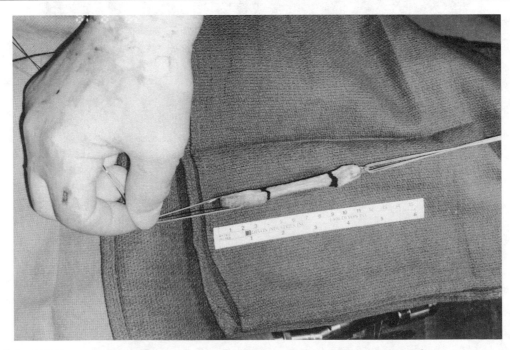

Figure 5–25 Graft for ACL Reconstruction. Intraoperative picture of bone-patellar tendon-bone autograft.

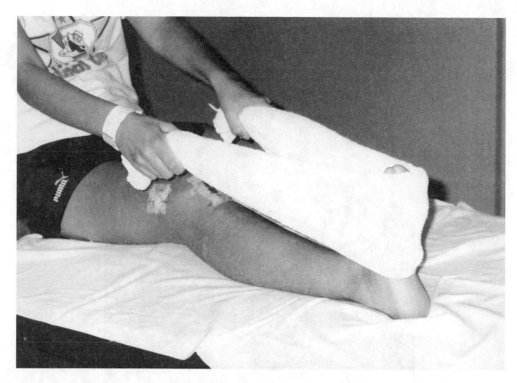

Figure 5–27 Gastroc-soleus Stretching after ACL Reconstruction.

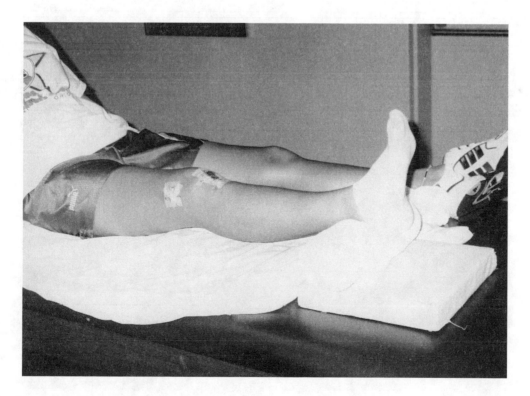

Figure 5–28 Quadriceps Isometrics after ACL Reconstruction.

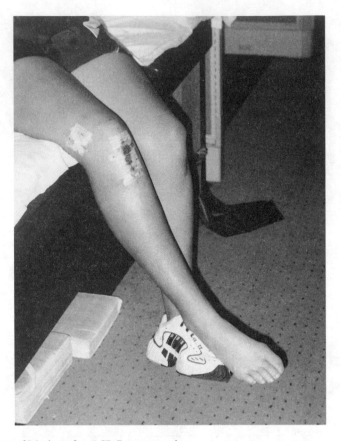

Figure 5–29 Active Assisted Range of Motion after ACL Reconstruction.

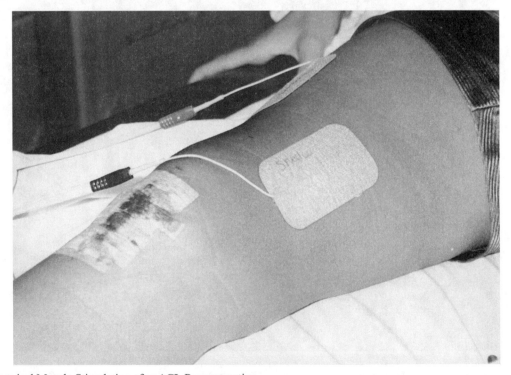

Figure 5–30 Electrical Muscle Stimulation after ACL Reconstruction.

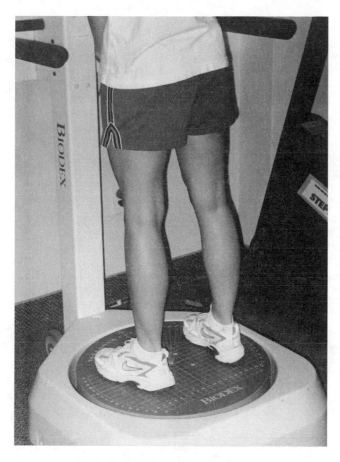

Figure 5–31 Balance after ACL Reconstruction to Improve Proprioception.

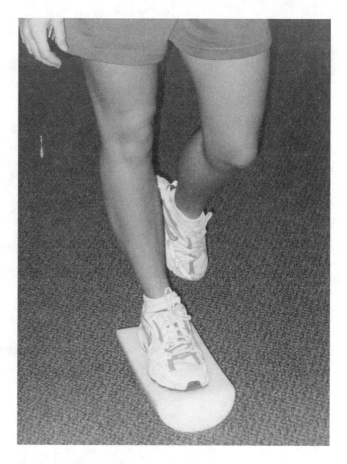

Figure 5–32 Single-Leg Balance for Proprioception after ACL Reconstruction.

an increase in posterior tibial translation when tested in 90° of flexion. Another test commonly performed is the 90° quadriceps active test (see Figure 5–33).[76] In this position, gravity displaces the tibia into a posterior position in a PCL-deficient knee. With quadriceps contraction, the tibia is displaced anterior to a reduced position and is noted as a positive test.

Treatment of PCL Injuries

Treatment of PCL injuries is controversial and is often based on the amount of posterior tibial translation. Isolated PCL injuries are often treated conservatively;[77] whereas combined ligament injuries involving the PCL are more aggressively treated with surgical reconstruction (see Figure 5–34).[78]

Medial Collateral Ligament Injury

The medial collateral ligament (MCL) is one of the most commonly injured knee ligaments in athletic injuries. Ana-

tomically, the MCL has two components, a superficial portion and deep portion. The MCL is the primary restraint against a valgus force at the knee (see Figure 5–35).

Injury to the medial collateral ligament occurs when a valgus stress is placed on the knee. These injuries can be confused with medial meniscus injuries, and the diagnosis is made on physical examination with MRI confirmation. The female athlete with an MCL injury will have tenderness to palpation on the medial aspect of the knee. The point of maximal tenderness may be at the femoral origin of the MCL or also at any point along the MCL to the insertion on the proximal medial tibia. The MCL is tested by applying a valgus stress to the knee at 0° and at 30° of knee flexion. The MCL injuries are categorized as grade 1, less than 5 mm of medial joint line opening with a valgus stress; grade 2, 5 to 10 mm of medial joint line opening; and grade 3, greater than 10 mm of joint line opening.

Isolated MCL injuries do not require surgical intervention. Pain is managed with ice and nonsteroidal anti-inflammatory drugs. Immediate physical therapy can begin with isometrics

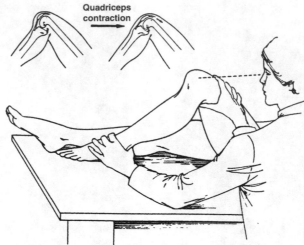

Figure 5–33 The 90° Quadriceps Active Test. Keeping the eyes at the level of the subject's flexed knee, the examiner rests the elbow on the table and uses the ipsilateral hand to support the subject's thigh and to confirm that the thigh muscles are relaxed. The foot is stabilized by the examiner's other hand, and the subject is asked to slide the foot gently down the table. Tibial displacement resulting from the quadriceps contraction is noted.

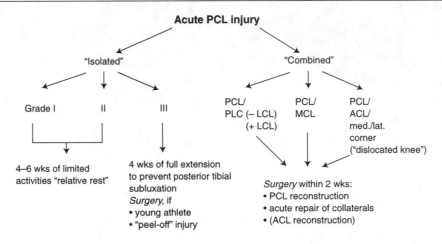

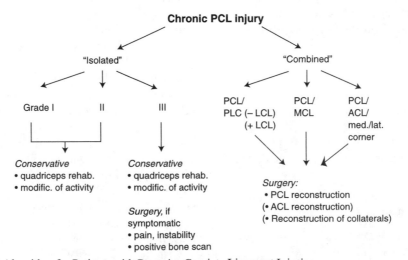

Figure 5–34 Treatment Algorithm for Patients with Posterior Cruciate Ligament Injuries.

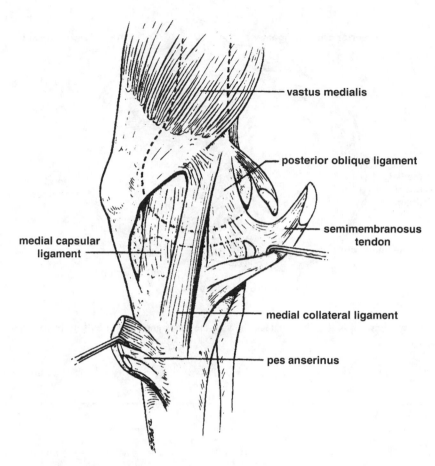

vastus medialis

posterior oblique ligament

semimembranosus tendon

medial capsular ligament

medial collateral ligament

pes anserinus

Figure 5–35 Anatomy of the Medial Structures of the Knee.

and strengthening of medial knee musculature. Bracing is often used symptomatically.

Lateral Collateral Ligament Injury

The lateral collateral ligament (LCL) is the primary restraint to a varus stress on the knee. Isolated LCL injuries are infrequent. The injury usually occurs when the foot is planted and there is a direct blow to the medial aspect of the knee. The LCL is often injured in combination with one or both cruciate ligaments. The LCL is tested by applying a varus stress to the knee at 0° and at 30° of knee flexion. Treatment is usually conservative, similar to that described for MCL injury.

MENISCUS INJURIES

The meniscus is a C-shaped structure between the femoral condyle and the tibial plateau of the knee (see Figure 5–36).[79] It is attached to the joint capsule and covers a portion of the tibial articular cartilage surface. The meniscus principally functions as a shock absorber and secondarily as a knee restraint to translational forces. The meniscus can be torn in an acute injury or as a result of a degenerative process.

History and Physical Examination

Athletic knee injuries often involve meniscus tears, and the athlete recounts a pop and swelling with decreased knee range of motion or locking. Pain is often localized to the joint line and may be exacerbated with knee hyperflexion.

Physical examination reveals tenderness with palpation along the involved joint line. Compression tests may also be painful, such as the Apley's maneuver or the McMurray's test. X-ray films are often negative, but MRIs are useful in providing a diagnosis (see Figure 5–37). Differential diagnosis of meniscus tears include patellofemoral chondromalacia, synovitis, fat pad inflammation, pathological plica,

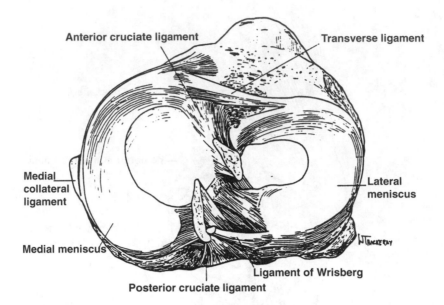

Figure 5–36 Meniscus Anatomy. Drawing of the tibial plateau showing the shape and attachments of the medial and lateral menisci.

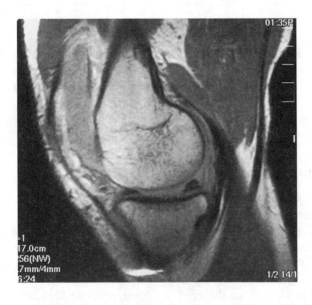

Figure 5–37 MRI of a Medial Meniscus Tear.

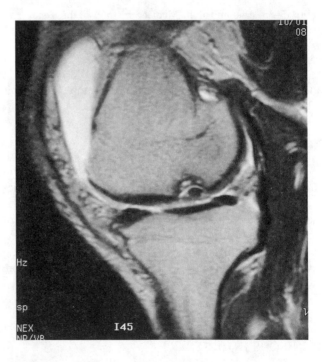

Figure 5–38 MRI of an Osteochondral Defect of the Medial Femoral Condyle with Loose Fragment.

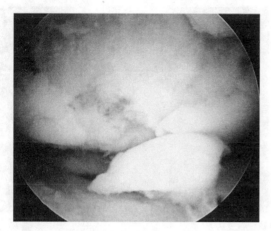

Figure 5–39 OCD with Loose Body. Arthroscopic picture of an osteochondral defect of the medial femoral condyle with nearby osteochondral loose body.

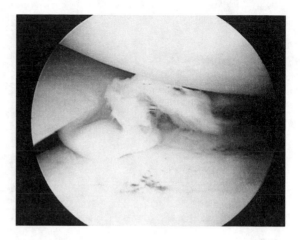

Figure 5–40 Nonrepairable Meniscus Tear. Intraoperative arthroscopic picture of a nonrepairable flap tear of the medial meniscus.

loose bodies, chondral lesions or fractures, osteochondritis dissecans (see Figures 5–38 and 5–39), ligament injuries, patellar subluxation or dislocation, and inflammatory arthritis.

Meniscus Tears Differential Diagnosis

- Patellofemoral chondromalacia
- Synovitis
- Fat pad inflammation
- OCD
- Loose bodies
- Ligament injuries
- Patellar subluxation
- Patellar dislocation
- Inflammatory arthritis

Clinical Guideline

Treatment of Meniscal Injuries

Meniscus tears (see Figure 5–40) often require arthroscopic surgical treatment. Meniscus surgery techniques[80] vary, but the goal is to preserve as much functioning meniscal tissue as possible, either by removing only the damaged portion (partial meniscectomy) or by repairing the torn meniscus with sutures (see Figure 5–41) or tacklike devices.

With improved surgical techniques, many meniscus tears can be repaired with little morbidity. Meniscal allografts are also available to try to restore some meniscal function.[81]

Meniscus—Surgical Treatment

- Partial meniscectomy
- Meniscal repair
  Sutures
  Arrows
  Screws
  Stingers, etc.
- Meniscal allografts

Clinical Guideline

INJURY PREVENTION

Recent studies have shown that women run, jump, and land differently than men when playing sports.[82,83] In female athletes there has been documentation as to gender differences in neuromuscular responses at the knee.[23] In particular, a different muscle recruitment order was noted at intermediate reflex response levels, with the quadriceps (ACL antagonists) initiated first in the female athlete group and the hamstrings (ACL antagonists) initiated first in the male athlete group. Women rely more on their quadriceps than their hamstrings, and this difference may be part of the reason that women have a higher ACL injury rate than men. Taking this information into account, there has been a push to retrain female athletes. More emphasis is being placed on performing athletic activities in a safety position: more crouched, bending the hips and knees, and avoiding knee extension and external tibial rotation (see Figure 5–42).[58,84] Hamstring strength has also been addressed in training programs for female athletes to avoid knee injuries.[28]

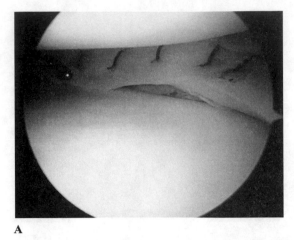
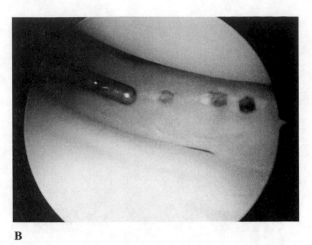

A   B

Figure 5–41 Repairable Meniscus Tears. A, intraoperative arthroscopic picture of a meniscus tear repaired with the inside-outside suture repair technique. B, intraoperative arthroscopic picture of a meniscus tear repaired with an all-inside technique using meniscal arrows.

Specific training programs, such as the Jump-Training Program, have been developed for female athletes to improve their jumping and landing mechanics (see Appendix 5–A), improve proprioception, center of gravity position, and decrease the impact of landing.[64] Plyometrics are essential to both rehabilitation and prevention of knee injuries.

Research suggests that female athletes also tend to have a slower muscle reaction time[23,82] compared with male athletes, and training and conditioning protocols are beginning to address this with specific drills including agility exercises.[75,85]

Neuromuscular control of the lower extremity is critical in dynamic knee stability and protection. Studies in subjects with ACL injuries have documented a decline in proprioceptive function on their knees.[32,34] Attention to balance and proprioception in training and rehabilitation programs should always be incorporated to enhance the female athlete's neuromuscular control and ultimately prevent injuries.

FUTURE RESEARCH

Knee injuries are common injuries in the female athlete. The causes of these injuries are multiple, and the ultimate

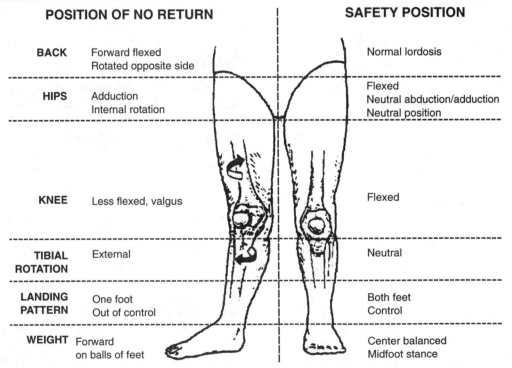

Figure 5–42 The Position-of-No-Return Mechanism for ACL Injury and the Safe Position.

outcome is related to an accurate anatomically and functionally based diagnosis. Appropriate rehabilitation is essential to outcome and prevention of reinjury. Protocols specific to females are becoming common; recently, even knee braces

specifically for female athletes have been introduced. Future studies and technological advances will continue to benefit the female athlete in the prevention and treatment of her knee injuries.

Jump-Training Program

Exercise	Repetitions or Time	
Phase I: Technique	Week 1	Week 2
1. Wall jumps	20 s	25 s
2. Tuck jumps*	20 s	25 s
3. Broad jumps stick land	5 reps	10 reps
4. Squat jumps*	10 s	15 s
5. Double-leg cone jumps*	30 s/30 s	30 s/30 s (side-to-side and back-to-front)
6. 180° jumps	20 s	25 s
7. Bounding in place	20 s	25 s
Phase II: Fundamentals	Week 3	Week 4
1. Wall jumps	30 s	30 s
2. Tuck jumps*	30 s	30 s
3. Jump, jump, jump, vert. jump	5 reps	8 reps
4. Squat jumps*	20 s	20 s
5. Bounding for distance	1 run	2 runs
6. Double-leg cone jumps*	30 s/30 s	30 s/30 s (side-to-side and back-to-front)
7. Scissor jump	30 s	30 s
8. Hop, hop, stick*	5 reps/leg	5 reps/leg
Phase III: Performance	Week 5	Week 6
1. Wall jumps	30 s	30 s
2. Step, jump up, down, vertical	5 reps	10 reps
3. Mattress jumps	30 s/30 s	30 s/30 s (side-to-side and back-to-front)
4. Single-legged jumps distance*	5 reps/leg	5 reps/leg
5. Squat jumps*	25 s	25 s
6. Jump into bounding*	3 runs	4 runs
7. Single-legged hop, hop, stick	5 reps/leg	5 reps/leg

Before jumping exercises, subjects did stretching (15–20 min), skipping (2 laps), and side shuffle (2 laps). After training, subjects did a cool down walk (2 min) and stretching (5 min). Each jump exercise was followed by 30-s rest period.
*These jumps performed on mats.

Clinical Guideline

Glossary of Jump-Training Exercises

1. 180° jumps: Two-footed jump. Rotate 180° in midair. Hold landing for 2 s, then repeat in reverse direction.
2. Bounding for distance: Start bounding in place and slowly increase distance with each step, keeping knees high.
3. Bounding in place: Jump from one leg to the other straight up and down, progressively increasing rhythm and height.
4. Broad jumps-stick (hold) landing: Two-footed jump as far as possible. Hold landing for 5 s.
5. Cone jumps: Double-leg jump with feet together. Jump side-to-side over cones quickly. Repeat forward and backward.
6. Hop, hop, stick: Single-legged hop. Stick second landing for 5 s. Increase distance of hop as technique improves.
7. Jump into bounding*: Two-footed broad jump. Land on single leg, then progress into bounding for distance.
8. Jump, jump, jump vertical: Three broad jumps with vertical jump immediately after landing the third broad jump.
9. Mattress jumps: Two-footed jump on mattress, tramp, or other easily compressed device. Perform side-to-side/back-to-front.
10. Scissors jump: Start in stride position with one foot well in front of the other. Jump up, alternating foot positions in midair.
11. Single-legged jumps distance*: One-legged hop for distance. Hold landing (knees bent) for 5 s.
12. Squat jumps*: Standing jump raising both arms overhead, land in squatting position touching both hands to floor.
13. Step, jump up, down, vertical: Two-footed jump onto 6- to 8-inch step. Jump off step with two feet, then vertical jump.
14. Tuck jumps: From standing position jump and bring both knees up to chest as high as possible. Repeat quickly.
15. Wall jumps (ankle bounces): With knees slightly bent and arms raised overhead, bounce up and down off toes.

*These jumps performed on mats.

Clinical Guideline

Stretching and Weight-Training Program

Stretches	*Weight-Training Exercises*
1. Calf stretch 1	1. Abdominal curl
2. Calf stretch 2: soleus	2. Back hyperextensions
3. Quadriceps	3. Leg press
4. Hamstring	4. Calf raises
5. Hip flexors	5. Pullover
6. Iliotibial band/lower back	6. Bench press
7. Posterior deltoids	7. Latissimus dorsi pulldowns
8. Latissimus dorsi	8. Forearm curls
9. Pectorals/biceps	9. Warm-down/short stretch

Clinical Guideline

REFERENCES

1. Morrey MA, Stuart MJ, Smith AM, Wiese-Bjornstal DM. A longitudinal examination of athletes' emotional and cognitive responses to anterior cruciate ligament injury. *Clin J Sports Med.* 1999;9:63–69.
2. Gomez E, DeLee JC, Farney WC. Incidence of injury in Texas girls' high school basketball. *Am J Sports Med.* 1996;24:684–687.
3. Zelisko JA, Noble HB, Porter M. A comparison of men's and women's professional basketball injuries. *Am J Sports Med.* 1982;10:297–299.
4. Nilsson S, Roaas A. Soccer injuries in adolescents. *Am J Sports Med.* 1978;6:358–361.
5. Levy AS, Wetzler MJ, Lewats M, Laughlin W. Knee injuries in women collegiate rugby players. *Am J Sports Med.* 1997;25:360–362.
6. Arendt EA, Agel J, Dick R. Anterior cruciate ligament injury patterns among collegiate men and women. *J Athletic Training.* 1999;34:86–92.

7. Arendt E, Dick R. Knee injury patterns among men and women in collegiate basketball and soccer: NCAA data and review of literature. *Am J Sports Med.* 1995;23:694–701.

8. Beachy G, Akau CK, Martinson M, Olderr TF. High school sports injuries: a longitudinal study at Punahou school: 1988 to 1996. *Am J Sports Med.* 1997;25:675–681.

9. Clarke KS, Buckley WE. Women's injuries in collegiate sports: a preliminary comparative overview of three seasons. *Am J Sports Med.* 1980;8:187–191.

10. DeHaven KE, Lintner DM. Athletic injuries: comparison by age, sport, and gender. *Am J Sports Med.* 1986;14:218–224.

11. Lindenfeld TN, Schmitt DJ, Hendy MP, Mangine RE, Noyes FR. Incidence of injury in indoor soccer. *Am J Sports Med.* 1994;22:364–371.

12. Putukian M, Knowles WK, Swere S, Castle NG. Injuries in indoor soccer: the Lake Placid dawn to dark soccer tournament. *Am J Sports Med.* 1996;24:317–322.

13. Gray J, Taunton JE, McKenzie DC, Clement DB, McConkey JP, Davidson RG. A survey of injuries to the anterior cruciate ligament of the knee in female basketball players. *Int J Sports Med.* 1985;6:314–316.

14. Lanese RR, Strauss RH, Leizman DJ, Rotondi AM. Injury and disability in matched men's and women's intercollegiate sports. *Am J Public Health.* 1990;80:1459–1462.

15. Messina DF, Farney WC, DeLee JC. The incidence of injury in Texas high school basketball: a prospective study among male and female athletes. *Am J Sports Med.* 1999;27:294–299.

16. Hutchinson MR, Ireland ML. Knee injuries in female athletes. *Sports Med.* 1995;19:222–302.

17. Decoster LC, Bernier JN, Lindsay RH, Vailas JC. Generalized joint hypermobility and its relationship to injury patterns among NCAA lacrosse players. *J Athletic Training.* 1999;34:99–105.

18. Ferretti A, Papandrea P, Conteduca F, Mariani PP. Knee ligament injuries in volleyball players. *Am J Sports Med.* 1992;20:203–207.

19. Malone TR, Hardaker WT, Garrett WE, Feagin JA, Bassett FH. Relationship of gender to anterior cruciate ligament injuries in intercollegiate basketball players. *J South Orthop Assoc.* 1993;2:36–39.

20. Haycock CE, Gillette JV. Susceptibility of women athletes to injury: myths vs reality. *JAMA.* 1976;236:163–165.

21. Heitz NA, Eisenman PA, Beck CL, Walker JA. Hormonal changes throughout the menstrual cycle and increased anterior cruciate ligament laxity in females. *J Athletic Training.* 1999;34:144–149.

22. Hunter LY. Women's athletics: the orthopedic surgeon's viewpoint. *Clin Sports Med.* 1984;3:809–827.

23. Huston LJ, Wojtys EM. Neuromuscular performance characteristics in elite female athletes. *Am J Sports Med.* 1996;24:427–436.

24. Micheli L. Female runners. In: D'Ambrosia R, ed. *Prevention and Treatment of Running Injuries.* Thorofare, NJ: Slack; 1982:199–208.

25. Tietz CC, Lind BK, Sacks BM. Symmetry of the femoral notch width index. *Am J Sports Med.* 1997;25:687–690.

26. Wojtys EM, Huston LJ, Lindenfeld TN, Hewett TE, Greenfield MLVH. Association between the menstrual cycle and anterior cruciate ligament injuries in female athletes. *Am J Sports Med.* 1998;26:614–619.

27. Barber-Westin SD, Noyes FR, Andrews M. A rigorous comparison between the sexes of results and complications after anterior cruciate ligament reconstruction. *Am J Sports Med.* 1997;25:514–526.

28. Hewett TE, Stroupe AL, Nance TA, Noyes FR. Plyometric training in female athletes: decreased impact forces and increased hamstring torques. *Am J Sports Med.* 1996;24:765–773.

29. Biedert RM, Stauffer E, Friederich NF. Occurrence of free nerve endings in the soft tissue of the knee joint: a histologic investigation. *Am J Sports Med.* 1992;20:430–433.

30. Johansson H, Sjolander P, Sojka P. A sensory role for the cruciate ligaments. *Clin Orthop Rel Res.* 1991;268:161–178.

31. Schultz RA, Miller DC, Kerr CS, Micheli L. Mechanoreceptors in human cruciate ligaments: a histological study. *J Bone Joint Surg Am.* 1984;66:1072–1076.

32. Beard DJ, Kyberd PJ, Fergusson CM, Dodd CAF. Proprioception after rupture of the anterior cruciate ligament: an objective indication of the need for surgery. *J Bone Joint Surg Br.* 1993;75:311–315.

33. Dye SF, Vaupel GL, Dye CC. Conscious neurosensory mapping of the internal structures of the human knee without intraarticular anesthesia. *Am J Sports Med.* 1998;26:773–777.

34. Barrack RL, Skinner HB, Buckley SL. Proprioception in the anterior cruciate deficient knee. *Am J Sports Med.* 1989;17:1–6.

35. Sanborn CF, Jankowski CM. Physiologic considerations for women in sport. *Clin Sports Med.* 1994;13:315–327.

36. Sady SP, Freedson PS. Body composition and structural comparisons of female and male athletes. *Clin Sports Med.* 1984;3:755–777.

37. Ciullo JV. Lower extremity injuries. In: Pearl AJ, ed. *The Athletic Female.* Champaign, IL: Human Kinetics; 1993:267–298.

38. Thein LA, Thein JM. The female athlete. *J Orthop Sports Phys Ther.* 1996;23:134–148.

39. Wiggins DL, Wiggins ME. The female athlete. *Clin Sports Med.* 1997;16:593–612.

40. Leblanc KE. The female athlete. *Comp Ther.* 1998;24:256–264.

41. Bourne MJ, Hazel WA Jr, Scott SG, Sim FH. Anterior knee pain. *Mayo Clin Proc.* 1988;63:482–491.

42. Ferkel RD. Lateral retinacular release. In: Fox JM, Del Pizzo W, eds. *The Patellofemoral Joint.* New York: McGraw-Hill; 1993:309–323.

43. Merchant AC. Radiography of the patellofemoral joint. *Oper Tech Sports Med.* 1999;7:59–64.

44. Blazina ME, Kerlan RK, Jobe FW, Carter VS, Carlson GJ. Jumper's knee. *Orthop Clin North Am.* 1973;4:665–678.

45. Ferretti A, Papandrea P, Conteduca F. Knee injuries in volleyball. *Sports Med.* 1990;10:132–138.

46. Puddu G, Cipolla M, Cerullo G, De Paulis F. Tendinitis. In: Fox JM, Del Pizzo W, eds. *The Patellofemoral Joint.* New York: McGraw-Hill; 1993:177–198.

47. Blackburn TA Jr, Eiland WG, Bandy WD. An introduction to the plica. *J Orthop Sports Phys Ther.* 1982;3:171–177.

48. Patel D, Laurencin CT, Tsuchiya A, Dutka M. Synovial folds-plicae. In: Fox JM, Del Pizzo W, eds. *The Patellofemoral Joint.* New York: McGraw-Hill; 1993:193–198.

49. McConnell J. Conservative management of patellofemoral problems. In: Grelsamer RP, McConnell J, eds. *The Patella—A Team Approach.* Gaithersburg, MD: Aspen Publishers; 1998:119–136.

50. Dye SF, Wojtys EM, Fu FH, Fithian DC, Gillquist J. Factors contributing to function of the knee joint after injury or reconstruction of the anterior cruciate ligament. *Instructional Course Lectures.* Vol 48. Rosemont, IL: AAOS; 1999:185–198.

51. McNerney J. Biomechanical management of patellofemoral pain and dysfunction with foot orthotic devices. In: Grelsamer RP, McConnell J, eds. *The Patella—A Team Approach.* Gaithersburg, MD: Aspen Publishers; 1998:177–227.

52. Natri A, Kannus P, Jarvinen M. Which factors predict the long-term outcome in chronic patellofemoral pain syndrome? A 7-yr prospective follow-up study. *Med Sci Sports Exerc.* 1998;30:1572–1577.

53. Halbrecht JL, Jackson DW. Acute dislocation of the patella. In: Fox JM, Del Pizzo W, eds. *The Patellofemoral Joint.* New York: McGraw-Hill; 1993:123–134.

54. Griffin LY. Rehabilitation of the knee extensor mechanism. In: Fox JM, Del Pizzo W, eds. *The Patellofemoral Joint*. New York: McGraw-Hill; 1993:279–290.

55. Molnar TJ. Patellofemoral rehabilitation. In: Fox JM, Del Pizzo W, eds. *The Patellofemoral Joint*. New York: McGraw-Hill; 1993:291–304.

56. Knortz KA, Reinhart RS. Women's athletics: the athletic trainer's viewpoint. *Clin Sports Med*. 1984;3:851–868.

57. Aronen JG, Chronister R, Regan K, Hensien MA. Practical, conservative management of iliotibial band syndrome. *Phys Sports Med*. 1993;21:59–69.

58. Ireland ML. Anterior cruciate ligament injury in female athletes: epidemiology. *J Athletic Training*. 1999;34:150–154.

59. Baker MM. Anterior cruciate ligament injuries in the female athlete. *J Women's Health*. 1998;7:343–349.

60. Bonci CM. Assessment and evaluation of predisposing factors to anterior cruciate ligament injury. *J Athletic Training*. 1999;34:155–164.

61. Harner CD, Paulos LE, Greenwald AE, Rosenbery TD, Cooley VC. Detailed analysis of patients with bilateral anterior cruciate ligament injuries. *Am J Sports Med*. 1994;22:37–43.

62. Beck JL, Wildermuth BP. The female athlete's knee. *Clin Sports Med*. 1985;4:345–366.

63. Rosene JM, Fogarty TD. Anterior tibial translation in collegiate athletes with normal anterior cruciate ligament integrity. *J Athletic Training*. 1999;34:93–98.

64. Rozzi SL, Lephart SM, Fu FH. Effects of muscular fatigue on knee joint laxity and neuromuscular characteristics of male and female athletes. *J Athletic Training*. 1999;34:106–114.

65. Loudon JK, Jenkins W, Loudon KL. The relationship between static posture and ACL injury in female athletes. *J Orthop Sports Phys Ther*. 1996;24:91–97.

66. Daniel DM, Stone ML, Sachs R, Malcom L. Instrumented measurement of anterior knee laxity in patients with acute anterior cruciate ligament disruption. *Am J Sports Med*. 1985;13:401–407.

67. Bach BR Jr, Warren RF, Flynn WM, Kroll M, Wickiewiecz TL. Arthrometric evaluation of knees that have a torn anterior cruciate ligament. *J Bone Joint Surg Am*. 1990;72:1299–1306.

68. Highgenboten CL, Jackson AW, Jansson KA, Meske NB. KT-1000 arthrometer: conscious and unconscious test results using 15, 20, and 30 pounds of force. *Am J Sports Med*. 1992;20:450–454.

69. Wroble RR, Van Ginkel LA, Grood ES, Noyes FR, Shaffer BL. Repeatability of the KT-1000 arthrometer in a normal population. *Am J Sports Med*. 1990;18:396–399.

70. Daniel DM, Stone ML, Dobson BE, Fithian DC, Rossman DJ, Kaufman KR. Fate of the ACL-injured patient. A prospective outcome study. *Am J Sports Med*. 1994;22:632–644.

71. Woods GW, Stanley RF Jr, Tullos HS. Lateral capsular sign: x-ray clue to significant knee instability. *Am J Sports Med*. 1979;7:27–33.

72. Larson RL, Taillon M. Anterior cruciate ligament insufficiency: principles of treatment. *J Am Acad Orthop Surg*. 1994;2:26–35.

73. Larson RV, Friedman MJ. Anterior cruciate ligament: injuries and treatment. *Instructional Course Lectures*. Rosemont, IL: AAOS; 1996:235–243.

74. Frank CB, Jackson DW. Current concepts review: the science of reconstruction of the anterior cruciate ligament. *J Bone Joint Surg Am*. 1997;79:1556–1576.

75. Wilk KE, Arrigo C, Andrews JR, Clancy WG Jr. Rehabilitation after anterior cruciate ligament reconstruction in the female athlete. *J Athletic Training*. 1999;34:177–193.

76. Daniel DM, Stone ML, Barnett P, Sachs R. Use of the quadriceps active test to diagnose posterior cruciate-ligament disruption and measure posterior laxity of the knee. *J Bone Joint Surg Am*. 1988;70:386–391.

77. Shelbourne KD, Davis TJ, Patel DV. The natural history of acute isolated, nonoperatively treated posterior cruciate ligament injuries: A prospective study. *Am J Sports Med*. 1999;27:276–283.

78. Harner CD, Hoher J. Evaluation and treatment of posterior cruciate ligament injuries. *Am J Sports Med*. 1998;26:471–482.

79. Warren R, Arnoczky SP, Wickiewicz TL. Anatomy of the knee. In: Nicholar JA, Hershman EB, eds. *The Lower Extremity and Spine in Sports Medicine*. Vol. 1. St. Louis, MO: Mosby; 1986:657–694.

80. DeHaven KE. Meniscectomy versus repair: clinical experience. In: Mow VC, Arnoczky SP, Jackson DW, eds. *Knee Meniscus: Basic and Clinical Foundations*. New York: Raven Press; 1992:131–139.

81. Jackson DW, Simon TM. Biology of meniscal allograft. In: Mow VC, Arnoczky SP, Jackson DW, eds. *Knee Meniscus: Basic and Clinical Foundations*. New York: Raven Press; 1992:141–152.

82. Shultz SJ, Perrin DH. Using surface electromyography to assess sex differences in neuromuscular response characteristics. *J Athletic Training*. 1999;34:165–176.

83. Rozzi SL, Lephart SM, Gear WS, Fu FH. Knee joint laxity and neuromuscular characteristics of male and female soccer and basketball players. *Am J Sports Med*. 1999;27:312–319.

84. McLean SG, Neal RJ, Myers PT, Walters MR. Knee joint kinematics during the sidestep cutting maneuver: potential for injury in women. *Med Sci Sports Exerc*. 1999;31:959–968.

85. Cook G, Burton L, Fields K. Reactive neuromuscular training for the anterior cruciate ligament-deficient knee: a case report. *J Athletic Training*. 1999;34:194–201.

Rehabilitation Protocols

Patellofemoral Protocols

A rehabilitation protocol for acute traumatic dislocation of the patella (nonoperative case) is outlined in the Clinical Guideline.

Rehabilitation for Acute Traumatic Dislocation of the Patella

Acute traumatic dislocation of the patella (nonoperative case)

Phase I: 24–48 hours
- Immobilization in knee immobilizer with lateral pad. Ace wrapped to hold patella against medial retinaculum; ice, electric stimulation unit, or other modalities to decrease swelling and pain
- Anti-inflammatory/analgesic (eg, ibuprofen, naproxen if needed)
- Crutches, bear weight as tolerated
- Attempt isometric quadriceps sets, hamstring sets, and hip abductor sets; hold each for count of 10; do 3 sets of 10 each
- May use neuromuscular stimulation unit to help retard atrophy, as well as decrease pain and swelling

Phase II: 1–3 wk
- May change to patellar-stabilizing brace under knee immobilizer
- Take immobilizer off 3 times a day for range of motion 0°–30°
- Continue ice, transcutaneous electrical stimulation (TENS), or neuromuscular stimulation unit to reduce atrophy and/or pain control
- Perform quadriceps setting in full extension
- Increase to full weight bearing
- Continue isometric exercises, as well as isotonic exercises in 0°–20°
- Can start short arc extensions 30°–0° using a rolled towel under the knee
- Continue isometrics for hamstrings
- Begin isotonic hip abduction and adduction exercises
- Progress to 3- to 5-lb weights and do 3 sets of 10 repetitions for each muscle group
- Do range of motion and strengthening for ankle (dorsi and plantar flexors, as well as invertors and everters)
- Do cross-leg biking for cardiovascular fitness and cross-training effort
- Passive and active assisted knee flexion exercises to 90°

Phase III: 3–6 wk
- Use patellar-stabilizing brace only when swelling and tenderness along medial retinaculum are resolved
- Do full range of motion exercises
- Do stretching exercises for hamstrings, quadriceps, hip abduction, hip adduction, flexion, and extension
- Advance isotonic quadriceps exercises (from 45° to 0°); progress to 3-lb weight; as can do 3 sets of 10 easily, advance by 2 lb up to 10–15 lb, depending on patient body weight and prior level of exercise
- Continue isotonic exercises for all other muscles of lower extremity
- Stair stepper with short steps, walking, or biking with elevated seat for cardiovascular fit-

ness when patient has 95°–100° of knee flexion passively and actively; begin fast stepping side to side and up and down a small step (4–6 inches)

Phase IV: 6 wk
- Achieve full range of motion
- Achieve strength equal to noninjured side by advancing isotonic exercises
- Work for muscular endurance and power by alternating long, slow workouts with short bursts of activity for each muscle group
- Continue cardiovascular fitness by biking, walking, or stair stepper
- May attempt to jog and increase running over next 4–6 wks if desired
- Add skills such as cut, squat
- Start jumping at 8–12 wks, depending on advancement of other parameters
- Develop proprioceptive skills in weeks 8–10
- Try step aerobics, functional sports skills, etc.
- Can return to full activity (anticipate 8–12 wk) if range of motion equal to opposite side; no swelling, no pain; strength 95%–100% of opposite extremity; can hop, skip, squat, and jump without difficulty

Clinical Guideline

Source: L.Y. Griffin, Rehabilitation of the Knee Extensor Mechanism, *The Patellofemoral Joint*, J.M. Fox and W. Del Pizzo, eds. pp. 279–290. Reproduced with permission of The McGraw-Hill Companies.

A rehabilitation protocol for patellofemoral stress syndrome is outlined in the Clinical Guideline.

Rehabilitation for Patellofemoral Stress Syndrome

Patellofemoral stress syndrome

Phase I: 1–2 days
- Knee immobilizer if acutely symptomatic
- Ice and oral anti-inflammatories to decrease inflammation and pain
- TENS unit if needed for pain control
- Begin quadriceps sets, straight leg raises when pain permits
- Hip adductor/abduction, flexion, and extension exercises

Phase II: Out of immobilizer
- Infrapatellar strap or patellar-stabilizing brace
- Continue ice, especially after exercise periods
- Continue TENS and oral anti-inflammatories if needed
- Straight leg raises, quadriceps sets, short arc extensions
- Flexibility exercises for quadriceps, hamstrings, iliotibial band, gastrocnemius, soleus

- Start to bike with seat elevated, swim (crawl only), use stair stepper (small steps done rapidly)
- Advance isotonic exercises for hip flexors, extensors, abductors, adductors, as well as muscles of the lower leg and foot, increasing weight as tolerated, doing 3 sets of 10 and increasing weight by 2 lb

Phase III: Use brace if needed
- Continue quadriceps isotonics from 30°–0°, increasing weight as tolerated to a maximum of 20 lb–30 lb
- Advance hamstring strengthening exercises
- Continue biking, swimming, stair stepper, or walking for cardiovascular and muscle endurance; increase duration, then speed
- Continue flexibility exercises

Phase IV: Add slow return to running if desired; increase distance, then speed
- Warm up well
- Ice after workout
- Continue to aerobically cross-train
- Start to jump, cut, half squats, kick, and other sport-specific skills if applicable
- Wear brace or tape for sport participation if desired

Clinical Guideline

Source: L.Y. Griffin, Rehabilitation of the Knee Extensor Mechanism, *The Patellofemoral Joint*, J.M. Fox and W. Del Pizzo, eds. pp. 279–290. Reproduced with permission of The McGraw-Hill Companies.

ACL Protocols

A rehabilitation protocol for accelerated rehabilitation for isolated ACL reconstruction using patellar tendon graft is outlined in the Clinical Guideline.

Accelerated Rehabilitation for ACL Patellar Tendon Graft (PTG) Reconstruction (Isolated)

I.   Preoperative phase

Goals
   Diminish inflammation, swelling, and pain
   Restore normal range of motion (especially knee extension)
   Restore voluntary muscle activation
   Provide patient education to prepare patient for surgery
Brace: Elastic wrap or knee sleeve to reduce swelling
Weight bearing: As tolerated with or without crutches
Exercises
   Ankle pumps
   Passive knee extension to zero
   Passive knee flexion to tolerance

Straight-leg raises

Quadriceps setting

Hip abduction and adduction raises

Closed kinetic chain exercises: minisquats, lunges, step-ups

Muscle stimulation: Electrical muscle stimulation to quadriceps during voluntary quadriceps exercises (4–6 n/d)

Cryotherapy/elevation: Apply ice 20 min of every hour; elevate leg with knee in full extension (knee must be above heart)

Patient education

Review postoperative rehabilitation program

Review instructional video (optional)

Select appropriate surgical date

II. Immediate postoperative phase (day 1–day 7)

Goals

Restore full passive knee extension

Diminish joint swelling and pain

Restore patellar mobility

Gradually improve knee flexion

Reestablish quadriceps control

Restore independent ambulation

Postoperative day 1:

Brace: EZ Wrap Brace (Professional Products, DeFunak Springs, FL) or immobilizer applied to knee locked in full knee extension during ambulation

Weight bearing: 2 crutches, weight bearing as tolerated

Exercises

Ankle pumps

Overpressure into full, passive knee extension

Active and passive knee flexion (90° by day 5)

Straight-leg raises

Quadriceps isometric setting

Hip abduction and adduction

Hamstring stretches

Closed kinetic chain exercises: minisquats, weight shifts

Continuous passive motion: As needed, 0°–45°–50° (as tolerated and as directed by physician)

Muscle stimulation: Use muscle stimulator during active muscle exercises (4–6 n/d)

Ice and elevation: Ice 20 min of every hour; elevate leg with knee in full extension

Postoperative days 2 to 3:

Brace: EZ Wrap Brace and immobilizer locked at zero

Weight bearing: 2 crutches as tolerated

Range of motion: Remove brace, perform range-of-motion exercises 4–6 times a day

Exercises

Multiangle isometrics at 90° and 60° (knee extension)

Knee extension 90°–40°

Patellar mobilization

Overpressure into extension

Ankle pumps

Straight-leg raises (3 directions)

Minisquats and weight shifts

Standing hamstring curls

Quadriceps isometric setting

Muscle stimulation: To quadriceps during exercises (6 n/d)

Continuous passive motion: 0°–90° as needed

Ice and elevation: Ice 20 min of every hour and elevate leg with knee in full extension

Postoperative days 4–7

Brace: EZ Wrap/immobilizer

Weight bearing: 2 crutches, weight bearing as tolerated

Range of motion: Remove brace, perform range-of-motion exercises 4–6 times per day/knee flexion 90° by day 5, approximately 100° by day 7

Exercise: Continue all exercises as listed in postoperative days 2–4, and progress proprioception and balance drills

Muscle stimulation: Apply to quadriceps during active exercises

Continuous passive motion: 0°–90° as needed

Ice and elevation: Ice 20 min of every hour and elevate leg with knee in full extension

III. Early rehabilitation phase (week 2–week 4)

Goals

Maintain full passive knee extension

Gradually increase knee flexion

Diminish swelling and pain

Muscle training

Restore proprioception

Patellar mobility

Criteria to progress to phase III

Quadriceps control/ability to perform good quadriceps set and straight-leg raises

Full passive knee extension

Passive range of motion from 9°–90°

Good patellar mobility

Minimal joint effusion

Independent ambulation

Week 2:

Brace: Discontinue brace or immobilizer at 2–3 wk

Weight bearing: As tolerated (goal is to discontinue crutches at 10 days)

Range of motion: Self-ROM stretching (4–8 times a day), emphasis on maintaining full, passive range of motion

KT-2000 test: 6.75-kg anterior-posterior test only

Exercises

Muscle stimulation to quadriceps during quadriceps exercises

Isometric quadriceps sets

Straight-leg raises (4 planes)

Leg press

Knee extension 90°–40°

Half-squats 0°–40°

Weight shifts

Front and side lunges

Hamstring curls

Bicycle
Proprioception training
Overpressure into extension
Passive range of motion from 0°–50°
Patellar mobilization
Well-leg exercises
Progressive resistance exercise program (begin with.45 kg, increase by .45 kg per wk)
Week 3:
Brace: Discontinue
Range of motion: Continue range-of-motion stretching and overpressure into extension
Exercises
Continue all exercises as in week 2
Passive range-of-motion exercises from 0°–115°
Bicycle for range-of-motion progression
Pool-walking program (if incision is closed)
Eccentric quadriceps program
Lateral lunges
Lateral step-ups
Front step-ups
Lateral step-overs (cones)
Stair-stepper machine
Progress proprioception and neuromuscular control drills

IV. **Intermediate phase (week 4–week 10)**
Goals
Restore full knee range of motion (0° –125°)
Improve lower extremity strength
Enhance proprioception, balance, and neuromuscular control
Improve muscular endurance
Restore limb confidence and function
Criteria to enter phase IV
Active range of motion from 0°–115°
Quadriceps strength 60% of contralateral side (isometric test at 60% of knee flexion)
Unchanged KT bilateral values
Minimal to no joint effusion
No joint line or patellofemoral pain
Brace: No immobilizer or brace; may use knee sleeve (Bauerfeind Comprifix brace, Bauerfeind USA, Kennesaw, GA)
Range of motion: Self-ROM 4–5 times per day (using the other leg to provide ROM)
KT-2000 Testing
Week 4: 9-kg test
Weeks 6 through 8: 9- and 13.5-kg tests
Week 4:
Progess isometric strengthening program
Leg press
Knee extension from 90°–40°
Hamstring curls
Hip abduction and adduction
Hip flexion and extension
Lateral step-overs
Lateral lunges
Front stcp-ups

Front step-downs
Wall squats
Vertical squats
Toe calf raises
Biodex stability system (balance, squats, etc)
Proprioception drills
Bicycle
Stair-stepper machine
Pool program (backward running, hip and leg exercises)
Week 6:
Continue all exercises
Pool running (forward) and agility drills
Balance on tilt boards
Progress to balance board throws
KT-2000 test (9- and 13.5-kg tests)
Week 8:
Continue all exercises listed in weeks 4–6
Plyometric leg press
Perturbation training
Isokinetic exercises (90°–40°) (120°–240°/s)
Walking program
Bicycle for endurance
Stair-stepper machine for endurance
KT-2000 test: 9- and 13.5-kg test
Week 10:
KT-2000 test (9- and 13.5-kg and manual maximum test)
Isokinetic test (test concentric knee extension and flexion at 180° and 300°/s)
Exercises
Continue all exercises listed in weeks 6, 8, and 10
Plyometric training drills
Continue stretching drills

V. **Advanced activity phase (week 10–week 16)**
Goals
Normalize lower extremity strength
Enhance muscular power and endurance
Improve neuromuscular control
Perform selected sport-specific drills
Criteria to enter phase V
Active range of motion from 0°–125° or greater
Quadriceps strength 70% of contralateral side knee flexor:extensor ratio of 70%–75%
No change in KT values (comparable with contralateral side, within 2 mm)
No pain or effusion
Satisfactory clinical examination
Satisfactory isokinetic test (values for females at 180°)
Quadriceps bilateral comparison 75%
Hamstrings equal bilateral
Quadriceps peak torque/body weight
Hamstrings/quadriceps ratio 66%–75%
Hop test (80% of contralateral leg)
Subjective knee scoring (modified Noyes System) 80 points or better
Continue all exercises listed in weeks 10–12

VI. Return-to-activity phase (week 16–week 22)

Goals

Gradual return to full unrestricted sports

Achieve maximal strength and endurance

Normalize neuromuscular control

Progress skill training

Criteria to enter phase VI

Full range of motion

Unchanged KT-2000 test (within 2.5 mm of opposite side)

Isokinetic test that fulfills criteria

Quadriceps bilateral comparison (80% or greater)

Hamstrings bilateral comparison (110% or greater)

Quadriceps torque/body weight ratio (55% or greater)

Hamstrings/quadriceps ratio 70% or greater

Proprioceptive test 100% of contralateral leg

Functional test 85% or greater of contralateral side

Satisfactory clinical examination

Subjective knee scoring (modified Noyes system: 90 points or better)

Tests: KT-2000, isokinetic, and functional tests before return

Exercises

Continue strengthening program

Continue neuromuscular control drills

Continue plyometric drills

Progress running and agility program

Progress sport-specific training

6-mo follow-up

Isokinetic test

KT-2000 test

Functional test

12-mo follow-up

Isokinetic test

KT-2000 test

Functional test

*PTG = patellar tendon graft.

Clinical Guideline

Special considerations and specific exercise drills for postoperative ACL rehabilitation in females are outlined in the Clinical Guideline.

Female ACL Rehabilitation: Special Considerations and Specific Exercise Drills

Hip musculature to stabilize knee

Lateral step-overs (regular, fast, very slow)

Step-overs with ball catches

Step-overs with rotation

Lateral step-ups on foam

Dip walk

Squats (foam) (Balance Master)

Front diagonal lunges onto foam

Retrain neuromuscular pattern hamstring control

Lateral lunges straight

Lateral lunges

Lateral lunges with rotation

Lateral lunges onto foam

Lateral lunges with ball catches

Squats unstable pattern

Lateral lunges jumping

Lateral unstable pattern

Coactivation balance through biofeedback

Slide board

Fitter (Fitter International, Calgary, Alberta, Canada)

Control valgus moment

Front step-downs

Lateral step-ups with Thera-Band (The Hygienic Corporation, Akron, OH)

Tilt board balance throws

Control hyperextension

Plyometric leg press

Plyometric leg press with 4 corners

Plyometric jumps

1 box

2 boxes

4 boxes

2 boxes rotation

2 boxes with catches

Bounding drills

Forward and backward step-over drills

High-speed training, especially hamstrings

Isokinetics

Backward lunging

Shuttle

Lateral lunges (fast jumps)

Resistance tubing for hamstring

Backward running

Neuromuscular reaction

Squats on tilt board

Balance beam with cords

Dip walk with cords

Balance throws

Balance throws perturbations

Lateral lunges with perturbations onto tilt board

Less-developed thigh musculature

Knee-extensor and -flexor strengthening exercises

Squats

Leg press

Wall squats

Bicycling

Poorer muscular endurance

Stair climbing

Bicycling

Weight training (low weights, high repetitions)

Cardiovascular training

Balance drills for longer durations

Clinical Guideline

CHAPTER 6

The Foot and Ankle

Carol Van Rossum De Costa, Alan A. Morris, and Nadya Swedan

INTRODUCTION

According to the American Academy of Orthopaedic Surgeons, 2.2 million people seek medical care for foot and ankle problems each year, with more than half of these visits for ankle sprains alone.[1] Foot and ankle injuries occur at higher rates than other lower extremity injuries.[2,3] An early study found that female athletes had significantly higher rates of injury than their male counterparts in sports such as basketball, gymnastics, and track and field.[4]

The foot experiences the full impact of bipedal weight bearing. As the most distal aspect of the kinetic chain, the foot and ankle complex is responsible for maintaining the upright position of the body and in achieving balance, mobility, and agility during athletic movements such as walking, running, and jumping. The foot and ankle must be able to function as a rigid lever for propulsion and as a torque converter to allow for the pelvic and lower extremity rotation necessary for many sports. Because ground reactive forces during running are approximately two to four times body weight and may reach five times body weight in jumping sports like basketball and volleyball, the foot and ankle complex must also function as a shock absorber.[5]

The female athlete has a high incidence of foot and ankle injuries, and many of these are noncontact in nature. In addition, many female athletes also complain of concomitant back, hip, and knee pain. These factors lend credence to a biomechanical origin for many of these injuries. Because the foot and ankle complex is the foundation of the kinetic chain, its biomechanical abnormalities may be the direct cause of injuries to the more proximal aspects of the chain. The sports medicine physician must be familiar with and able to address and correct these biomechanical abnormalities of the foot and ankle to fully treat their injured athletes.[4]

GENDER DIFFERENCES

Studies of the differences in anatomy and kinesiology between men and women have been controversial. Williams et al[6] found in their study that elite female distance runners had a similar anthropomorphic makeup to male athletes, with both groups having similar pelvic diameters and Q-angles. Hunter,[7] however, found differences in these same parameters and also showed that leg length made up a smaller percentage of overall height in women (51%) compared with men (56%). This difference in limb length resulted in an increase in the amount of foot-to-ground contact a female athlete must make to cover the same distances as her male counterparts.[8,9] The widened female pelvis is also cited as a reason for the high incidence of lower extremity injuries in female athletes. The wider pelvis has been linked to an increased valgus knee position and subsequent compensatory hyperpronation of the foot. Furthermore, the tendency for women to develop hallux valgus may be linked to biomechanical factors[10] and genetic factors such as ligamentous laxity. All of these factors may contribute to an increased incidence of foot and ankle injuries.[11]

BASIC ANATOMY OF THE FOOT AND ANKLE

The foot is composed of 28 bones and is generally divided into the forefoot, the midfoot, and the rearfoot. The forefoot consists of the five digits, each with three phalanges (except the hallux, which only has two), the five metatarsals, and the medial and lateral sesamoid bones. The midfoot, or tarsus, is made up of the navicular, the cuboid, and the medial, intermediate, and lateral cuneiforms. The calcaneus and talus form the rearfoot.

The forefoot and midfoot together form functional units known as rays. The first ray consists of the hallux, the sesamoids, the first metatarsal, and the medial cuneiform. The second and third rays are formed by their respective phalanges, metatarsals, and the intermediate (second ray) or lateral cuneiform (third ray). The fourth and fifth rays include the phalanges and metatarsals only. The first and fifth rays have independent ranges of motion, whereas the second, third, and fourth rays move as a unit.[12] The tarsometatarsal joint or Lisfranc's joint forms the transverse arch of the midfoot, and primary soft tissue support is provided by Lisfranc's ligament and the intercuneiform ligaments. The posterior tibial and peroneal tendons also help to reinforce this complex.[13]

Because the first metatarsophalangeal joint (MPJ) provides most of the push-off during running and jumping, its anatomy warrants further consideration. The first MPJ is made up of the proximal phalanx of the hallux, the head of the first metatarsal, the medial and lateral sesamoids, and a complex system of ligaments, including the medial and lateral collateral ligaments, the sesamoidal ligaments, and the intersesamoidal ligament. The first MPJ functions primarily in the sagittal plane to provide the 65° to 75° of dorsiflexion required for normal ambulation. In propulsion, the hallux needs to be stabilized against the ground to act as rigid lever for push-off. This is accomplished by the long and short flexors and the abductor hallucis. The sesamoids displace distally to allow the metatarsal to plantarflex, while the joint itself dorsiflexes.[14]

The calcaneus and talus make up the rearfoot. Although the calcaneus bears one-half of the body's weight, the talus serves as the foot's attachment point to the leg. The subtalar joint, which is actually three separate articulations between these two bones, allows for pronation and supination of the foot. The division of the midfoot and rearfoot is at the midtarsal joint, which is a functional unit made up of the calcaneal-cuboid and the talar-navicular joints. It also allows for pronation and supination. The plantar fascia, or aponeurosis, arises from the medial and lateral tubercles of the calcaneus. It is made up of medial, central, and lateral bands and inserts distally to both the skin and the flexor tendon sheaths. It serves to support the longitudinal arch.[15] The ankle joint is stabilized by the components of the deltoid ligament medially, the anterior talofibular and calcaneofibular ligaments laterally, and the posterior talofibular ligament posteriorly (Figures 6–1 and 6–2).

Motion of the foot and ankle is achieved by both intrinsic and extrinsic musculature. The foot itself has four layers of plantar intrinsic muscles. From superficial to deep these layers are as follows:

Layer 1: abductor hallucis, flexor digitorum brevis, and abductor digiti minimi

Layer 2: quadratus plantaris and lumbricales

Layer 3: adductor hallucis, flexor hallucis brevis, and flexor digiti minimi

Layer 4: dorsal and plantar interossei

The extrinsic muscles of the foot are divided into four groups on the basis of the compartment of the leg where they originate. The anterior group is made up of tibialis anterior, extensor digitorum longus, extensor hallucis longus, and peroneus tertius. These muscles are dorsiflexors and extensors. The superficial posterior group, also known as the triceps surae, plantarflexes the foot. Its muscles, the gastrocnemius and soleus, which together form the Achilles tendon, and the plantaris all insert into the posterior surface of the calcaneus. The deep posterior group, which also plantarflexes the foot, consists of tibialis posterior, flexor hallucis longus, and flexor digitorum longus. The tibialis posterior functions to invert the foot to slow pronation and to maintain the longitudinal arch. The lateral, or peroneal, group has two muscles, the peroneus longus and brevis. The brevis inserts into the base of the fifth metatarsal and is the major everter of the foot. The longus transverses the midfoot to insert at and plantarflex the first metatarsal.[15]

The dorsalis pedis and the posterior tibial arteries provide most of the foot's blood supply. The dorsalis pedis artery may be absent in up to 15% of the population, and many of these individuals may have a dorsal peroneal artery. Innervation of the foot is provided by branches of the peroneal and tibial nerves that arise from the division of the sciatic nerve (L4–S3). The exception to this is the saphenous nerve, which is a branch of the femoral nerve (L2–L4). The tibial nerve splits into the medial and lateral plantar nerves distal to the ankle after it passes through the tarsal tunnel. These nerves provide both motor and sensory innervation to the plantar aspect of the foot. The peroneal nerve has three component branches: the deep and superficial branches and the sural nerve. The superficial branch innervates the dorsal aspect of the foot, whereas the deep branch supplies the first interspace. The sural nerve provides sensory innervation to the lateral foot and ankle. The saphenous nerve innervates the medial aspect of the foot, including the first MPJ.

BIOMECHANICAL CONSIDERATIONS

In general, the foot can be classified as neutral, flat, or cavus. Each foot type lends itself to a unique set of injuries and treatment considerations. Although these classifications may help the sports medicine practitioner to diagnose and treat foot and ankle injuries, they should be used judiciously.

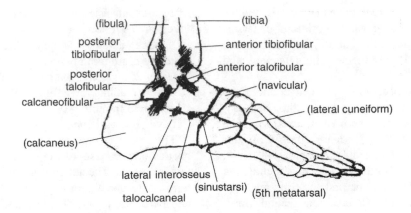

Figure 6–1 Lateral Ankle Ligaments. (Bones labeled in parentheses.) Illustration by Cheryl Burr, ATC.

Flat or pronated feet are also known as hypermobile feet. They may be congenital or traumatic in origin. The hypermobility is caused by increased subtalar and midtarsal joint range of motion that results from ligamentous laxity, anatomical malalignment, or biomechanical dysfunction. Athletes with hyperpronated feet often experience injuries associated with overuse such as tendinitis or injuries that result from excessive torque.

Cavus, or high-arched feet, generally have limited pronation and, as a result, decreased shock absorption. Cavus feet often have associated hammertoe deformities and an anterior displacement of the forefoot plantar fat pad. As a result, metatarsal and sesamoid injuries are more common in this foot type. In addition, because most cavus feet display a higher degree of rearfoot varus, lateral ankle injuries are also more common.[15]

Foot pain is not uncommon in athletes. Some types of sports predispose athletes to pain and injury in certain areas

of the lower extremities. Runners frequently have toe and foot symptoms. Ballet dancers often complain of foot and ankle pain resulting from overuse and trauma to the ankle and the tarsal-metatarsal joints. Martial artists and soccer players who rely on persistent direct contact to the foot complain of injuries to the soft tissues and bony structures of the foot and ankle joints. Stress fractures of the foot are also common and will be discussed in another section of this chapter.

HALLUX VALGUS

Moderate and severe hallux valgus can result in a painful bunion. This is a common problem in women of all ages. A previous study of a population of children revealed an incidence of hallux valgus in 36% of children ages 6 through 18, with 75% of that population studied being female.[16] The causes of hallux valgus include heredity, poor biomechanics,

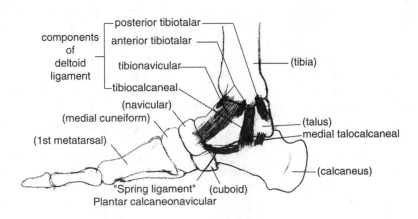

Figure 6–2 Medial Ankle Ligaments. (Bones labeled in parentheses.) Illustration by Cheryl Burr, ATC.

and poorly fitting shoes. Women have been noted to have this pathological condition to a greater degree than men. In athletes, hallux valgus has been associated with abnormal pronation of the subtalar joint.[17,18]

The athlete who has a bunion usually has a swollen, red, painful joint, and an obvious deformity (bunion) is noted at the first metatarsal head. Pain is reported with pressure, weight bearing, in shoes with a narrow forefoot, and sometimes at rest. Bullae can develop in the surrounding skin areas; both superficial and deep soft tissue infections can occasionally result. Clinical evaluation of hallux valgus can be performed by palpation of the medial and plantar aspects of the first metatarsal head at the junction with the first phalangeal joint. Pain is usually elicited on palpation and with movement. Radiological evaluation is a necessary tool to evaluate bone and joint integrity and determine the stage of the deformity. In addition, when evaluating a female athlete with foot pain, a complete history of the type of shoes worn for competition, training, and recreation should be obtained. It is also helpful for the athlete to bring her athletic and daily shoes into the office for inspection. Many clues can be attained by observing the wear pattern of the shoes and the location of calluses on the soles of the feet. Furthermore, the clinician can note the presence or absence of a supportive heel counter metatarsal pads, arch support, and the appropriateness of shoe type and size needed for a specific sport.

Treatment

Treatment of hallux valgus can be conservative or may involve surgery.[19,20] The classic treatment includes relative rest, ice, anti-inflammatory medications, and shoes with a wide toe box. Conservative management also includes physical therapy with modalities such as ultrasound, phonophoresis, fluidotherapy, and paraffin. Furthermore, abductor hallucis longus and intrinsic muscle strengthening and stretching are important in the rehabilitative process.

Orthoses are frequently used to treat hallux valgus by restoring the normal biomechanics and relieving direct stress to the area. Custom-molded orthoses may be rigid or semi-rigid and can be modified with first ray cutouts and metatarsal pads. Because women's dress shoes differ greatly from their athletic shoes, female patients may require two pairs of orthoses: one for their athletic shoes and one for their dress shoes. Other devices such as bunion shields and night splints may also help. Proper shoe wear in athletes with hallux valgus should include a wide toe box to accommodate widening of the forefoot area and to decrease direct pressure to the area. The clinician must also consider the shoes the athlete wears when not training; traditionally, these have narrow toe boxes and high heels. Shoes with high heels tend to transfer most of the pressure into the forefoot area and should be avoided.

Surgical intervention may be indicated for persistent complaints despite conservative treatment (see Table 6–1). Osteotomies performed at the distal aspect of the first metatarsal (the Chevron/Austin or Mitchell operation) have not been found to be advantageous to sprinters or dancers who plan to return to high-level performance[21(p 342)] and the Chevron/Austin procedure not to significantly alter foot mechanics in the middle- and long-distance runners.[20] Common risks of bunion surgery include lesser metatarsalgia or secondary metatarsal stress fracture, recurrence of the bunion, and first MPJ stiffness.

HALLUX RIGIDUS

Hallux limitus and rigidus is another injury that commonly affects the first MPJ of female athletes. Hallux limitus is the loss of normal range of motion of the first MPJ. The term "rigidus" is used when there is no range of motion (ROM) at the joint. This pathological condition occurs as a result of repetitive trauma to the first metatarsal joint in athletes involved in running, jumping, aerobics, and ballet dancing. It is usually associated with a metatarsus primus elevatus but may also be due to direct trauma. Hallux rigidus/limitus usually is seen as stiffness and pain at the first metatarsal joint. The athlete is usually concerned with the decrease in ROM, because it prevents her from achieving adequate push-off during running or performing.

On physical examination, there is pain on the dorsal aspect of the first metatarsal joint, with decreased and painful ROM (normal ROM of the joint is 65° of dorsiflexion). Crepitus is often present. Usually, a palpable bony protuberance is present on the dorsal aspect of the first MPJ. X-ray films can assist in confirming the diagnosis, and degenerative changes such as uneven joint space narrowing, subchondral sclerosis and cyst formation, and osteophytic proliferation are usually noted.

Conservative treatment includes oral anti-inflammatory medication, in addition to deep-heating modalities and active assistive and active ROM exercises. Mobilization of the joint with distraction and gliding of the joint is helpful in restoring proper functioning of the joint. Strengthening of the intrinsic muscles in the foot and hallux flexors and extensors is of paramount importance to the rehabilitation process. Correction of abnormal gait patterns can decrease the progression of the condition. A shoe with a large toe box will help to accommodate the bony protuberance. Shoe modifications such as stiff soles, metatarsal bars, and orthoses may decrease the load on the first MPJ during gait.

If conservative treatment is not successful, surgical intervention may become necessary for the athlete to return to her optimal level of activity. Surgical treatment includes excision of the osteophytes (cheilectomy) with chondroplasty, wedge osteotomy of the proximal phalanx, or metatarsal

Table 6–1 Evaluation and Treatment Hallux of Valgus (Bunion)

Painless Hallux Valgus	*Painful Hallux Valgus*

Evaluate shoes
  wide toe box
    adequate arch support
Consider orthotics
NSAIDs, ice
Strengthening/stretching exercises
	NSAIDs, ice
	Open-toed shoes/wide toe box
	Orthoses
	Physical therapy
	  modalities
	  strengthen
	  stretch
	  joint mobilization
	Consider surgery
	Consider changing sport or activity

osteotomies. Older athletes or those with severe deformity may require joint destructive procedures such as Keller arthroplasty. Implant arthroplasty of the first MPJ has a high complication rate and is controversial. The postsurgical rehabilitation should begin as soon as 1 day after the surgery, with edema control and gentle passive ROM as tolerated by the athlete.

Most athletes are able to return to prior levels of athletic performance after conservative therapy and after surgical intervention.

NAIL PATHOLOGY

Pathological conditions of the nail occur commonly in women involved in ballet dance and sports such as downhill skiing, skating, soccer, and running. Several common types of nail pathological conditions exist, including transverse ridging, bleeding around the nail bed, hematomas, and in-grown toenails.

The mechanism of injury varies depending on the activities in which the athlete is involved. A very important part of ballet dancing involves dancing on one's toes, en pointe (Figure 6–3), or dancing on the ball of the foot, demipointe (Figure 6–4). For male and female dancers, rising onto the ball of the foot (demipointe) is routinely choreographed. For selected female dancers the en-pointe position is frequently required. Because dancers practice the en-pointe position several hours during the course of the day, there is repetitive force placed on the great toe and its nail bed. As a result of the en-pointe position, the nail on the great toe can become hypertrophied, thickened, and discolored. Subungual hematoma and ingrown toenails may also occur as a result of the en-pointe position. Transverse ridging of the nail occurs as a result of repetitive trauma in sports such as soccer as a result of repetitive kicking.[22] Bleeding may occur in instances in which abrasions or loosening of the nails occurs.

The athlete usually presents with a complaint of changes in her nails, either insidious in cases of hypertrophy, ingrown

toenails, or ridging, or acute in cases of bleeding or hema-toma. Treatment of the ingrown toenail typically consists of wedge resection of the toenail. The treatment of other nail pathological conditions includes protection of the area to prevent infection and further trauma. Protective taping and soft wrapping can be helpful as well.

Prevention of some of these nail injuries can include instruction in proper technique in running, kicking, and dancing, taping, and use of protective shoes. Pointe shoes often wear out; therefore, the dancer must be able to evaluate the integrity of the shank along with the soft toe pad material. Dancers often have different shoes for performance and practice. Furthermore, runners should be aware of the quality of support and toe box size in their running shoes. Appropriate nail care, including proper hygiene and cutting the nail to follow the contour of the pulp, helps to prevent damage to nails.

SESAMOIDITIS

Sesamoiditis is common in athletes and dancers who perform activities that require repetitive weight bearing on the metatarsal head. Pain occurs in the area of the first metatarsal head. Runners often report increased pain during the push-off phase of the running cycle.

Predisposing factors to sesamoiditis include hyper-pronation, a common occurrence in female athletes. In addition, metatarsus varus and hallux valgus can contribute to these injuries. A mechanism of injury is direct trauma to the ball of the foot such as an improper landing. This can occur in dancers, leading to pain commonly in the medial sesamoid.[23(p 289)] In addition, soccer players and distance runners, who tend to hyperpronate their feet while running, develop sesamoid disorders. Sesamoids are also subject to stress fractures.[24(p 291)]

On physical examination, there is pain in the plantar aspect of the first metatarsal joint and pain on passive dorsi-flexion of the great toe. Diagnosis of sesamoiditis can be

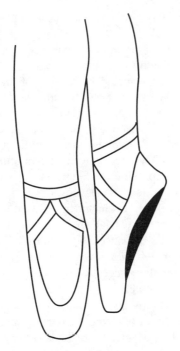

Figure 6–3 En-Pointe Dance Position in Ballet.

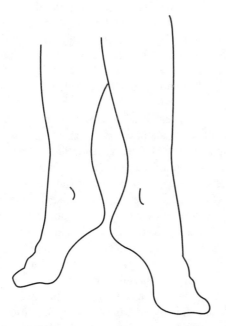

Figure 6–4 Demipointe Dance Position in Ballet.

made with the assistance of plain radiographs, tomograms, and bone scans. Fractures can sometimes be noted on X-ray examination, whereas stress fractures can be seen on short

tau inversion recovery (STIR) sequence magnetic resonance imaging (MRI) and bone scans.

Treatment of sesamoiditis includes refraining from jumping and sport activity for approximately 2 to 3 weeks. During this period, treatment should include relative rest, anti-inflammatory medication, and therapeutic modalities. Physical therapy, including strengthening of the intrinsic muscles and the flexor pollicis longus and brevis muscles, can improve and prevent symptoms. When the athlete is ready to return to her regular activities, orthoses are recommended. This is especially necessary for the runner and should be continued for a minimum of 6 months or indefinitely if symptoms return. Surgical intervention such as sesamoidectomies are rarely performed on athletes, because the biomechanical alignment may be affected, causing decreased performance ability.

PLANTAR FASCIITIS

The plantar fascia is the thick fan-shaped aponeurosis in the plantar aspect of the foot, which originates at the medial calcaneal tuberosity and inserts at the metatarsal phalangeal joints of the heads of the first to fifth metatarsals. The term "plantar fasciitis" is used to describe tenderness in the plantar fascia in the midfoot and hindfoot, including the medial longitudinal arch.

The injury and pain mechanism is usually repetitive stress to the plantar fascia, as seen in running and jumping. This is seen frequently in female runners, as they tend to be midfoot strikers.[6] Sprinters, because they mostly run on their toes, often complain of plantar fascial pain resulting from prolonged and repetitive stretching of the fascia. Microtears develop in the area, followed by inflammatory changes. In addition, a combination of biomechanical factors such as equinus, pes planus or unsupported pes cavus, and direct repetitive pressure also contributes to plantar fascial irritation. Inadequately cushioned, supported, or wornout shoes can also result in plantar fasciitis.

The presenting complaint is either heel or midfoot pain of insidious onset. The athlete usually reports pain on arising in the morning or on standing after a prolonged period of sitting. The pain usually subsides during the course of the day or as the athlete warms up. Those athletes involved in sports that require running, jumping, and prolonged weight bearing usually complain of pain after those activities. Calcaneal spurs can develop as a response to repetitive stress to the plantar fascia at the attachment on the calcaneus.

History is most important in making the diagnosis. On physical examination, pain can be elicited by palpation of the midfoot, in the area of the medial longitudinal arch, and at the base of the calcaneus. X-ray may reveal calcaneal spurring. In unremitting cases, MRI is more specific than bone scan in differentiating other sources of pain, such as calcaneal stress fractures.[24]

Treatment includes relative resting of the area and icing to decrease pain and inflammation. Nonsteroidal anti-inflammatory drugs (NSAIDs); physical therapy, including ultrasound or phonophoresis; and aggressive stretching of the plantar fascia and plantar flexors are also recommended. Pool running can allow the athlete to maintain cardiovascular fitness while decreasing the repetitive stress placed on the plantar fascia. Strengthening the intrinsic muscles of the foot helps to prevent recurrence of symptoms. The use of a dorsiflexion splint at night is an effective adjunct to the therapeutic process. Injection of corticosteroids into the area of maximal tenderness in the plantar fascia can decrease pain acutely; however, care must be taken to avoid injection directly into the fascia to decrease the risk of rupture. Repeat injections are *not* recommended.

The athlete may require a custom-molded orthotic with arches to support the weakened fascia. Heel cups are sometimes prescribed to relieve initial pain of impact but are not recommended long term. In rare instances of failure of conservative treatment, surgical release can be considered but is controversial.

POSTERIOR TIBIAL TENDINITIS

Posterior tibial tendinitis (PTT) is common in female athletes who are involved in sports that require agility, running, and cutting activities, such as basketball, soccer, and tennis. Hyperpronation of the foot and ankle with repetitive stress to the medial foot is the injury mechanism.[21] Female runners, who pronate their feet, are predisposed to PTT, along with dancers, who roll in as a compensation for inability to turn out at the hip, which causes eversion of the hindfoot and forced pronation of the midfoot and the forefoot (Figure 6–5). In addition, active supination as a compensatory mechanism to relieve pain from plantar fasciitis or a heel spur may result in PTT. In females older than 40, rupture of the posterior tibial tendon is more prevalent than in younger female athletes.[18]

Careful history and dynamic evaluation will help in diagnosing PTT. This evaluation may include observation of the athlete during walking or running exercises or, in the case of a dancer, observation of dance techniques such as turning out. On examination there is usually tenderness over the posterior tibial tendon, or with pain on palpation of an accessory navicular in the area of attachment of the posterior tibial tendon. Passive ankle pronation and abduction result in pain. Resisted plantarflexion and ankle inversion can also reproduce the pain.

The presence of an accessory navicular on plain X-ray with evidence of sclerotic bony changes supports the diagnosis. MRI can differentiate tenosynovitis from tendinitis, because tenosynovitis reveals normal tendon surrounded by fluid within the tendon sheath.[25] Tendinitis reveals abnormal signal within the tendon on T2 sequence. Clinical history can differentiate tendinitis from partial tear.

Treatment of PTT includes the use of the rest, ice, compression, and elevation (RICE) principle. Physical therapy, including ultrasound, phonophoresis, stretching, and strengthening of the posterior tibial musculotendinous unit, is recommended. Orthotics to correct hyperpronation or excessive supination will result in significant relief in associated symptoms. Improving the biomechanics of foot strike during running or athletic maneuvers is essential in preventing recurrence of PTT. This includes footwear and orthotics evaluation to improve subtalar alignment. In addition, correct techniques used by dancers to decrease hyperpronation of the foot and ankle can assist in preventing PTT. Taping the foot-ankle complex to decrease pronation can be adjunctive to training the athlete in proper techniques. If the pain persists despite therapy and orthotics, corticosteroid injection may be helpful in relieving the pain; surgical intervention is not usually warranted to treat this entity.

ANKLE INJURIES

Athletes on a whole experience ankle injuries to a greater degree than injuries to any other joint.[26] Lateral ankle sprains are most common in both genders, with basketball, volleyball, and soccer described as sports with significantly higher rates.[26] Most athletes have a history of inversion of the ankle. Hickey et al[27] found that the most frequent diagnosis of young elite female basketball players was ankle sprains.

The anatomical sites of these sprains are most commonly seen in the lateral ligament complex; most frequently anterior talofibula followed by the calcaneofibular ligament and the posterior talofibular ligament. Landing with inverted and plantarflexed feet is a common mechanism of injury to team sports players and dancers. In gymnasts, the mechanism tends to occur during a turn or when landing from a jump with an inverted ankle. Recurrent inversions result in chronic laxity and decreased proprioception, along with recurrent ankle sprains.[28] Furthermore, studies have shown that decreased movement or malalignment of the subtalar joint can lead to instability of the ankle joint.[29] The mechanism of injury to the medial ligaments is usually landing onto an excessively pronated foot. Injury to the deltoid ligament often occurs with eversion injuries or with severe lateral ankle sprains. Obtaining a history, including the mechanism of injury, aids in the diagnosis of ankle sprain type and severity.

The clinical presentation differs according to the grade of the sprain. There are four grades of ankle sprains. A grade I sprain is a mild ankle sprain, with microscopic tear of

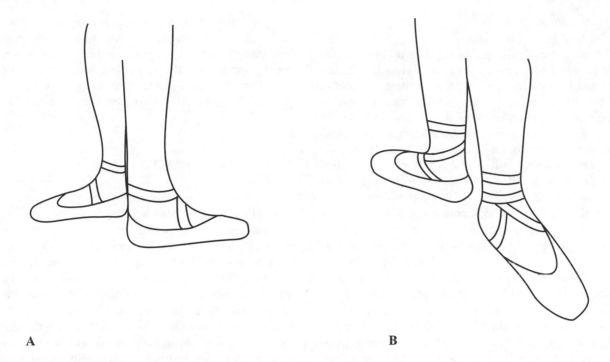

A   B

Figure 6–5 A, Turn-Out; Requires Hip External Rotation for Proper Foot Alignment; **B,** Turnout with Pronation To Compensate for Improper Hip Rotation.

the anterior talofibular ligament (ATFL) or calcaneofibular ligament. There is usually mild lateral edema, tenderness on palpation, and negative anterior drawer test and negative talar tilt test. The athlete is usually able to bear weight on the affected ankle.

In grade II sprains, there is evidence of laxity with inversion and positive anterior drawer test. The athlete usually reports difficulty weight bearing on the affected ankle. In grade IIIa sprains, there is a complete tear in the ATFL, usually involving the ankle capsule. There is usually marked edema in the lateral malleolar area and the peritendinous area of the Achilles tendon. There is usually a positive anterior drawer test with a negative talar tilt test (normal talar tilt is 3°–23°).

In a grade III sprain, there is rotatory laxity. As in a grade II sprain, the athlete usually reports difficulty weight bearing on the affected ankle. The talar tilt test is positive in a grade IIIb and IIIc sprain. Grade IV sprains are associated with fracture of the talus or the fibula.

Radiological studies should be used when appropriate. Leddy et al[30] performed a prospective study to evaluate the Ottawa ankle rules and introduced the new Buffalo rules.[30–32] These rules provide a systematic approach to determining

necessity of X-ray studies in clinical evaluation of ankle pain in trauma.

MRI can confirm ligamentous damage in ankle sprains. The MR criteria for diagnosis of acute ligament tears include discontinuity, detachment, or thickening of the ligament associated with increased intraligamentous signal intensity on T2-weighted images;[33] the absence of soft tissue suggests chronic tear. The deltoid ligaments are not as easily seen on MRI as the lateral ligaments. Arthrography can also aid in the assessment of ankle ligament integrity and aids in the diagnosis of osteochondral injury by improving the conspicuity of articular cartilage defect.

Differential Diagnosis of Lateral Ankle Pain

- Anterior talofibular ligament sprain
- Distal fibular fracture
- Base of 5th metatarsal fracture
- Fracture of the talar dome
- Peroneal tendinitis, tears, subluxation
- Sinus tarsi syndrome

Clinical Guideline

Treatment of Ankle Sprains

The treatment of ankle sprains depends on the grade of injury and whether the injury is acute or chronic. In acute grade I and II ankle injuries, RICE is instituted soon after the injury. With the exception of severe grade III and IV sprains, a rehabilitation program should begin as soon as possible. Early mobilization of the ankle joint is recommended to avoid untoward effects such as adhesions, synovitis, and reflex sympathetic dystrophy. The physical therapy program should include modalities such as ROM and isometrics progressing to active strengthening. The integrity of the subtalar joint should be evaluated as a biomechanical cause of the instability. If a biomechanical abnormality is present in the subtalar joint, it should be corrected as part of the rehabilitation process. Rubber tubing or elastic bands are frequently included in the home program to increase eversion and inversion strength (Figure 6–6). In addition, antigravity strengthening of the ankle muscles is recommended. Proprioceptive retraining is essential to prevent recurrent sprains.[28,34] A randomized controlled study of female athletes by Wedderkopp et al[35] revealed a significant decrease in traumatic and overuse ankle injuries in female athletes with the use of the ankle disk. Also known as balance or wobble boards, these are now commonly used to aid in restoring proprioceptive feedback and improving balance skills (Figure 6–7).

Agility drills, plyometric, and total body coordination exercises help the athlete to return to her previous level of activities. When strength and proprioception approach 90% of the uninvolved extremity, the athlete can return to her preinjury activity level. The athlete's readiness for return to play can be evaluated by the hop test. The athlete should be able to hop on one leg 10 times with the same height and cadence of the uninvolved leg. Proprioception can be tested by having the athlete stand on one leg with the arms abducted and eyes closed. On returning to play, the athlete may benefit from prophylactic taping, lace-up canvas, or other ankle support. The use of taping and bracing of ankles has been shown to decrease the incidence of reinjury among athletes.[36]

Treatment of medial sprains includes the basic treatment of lateral ankle sprains; however, recovery may be longer than that of the lateral ankle sprains and more challenging. Surgical intervention is usually considered when there is significant rotatory laxity as seen in grade III and IV ankle sprains. The goal of the surgery is restoration of ligament length to decrease the likelihood of long-term disability.[37] The postsurgical rehabilitation program is similar to that of the grade I and II sprains. Athletes with inadequately treated recurrent ankle sprains can develop osteoarthritic changes in the ankle joint.

Sinus tarsi syndrome is another complication of lateral ankle sprain. The athlete complains of pain after running or jumping. On physical examination there is pain on pronation of the ankle and palpation of the area of the sinus tarsi. Injection of a local anesthetic into the sinus tarsi can aid in differentiating sinus tarsi syndrome from subtalar dysfunction.

ACHILLES TENDINITIS

The likelihood of Achilles tendinitis developing in women is less than in men.[38] Still, Achilles tendinitis is seen in dancers with poor pointe techniques, in runners who wear shoes with soft heel counters and low heels, and court or field athletes who change training speed and distance rapidly. In addition, hill training can cause microtears and inflammation in the area of the Achilles tendon. Athletes with ankle equinus are prone to develop Achilles tendinitis.

Achilles tendinitis usually is initially seen with complaints of pain and swelling in the proximal aspect of the Achilles tendon. The onset can be insidious or acute after repetitive or rapid dorsiflexion of the ankle, in activities such as running, or while practicing the en-pointe or demipointe positions.

Diagnosis is made by eliciting pain on palpation of the area medial to the tendon insertion, as well as the proximal aspect of the calcaneus. Ultrasonography or MRI can help to determine evidence of a tear of the tendons or calcification in the peritendinous area in recurrent tenosynovitis. MRI is sensitive and specific for determining partial from complete tear.

Treatment of Achilles tendinitis includes relative rest, cryotherapy, NSAIDs, gentle progressive stretching of the Achilles tendon, and strengthening of the gastroc-soleus complex. In athletes with severe pain on ambulation and during sport activity, immobilization in a posterior splint set in slight plantar flexion decreases the stress on the Achilles tendon (this should be used for approximately 10 days). More practical recommendations include wearing heel cups or slightly high-heeled shoes. Physical modalities such as ultrasound help to increase the elasticity in the tendon, allowing for increased stretching and ROM of the tendon. Furthermore, the use of phonophoresis or iontophoresis assists in locally decreasing the inflammatory process. Corticosteroids and local anesthetic could be injected into the peritendinous area, but the practitioner should be aware that injection into the tendon can predispose the athlete to Achilles rupture. In cases of recurrent tendinitis, which is refractory to conservative management, surgical intervention may be warranted. Surgery is indicated if there is focal degeneration in the tendon on MRI; however, adhesions may result and become problematic.

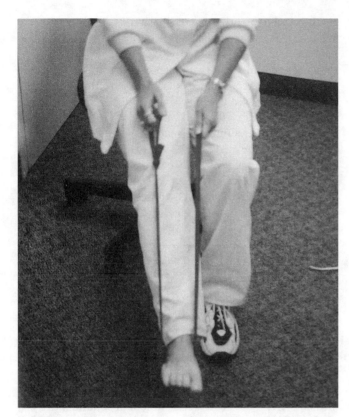

Figure 6–6 The Use of Elastic Bands To Increase Ankle Strength and Stability.

Achilles rupture is also reportedly uncommon in the female athlete. It occurs more frequently in middle-aged and older men[39(p 75)] or others after oral or injectable corticosteroids. Quinolone antibiotics are also associated with rupture. Achilles rupture usually occurs in the area of least blood supply in the tendon, approximately 2 to 6 cm proximal to its insertion to the calcaneus. The athlete usually has a history of running and/or cutting with rapidly accelerating or decelerating movements before Achilles tear (also known as "tennis leg"). The rupture occurs because of an increase in eccentric loading of the gastrocnemius complex. The athlete usually reports hearing or feeling a "pop." She may further report inability to push-off during walking and running.

A positive Thompson test assists in diagnosing Achilles rupture. The clinician performs this test by squeezing the gastrocnemius with the athlete in a prone position and the foot unsupported. Plantar flexion should occur if tendon is intact. There may, however, be false-negative results if there is an incomplete tear. Complete tears usually result in a muscular deformity seen in the posterior calf. In addition, the athlete will have difficulty performing toe raises on the involved extremity. There may be an increase in passive ankle dorsiflexion in comparison with the uninvolved ankle. MRI using a long relaxation time sequence is sensitive and specific for detecting

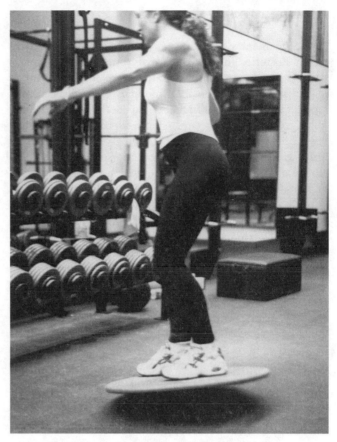

Figure 6–7 The Use of a Balance or Wobble Board To Increase Proprioception, Ankle Stability, Strength, and Balance.

a ruptured Achilles tendon.[25] Treatment of Achilles rupture includes casting and/or surgical repair; immobilization in a cast in plantar flexion for the initial 4 weeks with progression to neutral is standard treatment.

Rehabilitation after complete healing takes place should focus on ROM and strengthening exercises. Sports-specific exercises should not begin until 12 weeks after the repair. Jumping and agility drills should not begin until pain-free full ROM and strength have been achieved. When returning to play, heel cups and ankle supports may be helpful to prevent further strain on the tendon.

Signs of Achilles Rupture

- History of "pop" during activity
- (+) Thompson's test
- Excessive passive ankle dorsiflexion
- Prominent defect at the gastroc-calcaneal junction

Clinical Guideline

IMPINGEMENT SYNDROMES

Impingement syndromes can be both posterior and anterior. Posterior impingement syndromes are common in dancers, gymnasts, and ice skaters, who load their ankles in the plantar flexed position routinely. The mechanism is thought to be excessive plantar flexion of the ankle. Posterior impingement usually occurs in those dancers who frequently use the en-pointe position. In addition, extreme plantar flexion in kicking sports such as soccer is also a risk factor. The athlete usually presents with a complaint of insidious onset of pain during activities requiring plantar flexion.

In the posterior impingement syndrome, inflammation of the soft tissues can include capsular structures and tendinous structures (flexor hallucis longus or Achilles tendons). More commonly, bony structures such as osteophytes in the os trigonum, a large posterior process of the talus, or the posterior lip of the tibia can be impinged. The inflammatory process is exacerbated by repetitive plantarflexion of the ankle joint. Synovitis is often present in the affected joint.

On physical examination, there is pain on forced passive plantar flexion of the ankle. In addition, there may be pain on palpation of the area of the posterolateral aspect of the ankle joint in the area of the peroneal tendon posterior to the lateral malleolus. Diagnosis can be confirmed by injection of 1 to 2 mL of 1% lidocaine into the posterolateral ankle area. If the pain subsides, posterior impingement is likely the diagnosis. To detect osteophytes on the posterior lip of the tibia, a lateral X-ray film is recommended. MRI can reveal impingement of the flexor hallucis longus tendon and or retinacular tear or subluxation of the peroneal tendon.

Treatment of posterior impingement includes restriction of extreme plantar flexion, NSAIDs, and ice during the acute phase. Ankle orthoses can help to decrease impingement and pain. Local corticosteroid injection has also been helpful for local anti-inflammatory treatment. The physical therapy program should include modalities such as heat or ice, strengthening, soft tissue massage, proprioception, balancing, and ankle stabilizing exercises. Manual traction can also be beneficial. The athlete can return to her regular activities when she is pain free with usually aggravating positions. Initially, taping or bracing is recommended during dance performances or during sports activities to improve proprioceptive feedback.[28] In cases in which symptoms persist despite conservative treatment, surgery may be indicated. The aim of the surgery is to remove the impinged soft tissue or bony structure that causes the symptoms.

Anterior impingement syndrome is an injury similar to posterior impingement syndrome, except that it occurs with extreme dorsiflexion of the ankle joint. This entity is seen in ballet dancers,[40(p 895)] whose performances require use of the demi-plie position and competitive athletes such as softball catchers who spend extended periods squatting with the ankle in a dorsiflexed position. Soccer players also develop anterior impingement secondary to traction osteophytes.[41(p 56)] Soft tissue impingement includes scarred synovium and fragments of anterior tibiofibular ligament. Bony impingement may be caused by osteophytes on the anterior lip of the tibia and the neck of the talus.[42]

On physical examination, patients have pain on forced dorsiflexion of the ankle and may have tenderness and edema over the anterior talocrural line. The diagnosis and treatment are similar to posterior impingement; arthroscopy may be necessary to remove loose bony or soft tissue fragments.

MORTON'S NEUROMA

The most common clinical nerve entrapment syndrome in active and athletic women is Morton's neuroma, described as occurring 7–10 times more frequently in women than men.[41(p 54)] Most often causing focal pain between the second and third intermetatarsal space, neuromas can also occur at other locations. The athlete initially complains of focal or radiating pain with impact while wearing shoes, and can be symptom free while barefoot or in sandals or soft shoes. The pain can be sharp, burning, or radiating. Paresthesias can also be present. Associated foot structural abnormalities can include tight Achilles, hallux valgus, hallux rigidus, and pes cavus. On exam, focal tenderness is often present, or pain can be reproduced with forefoot squeezing or extending the affected metatarsals.

Conservative treatment of Morton's neuromas can be challenging, as it may require a reduction in athletic activity involving forefoot impact. Reinforcing the importance of wearing both athletic and dress shoes with a wide toe box and loose lacing cannot be overlooked. Physical therapy with soft tissue mobilization, corticosteroid iontophoresis or phonophoreses, ultrasound, and an emphasis on intrinsic muscle strengthening and stretching tight Achilles and calf musculature can be effective for symptom relief. Accommodating for cavus feet with arch support and insertion of metatarsal pads either separately or with full foot orthotics will relieve traction on the metatarsal heads and relieve pressure on the intermetatarsal space. Focal corticosteroid injection can be curative; occasionally surgical release or excision may be necessary.

PERONEAL NERVE INJURIES

Peroneal nerve injuries can develop in athletes who experience recurrent ankle inversion injuries.[43,44(p 83)] Because female athletes have been shown to have repetitive ankle sprains, the treating physician should be aware of peroneal nerve injury as a possible complication. The athlete may have a footdrop of acute onset. There may be pain with weakness of the ankle or ankle weakness alone. Footdrop can also result from compression of the nerve within the anterior compartment of the leg, as seen in chronic compartment syndrome. If a compartment syndrome is present, the athlete usually reports increased symptoms after a period of exercising and relief after resting. Diagnosis of compartment syndrome is made by measuring pre-exercise and postexercise compartmental pressure. In chronic compartment syndrome, usually both resting and exercising pressures are elevated with a delay in returning to pre-exercise levels (greater than 5–10 minutes).[45(p 286)]

Treatment of acute compartment syndrome is fasciotomy. A recent study of young female athletes who underwent fasciotomy suggested that they did not respond as favorably as their male counterparts.[46(p 27)] The exact reason for the differences in response to fasciotomy was not conclusive in that investigation. Fasciotomy is not recommended for chronic exercise-induced compartment syndrome.

Rehabilitation of Nerve Impingements

- Pressure relief in shoes
- Soft tissue mobilization
- Biomechanical analysis and correction
- Orthotics to support surrounding structures
- Modalities to decrease edema
- Strengthening surrounding muscles
- Patient evaluation to avoid impingement

Clinical Guideline

TARSAL TUNNEL SYNDROME

Tarsal tunnel syndrome describes the impingement of the tibial nerve in the fibro-osseous tunnel in the medial wall of the calcaneus. The nerve may also be impinged at the distal aspect of the gastrocnemius, the middle aspect of the medial tibia, or medial to the navicular bone, as in joggers foot. Entrapment of either the medial or lateral branches of this nerve must also be considered.

On physical examination, there is usually a positive Tinel's test over the area of the tarsal tunnel. There may be decreased sensation in the area of the great toe or along the medial or lateral longitudinal arch, corresponding to the area of impingement.

In persistent cases of nerve compromise, electrodiagnostic studies are recommended to rule out additional factors, including neuropathy, lumbar radiculopathy, tumors, or compression at the fibular head. Radiological studies can determine presence of a local or poximal tumor. The

nerve impingement could be due to a neuropraxia or an axonotmesis. Electrodiagnostic studies can determine the extent of the nerve damage and can solidify the diagnosis. Treatment can vary depending on the area of compression of the nerve. Surgical intervention can be helpful in some cases of peripheral nerve damage in the foot.[47] Conservative management includes pressure relief and modalities, along with soft tissue mobilization.

STRESS FRACTURES

Stress fractures result from repetitive submaximal trauma, which results in overloading otherwise healthy bones, or from episodic normal loading of abnormal bones. Female soldiers tend to experience greater numbers of metatarsal fractures than their male counterparts.[48] Athletes involved in high-impact activities including dance are more likely to sustain these fractures.

It has been proposed that because women tend to have smaller and narrower bones than men, there is less ability to absorb and redistribute the repetitive ground reaction forces during running, thus causing them to have stress fractures at a higher rate. The metatarsals are commonly involved in stress fractures in the foot.[49,50] In ballet dancers, there is commonly a spiral fracture in the proximal aspect of the fifth metatarsal bone, otherwise known as "dancers fracture."[51](This differs from the Jones fracture, which is an acute injury of the metaphyseal region of the fifth metatarsal.) Runners who wear poorly cushioned shoes or train on unforgiving terrain may also develop stress fractures. Athletes with increased pronation of the foot are more susceptible to tarsometatarsal fractures.[52] Although uncommon, fractures in the tarsal navicular have been reported, as well as the talus, in the female athletic population.

The presenting complaint is usually pain of insidious onset, with weight bearing, usually during a running or jumping activity. The pain usually subsides with rest. It is rare that the athlete pinpoints the specific precipitating event. When taking the history, the physician should focus on any change in the athletes' training schedule, change in shoe wear, or failure to change running shoes for a prolonged period. It is also important to inquire about a change in the terrain used for training. History of other factors, such as menstrual, and nutritional patterns should also be assessed to evaluate risk of the female athlete triad symptoms (see Chapter 19).

On physical examination, pain can be diffused or localized to bone. Pain with ultrasound and vibratory testing can be clinically suggestive of stress fracture. Although plain films are the initial radiological method of diagnosing acute fractures, bone scans are often required for diagnosis.[53] In some cases, further evaluation such as MRI[25,49] may be necessary. The STIR sequence of the MRI depicts low signal intensity areas, indicating a fracture line with periosteal edema and marrow edema.

Treatment of stress fractures involves rest from the impact sport activity in which the athlete is involved. A rest period of approximately 6 to 8 weeks is required in most cases for adequate healing to take place. Immobilization is usually not required. Physical therapy can include icing, transcutaneous electric nerve stimulation, isometric strengthening exercises, ROM, and pool exercises. The therapy program is recommended very early in the rehabilitative process.

To prevent stress fractures, athletes during screening examinations should be thoroughly evaluated by the physician for anatomical factors that may predispose a stress fracture. Kaufman et al[54] performed a study that focused on 18- to 29-year-old Navy Seal (sea air and land) candidates. They concluded that individuals with pes planus and pes cavus have been noted to have a higher incidence of stress fractures. Because these abnormalities can include hyperpronation of the foot, orthoses should be provided for athletes as a preventive measure. In addition, the athlete who is a runner should be counseled on avoiding sudden and frequent changes in the training regimen, including the terrain and avoidance of the use of old or nonsupportive running shoes. Athletes who are exceptionally thin, have a history of an eating disorder, or menstrual disruption should also be carefully screened.

CONCLUSION

As the sports physician and other practitioners become more informed of the causes of sports injuries in women, appropriate prevention strategies can be formulated to target those areas. This type of information is helpful to athletes, trainers, and physicians, who can use this information to prevent injuries in both female and male athletes. As researchers continue to focus on the female athlete, a significant impact will be made on the overall approach to managing this population.

A comprehensive rehabilitation program is imperative to correct biomechanical abnormalities. The athlete should be made aware of the importance of strengthening and proprioceptive training, which should continue even though she may be asymptomatic. Careful follow-up by the physician can be instrumental in helping the athlete to participate in an appropriate rehabilitation program to ensure proper recovery. The responsibility of the clinician treating the injured athlete goes beyond addressing the particular presenting complaint. The effect of biomechanical factors in the proximal areas of the kinetic chain should also be considered. Once a determination is made as to the cause of the complaint, steps must be taken to address, correct, and avoid repetition of the precipitating factors. When treating female athletes, factors that affect this population should always be considered to ensure comprehensive care.

REFERENCES

1. American Academy of Orthopaedic Surgeons. Correspondence. 1999.

2. Gross RH. Foot and ankle disorders. *Adolesc Med.* 1998;9:599–609.

3. Labowitz JM, Schweitzer ME, Larken UB, Solomon MG. Magnetic resonance imaging of ankle ligament injuries correlated with time. *J Am Podiatric Med Assoc.* 1998;88:387–393.

4. Clarke K, Buckley W. Women's injuries in collegiate sports. *Am J Sports Med.* 1980;8:187–191.

5. Young JL, Press JM. Rehabilitation of running injuries. In: Buschbacher RM, Braddom RL, eds. *Sports Medicine and Rehabilitation: A Sport Specific Approach.* Philadelphia: Hanley & Belfus; 1994:123–134.

6. Williams KR, Kavanagh PR, Ziff JL. Mechanical studies of elite female distance runners. *Int J Sports Med.* 1987;8:107–118.

7. Hunter LY. The female athlete. *Med Times.* 1981;109:48–57.

8. Hunter L. Aspects of injuries to the lower extremity unique to the female athlete. In: Nicholas JA, Hershman EB, eds. *The Lower Extremity and Spine in Sports Medicine.* St. Louis, MO: Mosby; 1986:90–111.

9. Beim G, Stone DA. Issues in the female athlete. *Orthop Clin North Am.* 1995;26:443–450.

10. Root ML, Orien WD, Weed JH, et al. *Normal and Abnormal Function of the Foot.* Los Angeles, CA: Clinical Biomechanics Corp; 1977.

11. Haycock CE, Gillette JV. Susceptibility of women athletes to injury: Myths vs. reality. *JAMA.* 1976;236:163–165.

12. Valmassy RL. *Clinical Biomechanics of the Lower Extremities.* St. Louis, MO: Mosby; 1996.

13. Trevino SG, Kodros S. Controversies in tarsometatarsal injuries. *Orthop Clin North Am.* 1995;26:229–237.

14. Lichiak JE. Hallux limitus in the athlete. *Clin Podiatr Med Surg.* 1997;14:407–426.

15. Subotnick SI. *Sports Medicine of the Lower Extremity.* 2nd ed. New York: Churchill Livingstone; 1999.

16. Yu G, Landers P, Lu K, et al. Foot and ankle disorders in children. In: Devalentines S, ed. *Juvenile and Adolescent Hallux Abducto Valgus Deformity.* New York: Churchill Livingstone; 1992:369–405.

17. Mann RA. *Biomechanics of the Foot and Ankle: Surgery of the Foot.* 5th ed. St. Louis, MO: Mosby; 1986.

18. Frey C, Sherriff MS. Tendon injuries about the ankle and athletes. *Clinics of Sports Med.* 1998;7:103–118.

19. Mann RA. Great toe disorders. In: Baxter DE, ed. *The Foot and Ankle in Sport.* St. Louis, MO: Mosby; 1995:245–258.

20. Lillich JS, Baxter DE. Bunionectomies and related surgery in the elite female and middle distance runner. *Am J Sports Med.* 1982;14:491–493.

21. Mitchell L. Foot and ankle injuries in the female athlete. In: Baxter DE. *The Foot and Ankle in Sports.* St. Louis, MO: Mosby; 1995:337–345.

22. Tanzi EL, Scher RK. Managing common nail disturbances in active patients and athletes. *Phys Sportsmed.* 1999;27:35–47.

23. Quirk R. Ballet injuries. In: Baxter DE, ed. *The Foot and Ankle in Sport.* St. Louis, MO: Mosby; 1995:287–303.

24. Kerr R, Forrester DM, Kingston S. Magnetic resonance imaging of foot and ankle trauma. *Orthop Clin North Am*. 1990;21:591–601.

25. Bencardino J. MR imaging of the foot and ankle. *Magn Reson Imaging*. 1999;7:131–149.

26. Garrick JG, Requa RK. The epidemiology of foot and ankle injuries in sports. *Clin in Podiatric Med Surg*. 1989;6:629–637.

27. Hickey GJ, Fricker PA, McDonald WA. Injuries of young elite female basketball players over a six-year period. *Clin J Sports Med*. 1997;7:252–256.

28. Rozzi SL, Lephart SM, Sterner R, Kuligowske L. Balance training for persons with functionally unstable ankles. *J Orthop Sports Phys Ther*. 1999;29:478–486.

29. Clanton TO, Porter DA. Primary care of foot and ankle injuries in the athlete. *Clin Sports Med*. 1997;16:435–466.

30. Leddy JJ, Smolinsky RJ, Lawrence J, Snyder JC, Priore RC. Prospective evaluation of the Ottawa Ankle Rules in a university sports medicine center with a modification to increase specificity for identifying malleolar fractures. *Am J Sports Med*. 1998;26:158–165.

33. Markert RJ, Walley ME, Guttman TG, Mehta R. A pooled analysis of the Ottawa ankle rules used on adults in the ED. *Am J Emerg Med*. 1998;16:564–567.

34. Steill IG, Greenberg GH, McKnight RD, Nair RC, et al. A study to develop clinical decision rules for the use of radiography in acute ankle injuries. *Ann Emerg Med*. 1992;21:384–390.

33. Schneck CD, Mesgarzadeh M, Bondakapour A. MR imaging of most commonly injured ankle ligaments Part 2. Ligament injuries. *Radiology*. 1992;184:507–512.

34. Briner WW Jr, Dacmar L. Common injuries in volleyball-mechanism of injury prevention and rehabilitation. *Sports Med*. 1997;24:419–429.

35. Wedderkopp N, Kaltoft M, Lungaard B, Rosenthal M, Froberg K. Injuries in young female players in European team handball. *Scand J Med Sci Sports*. 1997;7:342–347.

36. Cox JS. Surgical and non-surgical treatment of acute ankle sprains. *Clin Orthop*. 1985;198:118.

37. Gould N, Seligson D, Gassman J. Early and late repair of lateral ligaments of the ankle. *Foot Ankle*. 1980;1:84–89.

38. Soma CA, Mandelbaum BR. Achilles tendon disorders. *Clin Sports Med*. 1994;13:811–823.

39. Clain MR. The Achilles tendon. In: Baxter DE, ed. *The Foot and Ankle in Sports*. St. Louis, MO: Mosby; 1995:71–80.

40. Parkes JC II, Hamilton WG, Patterson AH, et al. The anterior impingement syndrome of the ankle. *J Trauma*. 1980;20:895–898.

41. Arendt EA, Tetiz CC. The lower extremities. In: Teitz CC, ed. *The Female Athlete*. Rosemont, IL: The American Academy of Orthopaedic Surgeons; 1997:45–62.

42. Basset FH III, et al. Talar impingement by the anterior inferior tibio-fibular ligament: A cause of chronic pain in the ankle after inversion sprain. *Am J Bone Joint Surg*. 1990;72:55–59.

43. Daghino W, Pasquadi M, Faletti C. Superficial peroneal nerve entrapment in young athlete: The diagnostic contribution of magnetic resonance imaging. *J Foot Ankle Surg*. 1997;36:170–172.

44. Kleinrensink GJ, Dijkstraa PDS, Boerboom AL, et al. Reduced motor conduction velocity of the peroneal nerve caused by inversion damage—a prospective longitudinal study. *Acta Orthop Scand*. 1996;67:83.

45. Reid DC. Exercise induced leg pain. In: Reid DC. *Sports Injury Assessment and Rehabilitation*. New York: Churchill Livingstone; 1992:269–300.

46. Micheli LJ, et al. Surgical treatment of chronic lower leg compartment syndrome in young female athletes. *Am J Sports Med*. 1999;27:197–201.

47. Barrett JP, Downey MS, Hillstrom HJ. Retrospective analysis of neuropraxia and axonotmesis injuries of select peripheral nerves of the foot and ankle and their conservative and surgical treatment (external neurolysis and neurectomy). *J Foot Ankle Surg*. 1999;38:185–193.

48. Protzman R, Griffis G. Stress fractures in men and women undergoing military training. *J Bone Joint Surg*. 1977;59:825.

49. Brukner P, Bennell K. Stress fractures in female athletes. Diagnosis, management and rehabilitation. *Sports Med*. 1997;24:65–71.

50. Monteleone GP. Stress fractures in the athlete. *Orthop Clin North Am*. 1995;24:423–432.

51. Hardaker WT. Foot and ankle injuries in classical ballet dancers. *Orthop Clin North Am*. 1989;20:21–27.

52. McBryde AM. Stress fractures. In: Baxter DE, ed. *The Foot and Ankle in Sport*. St. Louis: Mosby Yearbook; 1995:81–93.

53. Groshar D, Gorenbeg M, Ben-Haim S, Jerusalmi J, Liberson A. Lower extremity scintigraphy: The foot and ankle. *Semin Nucl Med*. 1998;28:62–67.

54. Kaufman KR, Brodine SK, Shafer RA, Johnson CW, Cullison TR. The effect of foot structure and range of motion on musculoskeletal overuse injuries. *Am J Sports Med*. 1999;27:585–593.

CHAPTER 7

Clinical Biomechanics—An Approach to Understanding Chronic Injuries in Women Athletes

Maxine Weyant

The evaluation and management of acute injuries in women athletes are usually straightforward. Generally, the mechanism of injury is fairly obvious, the examination required is usually limited to one region, and most acute injuries are self-limited conditions, requiring only rest and supportive care. With chronic injuries, in contrast, the causative mechanisms and perpetuating factors are often less apparent. The condition may have evolved over time as a consequence of or compensation for functional deficits proximal or distal to the site of symptoms, and the site of the presenting complaint may not be the site of the primary source of the problem.

When evaluating an injury, most physicians tend to hasten to reach the "diagnosis" and treat the "lesion." But the process of unraveling the causes and features of a chronic injury requires a more forensic approach to collecting all the data and allowing the story to unfold. Patients with chronic injuries usually have a combination of multiple functional deficits such as faulty alignment, muscle imbalances, congenital or acquired structural asymmetries, motion restrictions, laxity, or instability. Rather than asking: "What's the diagnosis?" we should ask: "What are all the functional deficits in the individual?" For if we simply treat the "lesion" on the magnetic resonance imaging scan or other imaging study, such as a rotator cuff tear or a lumbar disc herniation, we will not have corrected the underlying causes, and we will have failed to truly address the patient's problem.

Most chronic injuries are caused or perpetuated by mechanical factors.

Clinical Point

EVALUATION AND MANAGEMENT OF CHRONIC INJURIES

Most chronic injuries are caused or perpetuated by mechanical factors. The evaluation and management of these conditions require a more in-depth approach with a careful exploration of the history and a biomechanical approach to examination of the patient. This requires looking at all the functional linkages in the kinetic chain both statically and dynamically, assessing not only individual joint motion and stability but also how joints function together under static weight-bearing loads and during gait and other pertinent activities.

This biomechanical approach is especially important in evaluating women athletes because they tend to have a greater incidence of structural and alignment problems, greater flexibility, and ligamentous laxity, resulting in greater excursion of motion at all links in the kinetic chain. This can accelerate wear at joint surfaces and increase the risk of developing overuse injuries.

The patient history should carefully explore the nature of prior injuries, inquiring about actual symptoms rather than relying on presumptive diagnoses arrived at by the patient or the prior clinician. Clinicians should inquire about all activities (sport-specific, occupational, and recreational activities) and the conditions under which they are carried out (fatigue, stressful competition, faulty technique, poor posture, ground surfaces, equipment/ergonomic issues) to understand the functional demands of the athlete. We need to consider the possibility that training errors or conflicting concurrent activities have contributed to the chronicity of the injury.

We may need to recruit the assistance of trainers and coaches to look at an athlete's performance technique during sports and conditioning activities. Videotaped assessment is a valuable tool for analyzing athletic performance, not only because it can be used to improve technique but also because it can reduce the likelihood of injuries related to faulty technique. A vast array of motion assessment tools is available, including sophisticated computer software programs that use force plates, pressure pads, or slow-motion videography to analyze gait, jumping, swimming, and other activities. Many athletic trainers also incorporate a few functional static and dynamic tests as part of the preseason assessment of athletes to uncover areas of weakness and identify motion abnormalities that can be corrected by interventions such as physical therapy, gait retraining, or specific strength training.[1]

TREATMENT

After identifying the functional deficits, treatment of chronic, recalcitrant conditions is aimed at correcting the functional deficits, trying to optimize efficient postures and movement patterns, restoring normal physiological loads and motion at the joints, and re-establishing normal muscle length-tension relationships. The types of treatment used are, of course, specific to the deficits identified but may include joint or soft tissue mobilization, selective stretching and strengthening of certain muscles, functional closed kinetic chain training, proprioceptive and agility training, gait retraining, core trunk strengthening, and lumbopelvic stabilization. Treatment strategies may also incorporate the application of braces, tape, splints, or other techniques that unload the injured part, custom modification of equipment or shoes, and the use of devices such as heel lifts, wedges, arch supports, and custom orthoses. Custom orthoses (orthotics), in skilled hands, can not only support the arch but can also be made with posting and other features that can correct proximal dysfunctions such as excessive femoral internal rotation, lumbar lordosis, and can help unload the medial compartment of the knee. They can also include features that splint or protect injuries such as turf toe, sesamoiditis, or posterior tibial tendonitis. Orthotics can also improve stride efficiency in runners by providing a more functional lever to push off against.[2-4]

Rehabilitation of the competitive athlete should focus not only on resolution of symptoms and restoration of function, but also on maintenance of normal function during off-season training and prehabilitation before and during subsequent preseason training to prevent reinjury.

UNDERSTANDING FUNCTIONAL RELATIONSHIPS

Evaluating the patient from a biomechanical perspective requires not only a thorough understanding of functional anatomy but also an understanding of the functional relationships throughout the kinetic chain. Muscles function best within specific length-tension parameters. Contracting a muscle from a lengthened position not only produces a less effective contraction but can also cause injury to that muscle, especially if the load is significant or the action repetitive.[5] Similarly, joints function best within normal physiological ranges of motion and load-bearing forces. When loads are applied repeatedly at end range, within a restricted range of motion, or under conditions of faulty alignment, the direction and distribution of loading forces will cause accelerated wear of the joint surface. Instability or hypermobility will also increase joint surface shear. Articulations such as the hip and the lumbar vertebral segment are not designed to function at end range[6] and are extremely vulnerable to the effects of muscle imbalances such as tight hip flexors, adductors, or weak abdominal muscles or hamstrings.

Types of Functional Deficits

A woman with a chronic injury will usually have multiple functional deficits, some of which may be structural lesions such as rigid pes cavus, structural genu varum, congenital scoliosis, or tibial torsion; some may be consequences of a more proximal or distal problem, such as patellofemoral syndrome, resulting from excessive pronation at the subtalar joint or from wide femoral Q-angles. Other functional deficits may be functional compensations for another problem, such as functional pes planus or genu valgum occurring as a compensation for a leg length discrepancy on the side of the longer limb.

When evaluating patients from a biomechanical perspective, one should regard their functional deficits as points on a timeline and view these patients as if they are on a potential continuum of progressive dysfunction with respect to their likelihood for further progression of symptoms, further deterioration of joint surfaces, and further degradation of function proximally and distally. Identifying the causative and perpetuating factors and correcting the functional deficits, where possible, allow us not only to treat symptoms but to promote restoration of function and to potentially intervene in the process of further deterioration, thereby reducing the likelihood of injuries (both chronic and acute traumatic injuries) elsewhere along the kinetic chain.

Patients with chronic biomechanical injuries should be viewed as if they are on a timeline, on a potential continuum of progressive dysfunction. By promoting restoration of function, rather than simply treating the symptoms, we may be able to intervene in the process of further deterioration.

Clinical Point

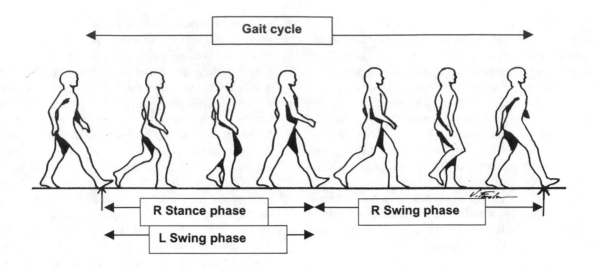

Figure 7–1 One Gait Cycle is the Interval between Initial Contact (Heel Strike) of One Foot and the Subsequent Initial Contact on the Same Foot. Each extremity passes through a stance phase and a swing phase. Traditional gait nomenclature breaks down the components of stance phase into specific actions: heel strike, foot flat, midstance, heel off, and toe off; and the swing phase components are acceleration, midswing, and deceleration. RLA terminology, developed at the Gait Laboratory of the Rancho Los Amigos Medical Center in California, describes the components of gait as events or time intervals rather than specific motions or actions. RLA components of stance phase are initial contact, loading response, midstance, terminal stance, and preswing; and swing phase consists of initial swing, midswing, and terminal swing.

The two sets of terms are not entirely interchangeable since not all the terms occur exactly during the same interval of time. Nonetheless, both systems are still widely used, and the terms are often intermingled in articles and texts, often even in the same sentence. Toe off is still the most useful term to describe forefoot motion in terminal stance, but the loading response (RLA) is a much more accurate term to describe the interval where subtalar motion occurs.

To illustrate the importance of these concepts, consider the impact of abnormal forefoot motion and other functional deficits, discussed in the following. Although a comprehensive review of biomechanics and functional relationships is well beyond the scope of this chapter, a discussion highlighting some of the most common areas of dysfunction may help illuminate how certain injury patterns evolve. Refer to Figure 7–1 for a summary of phases in gait.

Forefoot Motion

A lack of dorsiflexion at the forefoot will result in loss of propulsive forces of the foot during the toe-off portion of gait.[7,8] Over time, compensatory and substitution patterns emerge with a shortened stride length, perhaps a flexed-knee gait or forefoot abduction, and diminished hip extension at toe-off, along with lumbar sidebending motions to assist

propulsion and initiate swing phase. Eventually, hip extension may diminish altogether, and an individual will need to compensate by flexing the lumbar spine and leaning the upper torso forward. The abnormal distribution of loads to the lumbar spine and hips may result in accelerated degeneration, with the individual ultimately having the postural and gait patterns typical of most patients with lumbar spondyloarthropathy, with hip flexion contractures, a flattened lumbar curve, and a shortened stride pattern in which the legs remain out in front of the trunk throughout the gait cycle.

Foot Pronation/Supination

Normal subtalar pronation in gait is initiated just after heel strike and continues during the first 25% of the stance phase as body weight is shifted onto the foot. During pronation, the

Exhibit 7–1 Common Causes of Overpronation

Pes planus—congenital or acquired (ligamentous, tendon, joint, or neurological injury)
Forefoot varus
Chronic posterior tibial tendon dysfunction
Compensation for longer limb length

subtalar joint unlocks motion at the tarsal bones, allowing the foot to adapt to the supporting surface.[5(pp 379–418)] As the foot starts to push off, it resupinates, allowing for a more effective propulsion at toe-off. A coupled linkage exists between the subtalar joint and the tibia; for every degree of subtalar pronation that occurs, the tibia internally rotates 1°. Despite this coupling, however, the actual relationship of pronation to tibial rotation depends on what happens further distally in the foot and up the limb.

Excessive foot pronation may occur for a variety of reasons: as a consequence of posterior tibial tendon dysfunction, a structural forefoot varus, or as a compensation for a limb length discrepancy as a means of shortening the longer limb (a potential underlying cause for chronic unilateral plantar fasciitis) (see Exhibit 7–1). The resultant excessive internal rotation of the tibia can have an impact on all the surrounding structures. The patellar tendon insertion moves medially, increasing the likelihood of patellofemoral tracking problems. The strain on posterior tibialis can be significant, resulting in muscle injury, tendinitis, and gradual elongation of the tendon over time, rendering it completely dysfunctional, allowing the foot to pronate even more. Chronic Achilles tendonitis may sometimes result from excessive pronation causing traction along the medial side of the Achilles tendon. Excessive forefoot pronation sustained through toe-off is often a result of a structural forefoot varus, but it can also be associated with excessive femoral internal rotation at toe-off, causing eccentric firing of the hip external rotators after toe-off, resulting in chronic gluteal and lateral hip pain and weakness of the hip external rotators. The underlying cause may come from the foot, the hip, or elsewhere and, once again, may result from a structural abnormality, a compensation for, or consequence of another abnormality.

A rigid cavus foot that cannot pronate may result in a number of abnormalities as well. The foot may remain supinated throughout stance phase, or it may compensate by pronating in late midstance or at toe-off, causing a rotatory motion further up the limb. The presence of calluses beneath the hallux can sometimes reveal a shear pattern suggestive of this gait pattern. A rigid supinated foot often generates greater impact forces up the limb and can often be associated with insertional Achilles tendinitis. It may also contribute to varus angulation at the knee, causing increased wear at the medial compartment of the knee.

Limb Length Discrepancy

For decades, physicians have been taught that a limb length discrepancy (LLD) of less than 2 cm is not "clinically significant." Indeed, many practitioners believe that an LLD less than 3 cm is insignificant.[9] Although it may serve as a useful guideline for intervention when fracture healing has resulted in limb shortening or when stimulation of bone growth at the fracture site has resulted in lengthening, the prevailing opinion regarding what constitutes a "clinically significant" LLD may not be based on a realistic or systematic assessment of long-term functional outcomes. The prevailing opinion is based on the assumption that an LLD of 1 to 2 cm can be "absorbed" by the soft tissues of the body, both posturally and dynamically.[9] Although that assumption may be true, the functional adaptations to limb length differences will result in changes in muscle length-tension relationships and limb alignment, will have an impact on joint mechanics and load distribution, and can result in premature degeneration of articular surfaces and other structures.[5,6,10,11]

The body compensates for an LLD by trying to shorten the long limb and/or lengthen the shorter limb, depending on how much compensation is required and how well the various links in the chain can accommodate.[5(pp 448–495),7] The capacity to accommodate at various links in the chain depends on other structural factors such as alignment and flexibility, as well as factors such as age and gender. A woman athlete may have more soft tissue compliance and joint flexibility than a male athlete, but her structural features of a wider pelvis, larger Q angles, and lower extremity alignment tendencies may result in greater excursion of motion at some or all of the functional linkages, especially the pelvis and spine. A child has a narrower pelvis, greater overall flexibility and soft tissue compliance, and is less likely to be impacted by a structural asymmetry than an adult. Older adults have less soft tissue elasticity, less joint range of motion, and their stiffer limbs may transmit more of the asymmetry to their spine, making them more likely to have back pain with walking. Their lumbar discs and narrower joint spaces will be less tolerant of rotational and shear forces caused by the asymmetry.

The most typical compensations on the side of the long limb include pronating the foot and positioning the knee in slight valgus, which effectively shortens the limb (see Figure 7–2). On the short side, a typical compensation is to supinate the foot to lengthen the limb. A person with a rigid cavus foot cannot effectively pronate on the side of the long limb. Instead, she may compensate by standing with greater genu varum or recurvatum on the long side and may exhibit a varus thrust at the knee in gait during midstance.

An LLD also results in compensations elsewhere in the kinetic chain. The pelvis is tilted laterally, and the lumbar

- **Foot:** pronation of long limb, supination of short limb.

- **Knee:** genu valgum, varum, or recurvatum.

- **Hip:** adduction of long limb, abduction of short limb.

- **Pelvis:** Lateral tilt upward on long side, posterior ilial rotation on long side, anterior ilial rotation on short side.

- **Lumbar spine:** functional scoliosis, apex of curve toward short limb side, rotation of lower vertebrae toward short side.

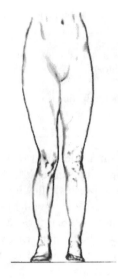

Figure 7–2 Functional Compensations for Limb Length Discrepancy (LLD).

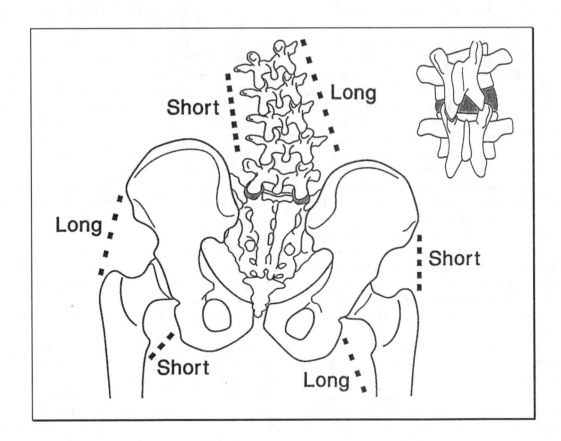

Figure 7–3 The Effects of Leg Length Asymmetry on Muscle Length, the Lumbar Spine, and Pelvis. In response to a leg length asymmetry, muscles will structurally lengthen or shorten to adapt to their position. A leg length asymmetry causes a pelvic tilt, a lateral flexion of the lumbar spine, and rotation of the lower lumbar segments toward the short side, resulting in asymmetrical compressive and torsional forces at the lumbar discs and facet joints.

spine is side-bent, with the apex of the curve pointing to the side of short limb.[11-14] The pelvic tilt not only results in lateral flexion of the lumbar spine, but it also rotates the lower lumbar segments toward the short side, resulting in asymmetric compressive and torsional forces across the lumbar discs and facet joints, especially during gait. In general, on the side of the long limb, the ilium will be rotated slightly posteriorly and the opposite ilium anteriorly, further increasing the rotatory motion at the lumbosacral junction during gait. At the hips, the long limb will be adducted relative to the pelvis and the short limb abducted (see Figure 7–3).

These asymmetries can be observed during the gait cycle. In swing phase, the pelvis usually tilts upward on the long side (hip hike) and the hip abducts and the femur swings out laterally (circumduction).[5(p 490)] As the short limb completes its swing phase, the pelvis may tilt down on the short side (hip drop). In stance phase, as the long limb proceeds through toe-off, the hip may internally rotate, which can fatigue the lateral hip and gluteal muscles by causing them to fire eccentrically.

Before we proclaim that a minor LLD is clinically insignificant, we should ask ourselves how much room there is in the lumbar facet joints and how much asymmetry of load distribution can be absorbed over time at the lumbar discs or the articular surfaces of the hips and knees.

Clinical Point

The repetitive mechanical stress on the soft tissues and skeleton associated with a mild LLD may be an underlying cause of unilateral overuse injuries such as stress fractures,[15] chronic posterolateral hip pain, trochanteric bursitis, iliotibial band tendinitis, and unilateral pain at the lumbosacral junction. The asymmetrical loads and shear forces may result in earlier breakdown of lumbar discs, facet joints, and articular surfaces of the hips and knees.

When contemplating whether an LLD as small as 0.5 to 1.5 cm is significant in an athlete with a chronic injury, we should consider the functional demands of the individual. A car slightly out of alignment may seem to do fine at low speeds and short distances, but when driven at 60 mph for longer durations, the minor malalignment will become more apparent and cause greater mechanical wear. Similarly, a long-distance runner, or any athlete who engages in repetitive impact activities, is more likely to be affected by a mild LLD than an individual who is sedentary or who engages in lower impact multiplanar activities.

When viewing the patient as if on a timeline or continuum of progressive dysfunction, the potential impact of asymmetry becomes more apparent. A 60-year-old who needs a unilateral total hip arthroplasty may have had a lifetime of asymmetrical loads from a mild LLD, but this etiological

Exhibit 7–2 Functional Deficits Associated with Chronic Shoulder Dysfunction

Postural dysfunctions
Forward head, upper cervical extension, lower cervical flexion
Thoracic kyphosis, scapular protraction, internal rotation of humerus
Lumbar lordosis (standing), lumbar flexion (sitting)

Muscle imbalances
Overactive upper trapezius, deltoids
Tight pecs, anterior scalenes
Weak scapular stabilizers, posterior rotator cuff muscles
Abnormal scapulohumeral rhythm
Capsular laxity or instability
Poor lumbopelvic/core trunk stability

factor will likely neither be apparent nor considered at the time of symptom presentation. Before we proclaim that a minor LLD is clinically insignificant, we should ask ourselves how much room there is in the lumbar facet joints and how much asymmetry of load distribution can be absorbed over time at the lumbar discs or the articular surfaces of the hips and knees.

Functional Relationships at the Shoulder and Spine

Chronic shoulder pain is one of the most difficult and frustrating conditions to treat. Whether the diagnosis is tendinitis, impingement syndrome, partial rotator cuff tear, adhesive capsulitis, instability, or degenerative joint disease, all patients with chronic shoulder problems have multiple functional deficits and abnormal patterns of muscle recruitment (see Exhibit 7–2).[16]

Their shoulder motions are often initiated and dominated by the upper trapezius and deltoid. The pain may cause them to splint, tonically contacting the upper trapezius, levator, rhomboids, and cervical muscles. Many patients with chronic shoulder injuries have cervical and thoracic postural dysfunction as a causative and perpetuating factor, which, in turn, is sustained by muscle guarding and substitution patterns as an adaptation to the injury.

Shoulder dysfunction can often result in more distal injuries.[17] Chronic tennis elbow has often been linked to excessive motions at the wrist, especially during the backhand swing in tennis. Often, however, the excessive wrist motion is a compensation for a weakness or other dysfunction at the shoulder.

The shoulder may also become injured as a result of functional deficits occurring more proximally, especially in the trunk and pelvis. In tennis and throwing sports, the pelvis acts as a differential in the transfer of ground reactive forces from the lower extremities to the trunk and shoulder.[18] If

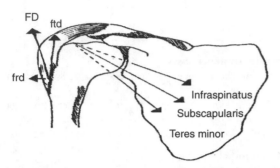

Figure 7–4 Summation of Forces at the Shoulder. Although the primary action of the deltoid is to abduct the arm, the summation of vectors of the action of the deltoid leads to elevation of the humeral head, an action offset by the depression forces coming from infraspinatus, subscapularis, and teres minor.

this transfer of energy at the pelvis is inefficient because of excessive motion or insufficient strength, the athlete may compensate at the shoulder, increasing the likelihood of injury.

The shoulder is essentially an unstable joint, requiring a delicate balance between stability and mobility. The muscles of the rotator cuff maintain stability by imparting a compressive force when they contract collectively and by the dynamic restraint each individual muscle imparts as it opposes motion initiated by other muscles.[5(pp 207–239),19]

The rotator cuff also opposes elevation of the humeral head by the deltoid. Although we think of the deltoid as a prime mover in flexion and abduction, the summation of forces resulting from contraction of the deltoid results in superior translation of the humeral head (see Figure 7–4).

This upward motion is normally opposed by downward and compressive forces that result from the co-contraction of subscapularis, teres minor, and infraspinatus. During abduction, teres minor and infraspinatus also externally rotate the humerus slightly, which keeps the greater tuberosity from impacting the acromion.

Normal rotator cuff function depends on optimal scapular positioning and scapular stability, which, in turn, depends on effective functioning of the scapular stabilizers—lower and middle trapezius, serratus anterior, rhomboids, all of which are impacted by the position of the spine.

Cervical and thoracic posture affects scapular positioning and shoulder function in a number of ways. Thoracic flexion causes elevation, abduction, and protraction of the scapula, lengthening the muscles of the back and posterior shoulder and rendering them less effective at stabilizing the scapula, the glenohumeral joint, and opposing the action of the deltoid. The typical chronic postural dysfunction of thoracic kyphosis, forward placement of the head, upper-cervical extension, results in tonically shortened chest, anterior scalene, and upper trapezius muscles, lengthened and weakened

thoracic extensors and upper cervical flexors, posterior cuff muscles, and scapular stabilizers. The forward head posture, over time, creates excessive wear on the midcervical discs and posterior elements, which can result in impairment of shoulder function as a result of referred pain patterns and neuromuscular weakness.[20] Excessive lumbar lordosis can also have an impact on shoulder function by impairing dynamic trunk stability.

Impingement syndrome[21] (see Chapter 2) is an excellent example of the interactions of multiple dysfunctions within and outside the shoulder. Impingement is often caused by or associated with postural dysfunction (especially in women), which, in turn, is made worse by guarding because of pain. Ironically, most of the functional adaptations to impingement syndrome seem to perpetuate the condition. The tonically contracted upper trapezius elevates the scapula out of the domain of the scapular stabilizers, and the overdominant deltoid elevates the humeral head, increasing the likelihood of impingement even further. The protracted position of the scapula orients the glenoid more anteriorly, which places the greater tuberosity more directly under the coracoacromial arch.[22]

Individuals with shoulder pain do not use their shoulder normally, even after the pain subsides and even during therapeutic exercise,[23] especially open kinetic chain resistance exercises. Over the years, we have come to realize that traditional tubing resistance exercises for a rotator cuff injury are like using knee extension machines for patellar tendinitis. It further loads the injured tissue and does little to restore functional patterns of muscle recruitment. Current trends in shoulder rehabilitation emphasize restoring scapular stability, correcting postural dysfunctions, and re-establishing normal patterns of muscle recruitment before proceeding with selective strengthening that uses traditional open chain resistance exercises. Under closed kinetic chain conditions, the limb is axially loaded as the rotator cuff and surrounding muscles are engaged submaximally within a pain-free arc, allowing normal patterns of co-contraction, muscle recruitment, and proprioception to be reestablished.[24,25]

Dynamic Trunk Stability

The pelvis, lumbar spine, and trunk musculature work in harmony to provide upright erect posture, to provide a column of torque to transfer kinetic energy to the upper body, and to provide a stable base of support for upper body motions. These structures also work together to maintain balance and dynamic stability of the body during collisions and other provocative challenges to balance and equilibrium. The integrity of this system as a functional linkage is affected by muscle imbalances at the hips, the pelvis, the lumbar spine, and abdomen, and by postural dysfunctions throughout the spine. Recent trends in rehabilitation of athletic injuries incorporate upright dynamic trunk and lumbopelvic stability training to improve the quality and efficiency of motion and strength at all the links in the kinetic chain.[26] These principles are especially important in the rehabilitation of all women with shoulder and back problems, not just athletes.

THE KINETIC CHAIN—TRAINING THE FEMALE ATHLETE FOR INJURY PREVENTION

Athletic performance requires a balance of stability and mobility, strength and flexibility. Activities such as running require distal stability and proximal mobility. Activities such as throwing and swinging a bat or racket require proximal stability and distal mobility. Motion can occur in the frontal, sagittal, or transverse plane or in a combination of planes (see Figure 7–5). Walking and running propel the body forward through the sagittal plane, whereas speedskating and rollerblading use mostly frontal plane motions to propel the body through the sagittal plane. Discus throwing and swinging a racket use motion in the transverse plane.

Most serious sports injuries such as anterior cruciate ligament tears occur during transverse plane motions, yet most strength and conditioning programs train primarily in sagittal and frontal planes.

Clinical Point

Most sports are multiplanar activities and require balance and stability in all three planes. The transverse plane poses the greatest challenge to balance and dynamic stability, and it is important to realize that many, if not most, serious sports injuries such as anterior cruciate ligament tears occur during transverse plane motions, yet most strength and conditioning programs use predominantly sagittal and frontal plane motions.[18] A current trend not only in rehabilitation but also in athletic training is to incorporate dynamic transverse plane activities into the training program with an emphasis on improving dynamic core trunk stability.[26] This results in more efficient energy transfer across the pelvis to the upper body, a greater ability to withstand collisions and other challenges to stability, and a reduction in the potential for injury. This type of training is especially important for women athletes in sports such as basketball, where the risk of serious injuries can be high and the ability to throw rapidly and with accuracy is highly dependent on lumbopelvic stability and trunk strength.

Another trend especially significant for women athletes is the addition of agility drills, combining speed, footwork, and multiplanar motions to enhance proprioception and neuromuscular conditioning with the goal of reducing the potential for injuries. These are especially important in basketball, soccer, volleyball, and martial arts.

Along with these trends is an emphasis at eliminating nonfunctional activities such as the supine bench press, which excludes the spine and trunk from the activity, does

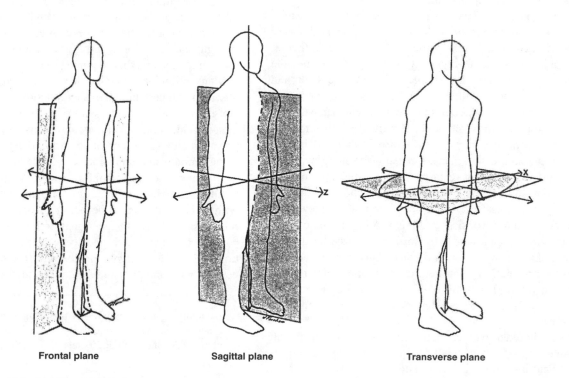

Frontal plane　　　　**Sagittal plane**　　　　**Transverse plane**

Figure 7–5 Three Principal Planes of Motion.

little to replicate any functional activity, and may actually increase the likelihood of injury such as osteolysis of the distal clavicle[27] compared with other, more functional, strengthening exercises, such as various types of pushups or upper body plyometric training.

From a biomechanical perspective, it becomes easy to understand why women may be more vulnerable to certain patterns of injury and overuse syndromes, perhaps even why women may not be able to generate as much force as men during certain activities such as throwing.

Women tend to have greater ligamentous laxity than men, and when this occurs at all links in the kinetic chain, the cumulative impact on stability, efficiency of gait, and the ability to generate torque across the pelvis is significant.

Clinical Point

Women have a lower center of gravity and appear to have less upper body strength and overall muscle bulk than men. The greater width of the pelvis in women results in larger Q angles, more frontal plane motion at the pelvis, and less mechanically efficient alignment from the ground up, as well as a more flexible, less efficient linkage from the pelvis to the lumbar spine and trunk.[28] Women also tend to have greater ligamentous laxity than men, and when this occurs at all links in the kinetic chain, the cumulative impact on stability, efficiency of gait, and the ability to generate torque across the pelvis is significant.

Women may also have a greater tendency to have certain postural dysfunctions such as thoracic kyphosis, forward head, and excessive lumbar lordosis (Exhibit 7–3). Whether this tendency is due to ligamentous laxity throughout the spine and shoulders, less upper body muscle bulk and strength, more pelvic tilt, or other factors such as a postural adaptation to breast or abdominal weight is unclear, but these postural patterns do contribute significantly to impaired strength and the tendency for injury in all individuals, both in athletics and in the workplace. A person who stands with pes planus, genu valgum or recurvatum, and especially femoral anteversion (all of which are common functional deficits in women) tends to settle into a stance that tilts the pelvis and increases lumbar lordosis, resulting also in a posterior shift of the thoracic spine and a forward shift of the head. This posture also results in forward placement of the shoulders, scapular protraction, lengthening of the posterior rotator cuff, and internal rotation of the humerus, increasing the likelihood of shoulder dysfunction, impingement, and overuse injuries.

In the shoulder, women also seem to have greater overall capsular laxity[29] and may have a greater likelihood of multidirectional instability[30] as a baseline characteristic, without any history of trauma or symptoms. This can increase the

Exhibit 7–3 Functional Deficits Prevalent among Female Athletes

---

Postural: cervicothoracic, scapulothoracic, lumbopelvic

Alignment: scoliosis, large Q angles, femoral anteversion, genu valgum, rearfoot valgus, pes planus, forefoot varus

Musculoligamentous: ligamentous laxity, poor dynamic core trunk/lumbopelvic stability, weak scapular stabilizers, overactive upper trapezius (both in initiating arm motion and as a compensation for proximal/distal weaknesses)

---

likelihood of tendon and ligament injury, because these structures are stretched to end range during motions such as a tennis backhand, overhand throwing, swimming strokes, rowing, and paddling a kayak. In aquatic sports such as swimming, water ballet, and kayaking/rowing, the resistance of the water creates a leverage torque on the proximal humerus, which, if unopposed by a firm capsule, a strong rotator cuff, and a well-stabilized scapula, can stretch the capsule and ligaments of the glenohumeral joint into end range, further increasing the amount of joint laxity and the likelihood of impingement and rotator cuff muscle injury.

Interestingly, the addition of upper body plyometric training[31] and closed chain shoulder strengthening exercises to the preseason strength and conditioning programs of female synchronized swimmers[29] was found to not only reduce the incidence of shoulder injuries and symptoms but also tended to eliminate their clinical findings of multidirectional instability and capsular laxity. Future trends will likely include a broader incorporation of these types of exercises into the strength and conditioning programs of all women in aquatic sports and in sports that require upper body strength.

Many clinicians who work with female athletes have observed that certain patterns of functional deficits (such as "miserable malalignment syndrome," weak trunk musculature, shoulder and postural dysfunctions) appear to be more prevalent among women or seem to be especially common among certain subpopulations of female athletes. It is hoped that in the not too distant future, more data will be available to allow clinicians, athletic trainers, and others who work with female athletes to be better informed regarding the relationship of certain functional deficits to specific injury patterns among women and to determine which interventions will most effectively prevent injuries, improve athletic performance, and prevent further decline of function.

By applying the principles of restoring and maintaining function, we may be able to intervene in the progressive physical decline of all our female patients.

Clinical Point

THE KINETIC CHAIN—IMPROVING AND MAINTAINING FUNCTION FOR ALL WOMEN

As previously discussed, it is helpful to view patients with chronic injuries on a potential timeline or continuum of progressive dysfunction. When we look at female athletes not only as individuals with a chronic injury but also as women who wish to remain athletically and recreationally active, the importance of restoring function and correcting postural deficits becomes clear. Likewise, if we view all our female patients, athletes and nonathletes, as individuals who wish to remain vital and functional as long as possible, we can see the value of restoring and maintaining function as a preventive strategy. By encouraging aerobic exercise, weight control, and exercises that help maintain core trunk stability and upright posture, we may be able to intervene in the progressive physical decline of women over time by reducing the incidence and morbidity of osteoporosis, the severity of degenerative processes in the spine and elsewhere, the incidence of falls in the elderly, and the consequences of deconditioning and inactivity.

REFERENCES

1. Gray G. *Lower Extremity Functional Profile.* Adrian, MI: Wynn Marketing; 1995.

2. Tomaro JE, Butterfield SL. Biomechanical treatment of traumatic foot and ankle injuries with the use of foot orthotics. *J Orthop Sports Phys Ther.* 1995;21(6):373–380.

3. Nawoczenski DA, Cook TM, Saltzman CL. The effect of foot orthotics on three-dimensional kinematics of the leg and rearfoot during running. *J Orthop Sports Phys Ther.* 1995;21(6):317–327.

4. McCulloch MU, Brunt D, Vander Linden D. The effect of foot orthotics and gait velocity on lower limb kinematics and temporal events of stance. *J Orthop Sports Phys Ther.* 1993;17(1):2–10.

5. Norkin C, Levangie P. *Joint Structure and Function: A Comprehensive Analysis.* 2nd ed. Philadelphia: FA Davis; 1992.

6. Jackson R. Postural dynamics: Functional causes of low back pain. In: D'Orazio BP, ed. *Low Back Pain Handbook.* Woburn, MA: Butterworth-Heinemann; 1999:159–191.

7. Dananberg HJ. Lower extremity mechanics and their effect on lumbosacral function. *Spine: State of the Art Reviews.* 1995;9(2):389–405.

8. Glasoe WM, Yack HJ, Saltzman CL. Anatomy and biomechanics of the first ray. *Phys Ther.* 1999;79:854–859.

9. Gross RH. Leg length discrepancy in marathon runners. *Am J Sports Med.* 1983;11:121–124.

10. Gofton JP, Trueman GE. Studies in osteoarthritis of the hip. II. Osteoarthritis of the hip and leg-length disparity. *Can Med Assoc J.* 1971;104(9):791–799.

11. Friberg O. Clinical symptoms and biomechanics of lumbar spine and hip joint in leg length inequality. *Spine.* 1983;8:643.

12. Giles LGF, Taylor JR. Lumbar spine structural changes associated with leg length inequality. *Spine.* 1982;7(2):159–162.

13. Gofton JP. Studies in osteoarthritis of the hip. IV. Biomechanics and clinical considerations. *Can Med Assoc J.* 1971;104(11):1007–1011.

14. Giles LG, Taylor JR. Low back pain associated with leg length inequality. *Spine.* 1981;6:510–521.

15. McCaw ST, Bates BT. Biomechanical implications of mild leg length inequality. *Br J Sports Med.* 1991;25(1):10–13.

16. Cavallo RJ, Speer KP. Shoulder instability and impingement in throwing athletes. *Med Sci Sports Exerc.* 1998;30:18–25.

17. Dilorenzo CE, Parkes JC II, Chmelar RD. The importance of shoulder and cervical dysfunction in the etiology and treatment of athletic elbow injuries. *J Orthop Sports Phys Ther.* 1990;11(9):402–409.

18. Gambetta V. *Building the Complete Athlete.* 4th ed. Presented at an instructional course; April 1998; Seattle, WA.

19. Kuhn JE. Biomechanics of glenohumeral stability. In: Norris TR, ed. *Orthopedic Knowledge Update: Shoulder and Elbow.* Rosemont, IL: American Academy of Orthopedic Surgeons; 1997.

20. Wells P. Cervical dysfunction and shoulder problems. *Physiotherapy.* 1982;68:66–73.

21. McCluskey III GM, Dellaero D. Special issues in athletes. In: Norris TR, ed. *Orthopedic Knowledge Update: Shoulder and Elbow.* Rosemont, IL: American Academy of Orthopedic Surgeons; 1997.

22. Zuckerman JD, Rokito AS, Cuomo F, Gallagher MA. Occupational shoulder disorders. In: Rockwood CA Jr, Matsen FA III, eds. *The Shoulder.* 2nd ed. Philadelphia: WB Saunders; 1998:1296–1312.

23. Babyar SR. Excessive scapular motion in individuals recovering from painful and stiff shoulders: Causes and treatment strategies. *Phys Ther.* 1996;76(3):226–238.

24. Kibler WB. Shoulder rehabilitation: Principles and practice. *Med Sci Sports Exerc.* 1998;30:40–50.

25. Wilk KE, Arrigo C. Current concepts in the rehabilitation of the athletic shoulder. *J Orthop Sports Phys Ther.* 1993;18:365–378.

26. Turner CE. Trunk control: Implications for rehabilitation. *Biomechanics.* 1999;6(9):16–22.

27. Turnbull JR. Acromioclavicular joint disorders. *Med Sci Sports Exerc.* 1998;30:26–32.

28. Sanborn CF, Jankowski CM. Physiologic considerations for women in sport. *Clin Sports Med.* 1994;13(2):315–327.

29. Chu DA. Athletic training issues in synchronized swimming. *Clin Sports Med.* 1999;18(2):437–445.

30. Pollock G. Multidirectional and posterior instability of the shoulder. In: *Ortho. Knowledge Update: Shoulder and Elbow.* Rosemont, IL: American Academy of Orthopedic Surgeons; 1997.

31. Chu DA. Plyometrics in sports injury rehabilitation and training. *Athletic Ther Today.* 1999;4(3):7–11, 32–33, 63.

CHAPTER 8

Sport for Women with Physical Disabilities

Carol A. Mushett, Benjamin F. Johnson, and Kenneth J. Richter

INTRODUCTION

Stephen Hawkings, renowned British physicist who has amyotrophic lateral sclerosis, opened the 1992 Paralympic Games in Barcelona, speaking the following words through his computer-generated voice, "Each one of us has within us a spark of fire, a creative force. Some of us have lost the use of parts of our bodies, through accident or illness, but that is really of minor significance. It is just a mechanical problem. The important thing is that we have the human spirit, the ability to create. This creativity can take many forms, from theoretical physics to physical achievement. The important thing is that one should be stretched to be outstanding in some field. These games provide an opportunity for that."

In remarks at the Third Paralympic Congress in Atlanta, August 16, 1996, Judith E. Heumann, Assistant US Secretary of Education, explained why Paralympic sport is important. "It gives disabled youth an opportunity to see people like themselves excel. It inspires disabled young people to believe that with hard work and talent, they can excel in their own chosen fields, just like the athletes excel in theirs. Most important, the Paralympics encourage the parents and families of disabled people to have high expectations for them."

She further elaborated on the role that sports can play in the lives of children with disabilities. "We should not be satisfied until all students are given the opportunities to participate in sports. Through sports, all students—disabled and nondisabled—can learn to work with others. Through sports, all students—disabled and nondisabled—can learn

that it takes persistent practice to learn new skills. Through sports, all students—disabled and nondisabled—can learn to make decisions in the midst of fast-paced action. Through sports, all students—disabled and nondisabled—can learn the joy that comes with success."

Sport is central to American life. Whether pursued in school yards, community facilities, or professional arenas, sport captures our attention and defines much of our American character. Participation in sports is held to be of particular importance in the physical, psychological, and social development of American youth.

The 1996 Surgeon General's Report on Physical Activity and Health clearly identified the link between regular physical activity and quality of life for individuals of all ages.[1] In 1992, the American Academy of Orthopaedic Surgeons issued a position statement strongly supporting the participation in sport of people of all ages with disabilities.[2]

In 1995, Juan Antonio Samaranch, President of the International Olympic Committee (IPC), stated, "Sports practice undeniably represents the important stimulus which disabled people need to overcome the many physical and psychological difficulties which hinder their daily lives. At the same time as offering the indispensable motivation which gives the strength to overcome obstacles and conquer adversity and pain on a solid foundation, sports guarantees everyone equal dignity and a spirit of fraternity, solidarity, and mutual understanding."[3]

Twenty percent of women ages 15 to 64 have a disability.[4]

Clinical Guideline

Special thanks to Jan Irving and Chris and Rita Hamilton.

According to the US Bureau of Census, people with disabilities are the largest minority group in the United States and include more than 49 million Americans. Five percent of all children less than age 18 have a disability. Nearly 14% of individuals 18 to 44 years of age are disabled.[4]

And yet, opportunities for children and adults with disabilities to participate in sport are few. The Carnegie Council on Adolescent Development estimated that more than 35 million children and youth without disabilities participated in organized sports in 1992.[5] In stark contrast, the United States Cerebral Palsy Athletic Association estimated that less than 10,000 youth with disabilities participated in organized sports that same year.[6] In 1993, the United States Disabled Sports Team estimated that only 400 organized programs for sport for athletes with physical disabilities were available throughout the United States.[7]

People with disabilities, often impeded by social stereotypes and misconceptions, continue to face numerous obstacles in their quest for full inclusion into American society. According to the records of the Congressional hearings on legislation regarding the Americans with Disabilities Act (1990), 43 million citizens with disabilities are relegated to a status that is economically, vocationally, educationally, and socially inferior.

For children with physical disabilities, exclusion begins early in life. Rarely is this exclusion manifested more than in the areas of physical education, recreation, and sport. The net results of this exclusion show that children with disabilities are denied the vital physical, social, and psychological benefits of physical activity.

IMPORTANCE OF SPORT

Sport is a term that encompasses a broad spectrum of experiences that include the social, recreational, and competitive. Physical activity is widely accepted as a necessary component for individual health. Over recent years, there has been increased emphasis on the role of sport and physical activity in enhancing health and quality of life of individuals with disability and chronic illness.[8]

Individuals with disability can generally receive the same health benefits from exercise and sport training as their able-bodied counterparts. These benefits include physical benefits (general fitness, cardiovascular conditioning, cardiopulmonary endurance, muscle strength, flexibility, postural control, balance, adaptation to impairments, optimal musculoskeletal functioning) as well as psychological benefits (improved motivation, self-confidence and self-esteem, personal adjustment, competitive spirit, reduced anxiety, and reduced tendency to withdraw.[8,9] Sport participation and intensive training has also been shown, similarly, to benefit individuals with neuromuscular impairment of cerebral origin.[10]

Physical Benefits of Sport

- General fitness
- Cardiovascular conditioning
- Cardiopulmonary endurance
- Muscle strength
- Flexibility
- Postural control
- Balance
- Adaptation to impairments
- Optimal musculoskeletal function

Clinical Guideline

During the last decade, sport for athletes with disabilities has moved away from a medical rehabilitation model, toward a competitive sports model. The relationship between sport and rehabilitation, however, continues to have relevance. Sport and physical activity can help in addressing some of the health and wellness needs of children and adults with disabilities. Sports can, and often do, provide appropriate physical interventions that reduce the incidence of medical complications and the onset of secondary disability, promote social integration, and enhance the quality of life of people with disabilities.

Psychological Benefits of Sport

- Improved motivation
- Self-confidence
- Self-esteem
- Personal adjustment
- Competitive spirit
- Reduced anxiety
- Reduced withdrawal

Clinical Guideline

Sport opportunities for women with disabilities range from recreational to highly competitive to elite paralympic sport. Athletes are classified or categorized by degree of impairment to ensure equitable competition. For example, athletes with visual impairment compete in three classes that vary in the amount of residual sight. Athletes with physical impairments such as spinal cord injury, cerebral palsy, or amputation are evaluated and placed in a sport-specific classification for competition. For competition, many sports, such as swimming, wheelchair basketball, and table tennis, use functional or integrated systems that allow athletes with a variety of disabilities to compete with each other (see Appendix 8–A). Some sports such as athletics, soccer, and cycling rely on disability-specific classification systems that evaluate both function and etiology of disability.

Sports can, and often do, provide appropriate physical interventions that reduce the incidence of medical complications and the onset of secondary disability.

Clinical Guideline

Jennings[11] stated, "To rehabilitate is to restore the power or capacity for living. Living does not signify merely biological life and function, but it takes on a qualitative dimension. It is the restoration of the power of living well, living meaningfully that rehabilitation seeks."[(p 402)] The World Health Organization defined health as "a state of complete physical, mental, and social well-being and not merely the absence of disease and infirmity."[12]

WOMEN IN SPORT

In 1998, the President's Council on Physical Fitness and Sports issued a research report that clearly identified several important findings related to girls in sport and physical activity. Highlights include the following:

- Exercise and sport can be used as a therapeutic or preventive intervention for enhancing physical and mental health for adolescent females
- Regular physical activity helps reduce symptoms of stress and depression among girls
- Sport participation enhances mental health in a variety of ways.[13]

In the joint meeting between the International Olympic Committee Executive Board and the National Olympic Committees, the Working Group on Women and Sport issued the following statement:[14]

Sport, whether competition sport or sport for all, has become a social force to be reckoned with, a major impact on the structure of society and the condition of women.[(p 1)]

Clinical Guideline

Great strides have been made by women in sport during the past decade. However, women with disabilities continue to be marginalized.[15] Sherrill[16] posited that women with disabilities "constitute a minority in the truest sense and are subject, perhaps more than any other individuals, to discrimination and oppression."[(p 52)]

In the 1996 Paralympic Summer Games held in Atlanta shortly after the Olympic Games, only 24% of the athletes were women. Forty-seven percent of the nations competing in the Games brought no women athletes.[17] In comparison, 13% of the nations competing in the Games of the XXVI

Olympiad in 1996 in Atlanta did not enter women athletes. The number and percentage of nations bringing no women to the Paralympic Games in 1996 reflected an alarming increase from 1992.[16] Similarly, only 21% of the athletes in the 1998 Paralympic Winter Games in Nagano were women.[18]

Paralympic Sport

- 1996 Summer Paralympic Games: 24% women athletes
- 1996 Summer Paralympic Games: 47% of nations totally male
- 1998 Winter Paralympic Games: 21% women athletes

Clinical Guideline

Little specific information is available about women in sport for athletes with disabilities. Anecdotally, women in paralympic sport report social factors, shortened sport careers, definitions of elitism, cultural implications of both gender and disability, and limited "grass roots" opportunities as factors limiting their participation in sport. However, further investigation is needed in this area.

IMPLICATIONS OF DISABILITY ON SPORT

Clearly, sport and physical activity are widely accepted and actively encouraged for women with disabilities (Figure 8–1); however, when training, one must consider the cause and implications of the individual's disability.[19] The position statement of the American Academy of Orthopaedic Surgeons[2] warned that when participating in sport, individuals with physical disabilities may need to take precautions. However, these precautions should be appropriate and without needless restrictions. There has been considerable confusion over the medical aspects of an athlete's disability and their implications on sport. Some of this has been due to a lack of research. However, important facts are emerging that sport medicine professionals, coaches, and athletes need to know. The following highlight key sport medicine concerns, which, depending on the athlete's disability, may warrant special consideration.

Temperature Regulation

Dysfunction of the sympathetic nervous system, which is of particular concern for athletes with a spinal cord injury (SCI) above the eighth thoracic level, may cause significant problems with the regulation of internal body temperature. These athletes may not sweat effectively or have vasodilation below the level of injury. This can result in the inability of the body's thermoregulatory system to cool itself through sweating or warm itself through shivering and vasodilation. Consideration should also be given to athletes with significantly

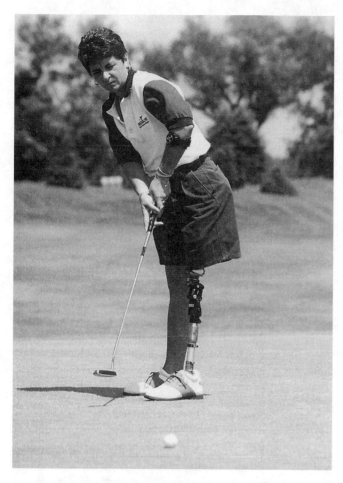

Figure 8–1 Donna Marie Garze wearing the Total Knee by Century XXII Innovations, Inc

reduced body surface such as an athlete with a bilateral amputation. Medications often used by individuals with disabilities, such as anticholinergics, sympathomimetics, diuretics, certain muscle relaxors, and thyroid replacement drugs, can also cause increased vulnerability to heat.[19]

Seizures

For more than 20 years, controversy has surrounded the issue of sport participation by athletes with seizure disorders. Seizures, a hypersynchronous discharge of the cerebral neurons, manifest in a variety of ways that range from Petit Mal to Grand Mal seizures.[20] Athletes with motor dysfunction of the cerebral origin, such as cerebral palsy, traumatic brain injury, and cerebral vascular accident, may also have a seizure disorder. Stress, hypoglycemia, dehydration, electrolyte imbalance, and hyperventilation have been found to trigger or increase the incidence of seizures.[19]

The athlete with a neurologic injury has a lowered threshold for seizure activity. However, there is a decrease in seizure activity among athletes due primarily to increased stability of neurologic membranes in an acidic pH rather than in an alkaline pH. Aerobic exercise results in a metabolic acidosis. The decrease in pH typically results in a decrease in seizures.[21] Clearly, however, appropriate nutritional and fluid intake, adequate rest, and compliance with prescribed antiseizure medications are important factors in controlling seizure activity.

Spasticity

Considerable discussion and debate surround the appropriateness of strength training and intense physical activity of individuals with spasticity of cerebral origin.[21] There is a long held concern that sport is inappropriate for people with spasticity of cerebral origin. The fear has been that intense sport or aggressive exercise will worsen the spasticity. Experience has not found this to be true.[10] In fact, it has been observed that the challenge of sport participation seems to lessen the impact of the participant's spasticity. This could be due to a resetting of the spasticity receptors, both centrally and peripherally, but research is needed to investigate this area.

Although athletes with spasticity may experience a transient increase, evidence does not substantiate a permanent or long-term increase in spasticity.[19] Flexion, especially in the upper extremities, often dominates over extension in athletes with cerebral palsy. Therefore, since muscular balance is important, strength training should focus primarily on extension and minimize flexion exercises.[21]

Autonomic Dysreflexia/Boosting

Typically, individuals with high SCI have a low baseline blood pressure with systolic often below 100 mm Hg. Autonomic dysreflexia is a syndrome that can occur in individuals with SCI higher than T6, and is characterized by marked elevation in blood pressure.[22] In a person with an intact spinal cord, the vasoconstriction reflexes are regulated by inhibitory impulses from the higher brain centers. However, in an individual with a high thoracic or cervical spinal injury, the injury blocks the descending regulatory impulses, allowing the blood pressure to go unchecked. The baroreceptors in the aortic arch and carotids may try to compensate; but, since the sympathetic pathways are blocked in the injured spinal cord, only the vagus can act. This may result in a bradycardia but cannot regulate the blood pressure. Headache, decrease in heart rate, goose pimples, shivering, and flushing result. During autonomic dysreflexia, the risk of seizures, cerebral hemorrhage, and even death exists.[22]

Boosting refers to the "intentional induction of autonomic dysreflexia among quadriplegic athletes for performance enhancement."[23] Athletes with high SCI have reported the use of tight leg straps, sharp objects, and, most commonly, over-distension of the bladder, in attempts to improve their sport performance. The practice of boosting has been compared to the use of performance-enhancing drugs, or "doping," because of the potential danger and the difficult ethical issues.

The IPC does not allow athletes to compete while in a boosted state. Competitors may be checked at the start of a race, but, for obvious reasons, not during competition. According to Dr. Michael Riding, medical officer of the IPC, the objective of the IPC's ban was to protect the competitors from the risks. However, he also points out that "we are deluding ourselves if we think that hypertension is solely the property of the boosted."[24] Some argue that boosting may be "only giving back to the competitors what they lost" and that "we have extrapolated a hospital situation to a sport situation."[24] At the VISTA 1999 Conference in Germany, Dr. Riding emphasized that the current IPC rules are an appropriate first step, but that additional research, which includes input from affected athletes, is essential.

Pressure Ulcers

Pressure ulcers are a common, yet preventable, problem for many athletes with SCI. The National Pressure Ulcer Advisory Panel defines a pressure ulcer as "an area of un-relieved pressure over a defined area, usually over a bony prominence, resulting in ischemia, cell death, and tissue necrosis."[25(p1057)] Pressure ulcers can develop as a result of prolonged or excessive time in one position. Incidence of pressure ulcers found in individuals with SCI is reported to be 30% during the 5 years post injury. The incidence is highest in individuals with complete quadriplegia and paraplegia.[25]

Key factors affecting the level of risk include intensity, duration, and tissue tolerance. That is to say that intense pressure over a short duration can do as much or more damage as less pressure over longer periods.[25] Athletes with SCI experience skin damage from both shearing forces and friction. The sacrum is the most common site of severe pressure ulcers. Other common problem areas include hips, buttocks, and heel.[25]

Prevention is the athlete's best defense against pressure ulcers. Wheelchair positioning for maximal sport perfor-mance often does not allow for proper distribution of pressure. When designing one's wheelchair for competition, athletes need to distribute weight and allow for weight relief. Support surfaces should also promote redistribution and reduction of pressure while minimizing shearing and friction.

Sport Injuries

Sport participation in general, and intense training for elite competition in particular, bring inherent risk of injury to the athlete. Many believe that athletes with disabilities are at greater risk than their nondisabled counterparts. However, epidemiologic studies of sport-related injuries reveal that athletes with disabilities experience injury rates similar to athletes without disabilities.[19]

The Athletes with Disabilities Injury Registry reported an injury rate of 7.23 per 1,000 exposures, which is consistent with rates reported in similar studies on athletes without disabilities.[19] Ferrara and Davis[26] reported that half of the sport-related injuries to wheelchair athletes were strains and muscular injuries to the upper extremities. The repetitive motion required for wheelchair propulsion puts repeated stress on the athlete's shoulder, wrist, and elbow. Wheelchair athletes are particularly susceptible to rotator cuff injuries and overuse injuries, such as impingement and bicipital tendinitis.

In addition to injuries typically sustained by athletes with-out a disability, amputee athletes may experience skin break-down or irritation during training. Athletes with lower-limb amputations may need specialized padding to protect the stump from injury. However, improvements in the design, materials, and technology of prosthetic devices have reduced the number and severity of sport-related injuries to amputee athletes.[19]

Pregnancy

Although there are unique issues of pregnancies in women with disability[27] and pregnancy has an impact on able-bodied women in sport, the literature is bereft of any data on the impact of sport and exercise in pregnant women with dis-abilities. Disabled women, such as women with high SCI, may have difficulties with pregnancy such as autonomic dysreflexia and precipitous labor.[28] Able-bodied women have been reported to use pregnancy as a sport-enhancing technique.[29] Most able-bodied women are encouraged to exercise;[30] however, the interrelationship of pregnancy with women with disabilities has not been studied. One of the reasons for this may be the barrier to women with disabilities that prevents them from participating in sport, as well as the small numbers of women with disabilities who actually do participate in sports. Although speculative, it is possible that pregnancy may be added as a last barrier to women with disabilities, which prevents participation in sports. Further research in this area is needed to clarify these issues, but one would expect that most women with disabilities would benefit from moderate exercise during pregnancy as their able-bodied counterparts do.

CONCLUSION

Sherrill summarized many of the challenges facing women with disabilities as they pursue sport:

Women with disability who aspire to high level sport competition may indeed face the greatest discrimination of all. Widespread individual differences in etiology, time of onset of disability, and unique manifestations of loss or reduction of functional ability combine with such variables as age, social class, education, race/ethnicity, and sexual preferences so that each individual keenly feels the aloneness of diversity.[16(p 53)]

As we contemplate the current status of women in disabled sport, we must learn from the progress and accomplishments of women in sport worldwide. In the 1996 International Olympic Committee Report of the Chairwoman of the Working Group on Women and Sport, we are reminded that "sport is a tremendous medium of communication and emancipation which has to a certain extent helped to build women's awareness and hence their role in society."[14(p 1)] We must also take inspiration from the inner strength revealed by women athletes with disabilities, not just on the playing fields but in their unrelenting spirit. Despite limited opportunities, often without coaching and with little technical support, they train and they compete. They win and they lose, with tenacity and with quiet resolve.

REFERENCES

1. United States Department of Health and Human Services. *Physical Activity and Health: A Report of the Surgeon General.* Atlanta, GA: US Department of Health and Human Services, Centers for Disease Control and Prevention, National Center for Chronic Disease Prevention and Health Promotion; 1996.

2. American Academy of Orthopaedic Surgeons. *Position Statement: Support of Sports and Recreation Programs for Physically Disabled People.* (Document Number: 1123). Rosemont, IL: AAOS; 1992.

3. Samaranch JA. *International Paralympic Committee Newsletter.* Fall issue, 1995.

4. McNeil J. *Americans with Disabilities 1991–92. Data from the Survey of Income and Program Participation.* Washington, DC: US Department of Commerce, Bureau of the Census; 1993.

5. Carnegie Council on Adolescent Development. *Fateful Choices: Healthy Youth for the 21st Century.* New York: Carnegie Corporation; 1992.

6. Mushett CA. Current trends in youth sports. *United States Cerebral Palsy Athletic Association Newsletter.* 1992;8:34.

7. Mushett CA, Richter KJ, Parliament CF. Sport for the disabled: A viable option for patients with neurologic injury. *Journal of Neuroscience Nursing.* 1993;25:372–374.

8. Goldberg B. *Sports and Exercise for Children with Chronic Health Conditions.* Champaign, IL: Human Kinetics; 1995.

9. McCann BC. Importance of sport for paraplegics. In: Vermeer A, ed. *Sports for the Disabled.* Arnhem, The Netherlands. RESPO, 1987:63–68.

10. Richter KJ, Gaebler-Spira D, Mushett CA. Annotation: Sport and the person with spasticity of cerebral origin. *Developmental Medicine and Child Neurology.* 1996;38:867–870.

11. Jennings B. Healing the self: The moral meaning of relationships in rehabilitation. *Am J Phys Med Rehabil.* 1993;72(6):401–404.

12. World Health Organization. *Constitution of the World Health Organization.* Geneva, Switzerland: World Health Organization; 1964.

13. The President's Council on Physical Fitness and Sports. *Physical Activity and Sport in the Lives of Girls: Physical and Mental Health Dimensions from an Interdisciplinary Approach. Executive Summary,* xiv. Washington, DC: The Council; 1998.

14. International Olympic Committee. *Report of the Chairwoman of the Working Group on Women and Sport.* Cancun: The Committee; 1996:14.

15. DePauw K. Presentation: VISTA '99. Cologne, Germany; 1999.

16. Sherrill C. Women with disability, Paralympics, and reasoned action contact theory. *WSPA J.* 1993;2(2):51–60.

17. Mushett CA. *Report to the Sports Council Executive Committee of the International Paralympic Committee.* Solleftea, Sweden: The Committee; 1997.

18. Mushett CA. *Report to the International Paralympic Committee Executive Committee.* Sydney, Australia: The Committee; 1999.

19. Richter KJ, Sherrill C, McCann CB, Mushett CA, Kaschalk S. Recreation and sport for people with disabilities. In: DeLisa JA, Gans B, eds. *Rehabilitation Medicine: Principles and Practice.* 3rd ed. Philadelphia: Lippincott-Raven; 1998:853–871.

20. Richter KJ. Seizures in athletes. *Journal of Osteopathic Sports Medicine.* 1989; 3:319–323.

21. Mushett CA, Wyeth DO, Richter KJ. Cerebral palsy. In: Goldberg B, ed. *Sports and Exercise for Children with Chronic Health Conditions.* Champaign, IL: Human Kinetics; 1995:123–133.

22. Freed MM. Traumatic and congenital lesions of the spinal cord. In: Kottke FJ, Lehmann JF, eds. *Krusen's Handbook of Physical Medicine and Rehabilitation,* 4th ed. Philadelphia: WB Saunders; 1990:717–748.

23. Burnham R, Wheeler G, Bhambhani Y, Belanger M, Eriksson P, Steadward R. Intentional induction of autonomic dysreflexia among quadriplegic athletes for performance enhancement: Efficacy, safety, and mechanisms for action. *Clinical Journal of Sport Medicine.* 1994;4:1 10.

24. Riding M. Boosting in paralympic sport: Some ethical considerations. *Proceedings: VISTA '99.* Cologne, Germany; in press.

25. O'Connor KC, Kirshblum SC. Pressure ulcers. In: DeLisa JA, Gans B, eds. *Rehabilitation Medicine Principles and Practice.* 3rd ed. Philadelphia: Lippincott-Raven; 1998:1057–1071.

26. Ferrara MS, Davis R. Injuries to elite wheelchair athletes. *Paraplegia.* 1990;28:335–341.

27. Pischke ME. Parenting with a disability. Special issue: Reproductive issues for person with physical disabilities. *Sex Dis.* 1993;11:3.

28. Charlifue SW, Gerhart KA, Menter RR, Menley MS. Sexual issues of women with spinal cord injuries. *Paraplegia.* 1992;30:192–199.

29. Warren MP, Shangold MM. *Sports Gynecology: Problems and Care of the Athletic Female.* Cambridge, MA: Blackwell Scientific Publications; 1997.

30. Artal R, Sherman C. Exercise during pregnancy: Safe and beneficial for most. *Phys Sportsmed.* 1999;24:89–95.

BIBLIOGRAPHY

1. American College of Sports Medicine. *Guidelines for Exercise Testing and Prescription*. Baltimore: Williams & Wilkins; 1995.

2. Brookins GK. Culture, ethnicity and bicultural competence: Implications for children with chronic illness and disability. *Pediatrics*. 1993;9:1056–1062.

3. Campbell E, Jones G. Psychological well-being in sport participants and nonparticipants. *Adapted Physical Activity Quarterly*. 1994;11:404–415.

4. Durstine LP, Painter P, Bloomquist LE. *Exercise Management for Persons with Chronic Diseases and Disabilities*. Indianapolis: American College of Sports Medicine; in press.

5. Fagan W, Sherrill C, French R. Locus of control quad rugby players and able-bodied men. *Clinical Kinesiology*. 1994;49:53–57.

6. Harvey D, Greenway AP. Congruence between mother and handicapped child's view of child's sense of adjustment. *The Exceptional Child*. 1982;29:111–116.

7. Hutzler Y, Bar-Eli M. Psychological benefits of sports for disabled people: A review. *Scandinavian Journal of Medical Science and Sports*. 1993;3:217–228.

8. LaPlante MP. Physical activity patterns and sports participation of people with disabilities. Presented at the Physical Activity and Health in Persons with Disabilities: A Research Symposium. 1996; Atlanta, GA.

9. Martin JJ, Mushett CA. Social support mechanisms among athletes with disabilities. *Adapted Physical Activity Quarterly*. 1996;13:74–83.

10. McCubbin J. Physical fitness assessment and program considerations for persons with cerebral palsy or amputations: A review of research. In: Steadward RD, Nelson ER, Wheeler GD, eds. *VISTA '93: The Outlook*. Edmonton, Canada: University of Alberta; 1994:58–70.

11. Nelson MA, Harris SS. The benefits and risks of sports and exercise for children with chronic health conditions. In: Goldberg B, ed. *Sports and Exercise for Children with Chronic Health Conditions*. Champaign, IL: Human Kinetics; 1995:14–19.

12. Peters DL, Raup CD. Developing the self-concept of the exceptional child. In: Yawkey TD, ed. *Self-Concept of the Young Child*. Provo, UT: Brigham Young University Press; 1980:167–186.

13. Rimmer JH. *Fitness and Rehabilitation: Programs for Special Populations*. Dubuque, IA: Brown & Benchmark; 1994.

14. Shephard RD. Exercise physiology and fitness in athletes with disabilities: An overview. In: Steadward RD, Nelson ER, Wheeler GD, eds. *VISTA '93: The Outlook*. Edmonton, Canada: University of Alberta; 1994:19–45.

15. Shephard RD. *Fitness in Special Populations*. Champaign, IL: Human Kinetics; 1994.

16. Sherrill C. Disability identity and involvement in sport and exercise. In: Fox K, ed. *The Physical Self: From Motivation to Wellbeing*. Champaign, IL: Human Kinetics; in press.

17. Sherrill C, Hinson M, Gench B, Kennedy SO. Self-concepts of disabled youth athletes. *Perceptual and Motor Skills*. 1990;70:1093–1098.

18. Sherrill C, Silliman L, Gench B, Hinson, M. Self-actualization of elite wheelchair athletes. *Paraplegia*. 1990;28:252–260.

19. Sherrill C, Williams T. Disability and sport: Psychological perspectives on inclusion, integration, and participation. *Sport Science Review*. 1996;5:42–64.

20. Weller RB, Truex WO. Assessing the effects of experimental studies on self-concept of pre-adolescent physically handicapped. *American Correctional Therapy Journal*. 1985;39:134–140.

21. Yeeger HEJ, Yahmed MH, VanderWoude IHV, Charpentree P. Peak oxygen uptake and maximum aerobic power output of Olympic wheelchair dependent athletes. *Medicine and Science in Sports*. 1996;67:1201–1209.

Athlete Profile

ANN CODY

Wheelchair Athlete

Sport has always played an important role in Ann Cody's life. Ann is the vice president of Sagamore Associates in Washington, DC, and a Paralympic gold, silver, and bronze medal winner.

Ann captured the gold medal and, with her teammates, set a new world record in the 4 × 100-m wheelchair relay sprint with a time of 1:05.51 in the Barcelona Paralympic Games in 1992. Ann also won a bronze medal in the 10,000-m wheelchair event with a time of 25:07.3 in these same Games. In Seoul, during the 1988 Paralympic Games, she won four silver medals. Ann has also competed at the elite level in wheelchair basketball and participates in many recreational sports.

At a Glance

Ann developed a T5–T6 complete spinal paralysis when a cold resulted in a viral infection in her spinal cord. A 16-year-old junior at Groton High School in New York, Ann initially thought that she would not be able to play sports again. "I was a big athlete," she said. "I did everything. It took me a couple of months to adjust. I realized that I missed sports terribly. That was really hard." Her high school coach made her aware that sport was still an option. At the University of Illinois, she found the facilities and encouragement that enabled her to become a top wheelchair athlete in both wheelchair racing and wheelchair basketball. As part of the University of Illinois women's wheelchair basketball team, Ann was a national all-tournament player for 6 years, and the team was national champions for 5 years. In 1990, she was voted the Wheelchair Athletics USA Female Athlete of the Year and the USA Track and Field Disabled Athlete of the Year. Ann won the wheelchair division of the Atlanta-based Peachtree Road Race in 1990. Ann has placed first in such events as the Los Angeles Marathon, the Chicago Marathon, the Toronto International Invitational, and the Mobil National Championship. In track events, she has set national records in the 1500-m event and has been national champion in 1988, 1990, and 1991 in a number of wheelchair racing events. Ann brought home a silver medal in the 1990 Goodwill Games for the 1500 m.

Ann earned her bachelor's degree in Painting in 1986 and a master of science in Leisure Studies in 1992 at the University of Illinois. "I enjoy most just pushing myself to greater performances. I think sports for people with disabilities, in general, are growing in acceptance," said Cody. "We're being provided with more opportunities to compete. Wheelchair racing is a great sport and it's an incredible way to stay in shape, but it takes hard work, time, and patience."

For more than 12 years, elite Paralympic sport played an extensive role in Ann Cody's life. Ann attributes her longevity as an elite athlete, nearly three times the average, primarily to the support of family, friends, and coaches. Fortunately, she has had no seriously limiting injuries. Ann has experienced several incidences of tendinitis of the wrist and shoulder and a rotator cuff problem. She also lost approximately 8 weeks of training because of a problem with a pressure sore from improper seating. Anecdotally, Ann reported that sport training actually helped to reduce injury, physical problems, and the onset of secondary health concerns, which often plague women with disabilities.

Ann is also acutely aware of the many challenges facing women athletes with disabilities. She reports "women's issues clearly affected my career...not only the lack of social encouragement but also the pressure of societal expectations was discouraging. Many times I was not taken seriously in sport environments. Training facilities and programs often disregarded methods or ideas to make reasonable accommodations so I could train. Sports businesses often have the attitude that a woman with a disability lacks commitment to sport or exercise." When asked what advice or insight she might give to emerging women athletes with disabilities, she offered the following encouragement:

Get to know yourself, your strengths and weaknesses, your talents and gifts, then learn how to use them. Discipline yourself and, most of all, believe in yourself because others will question your sacrifice, your investment in sport. I knew that in pursuing what I loved (sport) I was growing and challenging myself to be all I could be. I was learning discipline, building healthy relationships, and developing confidence. But, most of all, I encourage all women athletes to trust in your own inner knowledge.

Disabled Sport Organizations

The following sport organizations for athletes with disabilities are recognized as governing or coordinating bodies by the United States Olympic Committee:

Disabled Sports USA
DSUSA is a multisport organization providing year-round sports and recreation opportunities for people with disabilities.
451 Hungerford Drive, Ste. 100
Rockville, MD 20805
Tel: (301) 217–9838
Fax: (301) 217–0968
TDD: (301) 217–0963
Internet: http://www.dsusa.org/~dusa/dsusa.html
E-mail:dsusa@dsusa.org

Dwarf Athletic Association of America
The DAAA promotes and provides quality amateur level athletic opportunities for dwarf athletes in the United States.
418 Willow Way
Lewisville, TX 75067
Tel: (972) 317–8299
Fax: (972) 966–0184
Janet Brown, Executive Director,
JFBDA3@aol.com

Special Olympics International
SOI is a year-round sports training and athletic participation organization for children and adults with mental retardation.
1325 G Street, NW, Ste. 500
Washington, DC 20005–4709
Tel: (202) 628–3630
Fax: (202) 824–0200
Internet: http://www.specialolympics.org
E-mail: specialolympics@msn.com

US Association of Blind Athletes
USABA provides opportunities for sports participation and elite competition for blind/visually impaired athletes.
33 North Institute
Colorado Springs, CO 80903
Tel: (719) 630–0422
Fax: (719) 630–0616
Internet: http://www.usaba.org
E-mail: USABA@usa.net

USA Deaf Sports Federation
The USADSF (formerly American Athletic Association of the Deaf) provides organized competition for adult deaf and hearing-impaired athletes.
3607 Washington Blvd., Ste. 4
Ogden, UT 84403–1737
TEL/TTY: (801) 393–7916
Fax: (801) 393–2263
E-mail: USADSF@aol.com

United States Cerebral Palsy Athletic Association
The USCPAA offers competitive sports opportunities to persons with cerebral palsy, stroke, and traumatic brain injuries with acquired or congenital motor dysfunction.

25 West Independence Way
Kensington, RI 42881
Tel: (401) 792–7130
Fax: (401) 792–7132
Internet: http://www.uscpaa.org
E-mail: uscpaa@mail.bbsnet.com

Wheelchair Sports USA
WSUSA provides individuals who use wheelchairs the opportunity to participate in both recreational and competitive sports. WSUSA promotes competition at the regional, national, and international levels for athletes with permanent disabilities affecting mobility.
3595 East Fountain Boulevard, Ste. L-1
Colorado Springs, CO 80910
Tel: (719) 574–1150
Fax: (719) 574–9840
E-mail: wsusa@aol.com
Internet: http://www.wsusa.org

PART II

Across the Lifespan

CHAPTER 9

The Young Female Athlete

Karen Judy

INTRODUCTION

Young women benefit greatly from participation in sports. Early athletic involvement results in increased muscle strength and flexibility, improved lean body mass, greater cardiovascular efficiency, enhanced self-esteem and confidence, enhanced body image, greater ability to overcome adversity and cope with pressure, improved leadership skills, bonding with other children, and making new friends. Title IX has resulted in an explosion of participation in women's sports. During the 1980s women's sports participation increased by 700%.[1] Today 30 million children and adolescents participate in organized sports in the United States.[2]

PREADOLESCENCE

Growth

Growth velocity is similar for both boys and girls from the end of the first year of life until age 10, and only small differences are noted in body size and shape before puberty (see Figures 9–1 and 9–2 for growth velocities in boys and girls).[3]

Muscle strength is similar in girls and boys during the first decade of life. The difference in the strength of various muscle groups is only about 1 to 2 kg in favor of boys.[4] After puberty, however, boys demonstrate an increasingly greater muscle mass, particularly in the upper body.

The attainment of such motor skills as throwing, kicking, catching, jumping, hopping, and skipping during the first years of life is similar in boys and girls. Because boys and girls are equal in athletic abilities during childhood, they can compete together before puberty without concerns for safety.

Comparing genders in preadolescence, until age 10, boys and girls have similar growth and strength, allowing both sexes to compete together.

Clinical Guideline

Physiological Response to Exercise

Relatively little is known about the ways in which children respond physiologically to exercise. Ethical concerns regarding the use of children as research subjects along with the lack of techniques to disentangle the effects of training from the effects of growth and development contribute to the scarcity of knowledge regarding exercise in children.[5] It is known that young girls have a higher oxygen uptake while running or walking than adolescents or adult women. This means that at any walking or running speed, a young girl operates at a higher percentage of her maximal aerobic power and will fatigue earlier than an older girl or woman in endurance events.[6] This knowledge should be incorporated into training schedules and expectations of young girls in competitive events. More research is needed into the sports physiology of young competitive girls and how they compare with young male athletes.

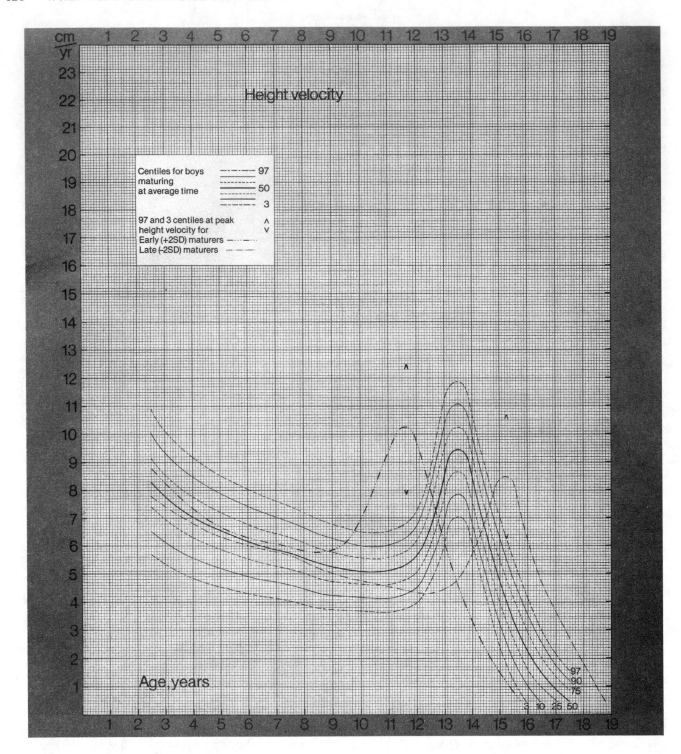

Figure 9–1 Growth Velocity Chart for Boys.

Heat and Cold Intolerance

Girls are less-effective thermoregulators when exercising in the heat and in the cold. Compared with women, prepubertal girls have a slower onset of sweating and a somewhat lower sweating rate (lower rate of output from each sweat gland) while exercising in the heat.[7] Because of this, young girls tolerate exercise in hot climates less effectively and are at greater risk for heat stress than adolescents or adult women. When young girls transition to a warm climate, their

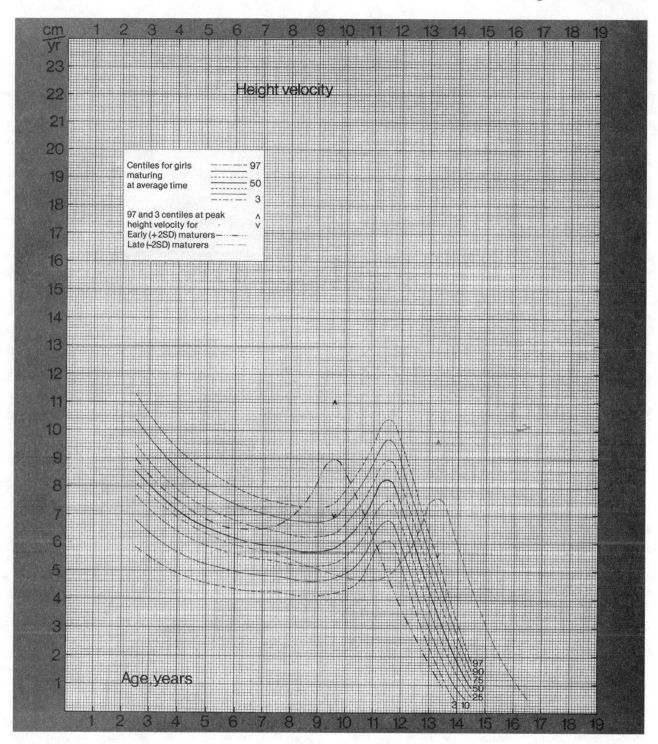

Figure 9–2 Growth Velocity Chart for Girls.

activities must be reduced in intensity and duration, then gradually increased.

Dehydration can lead to decreased concentration, coordination, strength, and stamina. Children must replace fluid losses. If exercise is less than 1 hour and the child is eu-volemic, there is no benefit to drinks containing sodium and chloride and carbohydrate compared with water.[2(p 1059)] Even with prolonged exercise, the effectiveness of carbohydrate-electrolyte solutions is controversial. To encourage consumption, fluids should be palatable.

No epidemiological evidence exists that young girls are more prone to hypothermia than older females are. Leaner girls have a greater heat loss than those who have a thicker, insulative subcutaneous fat layer. In cold winter sports this becomes important. A small, lean girl who is immersed in cold water is at a greater risk for hypothermia than a larger girl or one with thicker subcutaneous adipose tissue.[6]

Sports Readiness

Each youngster is a unique person. She varies in physical and psychological maturity, response to criticism, perception of what is stressful, and goals derived from sports. These differences play an important role in determining readiness for sports participation, degree of involvement, and enjoyment perceived from sport. Because of these variables, no specific best age can be given for all young athletes to begin sports competition. Perhaps the best indication of when a youth is ready to compete is when she, without adult interference, spontaneously expresses a desire to participate in a given sport. The initial intensity of competition should be low, increasing with skill and interest. If matched for size and maturity, most young athletes will find sports exhilarating, challenging, safe, and enjoyable.[8]

ADOLESCENCE

Growth

Adolescence is the beginning of the acceleration in the rate of growth before the attainment of sexual maturity (Figure 9–3). The adolescent growth spurt starts in some girls as early as 7 or 8 years of age and in others as late as 12 to 13 years. The pubertal growth spurt occurs on average 2 years earlier in girls than in boys, leading to a marked increase in height and weight. The maximal growth rate is achieved about 6 to 12 months before menarche (usually about age 13) and is maintained for only a few months (see Figures 9–1 and 9–2). Linear growth decelerates over the following 2 years. Most girls have achieved 90% to 95% of their ultimate adult height at the time of menarche.[5]

Muscular Strength

Muscular strength improves linearly with age from early childhood through about 15 years of age in girls, with no clear evidence of an adolescent spurt. After age 15, strength improves more slowly until age 30, when it plateaus. This pattern is in contrast to the marked acceleration of strength development during male adolescence, so that sex differences in muscular strength are considerable. Early maturing girls are slightly stronger than late maturing girls of the same chronological age during adolescence.

The differences between girls of contrasting maturity status, however, do not persist and are no longer evident by 14 to 15 years of age.[9] Women also have an increase in body fat (women have 25% body fat, men have 15% body fat); this is a disadvantage in sports in which body mass must be lifted (running, volleyball).[5] After puberty, gender differences persist because women have smaller hearts, smaller rib cages, smaller vital capacities, and greater respiratory rates than men.[5]

Hormonal

For a minority of young girls who exercise to excess, intense physical exercise can have adverse health consequences, including menstrual changes—delay in menarche, altered pubertal progression, anovulation, amenorrhea, and infertility.[10] Primary amenorrhea, or delayed menarche, is present when a young woman has not begun menses by 16 years of age. Secondary amenorrhea is defined as the absence of at least three to six consecutive menstrual cycles in girls who have begun menstruating. Many young athletes experience menarche at a later age than less active girls. In fact, infrequent or absent menses occurs in 10% to 20% of athletes in contrast to only 5% of the general population.[11] This appears to be particularly prevalent in sports that require high energy and low body weight such as running (less often in swimmers and cyclists).[12]

Although no physiological mechanism for this phenomenon has yet been found, one hypothesis is that the high energy demand of vigorous training prevents some girls from gaining sufficient body weight or fat to begin menstruation.[9] Another hypothesis is that a later age at menarche is associated with body characteristics that favor athletic performance and that the observed later age at menarche in athletes is simply a matter of natural selection.[13] Whether caused by physical training or merely an observational artifact, a later menarche appears to be associated with superior performance. The effects of heavy training on pubertal development and age at menarche must be assessed with regard to multiple factors, including genetics, nutritional status, socioeconomic status, family size, disease states, and the wide variation among individuals. This topic is one of considerable controversy and disagreement. In general, it is recommended that athletes who are 14 years of age and show no signs of puberty or those who have not experienced menses by the age of 16 years, regardless of secondary sexual characteristics, require a complete medical evaluation.[14]

Many possible medical causes exist for delay in menarche that must be ruled out before making the diagnosis of athletic amenorrhea. In addition, female athletes with amenorrhea experience reduced bone density and may be at risk for osteoporosis and fracture (refer to Chapters 18 and 19).

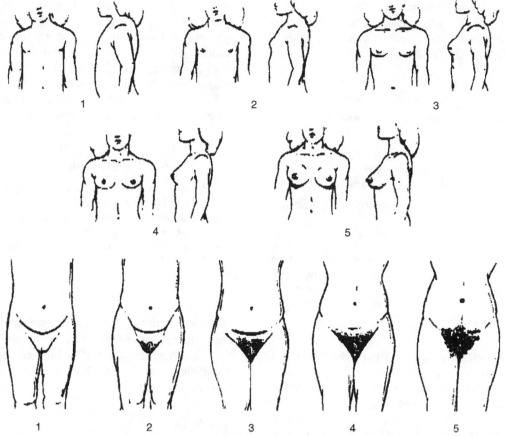

Figure 9–3 Stages of Female Sexual Maturation. Top and center, based on breast examination, stages are (1) prepubertal; no glandular tissue; (2) breast bud, small amount of glandular tissue; (3) breast mound and areola enlarged, no contour separation; (4) breast enlarged, areola and papilla form mound projecting from breast contour, and (5) mature, areola part of breast contour. Bottom, based on pelvic examination, stages are (1) no hair; (2) sparse, long, straight, lightly pigmented on labia majoria; (3) darker, beginning to curl, extend laterally; (4) coarse curly, abundant, less than adult; and (5) adult type and quantity, extending to medial thigh.

Measurable Factors That May Contribute to Late Menarche

- Nutritional status
- Socioeconomic factors
- Family size
- Disease states
- Exercise intensity
- Genetics

Clinical Guideline

Nutrition

Nutritional problems are more common in the female than the male athlete. The adequacy of the diet should be judged on foods eaten over a number of days to allow for natural fluctuations in appetite with special attention to iron, calcium, and caloric needs. Although children need to eat a variety of foods from all four food groups, it is not necessary that each meal or even day's meals be balanced.

Iron

Proper amounts of body iron are essential for optimizing athletic performance. Iron deficiency of a sufficient degree to cause anemia leads to easy fatigability and therefore an impaired physical work capacity. Gastrointestinal, neurological (mood and cognitive function), and immunological functions may also be negatively affected by low iron stores. Forty to 50% of adolescent female athletes demonstrate some degree of iron depletion, especially runners and swimmers.[15] The rapid growth, menstrual blood losses, and poor dietary habits of adolescent females place them at high risk for anemia. The American Academy of Pediatrics has recommended laboratory assessment of iron status in young females with "a serious commitment to exercise performance."[16]

Clinical Signs of Iron Deficiency Anemia

- Fatigue
- Decreased work capacity
- Impaired mood and cognition
- Decreased immunological function

Clinical Guideline

Given the prevalence of iron deficiency in adolescent female athletes, routine prophylactic iron supplementation (105 mg elemental iron a day) should be considered.[15]

Calcium

Inadequate calcium ingestion has been associated with stress fractures and shin splints.[17]

Most adolescent girls consume well below the 1200-mg recommended daily allowance of calcium.[18] A decreased consumption of milk and dairy products (sometimes in an effort to avoid high-fat foods, sometimes as a result of lactose intolerance) is often associated with an increased consumption of carbonated beverages. The high phosphorus content of these drinks may result in increased calcium excretion.[19] Providing teenage athletes with nutritional information regarding the variety of foods rich in calcium will allow them to select those foods that they prefer, and, hopefully, encourage them to assume responsibility for making wise food and beverage choices.

Weight Control

In general, it has been reported that 20% of all female athletes may have some degree of eating disorder. To control their weight, they use at least one of the following techniques for weight control: self-induced vomiting, laxatives, diet pills, diuretics, and bingeing.[17(p 1143)] A variety of factors may contribute to disordered eating patterns in the young athlete, including the pressure to optimize performance or meet inappropriate weight or body fat goals. Societal expectations and established norms for certain sports may encourage an athlete to attain a certain body shape, without regard to genetic predisposition, lack of appropriate coping skills to deal with stress, low self-esteem, and lack of sense of identity.[5(p 694–698)] Some sports place athletes at higher risk for these behaviors developing. These sports include (1)

those in which subjective judging encourages lean appearance, such as gymnastics, diving, figure skating, dance, and synchronized swimming; (2) sports that emphasize body leanness for optimal performance such as long distance running, swimming, and cross-country skiing; and (3) sports that use weight classifications such as rowing, body building, and martial arts.[5(pp 694–698)] Disordered eating may impair athletic performance and increase injury risk.

Sports with Higher Risks of Disordered Eating

- Aesthetic events: gymnastics, diving, figure skating, dance, and synchronized swimming
- Endurance activities: long distance running, swimming, cross-country skiing
- Weight classifications: rowing, body building, martial arts

Clinical Guideline

Athletes, parents, coaches, athletic administrators, training staff, and physicians need to be educated about the risks and warning signs of disordered eating, electrolyte disturbances, and cardiac dysrhythmias, menstrual dysfunction, and bone loss.

Steroid Use

Anabolic steroid use continues to increase among adolescent athletes and nonathletes alike. Prevalence of self-reported use of anabolic steroids has ranged from 5% to 11% of males and up to 2.5% of females.[20] Athletes seeking to add strength, bulk, muscle definition, or to improve their self-image must be considered to be at risk. Anabolic steroids cause myriad complications that are further discussed in Chapter 23.

STRENGTH TRAINING

Is strength training safe for children? Is it beneficial? Can it prevent injury? The purpose of strength training, according to a 1990 statement of the American Academy of Pediatrics Committee on Sports Medicine, is to "increase muscular strength, endurance, and/or power for sports participation or fitness enhancement."[21]

Strength training for prepubescent, pubescent, and postpubescent athletes is permissible if conducted by well-trained adults. The program should be appropriate to the youngster's stage of maturation, based on an objective medical assessment. In addition, repetitive use of maximal amounts of weight in strength training programs should be delayed until Tanner Stage 5 (full pubertal development).[22] At this time, all growth plates are closed. Repetition, even more than resistance, is the most important training principle, because endurance is of paramount concern. Low-resistance training is preferable, because it is less likely to produce fatigue and weakness.[22] Children may be expected to become stronger with appropriate strength training. Increased strength can enhance their performance in those athletic activities in which strength, power, or speed is required.[23] It may reduce the incidence and severity of overuse injury in sport. However, it cannot be expected to protect against serious acute injuries.[23] Close supervision is important in avoiding injuries, because trained adults are able to correct improper technique and resolve early musculoskeletal complaints.

Strength training for children and adolescents is not without risk. Proven medical concerns relate to back, shoulder, knee, and other joint injuries and to hypertension and related diseases. However, the rate of injury is probably rather low, comparable to many youthful activities that are considered safe. Also, the incidence and severity of injury can probably be minimized by attending to complaints about back, shoulder, knee, and other joint pain.[23] Rotation of muscle groups and types of strength training is recommended to prevent overuse.

Proper stretching is also necessary to prevent loss of flexibility. Stretching is probably the best way to increase muscle and tissue flexibility. It helps to relieve muscle tension, which in turn facilitates ease of movement, which can result in enhanced athletic performance.[1(p 87)] Joint hypermobility is more common in female subjects than in male subjects as demonstrated in many studies, but the clinical significance of this is not known. More research is needed in this area.

Maintaining Safe Preadult Strength Training

- Incorporate 5- to 10-minute cardiovascular warmup.
- Use low to medium resistance; *do not use maximum resistance.*
- Avoid resisted hyperflexion and hyperextension movements.
- Maintain strength training within functional range of motion.
- Change exercise program when strength training regimen becomes easy.
- Incorporate rest days; do not strength train similar muscle groups on consecutive days.
- Use cross-training to build strength and endurance.
- Resistance train *after* sports activity to prevent injury during play caused by fatigue.
- Use bodily resistance whenever possible (push-ups, pull-ups, squats).
- Carefully assess fit and range of motion of equipment, if used.
- Always finish strength training with stretching.
- Assess muscle soreness—soreness greater than 24 to 48 hours indicates overtraining.

Clinical Guideline

Psychological

The psychological benefits of athletic participation are numerous. When compared with nonathletes, some studies suggest that female athletes are more successful academically.[24] Girls involved in athletics are less likely to drop out of school, and they are more likely to attend college.[25] Among adolescent girls, there appears to be a correlation between athletic participation and older age of the first sexual experience, and an inverse relationship between involvement in sports and level of sexual activity and rate of pregnancy; furthermore, involvement in athletics programs is actually protective for young girls in regard to substance abuse.[25] Young women develop leadership skills, cooperativeness, teamwork, self-discipline, and coping skills in success and adversity, as well as respect for authority, competitiveness, sportsmanship, and self-confidence. They have opportunities for self-evaluation, peer comparison, and healthy competition, which helps to facilitate the development of positive self-esteem and self-control. Youth sports encourage socialization, social competence, family bonding, and facilitate the development of friendships across racial and ethnic groups. Youth sports also promote individual physical and psychological growth and health.[26] Female athletes tend to be more intrinsically motivated, assertive, achievement oriented, independent, and self-sufficient than nonathletic women.[27]

Sociological Benefits of Athletic Participation

- College attendance increased
- Delay of sexual relations and decreased rate of pregnancy
- Less substance abuse

Clinical Guideline

The psychological needs of young athletes are the same as for older athletes but to a greater degree. Young people require positive input and approval at frequent intervals, and competitive female athletes even more. The young athlete criticized in public by his coach learns nothing of positive value. Young females desire attention, praise, and opportunities to perform.[5(p 700)]

Positive reinforcement, encouragement, and sound technical instruction within a supportive environment are the best ways to facilitate motivation, morale, enjoyment, performance, physical competence, and group cohesion in sports.[26(p 708)] Motivation in sports for girls 8 to 18 years of age is related to improvement of skills, having fun, being challenged, learning new skills, and being physically fit.[28] A healthy goal is to encourage desired behaviors with positive reinforcement. This instills motivation and a desire to achieve instead of a fear of failure.

INJURIES

In the past decade, there has been a 700% increase in sports injuries in women; this increase parallels the increase in participation and competition in young women's athletics.[29,30] Sports injuries follow predictable patterns on the basis of age, sport, and training strategies. With the exception of knee and ankle injuries, injury rates for males and females are similar.[29,30] Sports injuries can be divided into two groups: isolated macrotrauma caused by a single event of impact or acceleration/deceleration; and repetitive microtrauma, generally referred to as chronic injury or overuse injury. Acute sports injuries include contusions, fractures, sprains, and strains. These injuries are three times more common during practice than during competition[31] and are more common in unsupervised than supervised sports. Injuries are also more common with increasing age, probably because of an increase in size, strength, and intensity of competition. The highest rate of serious skeletal injury occurs in Tanner stage III (midpubertal) athletes because of the relative growth plate weakness during maximal linear growth.[29] Acute traumatic injury to the extremity of the preadolescent and early adolescent is more likely to result in fracture through the epiphyseal plate than to cause ligament disruption, because the weakest point is at the growth plate.

Goals for preventing acute injury include supervised warmup and stretching, avoidance of reckless or illegal play, and use of developmentally appropriate equipment. Training should emphasize flexibility, strength, and endurance. Prehabilitation of weaker or "at-risk" joints is recommended. Competitors should be matched on the basis of weight and strength rather than on chronological age. Management of acute injury should include RICE—rest, ice, compression, and elevation—as well as nonsteroidal anti-inflammatory medications. Rehabilitation is paramount, with emphasis on obtaining full range of motion and strength before returning to competition. Incomplete rehabilitation increases risk of reinjury (refer to the Prologue).[32] Functional rehabilitation implies safe, pain-free return to sport with close follow-up by an athletic trainer, coach, therapist, and/or physician.

Repetitive microtrauma causes chronic overuse injury when the degree and frequency of the microtrauma outpace the athlete's repair mechanisms. These injuries are character-ized by mechanical pain (pain that increases with activity and decreases with rest) with no specific history of trauma.[33] Thirty to 50% of pediatric sports injuries are due to overuse.[34]

Chronic overuse injuries include avulsions, bursitis, tendinitis, apophysitis, long-bone stress fractures, and inflammation of the joints. These injuries are more common during growth spurts (Tanner stage III), because the soft tissue elongation lags behind bone growth, resulting in decreased joint flexibility.[35] Other predisposing factors in overuse injury include rotational and angular deformities, bone density, type of sport, training intensity and errors, and equipment.[35] The incidence of chronic overuse injuries can be minimized by optimizing the "six S's": shoes, surface, speed, structure, strength, and stretching.[1(p 104)] Properly sized equipment and well-maintained playing surfaces are important. Optimal training (speed) can be obtained by allowing no more than a 10% increase in training per week. Structural problems such as leg-length discrepancy, malalignment, and hyperpronation should be corrected with orthotics. Conditioning programs should emphasize strengthening and stretching, because muscular imbalance and decreased flexibility significantly increase the risk of injury.[29,30]

The knee is the most common area of injury in the young female athlete and is the most frequent complaint of young girls seen in a sports medicine practice. Commonly, patellofemoral pain/chondromalacia patella or patellar subluxation is diagnosed and often contributes to the discomfort and challenge of treating acute injuries to other knee joint structures. Adolescent and collegiate female basketball and soccer players have a higher risk for anterior cruciate ligament injuries and often have higher risks of tear than their male counterparts.[5(p 698)] Patellofemoral pain is more common in female athletes than in male athletes because of anatomical alignment and the resultant imbalance of musculotendinous units about the patella.[5(p 698)] Early treatment is most effective; prehabilitation in girls with excessive Q angles or patellar hypermobility is recommended. Assessment includes evaluation of ankle laxity, lower limb alignment including foot position, patellar glide, and patellar tilt. Rehabilitation is always recommended in athletes with persistent discomfort and is often curative. Refer to Appendix 5–A for guidelines on effective rehabilitation; this includes stretching, strengthening, proprioceptive training, and icing. Efficacy of prophylactic knee bracing is in doubt and not recommended by the American Academy of Pediatrics Committee on Sports Medicine,[36] although Mc-Connell taping can be quite helpful.

Ankle sprains are extremely common in all sports, at rates similar to the knee. Hip flexor tendinopathies are also prevalent, along with shoulder laxity and pain. The spine is also a common reported area of overuse injury in girls. The sports most likely to cause back pain are gymnastics, dance, riding, running, football, and ice hockey. Localized tenderness, kyphosis, step-off sign, and radicular signs combined with sports history and radiographs or bone scans can usually clarify the diagnosis.[35] Particular to sports involving repetitive extension, including diving and gymnastics, pars fractures and spondylolisthesis must be considered.

Management of both chronic and acute injury includes the use of nonsteroidal anti-inflammatory medication and ice for control of pain and inflammation. Supervised rehabilitation should emphasize stretching, strengthening, and using relative rest to optimize conditioning while avoiding activity that aggravates the injury. Maintaining athlete-team contact during rehabilitation is essential to the young athlete's sense of identity and anticipation of effective return to play.

PREVENTION OF INJURIES

The American College of Sports Medicine estimates that 50% of overuse injuries in children and adolescents are preventable.[37] Prevention of injuries involves keeping athletes properly hydrated before, during, and after events; monitoring intensity of training with gradual increases; enforcing preseason and postseason conditioning with prehabilitation as appropriate; providing appropriate medical coverage of sporting events; arranging proper officiating and safety rule enforcement for all competitive sporting events; maintaining proper equipment and field conditions[2]; and coach, trainer, parent, and athlete education of needs specific to female athletes.

In conclusion, young females gain considerably from participating in sports and should be encouraged to participate in as many forms of athletics as possible. Further research is greatly needed to define some of the physiological differences between young females compared with young males in the athletic arena. This research could improve young women's maximal performance in a wide range of athletics by allowing coaches and parents to learn the ideal training programs for competitive athletes of all ages.

REFERENCES

1. Schreiber LR. *The Parent's Guide to Kids Sports*. Boston: Time Inc Magazine Co; 1990:63–72.

2. Hergenroeder AC. Prevention of sports injuries. *Pediatrics*. 1998;101:1057–1063.

3. Tanner JM, Davis PSW. Clinical longitudinal standards for height and height velocity for North American children. *J Pediatrics*. 1985;107:317. Copyright owners: Castlemead Publications.

4. Malina RM. Growth, strength and physical performance. In: Shangold M, Mirkin G. *Women and Exercise: Physiology and Sports Medicine*. 2nd ed. Philadelphia: FA Davis; 1995:142–151.

5. Van De Loo DA, Johnson MD. The young female athlete. *Clin Sports Med*. 1995;24:689.

6. Bar-Or O. The prepubescent female. In: Shangold M, Mirkin G. *Women and Exercise: Physiology and Sports Medicine*. 2nd ed. Philadelphia: FA Davis; 1995:130–131.

7. Drinkwater BL, Kuppart IC, Denton JE, et al. Response of prepubertal girls and college women to work in the heat. *J Appl Physiol*. 1977;43:1046.

8. Cantu RC. *Sports Medicine in Primary Care*. Lexington, KY: Collamore Press; 1982:86–87.

9. Malina RM, Bouchard C. *Growth, Maturation, and Physical Activity*. Champaign, IL: Human Kinetics; 1991.

10. Baker ER. Menstrual dysfunction and hormonal status in women. *Fertil Steril*. 1981;36:691–696.

11. Schwartz B, Cumming DC, Riordan E, et al. Exercise-associated amenorrhea: A distinct entity? *Am J Obstet Gynecol*. 1981;141:662.

12. Sanborn CF, Martin BJ, Wagner WW. Is athletic amenorrhea specific to runners? *Am J Obstet Gynecol*. 1982;143:859.

13. Wells CL. *Women, Sport and Performance: A Physiological Perspective*. 2nd ed. Champaign, IL: Human Kinetics; 1991:85–96.

14. White CM, Hergenroeder AC. Amenorrhea, osteopenia, and the female athlete. *Pediatr Clin North Am*. 1990;37:1125–1137.

15. Rowland TW. Iron deficiency in the young athlete. *Pediatr Clin North Am*. 1990; 37:1153.

16. Smith NJ. *Sports Medicine: Health Care for Young Athletes*. Evanston, IL: American Academy of Pediatrics; 1983:1.

17. Loosli AR, Benson J. Nutritional intake in adolescent athletes. *Pediatr Clin North Am*. 1990;37:1143–1151.

18. Benardot D, Schwarz M, Heller DW. Nutrient intake in young, highly competitive gymnasts. *J Am Diet Assoc*. 1989;89:401–403.

19. Pearl AJ. *The Athletic Female: American Orthopaedic Society for Sports Medicine*. Champaign, IL: Human Kinetics; 1993:119–120.

20. American Academy of Pediatrics. Committee on Sports Medicine and Fitness. Adolescents and anabolic steroids: A subject review. *Pediatrics*. 1997;99:904–908.

21. American Academy of Pediatrics Committee on Sports Medicine. Strength training, weight and power lifting, and body building by children and adolescents. *Pediatrics*. 1990;86:801.

22. Alberta FG. Strength training vs "pumping iron." *Cont Pediatr.* 1993;10:36–52.

23. Webb DR. Strength training in children and adolescents. *Pediatr Clin North Am.* 1990;37:1187–1207.

24. Women's Sports Foundation Report. *Minorities in Sport.* East Meadow, NY: Women's Sports Foundation; 1989.

25. Bunker LK, Pradt K, eds. *The President's Council on Physical Fitness and Sports Report: Physical Activity and Sport in the Lives of Girls.* Washington, DC: US Department of Health and Human Services; 1997.

26. Stryer BK, Tofler IR, Lapchick R. A developmental overview of child and youth sports in society. *Child Adolesc Psych Clin North Am.* 1998;7:702.

27. Agostini R. *Medical and Orthopedic Issues of Active and Athletic Women.* Philadelphia: Hanley & Belfus; 1994:94.

28. Smith RE, Zane NWS, Smoll FL, et al. Behavioral assessment in youth sports: Coaching behaviors and children's attitudes. *Med Sci Sports Exerc.* 1983;15:208–214.

29. Stanitski CN. Common injuries in preadolescent and adolescent athletes: Recommendations for prevention. *Sports Med.* 1989;7:32–41.

30. Stanitski CN. Management of sports injuries in children and adolescents. *Orthop Clin North Am.* 1988;19:689–698.

31. Garrick JG, Requa RK. Girls' sports injuries in high school athletes. *JAMA.* 1978;239:2245–2248.

32. Micheli LJ. Pediatric and adolescent sports injuries: Recent trends. *Exerc Sport Sci Rev.* 1986;14:359–375.

33. O'Neill DB, Michele LJ. Overuse injuries in the young athlete. *Clin Sports Med.* 1988;7:591–610.

34. Difiori JP. Overuse injuries in children and adolescents. *Physician Sports Med.* 1999;27:1.

35. Molnar G. *Pediatric Rehabilitation.* 2nd ed. Baltimore: Williams & Wilkins; 1992:473–475.

36. American Academy of Pediatrics Committee on Sports Medicine. Knee brace use by athletes. *Pediatrics.* 1990;82:228.

37. Current comment from the American College of Sports Medicine. The prevention of sports injuries of children and adolescents. *Med Sci Sports Exerc.* 1993;25(Suppl 8):1–7.

Patellofemoral Rehabilitation and Strengthening Program

The following can be used as a guide for patellofemoral rehabilitation or prehabilitation. Stretches depicted are recommended as conditioning and preplay activity in multiple sports. Advanced quadriceps strengthening exercises demonstrated at the end of the pictorial can be incorporated into conditioning for athletes at all levels. Subject depicted is a 10-year-old white female soccer player, who had left knee pain develop. After an aggressive rehabilitation program incorporating the following stretches and exercises, along with a home program and icing after exercise and play, her pain resolved in 6 weeks.

Step 1: Assessment.

Figure 9–A1 On beginning therapy program, alignment should be assessed in relation to hip and foot. Foot and ankle alignment can also be observed and should be assessed in chronic conditions and with mistracking or significant malalignment. Q angle should be noted.

Figure 9–A2 Patellar tilt should be assessed. McConnell taping can be used if tilt is present as demonstrated in Figure 9–A3.

Figure 9–A3 McConnell taping aids in guiding the patella to appropriate tracking.

Step 2: Stretching—passive stretching shown; athletes should be taught self-stretches to do at home and before play.

Figure 9–A4 Hamstring stretch.

Figure 9–A5 Gastrocnemius stretch. Should also be done with bent knee to stretch soleus.

Figure 9–A6 Hip flexor stretch.

Figure 9–A7 Iliotibial band stretch.

Step 3: Strengthening

Figure 9–A8 Terminal knee extensions (pressing against pillow); can also be done isometrically against firm pillow with limited movement.

Figure 9–A9 Straight-leg raising.

Figure 9–A10 Terminal knee extensions with resistance.

Step 4: Advanced conditioning and maintenance

Figure 9–A11 Wall seats.

Figure 9–A12 Step ups.

Figure 9–A13 Balance and proprioception.

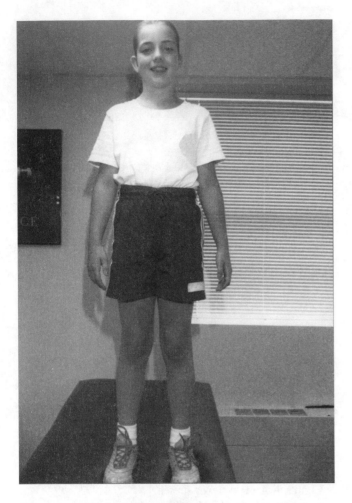

Figure 9–A1 Evaluating Alignment.

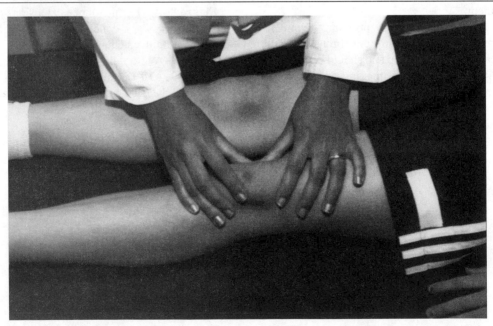

Figure 9–A2 Patellar Tilt.

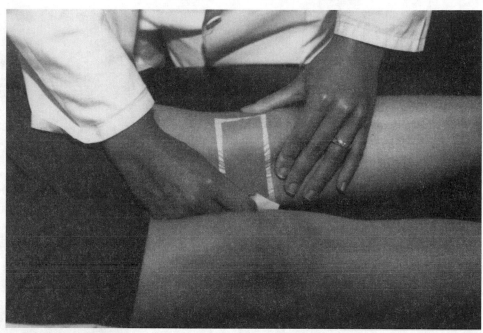

A

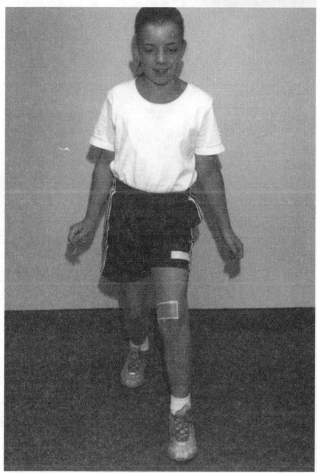

B

Figure 9–A3 McConnell Taping.

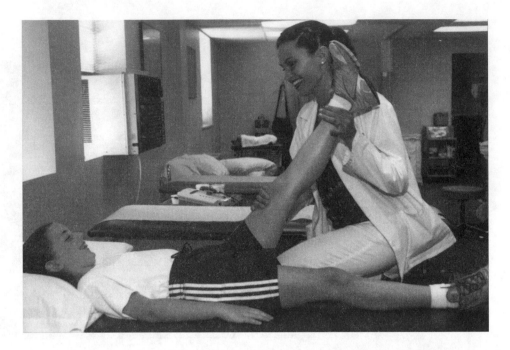

Figure 9–A4 Hamstring Stretch.

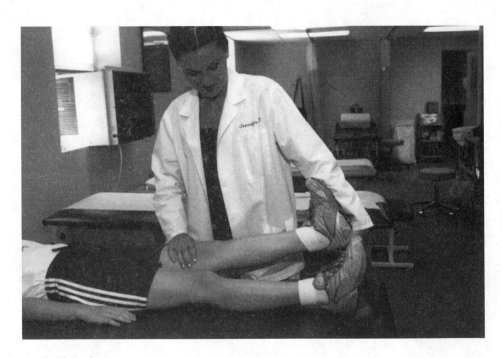

Figure 9–A5 Gastrocnemius Stretch.

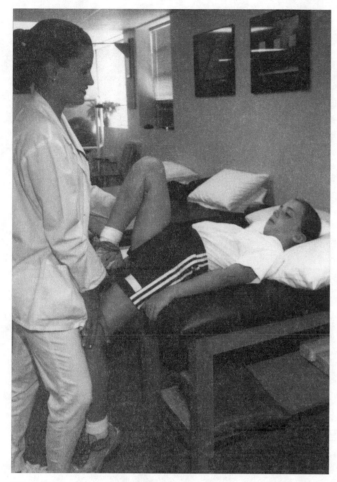

Figure 9–A6 Hip Flexor Stretch.

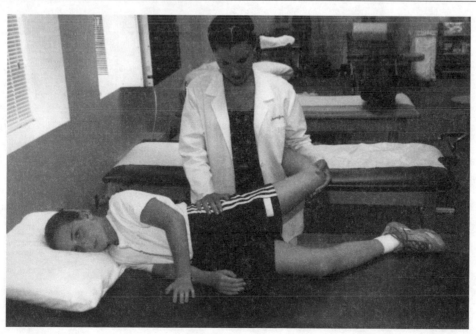

Figure 9–A7 Iliotibial Band Stretch.

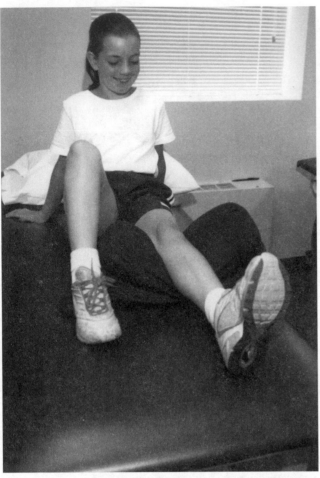

Figure 9–A8 Terminal Knee Extensions.

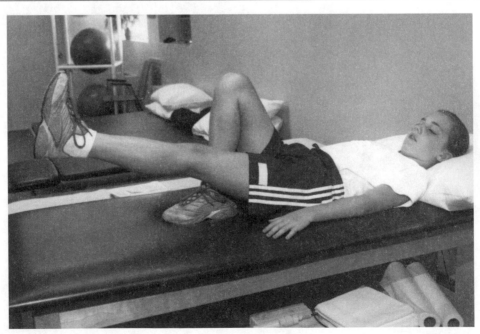

Figure 9–A9 Straight-Leg Raising.

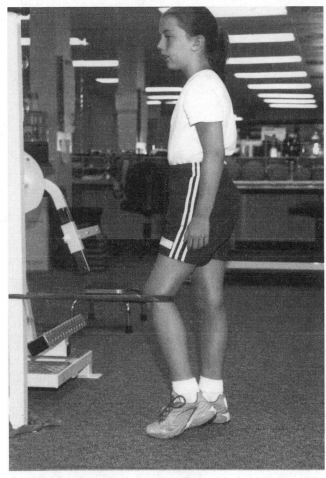

Figure 9–A10 Weightbearing Terminal Knee Extensions with Resistance.

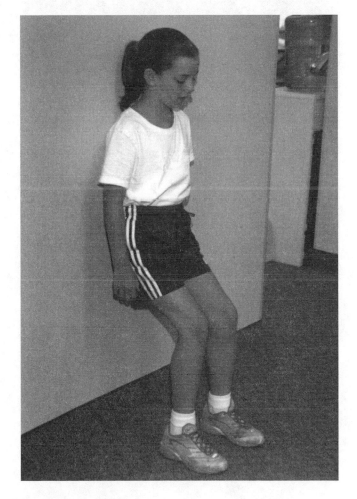

Figure 9–A11 Wall Seats.

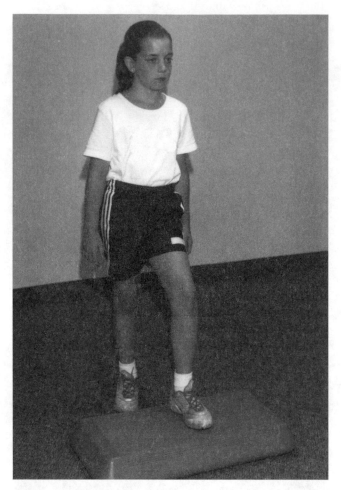

Figure 9–A12 Step Ups.

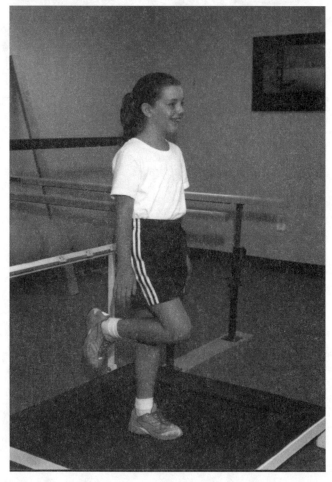

Figure 9–A13 Balance and Proprioception.

CHAPTER 10

Reproductive Cycles

Karen A. Carlberg

THE HUMAN MENSTRUAL CYCLE

Menstrual cycles occur in women between menarche, the first menstrual period, and menopause, the last menstrual period. In the United States, menarche occurs at an average age of 12 years, and menopause occurs at an average age of 51 years. Each menstrual cycle normally is associated with the ovulation of one egg and, therefore, one opportunity for a pregnancy.

On the average, each menstrual cycle lasts 28 days, although normal cycles may be as short as approximately 23 days or as long as about 35 days. In a "perfect" 28-day cycle, by convention the first day of a menstrual period is designated day 1. Ovulation occurs on day 14. Day 28 is the day before the next menstrual period begins.

The menstrual cycle can be divided into two phases: the follicular phase and the luteal phase. The follicular phase occurs on days 1 through 14. During these 2 weeks, ovarian follicles grow in preparation for ovulation. The ovum in the center of a follicle enlarges, and the follicular cells surrounding the ovum proliferate and grow. Of the several follicles that are developing in both ovaries early in the follicular phase, all but one normally die at some point during the follicular phase, and by about day 12, there is just one large developed follicle remaining in one ovary. This is called the graafian follicle and is destined for ovulation. At ovulation on day 14, the ovum is released from the ovary along with the layers of follicular cells immediately surrounding it. The remaining follicular cells stay in the ovary and transform themselves into a corpus luteum. This corpus luteum remains active in the ovary for about 10 days if a pregnancy does not occur. If a pregnancy does occur, the corpus luteum

remains active for most of the pregnancy. The luteal phase of a menstrual cycle is on days 15 through 28, when the corpus luteum is developing, active, and then regressing.

Although these events in the ovaries are essential to reproduction, other organs are essential as well. Ovarian activity is regulated by hormonal communications among the hypothalamus, anterior lobe of the pituitary gland, and ovarian follicles and corpora lutea, and by paracrine communications within the ovary. Regulation of ovarian activity by the brain and pituitary enables the brain to promote reproduction when the physical and emotional condition of the body as a whole is favorable for a pregnancy and to inhibit reproduction when the body's condition is not favorable for a pregnancy. In turn, hormones secreted by ovarian follicles and corpora lutea communicate to the uterine tubes, uterus, and mammary glands, causing them to prepare for ovulation, fertilization, and a potential pregnancy.

Figure 10–1 illustrates the fluctuations in blood concentrations of the major known reproductive hormones during a normal 28-day menstrual cycle. These include follicle-stimulating hormone (FSH) and luteinizing hormone (LH), which are called the gonadotropins and are secreted by the anterior lobe of the pituitary gland, estrogen (mainly 17β-estradiol), which is secreted by both ovarian follicles and corpora lutea, and progesterone, which is secreted mainly by the corpus luteum. Not shown in the figure is gonadotropin-releasing hormone (GnRH), which is secreted by the hypothalamus and not readily measurable in peripheral blood.

GnRH is secreted by neuroendocrine cells of the arcuate nucleus of the hypothalamus. These neuroendocrine cells secrete GnRH into capillaries of the hypothalamic-pituitary

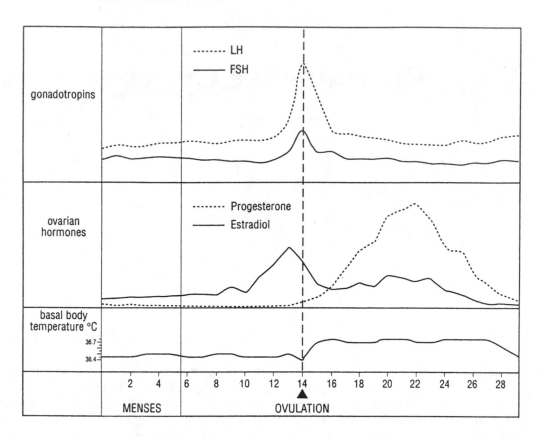

Figure 10–1 Fluctuations in Plasma Concentrations of Gonadotropins and Ovarian Hormones and in Basal Body Temperature during One Normal 28-Day Menstrual Cycle.

portal system, a system of blood vessels that then carries the GnRH directly to the anterior lobe of the pituitary gland, where GnRH molecules can diffuse out of the blood into the pituitary. Once in the pituitary, GnRH can bind to and stimulate gonadotropes, the anterior pituitary cells that secrete FSH and LH, which in turn stimulate the ovaries. The GnRH-secreting neuroendocrine cells probably are influenced by a variety of neurotransmitters and hormones, allowing their activity to be facilitated or inhibited by factors reflecting the physical and emotional condition of the body. When the GnRH-secreting neuroendocrine cells generate action potentials, they release GnRH from their axon terminals, just as any other type of neuron releases its neurotransmitter when it has action potentials. Instead of diffusing into a synaptic cleft, as most neurotransmitters do, GnRH diffuses into the capillaries that are located adjacent to the axon terminals. From these capillaries, the GnRH is carried by the bloodstream from the hypothalamus to the anterior pituitary. When GnRH molecules diffuse out of pituitary capillaries to gonadotropes, they bind to GnRH receptors on the gonadotropes, thus stimulating the pituitary cells to release FSH and LH. The regulation of FSH and LH secretion may involve other hormonal influences on the

gonadotropes as well, but those influences are not as well understood as those of GnRH.

Rather than generating action potentials continuously, the GnRH-secreting neuroendocrine cells generate brief, synchronous bursts of action potentials followed by periods of quiescence. Thus, GnRH is released in pulses. The time interval between pulses of GnRH may vary from about 1 to 2 hours during the follicular phase to about 4 hours or longer during the luteal phase. With each pulse of GnRH, there is a pulse of FSH secretion and a pulse of LH secretion. Figure 10–2 shows an example of the pulsations in blood concentration of LH, reflecting the pulses of GnRH and LH secretion. In Figure 10–1, average concentrations, rather than pulsations, of FSH and LH are shown. The pulses in FSH and LH concentrations are part of the communication from hypothalamus and pituitary to the ovaries.

When FSH and LH arrive at the ovaries, they stimulate ovarian activity, but in different ways. Both are essential for follicular maturation and ovarian hormone secretion. Follicles destined for ovulation begin developing a few months before ovulation, without requiring gonadotropin stimulation. About 2 to 3 weeks before ovulation, the follicles become dependent on gonadotropins. FSH stimulates

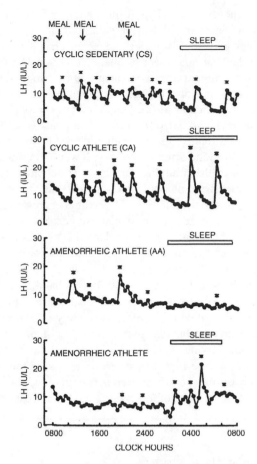

Figure 10–2 Serum LH Levels at 20-min Intervals for 24 h in a CS, a CA, and Two AA Women. A range of patterns was found in the AA women. The asterisks indicate pulses, as identified by the cluster pulse analysis program using a 2 × 1 cluster size and balanced T criteria of 2.1.

follicle growth, especially in the early follicular phase. The follicles have two layers of follicular cells surrounding the ovum: granulosa cells on the inside and theca cells around the periphery. FSH promotes proliferation and growth of the granulosa cells and stimulates these cells to synthesize and secrete estrogen. It causes granulosa cells to synthesize LH receptors. Also in the follicular phase, LH stimulates theca cells to synthesize and secrete androgens, which diffuse to the granulosa cells, where the androgens are precursors for estrogen synthesis. Thus, both gonadotropins participate in preparation of follicles for ovulation and in promoting estrogen secretion.

Figure 10–1 shows that estrogen concentrations are low early in the follicular phase and then rise to very high levels at the end of the follicular phase, reflecting granulosa cell activity. High levels of estrogen before ovulation are essential for ovulation to occur and for preparation of the reproductive tract for fertilization and implantation. Estro-

gen enhances uterine tube motility, promoting egg transport from ovary to uterus. It stimulates endometrial growth in preparation for implantation. It causes cervical epithelial cells to secrete a thin mucus that allows sperm penetration of the cervix.

High estrogen levels just before ovulation also stimulate the LH surge, which causes the graafian follicle to ovulate. This is a positive feedback action and is the way that the graafian follicle communicates to the hypothalamic-pituitary unit that the follicle is ready for ovulation. The very large amounts of LH stimulate maturation of the ovum and disintegration of the follicle wall, leading to release of the ovum from the ovary, along with the granulosa cells immediately surrounding the ovum.

After ovulation, most of the granulosa and theca cells remain in the ovary. The LH surge causes these cells to luteinize, forming the corpus luteum. Enzymatic changes in these cells result in their ability to secrete large amounts of progesterone and smaller amounts of estrogen. Therefore the luteal phase of the menstrual cycle is characterized by high levels of progesterone and moderate levels of estrogen.

The progesterone of the luteal phase is essential for a successful pregnancy. It promotes maturation of the endometrium, so that an embryo can implant in the uterus about a week after fertilization (which occurs within 24 hours of ovulation). It promotes quiescence of the smooth muscle in the uterine tube and myometrium. It causes the cervical epithelial cells to secrete a thick mucus that inhibits sperm movement through the cervix.

Unless a pregnancy occurs, the corpus luteum is short-lived. After about 12 days, it regresses and becomes a nonfunctional corpus albicans. As a result, concentrations of progesterone and estrogen fall precipitously on days 27 and 28 of the menstrual cycle.

In addition to the positive feedback action mentioned previously, there is a negative feedback relationship between the gonadotropins and ovarian hormones. Both estrogen and progesterone inhibit the secretion of GnRH, FSH, and LH. Therefore, except during the LH surge, there is a somewhat inverse relationship between the levels of gonadotropins and the levels of ovarian hormones.

A menstrual period results from the actions of estrogen and progesterone on the endometrium of the uterus. During the follicular phase, estrogen causes the endometrium to grow in thickness. The growth of endometrial glands and blood vessels is stimulated. In the luteal phase, progesterone causes a maturation, rather than a further growth in thickness, of the endometrium, preparing it for implantation. The endometrial glands begin synthesizing glycogen and other substances essential for successful implantation. When progesterone and estrogen concentrations fall at the end of the luteal phase, the endometrium responds by dying, disintegrating, and shedding. Over the course of about 3 to

5 days (days 1 through about 5 of the menstrual cycle), the shed endometrium leaves the uterine cavity as the menstrual flow. At the end of a menstrual period, only the deepest layer of the endometrium remains in the uterus. This remaining endometrium will grow and thicken with the next menstrual cycle.

In summary, a normal menstrual cycle results in the ovulation of one ovum on about day 14 of each cycle. Hormonal communications among the hypothalamus, anterior pituitary, ovarian follicles, and corpus luteum ensure that the ovarian follicles and reproductive tract develop and change in a sequence that will allow a successful pregnancy. If a pregnancy does not occur, the corpus luteum and endometrium die so that a new cycle, and a new opportunity for pregnancy, will ensue.

EFFECTS OF THE MENSTRUAL CYCLE ON EXERCISE PERFORMANCE

As described in the previous section, estrogen and progesterone promote changes in reproductive organs that are necessary for successful ovulation, fertilization, and implantation of an embryo. Once a pregnancy is established, the placenta secretes larger amounts of estrogen and progesterone than the ovaries do, and these hormones are important for creating adaptations in the mother's body that help her support the pregnancy. Many of these adaptations are in tissues other than reproductive organs. And many of these physiological effects have the potential to affect exercise performance. Therefore, it is reasonable to ask whether the fluctuations in estrogen and progesterone concentrations during a normal menstrual cycle affect exercise performance.

Several variables that are important to aerobic exercise performance may be influenced by ovarian hormones. These include ventilation, fluid volume homeostasis, body temperature regulation, and substrate metabolism.

Estrogen and progesterone influence ventilation, fluid volume homeostasis, body temperature regulation, and substrate metabolism. Each of these has the potential to affect exercise performance.

Clinical Guideline

Ventilation is stimulated by progesterone. This may be important during pregnancy when a mother must provide gas exchange for both herself and her fetus. In human subjects at rest, progesterone administration causes increased minute ventilation and arterial pH and reduced alveolar and arterial P_{CO_2}.[1,2] When progesterone levels are high during the luteal phase of the menstrual cycle, there may be a larger resting minute ventilation, lower alveolar P_{CO_2}, and increased ven-

tilatory response to both hypercapnia and hypoxia, but findings are inconsistent.[3–6] During submaximal exercise, the differences between follicular and luteal phases persist in some studies but not others. Schoene et al[3] found a higher minute ventilation for an equivalent submaximal exercise oxygen consumption (V_{O_2}) in the luteal phase compared with the midfollicular phase. Dombovy et al[7] reported that during submaximal exercise in the luteal phase, ventilation was increased relative to carbon dioxide production but not relative to V_{O_2}, and arterial P_{CO_2} was lower and arterial pH higher than in the midfollicular phase. Other investigators found no menstrual phase differences in minute ventilation during submaximal exercise.[6,8–10] Maximal exercise ventilation may be the same in the follicular and luteal phases[6,7,10,11] or higher in the luteal phase.[8] Beidleman et al[6] reported that arterial oxygen saturation during treadmill exercise was not affected by menstrual cycle phase at sea level, but was 2.4% higher in the luteal phase at 4300 m simulated altitude. If exercise ventilation is higher in the luteal phase than in the follicular phase, it could increase the energy cost of breathing during exercise but also provide more oxygen, eliminate more carbon dioxide, and reduce acid accumulation. Overall it appears that the high progesterone levels of the luteal phase may or may not affect exercise ventilation, but in any case do not seem to be of much functional significance.

Ventilation

- Stimulated by progesterone
- Higher during lateral phase
- Questionable functional significance

Clinical Guideline

Plasma volume can be increased by estrogen administration.[12,13] During pregnancy, plasma volume increases substantially, contributing to a mother's ability to circulate blood to the growing uterus and placenta. If plasma volume is higher during menstrual phases when estrogen levels are higher, this might provide a fluid reserve that could help a woman to maintain adequate blood pressure in the face of sweating-induced fluid loss. Unfortunately, there are few data on fluctuations in plasma volume with the normal menstrual cycle. Stephenson and Kolka[14] reported that resting plasma volume was about 5% lower in the midluteal phase than in the early follicular phase, but they did not study the late follicular phase, when estrogen levels are highest. A little more information exists on the effect of menstrual cycle phase on plasma volume changes during exercise and heat exposure. During exercise in the heat, loss of plasma volume is less during the midluteal phase than during the early follicular phase.[14,15] De Souza et al[16] suggested that plasma volume may be maintained better during the luteal phase because resting levels of aldosterone are higher and exercise-induced elevations in aldosterone are greater in the luteal phase. Stachenfeld et al[17] reported higher levels of aldosterone and plasma renin activity and lower levels of atrial natriuretic hormone in the midluteal phase compared with the early follicular phase, but no differences in body water loss during exercise in the heat. Neither Phillips[18] nor Lewandowski et al[19] found differences in systolic or diastolic blood pressures at the end of exercise during various menstrual phases. Thus, the ability to maintain plasma volume during exercise in the heat may or may not be better in the midluteal phase than in the early follicular phase; the late follicular phase apparently has not been studied. There is no indication that the ability to maintain adequate blood pressure varies with the menstrual cycle, although data are few.

Basal body temperature is about 0.2 to 0.6°C higher in the luteal phase than in the follicular phase of the menstrual cycle, as shown in Figure 10–1. This probably results from the action of progesterone on thermoregulatory neurons in the hypothalamus, causing an upward shift in the set point for body temperature. Exercise almost always results in a rise in body temperature. During exercise at moderate air temperatures, body temperature usually remains higher in the luteal phase than in the follicular phase.[20,21] Pivarnik et al[22] found that women exercising at room temperature in the luteal phase never reached a thermal equilibrium during 60 minutes of cycle ergometry, whereas their temperatures plateaued when they exercised in the follicular phase. Menstrual phase effects on body temperature usually persist during exercise in the heat,[23,24] although some investigators report no menstrual phase effects on body temperature during exercise in the heat.[25,26] During light exercise in uncompensable heat stress, that is, at 40°C in heavy protective clothing that restricted evaporative heat loss, Tenaglia et al[27] found that women could continue the experiment longer in the early follicular phase than in the midluteal phase, when they had a higher rectal temperature. Higher temperature thresholds for cutaneous vasodilation and sweating may lead to higher body temperatures during exercise in the luteal phase.[20,24] Kolka and Stephenson[28] found that forearm blood flow leveled off at a higher level and at a higher body temperature in the midluteal phase than in the early follicular phase during exercise in the heat; they suggested that an effect of estrogen on the vasculature was possible. However, Charkoudian and Johnson[29] presented evidence that the effect of estrogen and progesterone on the temperature threshold for cutaneous vasodilation is more likely to be in the central nervous system. Carpenter and Nunneley[23] concluded that menstrual phase differences in temperature regulation are small in magnitude and may have minimal practical significance for a woman's ability to exercise, even in the heat.

> Body temperature is higher during the luteal phase than in the follicular phase of the menstrual cycle. This difference persists during exercise.
>
> *Clinical Guideline*

Substrate availability may be a limiting factor for aerobic exercise if the exercise is prolonged. Muscle cells derive most of their energy from glucose and fatty acids, which may come from intramuscular, hepatic, or adipose stores of glycogen and triglyceride or from hepatic gluconeogenesis. During exercise, substrate mobilization is regulated by the autonomic nervous system and by exercise-induced elevations in circulating catecholamines, glucagon, glucocorticoids, and several other hormones, as well as inhibition of insulin secretion. If muscle and hepatic glycogen stores become depleted by prolonged exercise, the exercise no longer can continue at a high metabolic rate; the individual becomes exhausted. Estrogens and progesterone influence some aspects of substrate metabolism and its hormonal regulation. Muscle and hepatic glycogen deposition appear to be enhanced by both of the ovarian hormones.[30–32] Hackney[33] reported that resting muscle glycogen content was higher in the midluteal phase than in the midfollicular phase. These effects may result from an increase of the insulin/glucagon ratio.[31] During exercise, estrogens and progesterone may enhance fatty acid oxidation, reduce glucose oxidation, reduce muscle glycogen depletion, and therefore prolong maximal aerobic exercise duration.[34–37] Nicklas et al[38] exercised women to exhaustion 4 days after a glycogen depletion exercise bout followed by glycogen repletion. When the protocol was performed during the luteal phase, the magnitude of glycogen repletion was greater and time to exhaustion was slightly longer than during the follicular phase. Other studies found no menstrual phase effects on substrate use and its hormonal regulation during exercise[39] and no effect of estradiol administration to amenorrheic women on rate of muscle glycogen use and time to exhaustion in treadmill running.[40] Overall, the evidence suggests that during the luteal phase glycogen deposition may be enhanced, glycogen use reduced, and fat use increased. This would improve endurance for prolonged exercise by allowing glycogen stores to last longer. The data are not consistent, however, and differences in study designs make it difficult to predict how menstrual cycle phase will affect substrate use during exercise.

In general, there are only small effects of menstrual cycle phase or ovarian hormone concentrations on ventilation, plasma volume homeostasis, body temperature regulation, and substrate availability and use. In the follicular phase, there may a slight advantage in minimizing body temperature rise, whereas in the luteal phase there may be slight advantages in minimizing sweating-induced body fluid loss and glycogen depletion. Higher ventilation in the luteal phase could be either advantageous or disadvantageous. Whether these slight and opposing effects influence overall aerobic exercise performance depends on the nature and conditions of the exercise, such as whether the exercise occurs in the heat or whether the exercise is prolonged.

Aerobic exercise performance can be assessed directly in the laboratory by measuring maximal oxygen consumption (Vo_{2max}) or time to exhaustion at a heavy submaximal exercise load. Vo_{2max} and time to exhaustion are affected by the menstrual phase in some, but not all, studies, and when menstrual phase effects are found, results are contradictory. Schoene et al[3] found a lower Vo_{2max} and shorter time to exhaustion during the luteal phase compared with the follicular phase in nonathletic women, but no menstrual phase differences in athletic subjects. Lebrun et al[41] found a slightly lower Vo_{2max} in athletic subjects during the luteal phase compared with the follicular phase but no difference in endurance time at a high submaximal load. Higgs and Robertson[42] reported that time to exhaustion was lowest 2 days before and on the day of menstruation onset. On the other hand, Jurkowski et al[8] reported a longer time to exhaustion during the luteal phase compared with the follicular phase. Other investigators found no effects of menstrual phase on aerobic exercise performance.[6,7,10,11,21,43] Thus, there are no consistent findings of menstrual phase effects on aerobic exercise performance, as measured by Vo_{2max} or time to exhaustion. None of these studies were done in the heat.

Menstrual Cycle Phase

- No consistent findings of effects on aerobic exercise performance
- No effect on muscle strength
- Few studies on effect of athletic performance

Clinical Guideline

Another important aspect of exercise performance is muscle strength. Most studies have reported no effect of menstrual cycle phase on muscle strength. Grip strength and knee extension strength were the same in four menstrual phases studied by Higgs and Robertson.[42] Dibrezzo et al[44] reported that dynamic strength of the knee flexors and extensors was similar during menses, ovulation, and the luteal phase. Recreational weight lifters studied by Quadagno et al[45] showed no menstrual phase differences in maximum weight lifted in the bench press and leg press or number of repetitions at 70% of maximum weight. Lebrun et al.[41] reported no difference between early follicular and midluteal phases in isokinetic strength of the quadriceps and hamstring muscles. Gür[46] showed no difference between menstrual, late follicular and midluteal phases in either concentric or eccentric isokinetic peak torque of the quadriceps or hamstring muscles. A few studies have reported menstrual phase effects on muscle strength, although their findings are contradictory. Davies et al[47] found better handgrip strength and standing long jump performance during menses compared with the late follicular and midluteal phases. Sarwar et al[48] demonstrated higher maximum voluntary isometric strength for the quadriceps and handgrip at midcycle (late follicular to early luteal) than at four other stages of the menstrual cycle. Also at midcycle, they found a slower relaxation time and higher fatigability of the quadriceps muscles in response to single or tetanic electrical stimulation. They speculated that the high estrogen levels at midcycle may increase intramuscular inorganic phosphate concentration, which could cause the observed effects, although a mechanism by which this could occur is unknown. Because most studies show no menstrual phase effect on muscle strength, and those that do see an effect contradict one another, the best conclusion is that there is no practical effect of menstrual phase on strength.

Most important to athletes is the potential effect of menstrual cycle phase on performance in competition. Each sport uses a unique combination of variables related to aerobic capacity, strength, and other abilities that can be measured in the laboratory. Surprisingly, few studies have looked at menstrual phase effects in actual or simulated athletic competition. Brooks-Gunn et al[49] studied four highly trained teenage swimmers over a 4-month period. Only about half of the menstrual cycles studied appeared to be normal. Nevertheless, 100-yard swim times were consistently fastest during menstruation and slowest during the 4 days before menstruation onset. Bale and Nelson[50] found that 50-m swim times were fastest in the midfollicular phase, slowest on the first day of menstruation, and intermediate in the periovulatory and midluteal phases in 20 collegiate swimmers. Quadagno et al[45] found no differences among the premenstrual, menstrual, and postmenstrual phases in the swim times of 15 collegiate athletes.

A conclusion that can be drawn from all these studies is that there is no consistent, generalized effect of menstrual cycle phase on exercise performance. Some specific physiological variables, such as body temperature, ventilation, and aspects of substrate metabolism, are influenced by estrogen and progesterone. These effects may be important in certain activities or in certain environments. But under most circumstances, when these physiological variables are summed in sports competition, there are no predictable fluctuations in performance.

ORAL CONTRACEPTIVES AND EXERCISE PERFORMANCE

If fluctuations in estrogen and progesterone levels during a menstrual cycle affect physiological variables important to exercise performance, the same might be expected for oral contraceptives, which contain these hormones. The study of oral contraceptive effects is complicated by the fact that there are many different brands, with different specific synthetic hormones, different doses, and different regimens. This review includes only studies using relatively low doses, which are prescribed almost exclusively today, and studies in which all subjects were given the same preparation by the investigators.

Oral contraceptive pills usually contain both an estrogen and a progestin. The estrogen usually is ethinyl estradiol, at a dose of 20 to 50 μg per pill. The progestin may be norethindrone, norgestrel, or levonorgestrel, for example, and doses may be 0.05 to 2.5 mg per pill. Some brands are sequential, with either two or three different doses given over the course of a 3-week period to more closely simulate a natural menstrual cycle. In all cases, the pills are taken for 21 days and then discontinued or reduced with placebo for 7 days to allow a menstrual period to occur.

No one has studied the effect of oral contraceptive treatment on performance in actual athletic competitions. In the laboratory, maximal oxygen consumption, oxygen consumption at submaximal workloads, and physical working capacity have been affected by oral contraceptives in some studies but not others. Sandström et al[51] followed nonathletic women for 2 years while giving them 30 μg ethinyl estradiol and 0.15 mg levonorgestrel. Physical working capacity, defined as absolute work performed on a bicycle ergometer at a heart rate of 170 beats per minute, was unaltered by the medication. Heart volume also was unaltered, but there was a progressive increase in total hemoglobin. McNeill and Mozingo[52] reported that Vo_2 was higher for two submaximal workloads on a bicycle ergometer when 50 μg ethinyl estradiol and 1.0 mg norethindrone were used for 2 months. Notelovitz et al[53] found a reduced Vo_{2max} on a treadmill in moderately trained women who used 35 μg ethinyl estradiol and 0.4 mg norethindrone for 6 months. Oxygen pulse (volume of oxygen consumed per heart beat) also declined by the end of the treatment, but there were no effects on heart rate, minute ventilation, or tidal volume during either submaximal or maximal exercise. Bryner et al[54] saw no difference in Vo_{2max} or endurance time at 80% Vo_{2max} on a treadmill during the first month of treatment with 35 μg ethinyl estradiol and 1.0 mg norethindrone, although number of subjects was small.

A number of other studies have looked at women who already were taking oral contraceptives of varying types, doses, and durations that were not administered by the investigators and compared them with women not taking oral contraceptives. They examined variables such as exercise performance, cardiovascular responses to exercise, substrate metabolism during exercise, muscle function, and temperature regulation during exercise. In most cases they found no effects of oral contraceptives. Because the subjects had been taking different medications for different lengths of time, it cannot be known whether differing effects in different subjects canceled one another out or whether the oral contraceptives indeed had no effects. A few studies have documented effects of oral contraceptives, even though different subjects had been taking different preparations for differing lengths of time. These included less muscle soreness after exhaustive bench stepping[55] and reduced cyclic fluctuations in body temperature and sweating during exercise compared with control subjects[56] and higher body temperature and threshold for sweating onset during the third week of pill ingestion compared with the week without pill ingestion.[57]

There are too few well-controlled studies to make conclusions about the effects of oral contraceptives on exercise performance or exercise responses. Aerobic exercise performance may be decreased slightly or unaltered. A mechanism by which oral contraceptives might affect exercise performance is not established.

There are too few well-controlled studies to make conclusions about effects of oral contraceptives on exercise performance or exercise responses.

Clinical Guideline

No studies have been done on effects of other hormonal contraceptives on exercise performance. These include intramuscular injection of methoxyprogesterone acetate (Depo-Provera) and subcutaneous implants of levonorgestrel (Norplant).

EFFECTS OF EXERCISE TRAINING ON PREMENSTRUAL SYMPTOMS

Women with premenstrual syndrome (PMS) may have a variety of physical and affective symptoms that occur during the luteal phase, particularly the last few days before menstruation onset, but not during the follicular phase.[58,59] It is more common in women older than 30. The cause of PMS is not understood. The best explanation for PMS at present is that it results from interactions of ovarian steroids with central neurotransmitters, especially serotonin, but also endogenous opioids, alpha-adrenergic agonists, and gamma aminobutyric acid.

A large number of treatments for PMS have been advocated over the years. In her review, Johnson[59] categorizes these treatments as "not effective," "may be effective," and "are effective." Among the treatments in the "are effective" category are selective serotonin reuptake inhibitors and drugs that suppress ovulation.

Aerobic exercise is categorized as "may be effective" by Johnson.[59] This means that there are some small studies suggesting that aerobic exercise reduces symptoms of PMS, and there is no significant evidence against its effectiveness, but there are no large randomized trials clearly demonstrating its effectiveness.

There are some studies suggesting that aerobic exercise reduces symptoms of PMS, and there is no significant evidence against its effectiveness, but there are no large randomized trials clearly demonstrating its effectiveness.

Clinical Guideline

Very few studies have examined the effect of an exercise training program on symptoms of PMS in women who previously were sedentary. Prior et al[60] followed three groups of women for 6 months: sedentary women who started a running program, runners who increased their training in preparation for a marathon, and nonexercising women. Both groups of runners had reductions in some PMS symptoms after 6 months, including fluid-related symptoms and breast tenderness, along with a slight reduction in luteal phase length. Steege and Blumenthal[61] studied middle-aged women before and after 12-week training programs in either aerobic exercise or strength training. Premenstrual symptoms declined significantly in the aerobic training group but not in the strength training group, although some symptoms did improve in the strength training group. In neither study were premenstrual symptoms severe before the exercise training.

Other studies have compared premenstrual symptoms in habitually exercising women with those in sedentary women. Aganoff and Boyle[62] asked exercising and nonexercising women of widely ranging ages to complete questionnaires at three different menstrual phases. The exercising women had lower scores on all measures of negative affect and physical symptoms, but no difference in positive affect in the premenstrual phase, as well as the menstrual and intermenstrual phases. Choi and Salmon[63] found that women categorized as high exercisers had greater positive affect, lower negative affect, and fewer physical symptoms than sedentary women on the 5 days before menstruation onset. However, these beneficial effects of exercise were not seen in a group of competitive athletes. Neither study verified that menstrual cycles were ovulatory.

Another approach is to analyze data from questionnaires that include items on both premenstrual symptoms and exercise habits. Freeman et al[64] evaluated daily symptom reports and questionnaires from 60 women seeking treatment for moderate to severe PMS. They found that the severity of PMS was inversely correlated with the number of days of exercise per week.

In summary, although it commonly is believed that regular exercise can reduce premenstrual symptoms, there are few well-controlled studies demonstrating that this is true. This is an area in which more research is needed. No one has investigated a mechanism by which exercise may affect PMS.

EFFECTS OF EXERCISE TRAINING ON DYSMENORRHEA

Primary dysmenorrhea, or menstrual cramps, is lower abdominal pain that occurs during normal menstruation, especially on the first 1 to 2 days of menstrual bleeding.[65] In some women, the pain may radiate to the back or thighs. It is more common in younger women. The cause appears to be the effects of prostaglandins released by the disintegrating endometrium during menstruation. As progesterone levels fall at the end of the luteal phase, lysosomes in endometrial cells release phospholipase A_2, an enzyme that hydrolyzes phospholipids in cell membranes, forming arachidonic acid. The arachidonic acid may be converted to prostaglandins, which stimulate myometrial contraction, causing occlusion of small uterine blood vessels. The resulting ischemia stimulates uterine pain receptors. The effectiveness of prostaglandin synthesis inhibitors in alleviating dysmenorrhea provides good support for this explanation.

Secondary dysmenorrhea, on the other hand, is menstrual pain associated with uterine or pelvic pathological conditions. The cause of the pain and the age at which it occurs depend on the particular pathological condition.

It seems to be generally believed that exercise can reduce the symptoms of dysmenorrhea, but studies verifying this are few. Only a few studies have investigated the effects of exercise training programs on dysmenorrhea. Earlier studies[66–68] tested the effects of simple calisthenics and stretching exercises on college students or junior high school students with dysmenorrhea. On the average, girls performing the exercises regularly had a reduction or elimination of symptoms. These studies did not eliminate girls with secondary dysmenorrhea or anovulation. More recently, Isreal et al[69] studied women diagnosed with primary dysmenorrhea after eliminating volunteers with secondary dysmenorrhea. Half the women participated in a 12-week walk/jog program, and half served as controls. The walk/jog program almost eliminated symptoms of dysmenorrhea by the end of the study.

Other studies have used questionnaires to assess the relationship between exercise and dysmenorrhea. Results were variable. Izzo and Labriola[70] reported that dysmenorrhea was less common in adolescents who participated in athletic sports than in girls who exercised only occasionally and that adolescents who began sports activity after menarche noted a reduction in dysmenorrhea after they increased their exercise. Hightower[71] found that women who exercised at least once per week had lower pain intensity and less unpleasantness during menstruation than women who exercised less than once per week; half the women used oral contraceptives and half did not. Ronkainen et al[72] reported that national level runners and skiers were less likely than sedentary controls to have dysmenorrhea, but national level volleyball players did not differ from controls. Choi and Salmon[63] found that women categorized as competitive athletes or high exercisers had higher positive affect during menstruation than sedentary women, but the groups did not differ in physical symptoms, fatigue, or irritability during the menstrual period. Both Sundell et al[73] and Jarrett et al[74] found no relationship between frequency of physical exercise and severity of dysmenorrhea. Metheny and Smith[75] reported that nursing students who exercised three or more times per week had more severe symptoms of dysmenorrhea than sedentary students.

The only study of secondary dysmenorrhea and exercise was done by Cramer et al.[76] They interviewed infertile women with endometriosis and women admitted to hospitals for childbirth. Women with endometriosis were less likely to exercise regularly, less likely to have begun exercising at a young age, and less likely to exercise more than 2 hours per week.

Overall, the prospective training studies suggest that even mild exercise may reduce symptoms in young women diagnosed with primary dysmenorrhea. The varying methods and populations used in the questionnaire studies make their results difficult to interpret. It may be that regular exercise is helpful for women who are particularly prone to dysmenorrhea but less effective in most women with only mild dysmenorrhea. No one has investigated a mechanism by which exercise might affect dysmenorrhea.

Prospective training studies suggest that even mild exercise may reduce symptoms in young women diagnosed with primary dysmenorrhea.

Clinical Guideline

EFFECTS OF EXERCISE TRAINING ON MENSTRUAL CYCLES: SHORT LUTEAL PHASE, OLIGOMENORRHEA, AND AMENORRHEA

In the late 1970s people in the medical and sports communities began to realize that menstrual cycle irregularities were more common in athletes than in the general popula-

tion. The most obvious menstrual disorder was secondary amenorrhea or cessation of menstrual periods after they once had been established. Also noted were oligomenorrhea, or infrequent menstrual periods, and primary amenorrhea, or late menarche. Late menarche will be discussed in the next section. Another more subtle menstrual disturbance seen in athletes was the short luteal phase, in which the corpus luteum had a shorter lifespan than usual, so that there was a shorter than normal interval between ovulation and menstruation onset.

Secondary amenorrhea is present in about 2% to 5% of nonpregnant women of reproductive age.[77,78] In populations of athletes, 12% to 34% have secondary amenorrhea.[78–80] Distance runners are more likely to be amenorrheic than athletes in many other sports, but amenorrhea has been reported in women competing in swimming, cycling, skiing, weight lifting, bodybuilding, and several other sports,[78,81–85] as well as ballet dancers.[86]

Secondary amenorrhea may occur in 12% to 34% of athletes. Oligomenorrhea tends to be more common.

Clinical Guideline

The prevalence of amenorrhea and oligomenorrhea depends partly on the definitions that are used for these conditions. Secondary amenorrhea has been defined as the absence of menstrual periods for 3 months, 6 months, or fewer than four menstrual periods per year.[78,80–82] Definitions for oligomenorrhea or irregular menstruation vary even more but have included cycles differing in length by 9 days or more,[81] cycles longer than 35 days or shorter than 23 days,[78] or a few menstrual periods per year. In almost all studies, the prevalence of oligomenorrhea or irregular menstruation is greater than the prevalence of amenorrhea.

Amenorrhea and oligomenorrhea have been reported to be more common in athletes who exercise more, are younger, nulliparous, and had irregular menstrual cycles before becoming athletic.[78,79,87–90] Carlberg et al[91] reported that menstrual characteristics were similar in four out of five pairs of sisters with similar sports participation, suggesting a genetic component.

When amenorrhea occurs in an athlete, it is likely that there is little or no follicular development in the ovaries. This may result from reduced stimulatory activity by GnRH and gonadotropins. With little follicular activity in the ovary, there is not enough estrogen or progesterone to stimulate endometrial development in the uterus. If the endometrium does not grow, there can be no menstrual period. Endocrine studies in amenorrheic athletes support this explanation.

In amenorrheic athletes, it is likely that there is little or no follicular development in the ovaries. This may result from reduced stimulatory activity by GnRH and gonadotropins.

Clinical Guideline

Veldhuis et al[92] studied distance runners with none to three menstrual periods per year and normally menstruating sedentary women in the early follicular phase. Serial blood samples were taken at 20-minute intervals for 24 hours. Runners did not differ from controls in 24-hour mean serum LH concentration or LH pulse amplitude, but six of the nine runners had a decreased LH pulse frequency, with 1 to 6 LH pulses in 24 hours instead of the 8 to 15 LH pulses in 24 hours seen in the controls. Serum estradiol was 52 pg/mL in the runners compared to 81 pg/mL in the controls, a nonsignificant difference. After the first 24 hours, subjects received four graded doses of GnRH at 2-hour intervals. LH responses were significantly greater in the runners than in the controls, and estradiol responses were the same.

Yahiro et al[93] compared amenorrheic runners with eumenorrheic (normally menstruating) runners in the early follicular phase. The amenorrheic runners were similar to the eumenorrheic runners in basal serum levels of LH, FSH, and progesterone but had significantly lower levels of estradiol. In response to GnRH administration, the amenorrheic runners had higher responses of both LH and FSH.

Loucks et al[94] evaluated the reproductive axis in amenorrheic athletes (runners, cyclists, and triathletes), eumenorrheic athletes, and eumenorrheic sedentary women in the early follicular phase. The amenorrheic athletes had mean serum LH and FSH levels similar to those in eumenorrheic women but lower serum estradiol levels. LH pulse frequency over 24 hours was lower in eumenorrheic athletes than in controls and lower still in amenorrheic athletes; examples are shown in Figure 10–2. LH pulse amplitude was quite a bit higher than controls in some but not all athletes in both groups. In response to GnRH administration, amenorrheic athletes had significantly larger responses of both LH and FSH. Urinary estrone glucuronide and pregnanediol glucuronide, collected for one menstrual cycle or 30 days, showed the expected rises in the late follicular and midluteal phases, respectively, in the eumenorrheic subjects but consistently low levels in amenorrheic athletes (Figure 10–3).

Together, these three studies suggest strongly that the hypothalamic regulation of episodic GnRH secretion is the site of the defect in amenorrheic athletes. When the athletes are given GnRH, their pituitaries and ovaries can respond, and their pituitaries may be hypersensitive because of chronic understimulation by GnRH. The infrequent spontaneous LH pulses in amenorrheic athletes may be insufficient to stimulate much follicular development in the ovaries. As a result, estradiol and progesterone are at or below normal early follicular phase levels. Athletes may menstruate every few months if there is enough estrogen to stimulate some slow endometrial growth, followed by endometrial disintegration and bleeding.

Hypothalamic regulation of pulsatile GnRH secretion appears to be the site of the defect in amenorrheic athletes.

Clinical Guideline

Amenorrhea probably is the most extreme response of the reproductive system to strenuous exercise training. Oligomenorrhea, irregular menstruation, and short luteal phases are progressively less dramatic alterations in reproductive function. Some investigators have found that hypothalamic, pituitary, and ovarian activities have subtle abnormalities in athletes, even though menstrual periods may appear normal. A few studies have followed nonathletic women prospectively as they participate in a prescribed exercise training program, documenting changes in hypothalamic, pituitary, and ovarian function. Collectively these studies suggest that even moderate amounts of exercise training may alter hypothalamic function in some women, that these hypothalamic changes affect pituitary and ovarian function, and that as exercise training becomes more intense or more prolonged the reproductive aberrations become more severe. Some of these studies are described in the following paragraphs.

Hypothalamic, pituitary, and ovarian activities may have subtle abnormalities in athletes, even though menstrual periods may appear normal. Even moderate amounts of exercise training may alter hypothalamic function in some women, and as exercise training becomes more intense or more prolonged, the reproductive aberrations become more severe.

Clinical Guideline

Athletes with apparently normal menstrual periods actually may have subtle differences in hypothalamic, pituitary, and ovarian function. For example, Cumming et al[95] reported that normally menstruating runners, studied in the early follicular phase, had diminished LH pulse frequency, pulse amplitude, and area under the LH curve (a measure of total LH concentration over time) compared with sedentary controls (Figure 10–4). Loucks et al[94] found reduced LH pulse frequency and higher LH pulse amplitude in regularly menstruating athletes in the early follicular phase compared with controls.

Diminished gonadotropin stimulation during the follicular phase or midcycle may result in a corpus luteum that has

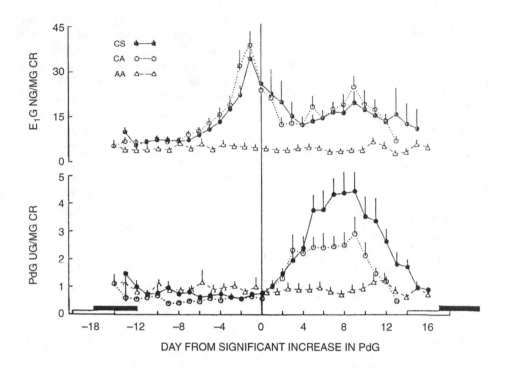

Figure 10–3 Mean (±SE) Daily Urinary Excretion of E_1G (*top*) and PdG (*bottom*) in CS (cyclic sedentary), CA (cyclic athletes), and AA (amenorrheic athletes) Women. Days are oriented from a significant increase in urinary PdG excretion, with day 1 being the day of the first significant increase. For urinary E_1G, 1.0 μg/mg creatinine (CR) = 2.134 pmol/mg CR; for PdG, 1.0 μg/mg CR = 2.014 nmol/mg CR. ■ Menses, CS; □ menses, CA.

lower secretory activity, and a shorter lifespan, than normal. This constitutes the "short luteal phase" condition, in which luteal phase progesterone levels are lower than normal, and the interval between ovulation and menstruation onset is up to several days shorter than normal. The follicular phase may be longer than normal, so that total menstrual cycle length appears normal. The short luteal phase and low luteal phase progesterone levels have been documented in a large number of "eumenorrheic" athletes.[94,96–99] De Souza et al[100] provided the most complete evaluation to date of luteal phase deficiencies in athletes. Measurement of urinary LH, FSH, estrone conjugates, and pregnanediol glucuronide over three menstrual cycles in 11 sedentary and 24 recreational runners revealed that all sedentary women consistently had ovulatory cycles with normal luteal phase lengths, but among the runners 43% of cycles showed luteal phase deficiencies and 12% of cycles were anovulatory. Cycles with luteal phase deficiencies had lower FSH levels during the last 5 days of the previous cycle, when newly developing ovarian follicles are being recruited, and lower mid-cycle LH levels. Apparently no one has investigated the effect of short luteal phases on fertility in athletes.

Athletes with apparently normal menstrual cycles may have a "short luteal phase" condition, with a long follicular phase, short luteal phase, and low midluteal progesterone levels.

Clinical Guideline

Several prospective studies have followed nonathletic women or moderate exercisers as they progressed through an exercise training program. Recreational runners who trained for a marathon by gradually increasing their weekly mileage by 30 miles/week, and then by 50 miles/week, had a gradual decline in midfollicular phase plasma estradiol levels, a nonsignificant decline in LH levels, and no change in FSH levels, all measured in a single blood sample.[101,102] LH and FSH responses to GnRH administration fell as weekly mileage increased. In other studies, untrained women who trained strenuously for two menstrual cycles had a high incidence of abnormalities develop, including delayed menses, lengthened follicular phases, short luteal phases, reduced luteal phase urinary progesterone, and loss of the LH surge.[103,104] Williams et al[105] studied untrained women who

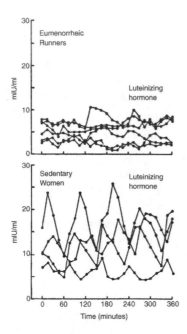

Figure 10–4 Serum LH Levels in Samples Obtained at 15-min Intervals over 6 hr in Six Eumenorrheic Runners (Top Panel) and Four Sedentary Controls (Lower Panel). The studies were performed in the early follicular phase of the menstrual cycle (days 3–6).

performed high-intensity exercise during just the late luteal and follicular phase or just the luteal phase of two menstrual cycles. Menstrual cycle lengths did not change, but about half the women in each group had changes such as smaller LH surges, shortened luteal phases, and reduced luteal urinary progesterone. No difference was found between women who exercised in the follicular phase compared with those who exercised during the luteal phase. All these studies demonstrate hormonal and menstrual changes that probably would not be noticed by a woman starting an exercise program or engaging in exercise of moderate intensity.

The mechanism by which strenuous exercise training may alter hypothalamic regulation of reproductive function still is unknown. The best evidence so far supports a role for inadequate energy availability relative to energy expenditure. In most but not all cases, this is accompanied by low body weight and low body fat. Inadequate energy availability may result from a combination of exercise and specific dietary practices or eating disorders.

The mechanism by which strenuous exercise training alters hypothalamic regulation of reproductive function still is unknown. The best evidence so far supports a role for inadequate energy availability relative to energy expenditure.

Clinical Guideline

Average body weight is lower in athletes with menstrual disturbances than in normally menstruating athletes in almost all studies.[78,86,88,90] In their prospective study of initially untrained women participating in an exercise program, Bullen et al[103] observed that women who lost weight during the training developed more menstrual disorders than women who maintained body weight.

Fat mass and percent body fat also are lower in athletes with menstrual disturbances than in menstruating athletes in most,[106,107] but not all,[108,109] studies. When hydrostatic weighing is used to evaluate body composition, percent body fat may be overestimated in amenorrheic athletes because of their low bone density,[110] reducing a difference between amenorrheic and menstruating athletes that actually may be there.

On average, amenorrheic athletes have lower body weight and less fat than menstruating athletes, but there is a lot of overlap between the groups.

Clinical Guideline

Frisch[111] argued for many years that there is a critical level of body fatness or a specific ratio of fat to lean mass that is necessary for ovulatory cycles to occur. The data from amenorrheic athletes suggest that, although the amount of fat or total body mass may play an important role, there are large differences among individual women in menstrual responses to changes in body weight, and there is a lot of overlap between amenorrheic athletes and menstruating athletes in fat mass and total body mass.

Dietary practices have been reported in a few studies to differ between amenorrheic and menstruating athletes, although findings have been inconsistent. Amenorrheic athletes may have higher intakes of fiber,[112] lower intakes of fat,[113] or a lower proportion of calories as protein.[106] For most measures of dietary intake, significant differences have not been found. Eating disorders have been reported in a subset of amenorrheic athletes by several investigators.[85,86,114,115]

In general, comparisons between amenorrheic and menstruating athletes in easily measured variables such as body weight, body composition, and dietary intake provide tantalizing but frustrating clues about what causes some athletes to become amenorrheic, because data are so inconsistent. A more fruitful approach seems to be examining effects of energy imbalance, that is, energy intake versus energy expenditure.

Loucks and her colleagues, as well as other investigators, have been working to understand interrelationships among energy balance, regulation of substrate metabolism and metabolic rate, and hypothalamic regulation of reproductive function. Loucks and Heath[116] found that food restriction (10 vs. 45 kcal/kg lean body mass per day), without a change in energy expenditure for 4 days in the follicular phase, caused a reduction in LH pulse frequency, an increase in LH pulse amplitude, and no change in 24-hour mean LH in normally menstruating sedentary women; food restriction also caused significant reductions in tri-iodothyronine (T_3), insulin, and insulin-like growth factor I (IGF-I). In a follow-up study, Loucks et al[117] differentiated the effects of low energy availability from the effects of exercise stress on LH secretion by asking eumenorrheic sedentary women to expend 30 kcal/kg lean body mass per day in intense exercise both with and without dietary compensation for the energy expenditure; each treatment was imposed for 4 days during a follicular phase. Intense exercise with energy compensation did not affect LH pulse frequency, LH pulse amplitude, or 24-hour mean LH. Intense exercise without energy compensation, that is, energy imbalance produced by excess energy expenditure, reduced LH pulse frequency and increased LH pulse amplitude, but these effects were not as pronounced as in the previous study of food restriction alone; this treatment also reduced T_3, insulin, and IGF-I. Together these two studies suggest that the alterations in LH secretion seen in amenorrheic athletes, that is, reduced pulse frequency and increased pulse amplitude, result more from low energy availability, induced by a combination of exercise and restrained eating, than from exercise per se.

Williams et al[118] had similar findings. When eumenorrheic recreational athletes were treated with 7 days of exercise plus calorie restriction (60% of calories for weight maintenance), LH pulse frequency declined, but when they were treated for 7 days with exercise plus a calorie supplement, LH pulse frequency was the same as during a control period.

Resting metabolic rate may be reduced in athletes with menstrual disorders as a response to inadequate energy intake relative to energy expenditure. Myerson et al[119] reported that amenorrheic runners had a lower resting metabolic rate, adjusted either for body weight or fat-free mass, than eumenorrheic runners or sedentary women. They also had lower T_3 levels. The investigators speculated that a lower resting metabolic rate allowed amenorrheic runners to maintain a stable body weight in the face of high energy expenditure. Lebenstedt et al[120] found that athletes with short luteal phases and low luteal progesterone levels had lower resting metabolic rates, adjusted for lean body mass, than athletes with normal luteal phases. They also had lower basal body temperatures, even during the follicular phase, and higher eating restraint scores.

If resting metabolic rate is reduced in amenorrheic athletes, it may be related to alterations in the thyroid hormone axis. Loucks et al[121] found low levels of T_3, thyroxine (T_4), and reverse T_3 in amenorrheic athletes without differences in thyroid-binding globulin or thyroid-stimulating hormone (TSH) concentrations. TSH response to thyrotropin-releasing hormone administration was blunted. In a study of eumenorrheic sedentary women, Loucks and Callister[122] looked at the effects of 4 days of food restriction with and without exercise and low- or high-intensity exercise with or without energy compensation on thyroid hormone levels. They found that negative energy imbalance, regardless of exercise treatment, resulted in declines in T_3 and increases in T_4 and reverse T_3, but exercise with energy compensation did not affect levels of these hormones. To further define the relationship between energy availability and thyroid physiology, Loucks and Heath[123] gave eumenorrheic nonathletic women four different levels of food intake for 4 days, while all groups expended 30 kcal/kg lean body mass per day in exercise, resulting in the four groups receiving no, one-quarter, one-half, or full dietary compensation for exercise energy expenditure. T_3 declined in the groups receiving one quarter or no dietary compensation for exercise energy expenditure, whereas free T_4 and reverse T_3 (but not T_4) increased in the groups receiving no dietary compensation, suggesting a threshold of energy availability necessary to maintain normal thyroid physiology.

Amenorrheic athletes might have an imbalance between energy intake and energy expenditure. They might compensate for this by alterations in the thyroid hormone axis and metabolic rate.

Clinical Guideline

Loucks suggests that the collective results of her studies indicate that amenorrheic athletes may be able to normalize their reproductive and thyroid axes by increasing their food intake to maintain an adequate energy availability. Reduction of exercise energy expenditure may not be necessary to achieve this goal.

Leptin, a recently discovered hormone,[124] may constitute a connection between body fatness, energy availability, and reproductive function in athletes. Leptin is secreted by adipose cells, and its plasma concentration may rise when either the total fat mass increases or there is a net deposition of stored nutrients rather than a net mobilization of nutrients in adipose cells.[125] Leptin communicates to the regions of the hypothalamus that regulate food intake and metabolic rate;[126] higher levels of leptin inhibit food intake and increase metabolic rate. It also seems to communicate to regions of the hypothalamus that regulate reproduction. There may be a threshold level of leptin that is required by the hypothalamus to allow GnRH secretion to occur normally.[127] For example, leptin injection into food-deprived mice restores estrous cycles and ovulation.[128] To date, only two studies have reported leptin levels in athletes with menstrual dysfunction.

Laughlin and Yen[129] found that leptin levels were lower in both amenorrheic and eumenorrheic athletes than in sedentary control subjects. The amenorrheic athletes differed from the eumenorrheic athletes in lacking a circadian rhythm for leptin. Tataranni et al[130] measured leptin in single fasting blood samples from sedentary and moderately trained women. Leptin concentration was highest in the sedentary controls, lowest in amenorrheic exercising women, and intermediate in exercising women with eumenorrhea or anovulation. Further investigation of leptin may help unravel the mechanism of exercise-induced menstrual disruption.

Leptin is secreted by adipose cells and communicates to areas of the hypothalamus that regulate food intake, metabolic rate, and reproduction. Further investigation of leptin may help unravel the mechanism of exercise-induced menstrual disruption.

Clinical Guideline

Several other hypotheses have been proposed to explain how exercise training can disrupt menstrual cycles. These include inhibition of GnRH secretion by hormones of the adrenocortical axis, β-endorphin, androgens, and prolactin. All these hormones are secreted in greater amounts during exercise, and all are known to inhibit GnRH secretion when in excess. In addition, psychological stress has been investigated as a link between competitive sports and menstrual dysfunction. None of these factors appears to be a primary causal factor for menstrual disturbances in athletes, although there may be some abnormalities in some athletes. Studies of these factors are described in the following paragraphs.

Exercise-Induced Possible Causes of Menstrual Dysfunction (None Are Explanatory)

- Elevated adrenocortical hormones
- Elevated β-endorphin
- Elevated androgens
- Elevated prolactin
- Elevated psychological stress

Clinical Guideline

The hypothalamic-pituitary-adrenocortical (HPA) axis includes corticotropin-releasing hormone (CRH), which is secreted by hypothalamic neuroendocrine cells in response to stress or exercise; adrenocorticotropic hormone (ACTH), secreted by the pituitary gland in response to CRH; and cortisol, secreted by the adrenal cortex in response to ACTH. These hormones induce a variety of physiological responses that contribute to the body's ability to adapt to stress or

exercise. They also inhibit reproductive functions at several levels, including inhibition by CRH of GnRH-secreting neuroendocrine cells and inhibition by cortisol of pituitary response to GnRH and endometrial response to estrogen.[131,132] Thus, it is reasonable to speculate that exercise-induced stimulation of the HPA axis could inhibit reproductive function in some athletes. Basal levels of cortisol have been modestly elevated in amenorrheic athletes, whereas ACTH levels and pulsatility are normal, and ACTH and cortisol responses to exercise, meals, or CRH injection are blunted.[94,133,134] Loucks et al[94] suggested that there is a resetting of the HPA axis in amenorrheic athletes. De Souza et al[134] found a normal dexamethasone suppression of cortisol in amenorrheic runners, suggesting that the HPA axis negative feedback system is normal, but speculated that an unknown extrapituitary factor might affect adrenocortical responsiveness to ACTH. Interestingly, some studies have shown an inhibitory effect of leptin on the HPA axis,[135,136] so low leptin levels might contribute to elevated HPA activity in amenorrheic athletes. Overall, it appears that the HPA axis may be slightly overactive in amenorrheic athletes, but there is no compelling evidence that HPA axis abnormalities play a central role in the development of exercise-induced menstrual cycle disruption.

β-endorphin is a hormone secreted by the pituitary gland in response to CRH, as well as a neurotransmitter. Among its many actions is an inhibition of LH secretion, presumably by an action on GnRH-secreting neuroendocrine cells.[132,137] Because plasma β-endorphin concentration rises during strenuous exercise,[138] investigators have hypothesized that it plays a role in exercise-induced inhibition of menstrual cyclicity. Although a few earlier studies reported higher basal β-endorphin levels in amenorrheic athletes, more recent studies found no difference between amenorrheic and menstruating athletes in β-endorphin at rest or after exercise.[139–141] β-endorphin response to either CRH[139] or an opioid receptor antagonist[140] did not differ between amenorrheic and menstruating athletes, although McArthur et al[142] reported that some oligoamenorrheic athletes responded to an opioid receptor antagonist with a higher mean amplitude of LH pulses.

Androgens in women are secreted by both the ovaries and the adrenal cortex. Because they inhibit GnRH secretion through a negative feedback mechanism and they rise in concentration during exercise,[143] their potential role in exercise-induced menstrual cycle disruption has been investigated. No evidence has been found that excess levels of androgens play a role. Loucks et al[94,144] found that amenorrheic athletes did not differ from eumenorrheic athletes in basal levels of testosterone or testosterone response to exercise, and basal androstenedione and androstenedione response to exercise were lower in amenorrheic athletes. De Souza et al[134] found no differences between amenorrheic and eumenorrheic runners in resting levels of testosterone, androstenedione, or dehydroepiandrosterone sulfate.

Prolactin is secreted by the pituitary gland in greater amounts during exercise,[145] and excess prolactin inhibits the hypothalamic-pituitary-gonadal axis.[146] Therefore, prolactin levels have been measured in amenorrheic athletes at rest and during exercise. There is good agreement that prolactin levels in amenorrheic and oligomenorrheic athletes at rest and during exercise are either the same or lower than those in menstruating athletes.[89,133,144,147,148] Boyden et al[149] followed women during an endurance running program that increased their training by 50 miles/week and found that basal prolactin levels declined significantly by the end of the program. Chang et al[150] found that 24-hour prolactin concentrations in oligomenorrheic runners were the same as in menstruating women and that prolactin suppression by dopamine infusion was the same as well. Therefore, there is no evidence that excess prolactin is responsible for exercise-induced menstrual disturbances.

Psychological stress is believed to increase the risk of menstrual dysfunction and infertility in the general population of women.[132] It might do so by enhancing secretion of one or more stress-responsive hormones, such as those of the HPA axis, which in turn could inhibit secretion of GnRH. Because some psychological stress may be associated with athletic competition, investigators have examined the possibility that it may contribute to exercise-induced menstrual disorders. Most studies have found that amenorrheic athletes do not differ from menstruating women in most measures of psychological characteristics or emotional stress.[106,115,144,151] Schwartz et al[106] found that, although amenorrheic runners had the same psychological profiles as other subjects, they reported more stress associated with running than other runners when asked to rate the stress from 0 to 10. Klock and De Souza[115] noted that, although mean scores for amenorrheic runners were in the normal range and not significantly different from other groups, there was a subset of amenorrheic runners whose test results indicated that they were mildly to moderately depressed.

In summary, it is well documented that menstrual disturbances are more common in athletes than in the general population. Disturbances range from short luteal phases in menstrual cycles of normal length to amenorrhea, a cessation of menstruation that may last for years. In all cases, apparently, there is some inhibition or aberration of GnRH secretion, which may range from slight to severe. In subtle disturbances, the major finding may be lower than normal progesterone levels during the luteal phase. In amenorrhea, estrogen and progesterone levels are low chronically. The mechanism by which exercise training affects menstrual cycles still is unknown. The most likely explanation appears to be related to reduced fat deposits and reduced energy intake relative to energy expenditure, and the metabolic

alterations consequent to this, but the precise mechanisms remain to be explained.

Other than infertility, the most important known health effect of exercise-induced menstrual disturbance is inadequate accretion of bone mineral in young athletes or loss of bone mineral in adult athletes. Even though exercise enhances bone strength, low estrogen levels result in a loss of bone similar to that seen in postmenopausal women. This is discussed in Chapter 18.

AGE AT MENARCHE IN ATHLETES

Menarche, the first menstrual period, occurs at a later age in athletes, on average, than in the general population. American girls experience menarche at an average age of between 12 and 13 years. In retrospective studies, average age at menarche has been 13.6 years in collegiate track and field athletes,[152] 14.0 years in elite figure skaters, 12.9 years in elite Alpine ski racers,[153] 14.2 years in Olympic volleyball candidates,[154] 13.4 years in competitive swimmers,[155] and 15.6 years in elite gymnasts.[156]

Average Age of Menarche in Various Sports (yr)

American average	12–13
Collegiate track & field	13.6
Elite figure skaters	14.0
Elite Alpine ski racers	12.9
Olympic volleyball candidates	14.2
Competitive swimmers	13.4
Elite gymnasts	15.6
Ballet dancers	13.4–15.4

Clinical Guideline

Ballet dancers also experience menarche at a late age. Frisch et al[157] surveyed a large group of ballet dancers and found that of the 77% who had experienced menarche, the average age was 13.7 years. Ten percent had primary amenorrhea, defined as no menarche by 16 years; these girls were significantly leaner than other dancers. Warren[158] followed pubertal progression for 4 years in 15 ballet dancers. During the course of the study, 13 dancers experienced menarche at an average of 15.4 years, whereas two still had primary amenorrhea at 18 years. The dancers were shorter and lighter for their ages than a control group, but heavier at menarche than the control group, who had menarche at an average of 12.5 years. Breast development was delayed in the dancers and frequently coincided with periods of rest because of vacation or injury, as did menarche.

A 5-year prospective study of gymnasts was conducted by Lindholm et al.[159] Twenty-five gymnasts experienced menarche during the study, at a mean age of 14.5 years compared with 13.2 years for a control group, and one had primary amenorrhea at 18 years. Growth in height was delayed in the gymnasts, and six had a final height shorter than expected according to the heights of their parents. Growth spurts often occurred during periods of reduced training as a result of injury.

If exercise, per se, delays menarche, then menarche should be late only in girls who train before menarche. Frisch et al[160] found this to be true among collegiate swimmers and runners. Menarche occurred at 15.1 years in athletes who trained before menarche and 12.8 years in athletes who began training after menarche. Stager et al[155] reported that menarche occurred at 13.5 years in competitive swimmers who trained before menarche and 12.7 years in those who began training after menarche.

There is a genetic determination of age at menarche in athletes, as well as in the general population. Some studies have found significant correlations between age at menarche in athletes and the age of menarche in the athletes' mothers and sisters.[161,162] The correlations were higher if the mothers or sisters also were athletes but still were significant if they were not athletes. Stager and Hatler[161] suggested that, although training before menarche may delay menarche, the genetically determined physical characteristics that predispose girls to success in sports also are those associated with later sexual maturation.

Stager et al[163] proposed that there may be statistical artifact in retrospective studies that examine the relation between age at onset of training and age at menarche. Using computer-generated "athletes" with random ages of menarche and onset of training, they demonstrated that, because there is overlap in the ages of these events, "athletes" with early onset of training are more likely to have an age of menarche that is later than that, and vice versa. So girls with a genetically determined late age of menarche are more likely to start training before menarche than girls with a genetically determined early age of menarche.

The only clear conclusion is that menarche occurs at a later age in athletes than in the general population. Causation is harder to demonstrate. Only prospective studies can provide convincing evidence for an effect of strenuous physical activity on pubertal development.

EXERCISE AND MENOPAUSE

Relationships between menopause and exercise have been studied only recently. Two kinds of questions can be asked: Does regular physical activity affect menopausal symptoms? Does the menopausal transition affect exercise performance?

Menopausal symptoms may or may not be affected by regular exercise. Hammar and colleagues found in two large questionnaire studies that physically active women were less likely than sedentary women to have moderate or severe hot flashes. In their first study, 22% of active postmenopausal women and 44% of a control group reported moderate or severe hot flashes or sweating.[164] In their second study, severe vasomotor symptoms were reported by 5% of women who exercised more than 2 hours/week, 14% of women who exercised 1 to 2 hours/week, and 16% of women who did not exercise.[165] On the other hand, Sternfeld et al[166] found no relationship between physical activity and vasomotor symptoms. They did a case-control study of recently menopausal women who had hot flashes or night sweats either at least once per day or less than once per week and found no difference between the groups in amounts of recreational, household, or occupational activity.

There are too few data to know whether regular physical activity affects menopausal symptoms, such as hot flashes.

Clinical Guideline

One study suggested that women with frequent hot flashes are likely to have hot flashes during exercise. Freedman and Krell[167] reported that women with five or more hot flashes per day all had a hot flash during ergometer exercise as soon as rectal temperature reached a mean of 37.4°C, whereas women who had never had a hot flash did not have one under these conditions. The women with frequent hot flashes also had lower sweating thresholds, smaller zones between sweating and shivering thresholds, and higher sweat rates.

Little information exists as to whether the menopausal transition affects exercise performance. Phillips et al[168] reported that specific force (maximum voluntary force per cross-sectional area) of the adductor pollicis muscle was similar in premenopausal women and men of the same age, but around the time of menopause it declined dramatically in women but not in men. Bassey et al,[169] on the other hand, found no differences in handgrip strength, isometric quadriceps strength, or leg extensor power among women aged 45 to 54 years, who had regular menstrual periods, irregular periods, or were postmenopausal.

Too few data are available to know whether the menopausal transition affects exercise performance.

Clinical Guideline

There has been a larger number of studies on the effects of hormone replacement therapy (HRT) on exercise performance and exercise responses in postmenopausal women.

Variables that have been studied include muscle strength, temperature regulation, aerobic capacity, and cardiovascular responses to aerobic exercise in postmenopausal women with cardiac disease.

Muscle strength may or may not be affected by HRT. Phillips et al[168] reported that the reduction in specific force of the adductor pollicis muscle that they saw in women around the time of menopause was prevented by HRT. Heikkinen et al[170] found that sequential treatment with estradiol valerate and medroxyprogesterone acetate resulted in increased isometric strength of back extensor muscles but not back or hip flexion. Several other studies found no effect of HRT on muscle strength. Bassey et al[169] found no differences between women taking HRT and either premenopausal or postmenopausal women in handgrip strength, isometric quadriceps strength, or leg extensor power. Taaffe et al[171] saw no effect of HRT on dynamic muscle strength in five different measures of major lower body muscle groups. Brown et al[172] studied postmenopausal women during an 11-month weight-bearing exercise program; half the women were given conjugated estrogens and medroxyprogesterone acetate during the training. All exercising women improved in several measures of lower body strength, without an effect of HRT. Armstrong et al[173] gave either conjugated estrogens plus calcium or calcium alone for 48 weeks to postmenopausal women with recent wrist fractures. HRT did not affect grip strength, walking speed, or balance.

Temperature regulation was affected by HRT in subjects studied by Brooks et al[174] During bicycle ergometer exercise in the heat, rectal temperature was lower in postmenopausal women who had been taking estrogens alone for at least 2 years, but women who had been taking an estrogen plus a progestin had rectal temperatures similar to those in subjects taking no hormones. Forearm vascular resistance increased at a lower body temperature in the women taking estrogen alone. The authors speculated that estrogen altered temperature regulation by acting on either hypothalamic thermoregulatory neurons or peripheral vasculature and that progestin inhibited these effects but was not in high enough concentration to cause an increase in body temperature.

In healthy postmenopausal women, most aspects of aerobic exercise performance have not been affected by HRT. Snabes et al[175] gave micronized estradiol or placebo to women for 12 weeks, had a 6-week washout period, then reversed treatments for another 12 weeks. During treadmill exercise, estradiol treatment had no effect on maximal oxygen uptake, total exercise time, systolic or diastolic pressures, or any ventilatory parameters. Heart rate was somewhat lower both at rest and during exercise in the estradiol condition. Albertsson et al[176] found that 24-hour treatment with transdermal estradiol did not affect exercise time on a bicycle ergometer, maximal workload, heart rate, or blood pressure compared with a placebo condition. Lee et al[177] reported that 30-day treatment with conjugated estrogen did not affect exercise duration, heart rate, blood pressure, or electrocardiogram during treadmill exercise compared with a drug-free period. Brown et al[172] reported that conjugated estrogen and medroxyprogesterone acetate given during an 11-month weight-bearing exercise program did not affect the gain in Vo_{2max}. Green et al[178] studied endurance-trained women who had been taking estrogen or estrogen plus progesterone, as well as endurance-trained women who had not taken hormones. During graded treadmill exercise, the hormone-treated women had the same Vo_2 peak and peak heart rate but higher peak cardiac index (peak cardiac output divided by body surface area) and peak stroke volume index and lower total peripheral resistance and arteriovenous oxygen difference at peak exercise. The authors speculated that estrogen reduced vascular tone by direct actions on smooth muscle, causing the alterations in cardiac function. Taken together, these studies suggest that HRT does not affect overall aerobic performance very much in healthy women but might allow women to achieve a given Vo_2 with less cardiac work because of a reduction in vascular tone.

In postmenopausal women with cardiac disease, HRT may benefit aerobic exercise performance more than it does in women without cardiac disease. Albertsson et al[176] reported that 24-hour treatment with transdermal estradiol resulted in higher maximal workload, longer exercise time, less angina pain, and fewer electrocardiographic abnormalities compared with placebo treatment in women with exercise-induced angina pectoris and ST segment depression. Webb et al[179] treated women with atherosclerotic coronary heart disease with transdermal estradiol or placebo in a cross-over design for 8 weeks per treatment. During treadmill exercise, estradiol treatment resulted in lower heart rate at peak exercise and longer exercise time before electrocardiographic abnormalities but no difference in total exercise time, time to angina, or number of angina episodes. Holdright et al,[180] on the other hand, found no effect of transdermal estradiol vs placebo for 24 hours on total exercise time on a treadmill, time to angina, or time to electrocardiographic abnormalities in women with coronary artery disease and angina.

Exercise is very important for bone health and cardiovascular health in postmenopausal women. This is discussed in Chapter 12.

In summary, menopause may have little effect on exercise performance, although very few studies have been done. HRT has few effects on exercise performance in healthy women, but in women with cardiac disease the vascular effects of estrogen may improve aerobic exercise capacity. Little is known about whether regular exercise affects menopausal symptoms such as hot flashes.

HRT has few effects on exercise performance in healthy women, but in women with cardiac disease the vascular effects of estrogen may improve exercise capacity.

Clinical Guideline

CONCLUSION

The hormonal fluctuations of the menstrual cycle (as well as the cessation of menstrual cycles at menopause) appear to have little consistent effect on exercise performance, even though estrogen and progesterone influence several physi-

ological variables that are important to exercise. Hormonal contraceptives have not been found to have major effects on exercise performance.

On the other hand, exercise training does affect the menstrual cycle. Athletic women often have aberrations in the hypothalamic regulation of menstrual cycles, resulting in symptoms ranging from short luteal phases to secondary amenorrhea. The cause for this still is unknown, but may be related to an imbalance of energy intake and energy expenditure.

Exercise training may have some beneficial effects on premenstrual symptoms, dysmenorrhea, or menopausal symptoms. However, more well-controlled studies are needed in each of these areas.

REFERENCES

1. Goodland RL, Reynolds JG, McCoord AB, Pommerenke WT. Respiratory and electrolyte effects induced by estrogen and progesterone. *Fertil Steril.* 1953;4:300–317.
2. Bonekat HW, Dombovy ML, Staats BA. Progesterone-induced changes in exercise performance and ventilatory response. *Med Sci Sports Exerc.* 1987;19:118–123.
3. Schoene RB, Robertson HT, Pierson DJ, Peterson AP. Respiratory drives and exercise in menstrual cycles of athletic and nonathletic women. *J Appl Physiol.* 1981;50:1300–1305.
4. Dutton K, Blanksby BA, Morton AR. CO_2 sensitivity changes during the menstrual cycle. *J Appl Physiol.* 1989;67:517–522.
5. Regensteiner JG, McCullough RG, McCullough RE, Pickett CK, Moore LG. Combined effects of female hormones and exercise on hypoxic ventilatory response. *Resp Physiol.* 1990;82:107–114.
6. Beidleman BA, Rock PB, Muza SR, Fulco CS, Forte VA, Cymerman A. Exercise V_E and physical performance at altitude are not affected by menstrual cycle phase. *J Appl Physiol.* 1999;86:1519–1526.
7. Dombovy ML, Bonekat HW, Williams TJ, Staats BA. Exercise performance and ventilatory response in the menstrual cycle. *Med Sci Sports Exerc.* 1987;19:111–117.
8. Jurkowski JEH, Jones NL, Toews CJ, Sutton JR. Effects of menstrual cycle on blood lactate, O_2 delivery, and performance during exercise. *J Appl Physiol.* 1981;51:1493–1499.
9. Stephenson LA, Kolka MA, Wilkerson JE. Perceived exertion and anaerobic threshold during the menstrual cycle. *Med Sci Sports Exerc.* 1982;14:218–222.
10. Bemben DA, Salm PC, Salm AJ. Ventilatory and blood lactate responses to maximal treadmill exercise during the menstrual cycle. *J Sports Med Phys Fitness.* 1995;35:257–262.
11. De Souza MJ, Maguire MS, Rubin KR, Maresh CM. Effects of menstrual cycle phase and amenorrhea on exercise performance in runners. *Med Sci Sports Exerc.* 1990;22:575–580.
12. Friedlander M, Laskey N, Silbert S. Effect of estrogenic substance on blood volume. *Endocrinology.* 1936;20:329–332.
13. Witten CL, Bradbury JT. Hemodilution as a result of estrogen therapy.

Estrogenic effects in the human female. *Proc Soc Exp Biol Med.* 1951;78:626–629.
14. Stephenson LA, Kolka MA. Plasma volume during heat stress and exercise in women. *Eur J Appl Physiol.* 1988;57:373–381.
15. Gaebelein CJ, Senay LC. Vascular volume dynamics during ergometer exercise at different menstrual phases. *Eur J Appl Physiol.* 1982;50:1–11.
16. De Souza MJ, Maresh CM, Maguire MS, Kraemer WJ, Flora-Ginter G, Goetz KL. Menstrual status and plasma vasopressin, renin activity, and aldosterone exercise responses. *J Appl Physiol.* 1989;67:736–743.
17. Stachenfeld NS, DiPietro L, Kokoszka CA, Silva C, Keefe DL, Nadel ER. Physiological variability of fluid-regulation hormones in young women. *J Appl Physiol.* 1999;86:1092–1096.
18. Phillips M. Effect of the menstrual cycle on pulse rate and blood pressure before and after exercise. *Res Quart.* 1968;39:327–333.
19. Lewandowski J, Pruszczyk P, Elaffi M, et al. Blood pressure, plasma NPY and catecholamines during physical exercise in relation to menstrual cycle, ovariectomy, and estrogen replacement. *Regul Pept.* 1998;75–76:239–245.
20. Hessemer V, Brück K. Influence of menstrual cycle on thermoregulatory, metabolic, and heart rate responses to exercise at night. *J Appl Physiol.* 1985;59:1911–1917.
21. Stephenson LA, Kolka MA, Wilkerson JE. Metabolic and thermoregulatory responses to exercise during the human menstrual cycle. *Med Sci Sports Exerc.* 1982;14:270–275.
22. Pivarnik JM, Marichal CJ, Spillman T, Morrow JR. Menstrual cycle phase affects temperature regulation during endurance exercise. *J Appl Physiol.* 1992;72:543–548.
23. Carpenter AJ, Nunneley SA. Endogenous hormones subtly alter women's response to heat stress. *J Appl Physiol.* 1988;65:2313–2317.
24. Stephenson LA, Kolka MA. Menstrual cycle phase and time of day alter reference signal controlling arm blood flow and sweating. *Am J Physiol.* 1985;249:R186–R191.
25. Horvath SM, Drinkwater BL. Thermoregulation and the menstrual cycle. *Aviat Space Environ Med.* 1982;53:790–794.

26. Wells CL, Horvath SM. Responses to exercise in a hot environment as related to the menstrual cycle. *J Appl Physiol.* 1974;36:299–302.

27. Tenaglia SA, McLellan TM, Klentrou PP. Influence of menstrual cycle and oral contraceptives on tolerance to uncompensable heat stress. *Eur J Appl Physiol.* 1999;80:76–83.

28. Kolka MA, Stephenson LA. Effect of luteal phase elevation in core temperature on forearm blood flow during exercise. *J Appl Physiol.* 1997;82:1079–1083.

29. Charkoudian N, Johnson JM. Modification of active cutaneous vasodilation by oral contraceptive hormones. *J Appl Physiol.* 1997;83:2012–2018.

30. Matute ML, Kalkhoff RK. Sex steroid influence on hepatic gluconeogenesis and glycogen formation. *Endocrinology.* 1973;92:762–768.

31. Mandour T, Kissebah AH, Wynn V. Mechanism of oestrogen and progesterone effects on lipid and carbohydrate metabolism: Alteration in the insulin:glucagon molar ratio and hepatic enzyme activity. *Eur J Clin Invest.* 1977;7:181–187.

32. Carrington LJ, Bailey CJ. Effects of natural and synthetic estrogens and progestins on glycogen deposition in female mice. *Horm Res.* 1985;21:199–203.

33. Hackney AC. Effects of the menstrual cycle on resting muscle glycogen content. *Horm Metab Res.* 1990;22:647.

34. Hatta H, Atomi Y, Shinohara S, Yamamoto Y, Yamada S. The effects of ovarian hormones on glucose and fatty acid oxidation during exercise in female ovariectomized rats. *Horm Metab Res.* 1988;20:609–611.

35. Kendrick ZV, Ellis GS. Effect of estradiol on tissue glycogen metabolism and lipid availability in exercised male rats. *J Appl Physiol.* 1991;71:1694–1699.

36. Ellis GS, Lanza-Jacoby S, Gow A, Kendrick ZV. Effects of estradiol on lipoprotein lipase activity and lipid availability in exercised male rats. *J Appl Physiol.* 1994;77:209–215.

37. Hackney AC, McCracken-Compton MA, Ainsworth B. Substrate responses to submaximal exercise in the midfollicular and midluteal phases of the menstrual cycle. *Int J Sport Nutr.* 1994;4:299–308.

38. Nicklas BJ, Hackney AC, Sharp RL. The menstrual cycle and exercise: Performance, muscle glycogen, and substrate responses. *Int J Sports Med.* 1989;10:264–269.

39. Kanaley JA, Boileau RA, Bahr JA, Misner JE, Nelson RA. Substrate oxidation and GH responses to exercise are independent of menstrual phase and status. *Med Sci Sports Exerc.* 1992;24:873–880.

40. Ruby BC, Roberts RA, Waters DL, Burge M, Mermier C, Stolarczyk L. Effects of estradiol on substrate turnover during exercise in amenorrheic females. *Med Sci Sports Exerc.* 1997;29:1160–1169.

41. Lebrun CM, McKenzie DC, Prior JC, Taunton JE. Effects of menstrual cycle phase on athletic performance. *Med Sci Sports Exerc.* 1995;27:437–444.

42. Higgs SL, Robertson LA. Cyclic variations in perceived exertion and physical work capacity in females. *Can J Appl Sport Sci.* 1981;6:191–196.

43. De Bruyn-Prevost P, Masset C, Sturbois X. Physiological response from 18–25 years women to aerobic and anaerobic physical fitness tests at different periods during the menstrual cycle. *J Sports Med Phys Fitness.* 1984;24:144–148.

44. Dibrezzo R, Fort IL, Brown B. Dynamic strength and work variations during three stages of the menstrual cycle. *J Orthop Sports Phys Ther.* 1988;10:113–116.

45. Quadagno D, Faquin L, Lim GN, Kuminka W, Moffatt R. The menstrual cycle: Does it affect athletic performance? *Phys Sportsmed.* 1991;19:121–124.

46. Gür H. Concentric and eccentric isokinetic measurements in knee muscles during the menstrual cycle: A special reference to reciprocal moment ratios. *Arch Phys Med Rehabil.* 1997;78:501–505.

47. Davies BN, Elford JCC, Jamieson KF. Variations in performance in simple muscle tests at different phases of the menstrual cycle. *J Sports Med. Phys Fitness.* 1991;31:532–537.

48. Sarwar R, Niclos BB, Rutherford OM. Changes in muscle strength, relaxation rate and fatigability during the human menstrual cycle. *J Physiol.* 1996;493:267–272.

49. Brooks-Gunn J, Gargiulo JM, Warren MP. The effect of cycle phase on the performance of adolescent swimmers. *Phys Sportsmed.* 1986;14:182–192.

50. Bale P, Nelson G. The effects of menstruation on performance of swimmers. *Aust J Sci Med Sport.* 1985;March:19–21.

51. Sandström B, Backman C, Dahlström JA, Zador G. Adjustments of circulation including blood pressure to orthostatic reaction and physical exercise during application of a low estrogen dose steroid oral contraceptive. *Acta Obstet Gynecol Scand Suppl.* 1979;88:49–55.

52. McNeill AW, Mozingo E. Changes in the metabolic cost of standardized work associated with the use of an oral contraceptive. *J Sports Med Phys Fitness.* 1981;21:238–244.

53. Notelovitz M, Zauner C, McKenzie L, Suggs Y, Fields C, Kitchens C. The effect of low-dose oral contraceptives on cardiorespiratory function, coagulation, and lipids in exercising young women: A preliminary report. *Am J Obstet Gynecol.* 1987;156:591–598.

54. Bryner RW, Toffle RC, Ullrich IH, Yeater RA. Effect of low dose oral contraceptives on exercise performance. *Br J Sports Med.* 1996;30:36–40.

55. Thompson HS, Hyatt JP, DeSouza MJ, Clarkson PM. The effects of oral contraceptives on delayed onset muscle soreness following exercise. *Contraception.* 1997;56:59–65.

56. Grucza R, Pekkarinen H, Titov EK, Kononoff A, Hänninen O. Influence of the menstrual cycle and oral contraceptives on thermoregulatory responses to exercise in young women. *Eur J Appl Physiol.* 1993;67:279–285.

57. Rogers SM, Baker MA. Thermoregulation during exercise in women who are taking oral contraceptives. *Eur J Appl Physiol.* 1997;75:34–38.

58. Mortola JF. Premenstrual syndrome. *Trends Endocrinol Metab.* 1996;7:184–189.

59. Johnson SR. Premenstrual syndrome therapy. *Clin Obstet Gynecol.* 1998;41:405–421.

60. Prior JC, Vigna Y, Sciarretta D, Alojado N, Schulzer M. Conditioning exercise decreases premenstrual symptoms: A prospective, controlled 6-month trial. *Fertil Steril.* 1987;47:402–408.

61. Steege JF, Blumenthal JA. The effects of aerobic exercise on premenstrual symptoms in middle-aged women: A preliminary study. *J Psychosom Res.* 1993;37:127–133.

62. Aganoff JA, Boyle GJ. Aerobic exercise, mood states and menstrual cycle symptoms. *J Psychosom Res.* 1994;38:183–192.

63. Choi PY, Salmon P. Symptom changes across the menstrual cycle in competitive sportswomen, exercisers and sedentary women. *Br J Clin Psychol.* 1995;34:447–460.

64. Freeman EW, Sondheimer SJ, Rickels K. Effects of medical history factors on symptom severity in women meeting criteria for premenstrual syndrome. *Obstet Gynecol.* 1988;72:236–239.

65. Golomb LM, Solidum AA, Warren MP. Primary dysmenorrhea and physical activity. *Med Sci Sports Exerc.* 1998;30:906–909.

66. Lundquist C. Use of the Billig exercise for dysmenorrhea for college women. *Res Quart.* 1947;18:45–53.

67. Hubbell JW. Specific and non-specific exercises for the relief of dysmenorrhea. *Res Quart.* 1949;20:378–386.

68. Golub LJ, Menduke H, Lang WR. Exercise and dysmenorrhea in young teenagers: A 3-year study. *Obstet Gynecol.* 1968;32:508–511.

69. Isreal RG, Sutton M, O'Brien KF. Effects of aerobic training on primary dysmenorrhea symptomatology in college females. *J Am Coll Health.* 1985;33:241–244.

70. Izzo A, Labriola D. Dysmenorrhea and sports activities in adolescents. *Clin Exp Obstet Gynecol.* 1991;18:109–116.

71. Hightower M. Effects of exercise participation on menstrual pain and symptoms. *Women Health.* 1997;26:15–27.

72. Ronkainen H, Pakarinen A, Kauppila A. Pubertal and menstrual disorders of female runners, skiers and volleyball players. *Gynecol Obstet Invest.* 1984;18:183–189.

73. Sundell G, Milsom I, Andersch B. Factors influencing the prevalence and severity of dysmenorrhoea in young women. *Br J Obstet Gynaecol.* 1990;97:588–594.

74. Jarrett M, Heitkemper MM, Shaver JF. Symptoms and self-care strategies in women with and without dysmenorrhea. *Health Care Women Int.* 1995;16:167–178.

75. Metheny WP, Smith RP. The relationship among exercise, stress, and primary dysmenorrhea. *J Behav Med.* 1989;12:569–586.

76. Cramer DW, Wilson E, Stillman RJ, et al. The relation of endometriosis to menstrual characteristics, smoking, and exercise. *JAMA.* 1986;255:1904–1908.

77. Bachmann GA, Kemmann E. Prevalence of oligomenorrhea and amenorrhea in a college population. *Am J Obstet Gynecol.* 1982;144:98–102.

78. Carlberg KA, Buckman MT, Peake GT, Riedesel ML. Survey of menstrual function in athletes. *Eur J Appl Physiol.* 1983;51:211–222.

79. Dale E, Gerlach DH, Wilhite AL. Menstrual dysfunction in distance runners. *Obstet Gynecol.* 1979;54:47–53.

80. Glass AR, Deuster PA, Kyle SB, Yahiro JA, Vigersky RA, Schoomaker EB. Amenorrhea in Olympic marathon runners. *Fertil Steril.* 1987;48:740–745.

81. Frisch RE, Gotz-Welbergen AV, McArthur JW, et al. Delayed menarche and amenorrhea of college athletes in relation to age of onset of training. *JAMA.* 1981;246:1559–1563.

82. Sanborn CF, Martin BJ, Wagner WW. Is athletic amenorrhea specific to runners? *Am J Obstet Gynecol.* 1982;143:859–861.

83. Elliot DL, Goldberg L. Weight lifting and amenorrhea. *JAMA.* 1983;249:354.

84. Ronkainen H, Pakarinen A, Kauppila A. Pubertal and menstrual disorders of female runners, skiers and volleyball players. *Gynecol Obstet Invest.* 1984;18:183–189.

85. Walberg JL, Johnston CS. Menstrual function and eating behavior in female recreational weight lifters and competitive body builders. *Med Sci Sports Exerc.* 1991;23:30–36.

86. Brooks-Gunn J, Warren MP, Hamilton LH. The relation of eating problems and amenorrhea in ballet dancers. *Med Sci Sports Exerc.* 1987;19:41–44.

87. Feicht CB, Johnson TS, Martin BJ, Sparkes KE, Wagner WW Jr. Secondary amenorrhoea in athletes. *Lancet.* 1978;2:1145–1146.

88. Speroff L, Redwine DB. Exercise and menstrual function. *Phys Sportsmed.* 1980;8(5):41–52.

89. Baker ER, Mathur RS, Kirk RF, Williamson H. Female runners and secondary amenorrhea: Correlation with age, parity, mileage, and plasma hormonal and sex-hormone-binding globulin concentrations. *Fertil Steril.* 1981;36:183–187.

90. Shangold MM, Levine HS. The effect of marathon training upon menstrual function. *Am J Obstet Gynecol.* 1982;143:862–869.

91. Carlberg KA, Peake GT, Buckman MT. Familial susceptibility to athletic amenorrhea. *Ann Sports Med.* 1983;1:115–116.

92. Veldhuis JD, Evans WS, Demers LM, Thorner MO, Wakat D, Rogol AD. Altered neuroendocrine regulation of gonadotropin secretion in women distance runners. *J Clin Endocrinol Metab.* 1985;61:557–563.

93. Yahiro J, Glass AR, Fears WB, Ferguson EW, Vigersky RA. Exaggerated gonadotropin response to luteinizing hormone-releasing hormone in amenorrheic runners. *Am J Obstet Gynecol.* 1987;156:586–591.

94. Loucks AB, Mortola JF, Girton L, Yen SSC. Alterations in the hypothalamic-pituitary-ovarian and the hypothalamic-pituitary-adrenal axes in athletic women. *J Clin Endocrinol Metab.* 1989;68:402–411.

95. Cumming DC, Vickovic MM, Wall SR, Fluker MR. Defects in pulsatile LH release in normally menstruating runners. *J Clin Endocrinol Metab.* 1985;60:810–812.

96. Shangold M, Freeman R, Thysen B, Gatz M, The relationship between long-distance running, plasma progesterone, and luteal phase length. *Fertil Steril.* 1979;31:130–133.

97. Prior JC, Cameron K, Yuen BH, Thomas J. Menstrual cycle changes with marathon training: Anovulation and short luteal phase. *Can J Appl Sport Sci.* 1982;7:173–177.

98. Ellison PT, Lager C. Moderate recreational running is associated with lowered salivary progesterone profiles in women. *Am J Obstet Gynecol.* 1986;154:1000–1003.

99. Pirke KM, Schweiger U, Broocks A, Tuschl RJ, Laessle RG. Luteinizing hormone and follicle stimulating hormone secretion patterns in female athletes with and without menstrual disturbances. *Clin Endocrinol.* 1990;33:345–353.

100. De Souza MJ, Miller BE, Loucks AB, et al. High frequency of luteal phase deficiency and anovulation in recreational women runners: Blunted elevation in follicle-stimulating hormone observed during luteal-follicular transition. *J Clin Endocrinol Metab.* 1988;83:4220–4232.

101. Boyden TW, Pamenter RW, Stanforth P, Rotkis T, Wilmore JH. Sex steroids and endurance running in women. *Fertil Steril.* 1983;39:629–632.

102. Boyden TW, Pamenter RW, Stanforth PR, Rotkis TC, Wilmore JH. Impaired gonadotropin responses to gonadotropin-releasing hormone stimulation in endurance-trained women. *Fertil Steril.* 1984;41:359–363.

103. Bullen BA, Skrinar GS, Beitins IZ, von Mering G, Turnbull BA, McArthur JW. Induction of menstrual disorders by strenuous exercise in untrained women. *N Engl J Med.* 1985;312:1349–1353.

104. Beitins IZ, McArthur JW, Turnbull BA, Skrinar GS, Bullen BA. Exercise induces two types of human luteal dysfunction: Confirmation by urinary free progesterone. *J Clin Endocrinol Metab.* 1991;72:1350–1358.

105. Williams NI, Bullen BA, McArthur JW, Skrinar GS, Turnbull BA. Effect of short-term strenuous endurance exercise upon corpus luteum function. *Med Sci Sports Exerc.* 1999;31:949–958.

106. Schwartz B, Cumming DC, Riordan E, Selye M, Yen SSC, Rebar RW. Exercise-associated amenorrhea: A distinct entity? *Am J Obstet Gynecol.* 1981;141:662–670.

107. Carlberg KA, Buckman MT, Peake GT, Riedesel ML. Body composition of oligo/amenorrheic athletes. *Med Sci Sports Exerc.* 1983;15:215–217.

108. Loucks AB, Horvath SM, Freedson PS. Menstrual status and validation of body fat prediction in athletes. *Hum Biol.* 1984;56:383–392.

109. Sanborn CF, Albrecht BH, Wagner WW. Athletic amenorrhea: Lack of association with body fat. *Med. Sci Sports Exerc.* 1987;19:207–212.

110. Bunt JC, Going SB, Lohman TG, Heinrich CH, Perry CD, Pamenter RW. Variation in bone mineral content and estimated body fat in young adult females. *Med Sci Sports Exerc.* 1990;22:564–569.

111. Frisch RE. Fatness, menarche, and female fertility. *Perspec Biol Med.* 1985;28:611–633.

112. Lloyd T, Buchanan JR, Bitzer S, Waldman CJ, Myers C, Ford BG. Interrelationships of diet, athletic activity, menstrual status, and bone density in collegiate women. *Am J Clin Nutr.* 1987;46:681–684.

113. Deuster PA, Kyle SB, Moser PB, Vigersky RA, Singh A, Schoomaker EB. Nutritional intakes and status of highly trained amenorrheic and eumenorrheic women runners. *Fertil Steril.* 1986;46:636–643.

114. Gadpaille WJ, Sanborn CF, Wagner WW. Athletic amenorrhea, major affective disorders and eating disorders. *Am J Psychiatry.* 1987;144:939–942.

115. Klock SC, DeSouza MJ. Eating disorder characteristics and psychiatric symptomatology of eumenorrheic and amenorrheic runners. *Int J Eat Disord.* 1995;17:161–166.

116. Loucks AB, Heath EM. Dietary restriction reduces luteinizing hormone (LH) pulse frequency during waking hours and increases LH pulse amplitude during sleep in young menstruating women. *J Clin Endocrinol Metab.* 1994;78:910–915.

117. Loucks AB, Verdun M, Heath EM. Low energy availability, not stress of exercise, alters LH pulsatility in exercising women. *J Appl Physiol.* 1998;84:37–46.

118. Williams NI, Young JC, McArthur JW, Bullen B, Skrinar GS, Turnbull B. Strenuous exercise with caloric restriction: Effect on luteinizing hormone secretion. *Med Sci Sports Exerc.* 1995;27:1390–1398.

119. Myerson M, Gutin B, Warren MP, et al. Resting metabolic rate and energy balance in amenorrheic and eumenorrheic runners. *Med Sci Sports Exerc.* 1991;23:15–22.

120. Lebenstedt M, Platte P, Pirke KM. Reduced resting metabolic rate in athletes with menstrual disorders. *Med Sci Sports Exerc.* 1999;31:1250–1256.

121. Loucks AB, Laughlin GA, Mortola JF, Girton L, Nelson JC, Yen SSC. Hypothalamic-pituitary-thyroidal function in eumenorrheic and amenorrheic athletes. *J Clin Endocrinol Metab.* 1992;75:514–518.

122. Loucks AB, Callister R. Induction and prevention of low-T$_3$ syndrome in exercising women. *Am J Physiol.* 1993;264:R924–R930.

123. Loucks AB, Heath EM. Induction of low-T$_3$ syndrome in exercising women occurs at a threshold of energy availability. *Am J Physiol.* 1994;266:R817–R823.

124. Zhang Y, Proenca R, Maffei M, Barone M, Leopold L, Friedman JM. Positional cloning of the mouse obese gene and its human homologue. *Nature.* 1994;372:425–432.

125. Levine AS, Billington CJ. Do circulating leptin concentrations reflect body adiposity or energy flux? *Am J Clin Nutr.* 1998;86:761–762.

126. Coleman RA, Herrmann TS. Nutritional regulation of leptin in humans. *Diabetologia.* 1999;42:639–646.

127. Cunningham MJ, Clifton DK, Steiner RA. Leptin's actions on the reproductive axis: Perspectives and mechanisms. *Biol Reprod.* 1999;60:216–222.

128. Ahima RS, Prabakaran D, Mantzoros C, et al. Role of leptin in the neuroendocrine response to fasting. *Nature.* 1996;382:250–252.

129. Laughlin GA, Yen SSC. Hypoleptinemia in women athletes: Absence of a diurnal rhythm with amenorrhea. *J Clin Endocrinol Metab.* 1997;82:318–321.

130. Tataranni PA, Monroe MB, Dueck CA, et al. Adiposity, plasma leptin concentration and reproductive function in active and sedentary females. *Int J Obes.* 1997;21:818–821.

131. Chrousos GP, Torpy DJ, Gold PW. Interactions between the hypothalamic-pituitary-adrenal axis and the female reproductive system: Clinical implications. *Ann Intern Med.* 1998;129:229–240.

132. Ferin M. Stress and the reproductive cycle. *J Clin Endocrinol Metab.* 1999;84:1768–1774.

133. De Souza MJ, Maguire MS, Maresh CM, Kraemer WJ, Rubin KR, Loucks AB. Adrenal activation and the prolactin response to exercise in eumenorrheic and amenorrheic runners. *J Appl Physiol.* 1991;70:2378–2387.

134. De Souza MJ, Luciano AA, Arce JC, Demers LM, Loucks AB. Clinical tests explain blunted cortisol responsiveness but not mild hypercortisolism in amenorrheic runners. *J Appl Physiol.* 1994;76:1302–1309.

135. Heiman ML, Ahima RS, Craft LS, Schoner B, Stephens TW, Flier JS. Leptin inhibition of the hypothalamic-pituitary-adrenal axis in response to stress. *Endocrinology.* 1997;138:3859–3863.

136. Jessop DS. Central non-glucocorticoid inhibitors of the hypothalamo-pituitary-adrenal axis. *J Endocrinol.* 1999;160:169–180.

137. Seifer DB, Collins RL. Current concepts of β-endorphin physiology in female reproductive dysfunction. *Fertil Steril.* 1990;54:757–771.

138. Goldfarb AH, Jamurtas AZ. ß-endorphin response to exercise: An update. *Sports Med.* 1997;24:8–16.

139. Hohtari H, Salminen-Lappalainen K, Laatikainen T. Response of plasma endorphins, corticotropin, cortisol, and luteinizing hormone in the corticotropin-releasing hormone stimulation test in eumenorrheic and amenorrheic athletes. *Fertil Steril.* 1991;55:276–280.

140. Samuels MH, Sanborn CF, Hofeldt F, Robbins R. The role of endogenous opiates in athletic amenorrhea. *Fertil Steril.* 1991;55:507–512.

141. Harber VJ, Sutton JR, MacDougall JD, Woolever CA, Bhavnani BR. Plasma concentrations of β-endorphin in trained eumenorrheic and amenorrheic women. *Fertil Steril.* 1997;67:648–653.

142. McArthur JW, Turnbull BA, Pehrson J, et al. Nalmefene enhances LH secretion in a proportion of oligo-amenorrheic athletes. *Acta Endo.* 1993;128:325–333.

143. De Crée C. Sex steroid metabolism and menstrual irregularities in the exercising female: A review. *Sports Med.* 1998;25:369–406.

144. Loucks AB, Horvath SM. Exercise-induced stress responses of amenorrheic and eumenorrheic athletes. *J Clin Endocrinol Metab.* 1984;59:1109–1120.

145. Shangold MM, Gatz ML, Thysen B. Acute effects of exercise on plasma concentrations of prolactin and testosterone in recreational women runners. *Fertil Steril.* 1981;35:699–702.

146. Healy DL, Pepperell RJ, Stockdale J, Brenner WJ, Burger HG. Pituitary autonomy in hyperprolactinemic secondary amenorrhea: Results of hypothalamic-pituitary testing. *J Clin Endocrinol Metab.* 1977;44:809–819.

147. Wakat DK, Sweeney KA, Rogol AD. Reproductive system function in women cross-country runners. *Med Sci Sports Exerc.* 1982;14:263–269.

148. Horgan F, Kerstetter T. Reduced prolactin responses to exercise in amenorrheic athletes. *J. Sports Sci.* 1983;1:227–234.

149. Boyden TW, Pamenter RW, Grosso D, Stanforth P, Rotkis T, Wilmore JH. Prolactin responses, menstrual cycles, and body composition of women runners. *J Clin Endocrinol Metab.* 1982;54:711–714.

150. Chang FE, Richards SR, Kim MH, Malarkey WB. Twenty four-hour prolactin profiles and prolactin responses to dopamine in long distance running women. *J Clin Endocrinol Metab.* 1984;59:631–635.

151. Galle PC, Freeman EW, Galle MG, Huggins GR, Sondheimer SJ. Physiologic and psychologic profiles in a survey of women runners. *Fertil Steril.* 1983;39:633–639.

152. Malina RM, Harper AB, Avant HH, Campbell DE. Age of menarche in athletes and non-athletes. *Med Sci Sports.* 1973;5:11–13.

153. Ross WD, Brown SR, Faulker RA, Savage MV. Age of menarche of elite Canadian skaters and skiers. *Can J Appl Sport Sci.* 1976;1:191–193.

154. Malina RM, Spirduso WW, Tate C, Baylor AM. Age at menarche and selected menstrual characteristics in athletes at different competitive levels and in different sports. *Med Sci Sports.* 1978;10:218–222.

155. Stager JM, Robertshaw D, Miescher E. Delayed menarche in swimmers in relation to age at onset of training and athletic performance. *Med Sci Sports Exerc.* 1984;16:550–555.

156. Claessens AL, Malina RM, Lefevre J, et al. Growth and menarcheal status of elite female gymnasts. *Med Sci Sports Exerc.* 1992;24:755–763.

157. Frisch RE, Wyshak G, Vincent L. Delayed menarche and amenorrhea in ballet dancers. *N Engl J Med.* 1980;303:17–19.

158. Warren MP. The effects of exercise on pubertal progression and reproductive function in girls. *J Clin Endocrinol Metab.* 1980;51:1150–1157.

159. Lindholm C, Hagenfeldt K, Ringertz BM. Pubertal development in elite juvenile gymnasts. Effects of physical training. *Acta Obstet Gynecol Scand.* 1994;73:269–273.

160. Frisch RE, Gotz-Welbergen AV, McArthur JW, et al. Delayed menarche and amenorrhea of college athletes in relation to age of onset of training. *JAMA.* 1981;246:1559–1563.

161. Stager JM, Hatler LK. Menarche in athletes: The influence of genetics and prepubertal training. *Med Sci Sports Exerc.* 1988;20:369–373.

162. Malina RM, Ryan RC, Bonci CM. Age at menarche in athletes and their mothers and sisters. *Ann Human Biol.* 1994;21:417–422.

163. Stager JM, Wigglesworth JK, Hatler LK. Interpreting the relationship between age of menarche and prepubertal training. *Med Sci Sports Exer.* 1990;22:54–58.

164. Hammar M, Berg G, Lindgren R. Does physical exercise influence the frequency of postmenopausal hot flushes? *Acta Obstet Gynecol Scand.* 1990;69:409–412.

165. Ivarsson T, Spetz AC, Hammar M. Physical exercise and vasomotor symptoms in postmenopausal women. *Maturitas.* 1998; 29:139–146.

166. Sternfeld B, Quesenberry CP, Husson G. Habitual physical activity and menopausal symptoms: A case-control study. *J Women's Health.* 1999;8:115–123.

167. Freedman RR, Krell W. Reduced thermoregulatory null zone in postmenopausal women with hot flashes. *Am J Obstet Gynecol.* 1999;181:66–70.

168. Phillips SK, Rook KM, Siddle NC, Bruce SA, Woledge RC. Muscle weakness in women occurs at an earlier age than in men, but strength is preserved by hormone replacement therapy. *Clin Sci (Colch).* 1993;84:95–98.

169. Bassey EJ, Mockett SP, Fentem PH. Lack of variation in muscle strength with menstrual status in healthy women aged 45–54 years: Data from a national survey. *Eur J Appl Physiol Occup Physiol.* 1996;73:382–386.

170. Heikkinen J, Kyllönen E, Kurttila-Matero E, et al. HRT and exercise: Effects on bone density, muscle strength and lipid metabolism. A placebo controlled 2-year prospective trial on two estrogen-progestin regimens in healthy postmenopausal women. *Maturitas.* 1997;26:139–149.

171. Taaffe DR, Luz Villa M, Delay R, Marcus R. Maximal muscle strength of elderly women is not influenced by oestrogen status. *Age Ageing.* 1995;24:329–333.

172. Brown M, Birge SJ, Kohrt WM. Hormone replacement therapy does not augment gains in muscle strength or fat-free mass in response to weight-bearing exercise. *J Gerontol A Biol Sci Med Sci.* 1997;52:B166–170.

173. Armstrong AL, Oborne J, Coupland CA, Macpherson MB, Bassey EJ, Wallace WA. Effects of hormone replacement therapy on muscle performance and balance in post-menopausal women. *Clin Sci (Colch).* 1996;91:685–690.

174. Brooks EM, Morgan AL, Pierzga JM, et al. Chronic hormone replacement therapy alters thermoregulatory and vasomotor function in postmenopausal women. *J Appl Physiol.* 1997;83:477–484.

175. Snabes MC, Herd JA, Schuyler N, Dunn K, Spence DW, Young RL. In normal postmenopausal women physiologic estrogen replacement therapy fails to improve exercise tolerance: A randomized, double-blind, placebo-controlled, crossover trial. *Am J Obstet Gynecol.* 1996;175:110–114.

176. Albertsson PA, Emanuelsson H, Milsom I. Beneficial effect of treatment with transdermal estradiol-17-beta on exercise-induced angina and ST segment depression in syndrome X. *Int J Cardiol.* 1996;54:13–20.

177. Lee M, Giardina EG, Homma S, DiTullio MR, Sciacca RR. Lack of effect of estrogen on rest and treadmill exercise in postmenopausal women without known cardiac disease. *Am J Cardiol.* 1997;80:793–797.

178. Green JS, Crouse SF, Rohack JJ. Peak exercise hemodynamics in exercising postmenopausal women taking versus not taking supplemental estrogen. *Med Sci Sports Exerc.* 1998;30:158–164.

179. Webb CM, Rosano GM, Collins P. Oestrogen improves exercise-induced myocardial ischaemia in women. *Lancet.* 1998;351:1556–1557.

180. Holdright DR, Sullivan AK, Wright CA, Sparrow JL, Cunningham D, Fox KM. Acute effect of oestrogen replacement therapy on treadmill performance in postmenopausal women with coronary artery disease. *Eur Heart J.* 1995; 6:1566–1570.

The Pregnant Athlete

Gloria C. Cohen and Nadya Swedan

INTRODUCTION

Many women would like to continue to exercise during pregnancy. Other women who have not been following a regular exercise program before pregnancy would like to begin exercising during pregnancy. When prescribing an exercise program during pregnancy, one must consider the individual woman, the physiological and anatomical issues unique to pregnancy, and the appropriateness of various forms of exercise.

This chapter covers the maternal and fetal responses to exercise and the types of exercise that the pregnant athlete with an uncomplicated pregnancy can participate in. Labor and delivery and the postpartum period for the active female are also discussed.

PHYSIOLOGICAL AND ANATOMICAL ISSUES UNIQUE TO PREGNANCY

When considering exercise during pregnancy, one must evaluate both maternal and fetal responses to the activity. In addition, the pregnant athlete must consider the anatomical and musculoskeletal changes that occur as the pregnancy progresses.

Maternal Responses

1. The cardiovascular system of the pregnant woman undergoes significant adaptations with increased heart rate, cardiac output, and blood volume. Resting cardiac output in normal pregnancy is increased by 30% to 50% above nonpregnant values. This increase is primarily due to an increase in stroke volume. Heart rate also has a tendency toward elevation and variability, particularly in the third trimester. This change may also affect further alterations in cardiac output. The resting heart rate may increase by 15 beats per minute in the second and third trimesters. Given these cardiovascular dynamics, heart rates cannot be used as reliable predictors of fitness or exercise intensity during pregnancy.

2. Cardiac output distribution relates to the duration, type, and intensity of exercise. As the pregnant woman exercises, oxygen-rich blood is diverted away from the uterus to the working tissues of the mother. In addition, there is an increased release of norepinephrine and epinephrine during exercise,[1] both of which may not only further decrease uterine blood flow by vasoconstriction but may also increase uterine activity.

   Maternal body position may also affect cardiac output, particularly so in the supine position after 20 weeks' gestation. This position can cause a 9% decrease in cardiac output.[2] This decrease is related to compression of the vena cava by the enlarging uterus and a relative obstruction of venous return. This may lead to maternal hypotension and a decrease in blood supply to the fetus.

3. There is an absolute increase in oxygen consumption. The maximum oxygen consumption (L/min) at term is 16% to 32% increased over the nonpregnant female.[3] The increase in oxygen consumption is closely related to the increase in body weight.[4] It is therefore not surprising that pregnant women find it

gradually more difficult to perform muscular activity, especially when weight bearing or lifting is involved.

4. The respiratory system is affected by physiological and anatomical changes that occur during pregnancy. The pregnant woman tends to hyperventilate, causing an increase in the minute ventilation and a decrease in the arterial carbon dioxide tension. This is due to increased plasma progesterone and an increased sensitivity to carbon dioxide.[5] In addition, she must work hard during inspiration to displace the enlarging uterus downward.

5. Hyperthermia resulting from febrile illness in the first trimester has been associated with intrauterine growth retardation, intrauterine death, and central nervous system abnormalities such as neural tube defects.[2,6,7] Therefore, concern exists that exercise-induced hyperthermia may also result in these fetal problems, but no prospective studies to date have found any association between maternal temperature elevated by exercise and congenital malformations.[8–10]

The metabolic rate increases during both exercise and pregnancy, thereby resulting in greater heat production. The intensity and duration of the exercise affect the heat production. With moderate aerobic exercise, the mother is able to dissipate heat effectively. This efficient heat dissipation during pregnancy may be a result of pregnancy-associated physiological changes such as increased blood volume and skin blood flow.[11] In both the pregnant and nonpregnant states, the conditioned athlete's body seems to have an improved ability to dissipate heat.

The pregnant athlete must be aware of environmental conditions and should be aware of the problem of dehydration, which can adversely affect thermoregulation. Dehydration can cause uterine irritability and preterm labor during late pregnancy.[12] The exercising pregnant woman must hydrate before, during, and after exercise.

Maternal Physiological Adaptations to Exercise

- Increased stroke volume
- Increased heart rate
- Increased cardiac output
- Increased blood volume
- Increased oxygen consumption
- Increased respiratory rate
- Increased metabolic rate
- Increased heat production

Clinical Guideline

Fetal Responses

1. The fetal heart rate response during and after exercise is quite variable. Studies have reported either an in-crease[13,14] or decrease[15–17] in the fetal heart rate. An increased fetal heart rate of 10 to 30 beats per minute usually returns to normal within 15 minutes in women performing mild to moderate exercise. Transient fetal bradycardia during and after exercise has been attributed to monitoring artifact[17] but may also indicate fetal distress, particularly in a complicated pregnancy. It is imperative to remember that such bradycardias may be a symptom of uteroplacental insufficiency.

2. The fetal body temperature under normal resting conditions is approximately 0.5°C greater than the maternal temperature,[18,19] primarily because of the higher fetal and placental metabolic rates from growth and development. This temperature gradient provides a mechanism by which the fetus can transfer heat to the mother. With exercise this gradient is temporarily reversed as the maternal temperature rises. Fetal temperature may take more than 1 hour to return to normal after 40 minutes of vigorous exercise at 70% Vo_{2max}.[20]

CAUTIONS

As the pregnant athlete exercises, blood carrying oxygen for the fetus is diverted from the uterus to the working tissues of the muscle, skin, and heart. This may decrease fetal oxygen availability and placental diffusing capacity.[5] Maternal and fetal reserves may compensate for this transient unfavorable effect from moderate exercise. Altered fetal growth and development, however, may result from repeated exposure to extensive exercise stress.[21]

Exercising in the supine position after 20 weeks' gestation causes the enlarging uterus to fall back onto the vena cava and may cause maternal hypotension and a subsequent decrease in the blood supply to the fetus. Many physicians believe that a woman with an uncompromised pregnancy can exercise briefly in this position without adverse consequences.[22,23]

Maternal or fetal hypoglycemia may occur under conditions of prolonged exercise. In a study involving pregnant women in their third trimester, the results indicated that their blood glucose levels decreased at a faster rate and to a significantly lower level after exercise than the nonpregnant women in response to 1 hour of prolonged moderate intensity exercise (at 55% of their Vo_{2max}).[24] Glucose is an essential nutrient for the developing fetus. The pregnant athlete must consume adequate extra calories to meet the metabolic requirements of pregnancy and exercise. The demands of the activity depend on the intensity and duration of the exercise.

The musculoskeletal changes that occur during pregnancy can lead to injury if the pregnant athlete does not appreciate these adjustments. The center of gravity becomes lower because of the increased weight gain and enlarging abdominal girth. This results in the pregnant athlete experiencing biomechanical alterations as balance becomes challenged. There is also ligamentous laxity and increased joint flexibility from the release of the hormones relaxin and progesterone.[25] The combination of increased body weight and increased laxity can increase the risk of overuse injuries and muscle/tendon stress. It is therefore important to avoid severe ballistic movements (jerky and bouncing) when stretching and exercising.

Exercise Precautions during Pregnancy

- Temperature regulation—prevent overheating
- Position—avoid supine position
- Glucose homeostasis
- Balance and flexibility alterations

Clinical Guideline

CONTRAINDICATIONS

There are several conditions in which exercise in pregnancy is contraindicated because of the risk of compromising the fetus and the mother. Medical contraindications include cardiovascular or respiratory conditions, infection, anemia, and thyrotoxicosis. Poor obstetrical history (eg, intrauterine growth retardation, prematurity, more than one previous miscarriage) and high-risk current obstetrical status (eg, hypertension, uterine bleeding, premature rupture of membranes, cervical cerclage, intrauterine growth retardation, anticoagulant treatment) are also contraindications to exercise in pregnancy.

Contraindications to Exercise during Pregnancy

- Medical (cardiovascular, respiratory, infection, anemia, thyrotoxicosis)
- Poor obstetrical history
- Current obstetrical status high risk
- Environmental stress

Clinical Guideline

BACK AND PELVIC ISSUES IN PREGNANCY AND EXERCISE

While to date there are no studies documenting incidence of back and pelvic pain in active versus inactive women, the overall prevalence of back pain in pregnancy, 50%, merits attention.[26–30] (In comparison, frequency of back pain in nonpregnant women is approximately 20% to 25%.[27,31]) Back pain of pregnancy can cause frustration and limit function, evidenced by reports of work impairment and disability both during and after pregnancy.[27,31–32] Parity, age, smoking, stature, work, and activity levels have all been investigated as predictors of back pain with contradictory evidence. However, most clinicians agree that the occurrence of back pain is lower in incidence and severity in athletic, active women secondary to increased abdominal and paraspinal strength and stability.

Back pain of pregnancy is usually multifactorial. As Kristiansson and colleagues describe: "hormonal, biomechanical, circulatory, and psychological changes"[31(p 707)] all play a role in the nature and cause of pain. Hormonal changes of pregnancy lead to water retention of connective tissues, which may increase musculoskeletal pain. Neuropeptide changes and progesterone have also been implicated as generators and modulators of pain in pregnancy.[33] Relaxin, an insulin-like hormone resulting in the pelvic ligamentous laxity necessary for birth, has been identified as an important factor in research of musculoskeletal conditions.

As a result of the effects of relaxin on collagen, there is an increase in sacroiliac joint movement and symphysis pubis widening. Sacroiliac anterior and posterior longitudinal ligaments also increase in laxity. This compromises pelvic stability (see Figure 11–1). Studies show this relaxin mediated laxity occurring in the first half of pregnancy.[30,34] A study by Kristiansson in 1996 measured levels of serum relaxin in pregnancy and found relatively higher levels corresponding with incidence of both symphyseal and low back pain;[30] combination pain patterns were associated with the highest levels of serum relaxin. Kristiansson and colleagues further suggested that, in combination with estrogen, relaxin's effects on cartilage remodeling within the ligaments are also pain generators.

Posture has been implied as a cause of back pain. After the twelfth week, the uterus expands superiorly, anteriorly, and laterally. A posterior posture is the most common—75% of pregnancies result in uterine weight carried posterior to the center of gravity.[28(p 331)] Anterior posture, the remaining 25%, has been proposed to be associated with pubic symphysis problems. However, of all pregnant women with back pain, the majority begin to experience back pain at the twelfth week;[35] therefore, postural theories of back pain have been challenged. Recent studies have found less reliable relationships between lordosis and back pain.[29]

The common occurrence of pain worsening later in the day suggests a component of fatigue. Some women alter their gait and movement patterns as a result of pregnancy, which further alters pressure on spine-supporting soft tissues. Pain-sensitive structures include intervertebral discs, facet joints, paraspinal muscles, and ligaments, in particular

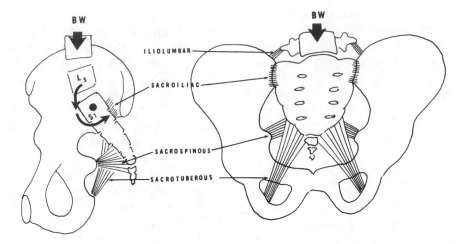

Figure 11-1 Ligamentous Support of the Pelvis. Left, a side view of the pelvis indicates the body weight (BW) on L5 vertebra causes rotation of the sacrum (curved arrows). Right, anterior-posterior view of pelvis.

anterior and posterior longitudinal ligaments.[26(p 90)] Muscle imbalances resulting from laxity, weakness, or center of gravity changes can generate pain. Abdominal muscles, important contributors to both spinal and uterine posture, become lax, stretched, and thereby weakened,[36] further decreasing the ability to stabilize the spine and moderate back pain. Relaxin can also result in diastasis recti, further weakening abdominal muscles.

PATTERNS OF BACK PAIN IN PREGNANCY

Patterns of back pain in pregnancy are most commonly classified as posterior pelvic pain (PPP) and lumbar pain. Less commonly described patterns are sciatic and nocturnal. History of pain can often distinguish the source and type. Again, the practitioner should remember that pain can be due to more than one cause, which may make the diagnosis and treatment challenging. Identifying the pain pattern aids in effective treatment.[37–39]

The most commonly described pattern attributed to pregnancy back pain is PPP with occurrence thought to be as great as two to four times more frequent than other patterns of pregnancy-related back pain.[37–41] Symptoms can be quite bothersome, and this pain pattern may be less responsive to therapy and overall fitness.[42(p 898)] Östgaard, in a study published in *Spine* in 1996, found one in three of all pregnant women to have PPP.[43] PPP is often activity-related, including stepping off a curb, turning in bed, stair climbing, or walking on uneven surfaces. Pain can be unilateral or bilateral; sharp and across the lower back; into the buttock, hip, or groin; and occasionally into the thigh. Generally, it is described as distal and lateral to LS-SI[42(p 895)] (see Figure 11-2).

Symptoms describing subluxation can also be present, including symphysiolysis.[41(p 74)] A Norwegian study in 1999 describes this as "symptom giving pelvic girdle relaxation" (PGR),[44] a term suggested by the Norwegian Medical Association in 1991 as function-impairing pain associated with pelvic instability. This study also suggested that women with a history of low back pain had PGR earlier in pregnancy, and that those who had the symptoms develop earlier in pregnancy also have it for longer durations during the day.[44(p 114)] "Pelvic insufficiency" has also been used to describe the combination of laxity and pain.

The posterior pain provocation test has been recognized as a reliable method to detect this type of pain. This test is done with the patient supine, with the hip and knee on the painful side flexed. While stabilizing the pelvis by holding the opposite iliac crest, a vertical downward force is applied to the flexed hip. If this maneuver reproduces the patient's pain, PPP is contributing[26(p 91),42(p 896)] (see Figure 11-3).

Lumbar pain, similar to lumbar pain in nonpregnant women, frequently is described as worse in prolonged sitting or standing, bending, and with lifting. The nature of the pain is usually dull and achy. It is described as an ache around the mid low to upper back, often worse at the end of the day. This pain pattern is often due to muscular spasm, strain, and fatigue, along with postural and abdominal weakness, and is associated with paraspinal tenderness. Location of discomfort is more midline and proximal than that of PPP.

Sciatic pain can be due to either sacroiliac or lumbar causes and can also be secondary to piriformis syndrome, spondylolysis, or spondylolisthesis, or disc or facet pathological conditions and radiculopathy. "True sciatica" has been reported to occur in only 1% of pregnancies;[35] inci-

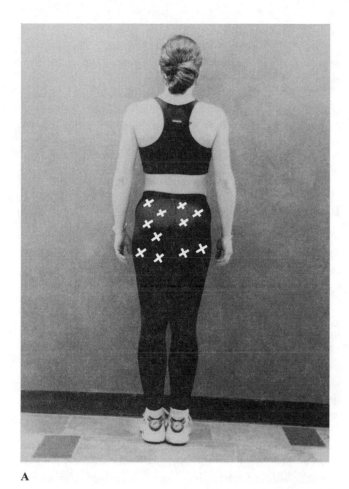 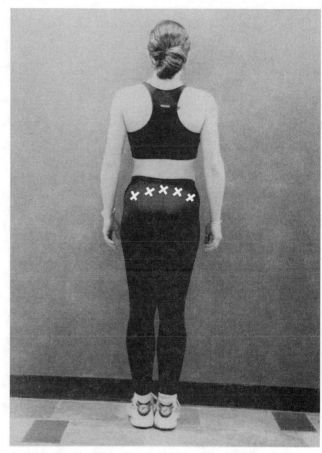

Figure 11–2 Pain Distributions. (A) Common distribution of posterior pelvic pain, (B) common distribution of lumbar pain.

dence of clinically significant disc herniation is also reported as extremely rare (1:10,000).[45] If neurological symptoms are present, a thorough evaluation is warranted. Although there have only been a limited number of lumbar spine magnetic resonance studies on pregnant women to date, there have been no documented effects of specific fetal harm;[46,47] however, this must be used judiciously with consent from the obstetrician and a well-informed mother.

Overall frequency of back pain at night during pregnancy is approximately one third.[48(p 368)] (This includes both combination pain patterns along with pain occurring only at night.) True "nocturnal" pain of pregnancy is unique in its history of *not* worsening with turning in bed. The pain is described as a cramping and often awakens women at night, attributed to vascular engorgement of vena caval structures by both hypervolemia and by the weight of the fetus. This has been proposed to cause pain due to hypoxia of nerves, particularly those near epidural veins.[48(p 370)] Engorgement of neurovascular structures supplying paraspinal muscles and lumbopelvic ligaments is also theorized to cause pain.

Back pain at night can also result from day-long fatigue and gravity-related biomechanical stress.[26(p 91)]

Common Causes of Back Pain in Pregnancy

- Posterior pelvic
- Lumbar
- Nocturnal
- Sciatic
- Osteoporosis
- Diastasis recti

Clinical Guideline

A less frequent, although notable, cause of back pain occurring with equal frequency during the third trimester and in the postpartum period[49(p 148)] is osteoporosis, with most cases occurring in first pregnancies. Because of the contraindicated and limited use of X-rays during pregnancy,

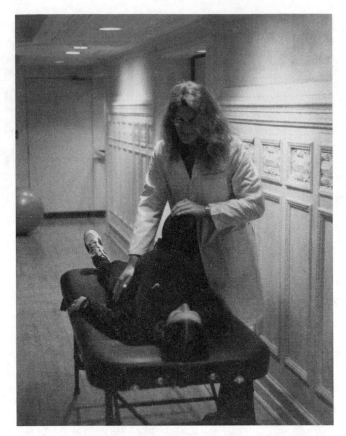

Figure 11–3 The Posterior Pain Provocation Test. While stabilizing the pelvis by holding the opposite iliac crest, a vertical force is applied to the flexed hip. If this maneuver reproduces the patient's pain, posterior pelvic pain is contributing.

osteoporosis is speculated to be more prevalent than documented. Transient osteoporosis of the hip has also been described and should also be considered in cases of hip or groin pain.[50] Calcium supplementation with adequate vitamin D intake must be encouraged, especially in patients eating a low-fat diet. If significant osteoporosis is documented, breast-feeding is not recommended. Pregnancy is known to further decrease bone mineral density by inducing trabecular bone loss, and lactation is known to affect cortical loss.[51]

Cautions

Back pain can also be a sign of fetal and/or maternal distress. If accompanied by vaginal discharge, bleeding, burning, or itching, the patient should see her obstetric-care physician at once. Back pain associated with contractions and bleeding or fluid leaks is an emergency. Other internal causes that can lead to back pain include urinary tract infections and disease; gastrointestinal disease, including constipation; cardiovascular disease; and tumors, including

fibroids. Sickle cell anemia and rheumatological diseases can also be first seen as back pain. Persistent, nonpositional pain that is unrelated to activity or rest is an indication that causes other than musculoskeletal should be investigated. Neurological symptoms, including numbness, weakness, and loss of reflexes, require close medical supervision. Cauda equina symptoms, including impaired bowel and bladder function and altered sensation, warrant emergency medical care, magnetic resonance imaging investigation, and surgical consideration.

Treatment

Treatment of back pain in pregnant women is not dissimilar from treatment in nonpregnant women; overall analysis and education on posture, positioning, adequate rest, activity modification, and lumbar and pelvic supports are beneficial. Lifting and bending should be minimal. Comfortable, low-heeled shoes should be recommended. Sacroiliac belts, such as the "prenatal cradle" or "maternal SI lock," (Figure 11–14) have also been successful at reducing PPP. Positioning, including using a lumbar support cushion while seated, and a wedge-shaped pillow to support the abdomen while side-lying, can be helpful. Relaxation and brief localized warm or cold modalities can be helpful. Physical therapy can be prescribed for abdominal and pelvic strengthening, increased spinal stability, and increased hip and lower extremity flexibility. Exercises with abdominal countersupport using the hands of patient or therapist to reinforce abdominal musculature are beneficial. Exercise maintains mobility, strength, and posture, all of which prevent and decrease the intensity of low back pain. Each woman should be treated individually when prescribing exercise modalities and be advised to stop certain activities that may actually worsen her pain.

A 1999 study by Kihlstrand et al[27] on water gymnastics revealed significant reduction in the intensity of back pain during the second half of pregnancy; massage in the side-lying position has also been proven to be beneficial in studies. Side-lying manual traction[40] and gentle patient- or therapist-guided manipulation[38] have been described as effective. Alternative therapies include acupuncture, acupressure, and biofeedback. Whirlpool baths, Jacuzzis, prolonged heat, and electrical modalities, including electrical stimulation and ultrasound, are contraindicated in treatment of back pain in pregnancy.

For pharmacological pain control during later pregnancy, acetaminophen can usually be taken for brief periods with the approval of the obstetric-care physician. Aspirin and other nonsteroidal anti-inflammatory medications are not advised, due to the increased risk of fetal patent ductus arteriosis and increased maternal bleeding, especially during delivery.

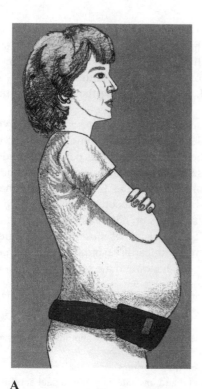 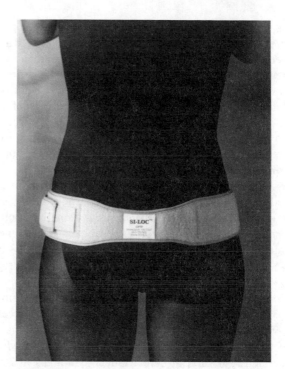

A **B**

Figure 11–4 (A) Maternity SI-LOC Side View. (B) SI-LOC Posterior View.

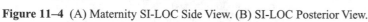

Common Management of Low Back Pain in Pregnancy

- Postural reeducation
- Lumbar and abdominal support cushions
- Frequent repositioning
- Sacroiliac belts
- Relaxation
- Physical therapy
- Moderate exercise
- Stretching programs
- Side-lying massage

Clinical Guideline

POSTPARTUM BACK PAIN

Most women with postpartum back pain had a history of posterior pelvic or lumbar back pain during or before pregnancy.[33(p 406)] Östgaard, in a study published in *Spine*, 1996, suggests that intensity of and disability from back pain in pregnancy are predictive of persistent postpartum pain.[43] Östgaard's studies also suggest that lumbar pain patterns are prevalent more than during pregnancy, although a 1999 study by Nilsson-Wikmar[52] revealed a higher percentage of posterior pelvic and sacroiliac pain. Younger age and multi-

parity have also been described as predictors of postpartum back pain.[53]

It is generally believed that laxity due to relaxin remains present for 3–4 months postpartum.[34] In PPP that persists postpartum, strenuous and high-impact activities should be avoided because of the possibility of pelvic instability.[37(p 67)] Occasionally, coccydynia results after delivery as a result of laxity and movement at the sacrococcygeal joint. This is a very painful condition and can be quite limiting. Epidural anesthesia has also been described as a cause of postpartum back pain; however, recent studies have suggested this lasts only the first day after delivery and declines thereafter.[54]

Treatment addresses the underlying cause. Gynecological sources of persistent low back and pelvic pain should always be considered. Although most postpartum back pain is self-limited,[52] patients should be actively managed to prevent progression into chronic back pain. The reader is referred to Chapters 3 and 4 for further evaluation and management guidelines.

NEUROPATHIES IN PREGNANCY

Active and athletic pregnant women may be more likely to experience symptoms of overuse neuropathies. Although neuropathies and nerve compression syndromes during pregnancy are discussed as frequent, literature describing specific patterns is limited. Various case studies have been published, including bilateral femoral neuropathy,[55] isolated and unilateral femoral neuropathy,[56,57] obturator neuropathy,[58] and neuropathy and gastropathy associated with diabetes.[59] On discussion with obstetricians, many will relate a notable number of patients who complain of tingling and numbing sensations in their extremities. Frequently, meralgia paresthetica occurs; tarsal tunnel syndrome and syndrome of the rectus abdominis muscle also occur.[58] Carpal tunnel syndrome is most frequently described.

Onset of carpal tunnel syndrome has actually been attributed by some to fluid changes in pregnancy.[60(p 303)] One of the most common neuropathies, carpal tunnel syndrome is described as occurring overall more frequently in women than men (3:1).[61(p 1284)] A comprehensive study in 1998 by Stolp-Smith et al[62] revealed an incidence of 34% in pregnancy, with 50% of the cases diagnosed in the third trimester. Nocturnal hand pain was described as very common, along with bilateral hand paresthesias. Eighty-six percent improved spontaneously after pregnancy or with conservative treatment. Another study by Courts,[63] published in 1995, found resolution of carpal tunnel symptoms in 76% of women by 1 month postpartum with the use of hand splints. In addition to neutral or cock-up wrist splinting (Figure 11–5), conservative management of this disorder includes repositioning, stretching, and icing. Corticosteroid injections can also be considered. Physical therapy should be prescribed in unremitting cases. Pyridoxine hydrochloride, vitamin B_6, is also helpful in relieving symptoms of paresthesias.

Compression neuropathies resulting from labor and delivery can occur and include femoral neuropathy, peroneal neuropathy, and obturator neuropathy. These are most likely positional or caused by prolonged traction or compression forces. They can also be due to hematomas. Peroneal neuropathy resulting in footdrop has been reported, as secondary to prolonged lying on one side and squatting.[64]

In active women, foot and toe neuropraxias can be avoided by accommodating shoe size to the increase due to fluid retention. Patients should be educated on positioning, stretching, and changing routines to prevent overuse neuropathies. Referral to a physiatrist or neurologist for persistent complaints, especially symptoms of weakness, is prudent. Physical therapy is often beneficial. Although most symptoms are self-limited, follow-up during the postpartum period is advised.

The American College of Obstetricians and Gynecologists (ACOG) 1985 guidelines[65] cautioned against exceeding a maternal heart rate of 140 beats per minute and recommended exercise of no longer than 15 minutes and a core temperature not to exceed 38°C. These guidelines were revised in 1994,[66] and the recommendation was modified with previous guidelines on heart rate and duration of exercise removed. It now reads that most women "can exercise moderately to maintain cardiorespiratory and muscular fitness throughout pregnancy and the postpartum period."

The Prenatal Workout

A recommended prenatal workout should include the following:
1. A 10- to 15-minute warmup.
2. An abbreviated and low-intensity, nonimpact aerobic portion (20 to 30 minutes).
3. Careful heart rate monitoring.
4. A cool-down period with gentle stretching. The aerobic activity should be gradually slowed down over a 5-minute period, followed by 5 to 10 minutes of gentle stretching.

Clinical Guideline

There is a scarcity of research on the elite-level athlete and recommendations for exercise intensity during pregnancy. With the elite-level athlete, there is often a desire to achieve a high level of fitness while maintaining a training schedule that will not harm the developing fetus or the mother.[67] At this time, the physician should advise the pregnant athlete to maintain a lower level of exercise program than is usual for her to avoid any unnecessary consequences to the fetus. The physician must also review the athlete's exercise program with her on a regular basis and, when indicated, with her coach as well.

PSYCHOLOGICAL ASPECTS

Exercise has been associated with a sense of enhanced psychological well-being. This is particularly relevant in pregnancy when the woman is adjusting to the alterations in her body image and mood changes. These mood changes can range from mild transient moodiness to prolonged depression and anxiety. A number of studies have shown that exercise is associated with reduced anxiety and depression.[68–70]

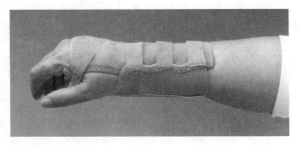

Figure 11–5 Neutral Wrist Splint Used To Alleviate Symptoms of Carpal Tunnel Syndrome.

Koltyn and Schultes[71] studied the effect of exercise on mood changes in the postpartum period in women who exercised compared with those who did not. They found that exercise and quiet rest decreased anxiety and depression, but that with exercise there was both a decrease in total mood disturbance and an increase in vigor.

It is important to recognize the exercise-dependent pregnant athlete who indulges in excessive repetitive exercise. This exercise dependence may be a sign of psychological dysfunction. This individual must be assessed by her physician, counseled about a balanced moderate training program, and regularly monitored.

SPECIFIC SPORTS RECOMMENDATIONS

The exercise program for a pregnant woman needs to be individualized. The best form of activity is one she enjoys, will continue, and that is appropriate for her to pursue for the long term. Those women who led sedentary lifestyles before pregnancy should begin with physical activity of very low intensity and progress gradually. Many women who have been exercising before pregnancy choose to continue their previous type of activity and to modify intensity and duration of exercise throughout the pregnancy.

Some general sport guidelines (provided there are no contraindications to exercise) follow:

Running/jogging—If a woman has been running before her pregnancy, she may continue to do so but should modify the intensity and duration.[72] It is not recommended that a woman start a running program during pregnancy.

Cycling—Changes in the body's center of gravity can affect balance. A stationary bicycle is usually a safer choice (Figure 11–6). Cycling is a sport that can be started during pregnancy. Elite-level cyclists may want to change from a racing bike to a mountain bike for more shock absorption and an upright position on the bike.

Aerobics—The pregnant athlete is advised to avoid bouncing movements and extended periods of time in the supine position (especially after 20 weeks' gestation). Low-impact aerobics is recommended as the pregnancy progresses.

Swimming—This sport can be initiated during pregnancy. Diving and jumping into the pool are not advisable, and extremes of water temperature need to be avoided. Swimming is not advisable if there is any fluid leak.

Weight training—The goal is strength maintenance. Routines should be modified with lighter weight and fewer repetitions with no straining. Proper breathing technique is important to avoid breath-holding and the Valsalva maneuver. The latter can decrease splanchnic blood flow and uterine perfusion and lead to hypertension. Exercises usually performed in the supine position should be changed to seated or upright positions. The pregnant athlete should avoid heavy weights to decrease the risk of sustaining muscle strain. It is not recommended that this activity be started during pregnancy.

Racquet sports—The pregnant athlete can continue to play, but she must play conservatively given the changes in center of gravity and coordination.

Cross-country skiing—This sport should not be initiated during pregnancy. It is a good aerobic activity to continue for the experienced skier.

The pregnant athlete must appreciate that there is a risk of falling with any of the preceding activities. In addition, she must regularly reevaluate the exercise program with her physician as her pregnancy progresses.

ACTIVITIES NOT RECOMMENDED

High-risk sports and contact sports are not recommended during pregnancy. There is increased potential for falls and trauma and risk of abdominal trauma, particularly with the contact sports.

Activities Not Recommended

High-risk sports (increased potential for falls/trauma)
- Downhill skiing
- Skating
- Water skiing
- Scuba diving
- Gymnastics
- Hang gliding
- Horseback riding

Contact sports (increased risk of abdominal trauma)
- Hockey (field and ice)
- Basketball
- Soccer
- Boxing
- Wrestling
- Football

Clinical Guideline

Scuba diving occurs in a compressed air environment. There is risk of decompression sickness in the mother, maternal acid-base and nitrogen imbalances, and intravascular air embolism in the fetus.[18] The possibility of increased risk of fetal anomalies occurs with deep dives. The fetus is not protected from decompression problems compared with the mother. In addition, hyperoxia might cause additional problems for the fetus. Some physicians recommend to women divers when they are trying to conceive that they refrain from diving because of the risk to the developing fetus.

In horseback riding, aside from the risk of injury from a fall, the pregnant athlete is prone to tenosynovitis of the

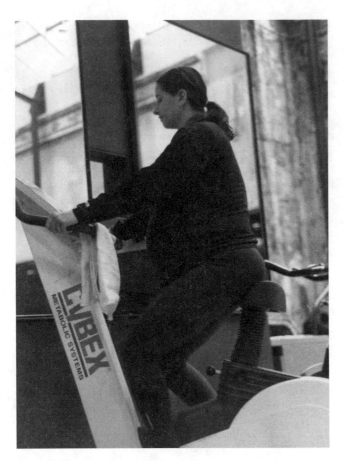

Figure 11–6 Upright Stationary Cycling is a Good Form of Aerobic Exercise during Pregnancy.

adductor longus. This may be seen with symptoms of vulvar point tenderness. This activity may also cause increased movement of the pubic symphysis.

Physical activity at altitude needs to be considered on an individual basis, keeping in mind that advice is based only on isolated observations and limited studies. Exercise at altitude increases the demands on the body and, for the pregnant athlete, requires adaptation to the combined stresses of altitude (with relative hypoxemia) and pregnancy. Guidelines for short-term altitude exposure and exercise at altitude during pregnancy advise not exceeding altitudes of 2500 m (8250 ft) in the first 4 to 5 days.[73,74] If the pregnant athlete wishes to exercise directly after altitude exposure, she should do so at a lower altitude. It is preferable that she spend a few days at rest at altitude to allow for acclimatization. There is still the possibility of occurrence of mild altitude illness. The preceding guidelines exclude hypoxic conditions such as maternal smoking and anemia and intrauterine growth retardation.

NUTRITIONAL DEMANDS

Pregnancy can be a time of excitement, anxiety, and stress. Adding to society's pressures on women to be thin, fit, and successful, fear of weight gain may drive harmful behaviors such as restrictive eating and overexercising. It is quite common for weight to be a major concern during a woman's first pregnancy and can also recur if a woman feels she had gained too much weight during a prior pregnancy. Restricting diets in calories or food categories, including fat or carbohydrates, has become common practice and must be prohibited during pregnancy, particularly in athletic women. It is important to remind each patient that pregnancy is *not* a time to change body shape—weight gain parameters can be established with the following guidelines for total weight increase over 40 weeks: underweight women, 30 to 40 lb; normal weight, 25 to 35 lb; overweight, 15 to 25 lb.[12(p 194)] Increase in fat stores and distribution is a natural occurrence of pregnancy; therefore, body fat should *not* be monitored during pregnancy.

As with all medical issues, the discussion of nutrition in pregnancy begins with a thorough history, including medical; gynecological; and obstetric, family, social, and exercise. Evaluating the woman's prepregnancy health is crucial in recommending nutrition. Guidelines should be clear. The sensation of nausea and or vomiting, particularly during the first trimester, may make proper nutrition a challenge. Other obstacles to adequate nutrition include pica, lactose intolerance, constipation, and caffeine intake.[75]

Because pregnancy is a hypermetabolic state, increased caloric intake is required. Athletic pregnant women have even higher caloric needs. Nutrition and caloric intake should be within appropriate guidelines to meet the additional demands of pregnancy and exercise; one cannot assume that exercise increases appetite.

Proper nutrition, as with all pregnant mothers, is essential to efficient exercise. A well-balanced diet with adequate protein and rich in fruits and vegetables is ideal. In exercisers, in particular, prenatal vitamins are highly recommended. Although no specific guidelines exist for exercise-increased needs in specific elements of nutrition, daily needs of pregnancy are fairly well established (see Clinical Guideline). Fat-soluble vitamin supplementation, specifically vitamins A and D, must be monitored, because birth defects can occur with oversupplementation.[12(p 194)] Excessive use of vitamin and or mineral supplements is not advised; referral to a nutritionist is prudent if concerns are present.

Exercise-induced iron loss has been described.[76] Additional mineral insufficiencies prevalent in active women include calcium and zinc.[77(p 76)] Calcium needs increase during pregnancy, and absorption is increased.[77(p 82)] Vitamin D and phosphorus intake should also be adjusted to further maximize calcium absorption. Some clinicians suggest that to facilitate bony absorption, calcium should be taken at night, without caffeine, and vitamin D taken in the morning. Although exercise is also protective of bony mass, cases of osteoporosis in pregnancy have been described;[49–50] therefore, the possibility of stress fractures in active pregnancies must also be considered.

Caloric intake increases proportionate to activity—at least 250 additional daily calories are needed for exercise in addition to the increased needs of pregnancy. Caloric needs increase through pregnancy proportionate to fetal and placental growth; after the first trimester by approximately 300 additional calories a day.[78(p 91)] This increase should be proportionate to metabolic demands and exercise intensity, with an emphasis on adequate protein.[79(p 182)] In breast-feeding mothers, caloric and nutritional needs remain elevated; 500 kcal daily are attributed solely to breast-milk production;[80(p 110)] dosages of vitamins and minerals in lactating women are recommended at levels even higher than that of pregnancy (refer to Chapter 21).

Daily Nutritional Needs of Pregnancy

- 30–60 mg iron (with vitamin C source)
- 1200–1500 mg calcium
- 1.5 mg thiamine (B_1)
- 18 mg niacin
- 1.6 mg riboflavin (B_2)
- 2.2 mg pyridoxine (B_6)
- 3 μg cyanocobalamin (B_{12})
- 6 mg pantothenic acid
- 400–600 μg folate
- 60–80 g protein
- 70 mg vitamin C
- 360 mg magnesium
- 10 μg vitamin D
- 800 μg vitamin A
- 1200 mg phosphorus

Clinical Guideline

In prolonged or excessive exercise, particularly in a relative fasting state, hypoglycemia and ketosis may result, although regular exercise makes hypoglycemia and hyperglycemia, as well as ketosis, less likely. Exercise increases the mobilization of carbohydrates and fats up to sixfold; however, in pregnancy, the normal catecholamine response is "blunted," particularly in the second and third trimesters.[19(p 116–117)] Pregnant exercisers use carbohydrates preferentially secondary to decreased Vo_{2max}; therefore, it is recommended that duration of exercise not exceed 45 minutes.[81(p 52)] Conservative clinicians recommend glucose monitoring in all pregnant women who exercise.[82(p 183–184)] This is especially prudent in women who participate in more intense forms of exercise. This can easily be done using prescribed glucose monitors, stylets, and strips both during and after exercise periodically through stages of pregnancy.

The benefits of exercise in gestational diabetes have been well supported.[83] Moderate, monitored exercise in pregnancy helps to maintain normal blood glucose by increasing peripheral insulin sensitivity. The athlete with gestational diabetes should be working with a certified diabetes educator to determine appropriate dietary needs and exercise allowance. Hydration is crucial in gestational diabetes.

Fluid needs are extremely important, particularly in the exercising pregnant woman. A loss of 1% body weight can interfere with thermoregulation, an important function of pregnancy. Water loss of 3% to 5% leads to oxygenation impairment; a loss of 7% body weight can result in collapse.[77(p 110)] The thirst response (beginning at approximately 1% loss) occurs after the fluid is already lost (aftereffect). During the late third trimester, dehydration can cause uterine irritability and even preterm labor.[12(p 195)] Therefore, fluid intake *during* exercise is extremely important. Fluid loss is a very simple parameter to measure. The pregnant woman should weigh herself before and after exercise. In general, 16 oz of fluid are required to replace each pound lost. Clapp recommends no greater than a 3-lb weight loss during exercise.[82(p 182)]

LABOR AND DELIVERY

No conclusive evidence exists that exercise has a beneficial or detrimental effect on labor and delivery. Some studies have found that maternal exercise during pregnancy decreased the duration of the active stage of labor and the incidence of some obstetric complications during delivery.[84–85] Other investigators, however, did not find any difference in duration of labor between women who continued their exercise program during pregnancy and those who had reduced their training during pregnancy.[86] Anecdotal reports and some data support the belief that highly trained elite athletes tolerate the workload of labor, particularly prolonged labor, better than the untrained or recreational athlete.[87]

POSTPARTUM/LACTATION

The timing for resuming exercise will depend on the type of delivery, vaginal or Caesarean, and whether there were any complications. Women who have had an uncomplicated vaginal delivery return to exercise sooner than those who have had an operative procedure. A gradual return to exercise should be emphasized, and high-impact sports (running, aerobics) should not be resumed until after the 6-week postpartum checkup. Uterus involution takes 6 weeks to revert to the nonpregnant state. Water sports should be avoided until vaginal bleeding has ceased and the episiotomy or incision has healed.

The lactating woman can continue to exercise provided she maintains adequate breast support and hydration and consumes an appropriate diet with sufficient caloric intake. Moderate intensity exercise does not increase breast-milk lactic acid.[88]

CAN MATERNITY MAKE A WOMAN A BETTER ATHLETE?

Pregnancy itself is a training state. In a study by Kulpa et al[89] of low-risk pregnant subjects, the subjects improved or maintained their level of fitness during pregnancy and postpartum. The control and exercise groups differed only in the frequency of aerobic exercise. Compared with the control group, the exercisers showed a significant training effect. There are also anecdotal reports of elite athletes improving their performances by the end of the first year after childbirth.

GENERAL PRINCIPLES

1. Pregnancy is not the time to improve cardiovascular fitness or to first embark on a strenuous exercise program. Simple maintenance should be the goal.
2. High-risk obstetrical patients for whom exercise is not advisable should be identified.
3. Women with uncomplicated pregnancies should be counseled on their exercise programs.

4. The pregnant athlete/active woman requires more calories in her diet than does a sedentary woman. Proper nutrition with adequate calories and hydration is essential for exercise.
5. Proper athletic equipment/clothing, appropriate footwear, and a supportive bra should be used. The bra should be firm enough to control breast motion, but not so tight as to interfere with breathing.

FUTURE DIRECTIONS

It is important to continue to clarify safe limits of exercise in pregnancy. Further studies are required to assess the effects of short- and long-term exercise on the normal physiological adaptation to pregnancy, labor, the postpartum period, and lactation. It would be beneficial to have more specific guidelines for exercise during pregnancy, but investigations in this area are difficult given the high risks involved with human maternal-fetal studies.

At this time, it is reasonable to guide the woman through her pregnancy with practical advice regarding exercise. The pregnant athlete and her developing fetus are the focus of her "support team," which in addition to the physician may consist of trainer, coach, therapist, and nutritionist. Regular communication among the team members and monitoring of the pregnant athlete are essential to an enjoyable and healthy pregnancy and ultimately a positive outcome—a healthy mother and normal healthy child(ren).

REFERENCES

1. Winder WW, Hagberg JM, Hickson RC, Ehsani AA, McLane JA. Time course of sympathoadrenal adaptation to endurance exercise training in man. *J Appl Physiol.* 1978;45:370–374.
2. Clark SL, Cotton DB, Pivarnik JM, Lee W, Hankins GD, Benedetti TJ. Position change and central hemodynamic profile during normal third-trimester pregnancy and post partum. *Am J Obstet Gynecol.* 1991;164:883–887.
3. Lotgering FK, Gilbert RD, Longo LD. Maternal and fetal responses to exercise during pregnancy. *Physiol Rev.* 1985;65:1–36.
4. Gorski J. Exercise during pregnancy: Maternal and fetal responses. A brief overview. *Med Sci Sports Exerc.* 1985;17:407–416.
5. McMurray RG, Mottola MF, Wolfe LA, Artal R, Millar L, Pivarnik JM. Brief review: Recent advances in understanding maternal and fetal responses to exercise. *Med Sci Sports Exerc* 1993;25(12):305–321.
6. Cohen GC. Exercise in pregnancy. *Sports Science Exchange. Gatorade Sports Science Institute.* 1991;3(31).
7. Araujo D. Expecting questions about exercise and pregnancy? *Physician Sportsmed.* 1997;259(4):85–93.
8. Stevenson L. Exercise in pregnancy. Part 1: Update on pathophysiology. *Can Fam Phys.* 1997;43:97–104.
9. Clarren SK, Smith DW, Harvey MAS, Ward RH, Myrianthopoulos NC. Hyperthermia—a prospective evaluation of a possible teratogenic agent in man. *J Pediatr.* 1979;95(1):81–82.
10. Jones RL, Botti JJ, Anderson WM, Bennett NL. Thermoregulation during aerobic exercise in pregnancy. *Obstet Gynecol.* 1985;65(3):340–345.
11. Clapp JF III, Wesley M, Sleamaker RH. Thermoregulatory and metabolic responses to jogging prior to and during pregnancy. *Med Sci Sports Exerc.* 1987;19(2):124–130.
12. Kulpa P. Exercise during pregnancy and post partum. In: Agostini R, ed. *Medical and Orthopedic Issues of Active and Athletic Women.* Philadelphia: Hanley & Belfus; 1994:191–199.
13. Collings C, Curet LB. Fetal heart rate response to maternal exercise. *Am J Obstet Gynecol.* 1985;151:498–501.
14. Hauth JC, Gilstrap LC, Widmer K. Fetal heart rate reactivity before and after maternal jogging during the third trimester. *Am J Obstet Gynecol.* 1982;142:545.
15. Artal R, Romem Y, Paul RH, Wiswell R. Fetal bradycardia induced by maternal exercise. *Lancet.* 1984;2:258–260.
16. Carpenter MW, Sady SP, Hoegsberg B, et al Fetal heart rate response to maternal exertion. *JAMA.* 1988;259:3006–3009.
17. Paolone AM, Shangold M, Paul D, Minnitti J, Weiner S. Fetal heart rate measurement during maternal exercise—avoidance of artifact. *Med Sci Sports Exerc.* 1987;19:605–609.
18. Mullinax KM, Dale E. Some considerations of exercise during pregnancy. *Clin Sports Med.* 1986;5:559–570.

19. Warren MP, Shangold MM. The pregnant athlete. In: *Sports Gynecology: Problems and Care of the Athletic Female.* Cambridge: Blackwell Science; 1997:113–135.

20. Lotgering FK, Gilbert RD, Longo LD. Exercise responses in pregnant sheep: Blood gases, temperatures and fetal cardiovascular system. *J Appl Physiol.* 1983;55:842–850.

21. Wolfe LA, Ohtake PJ, Mottola MF, McGrath MJ. Physiological interactions between pregnancy and aerobic exercise. *Exerc Sport Sci Rev.* 1989;17:295–351.

22. Bergfeld JA, Martin MC, Shangold MM, Warren MP. Women in athletics: Five management problems. *Patient Care.* 1987;21:60–64, 73–74, 76–80, 82.

23. Paisley JE, Mellion MB. Exercise during pregnancy. *Am Fam Physician.* 1988;38:143–150.

24. Soultanakis HN, Artal R, Wiswell RA. Prolonged exercise in pregnancy: Glucose homeostasis, ventilatory and cardiovascular responses. *Sem Perinatol.* 1996;20(4):315–327.

25. Artal R, Friedman MJ, McNitt-Gray JL. Orthopedic problems in pregnancy. *Physician Sportsmed.* 1990;18:93–105.

26. Colliton J. Back pain and pregnancy: Active management strategies. *Physician Sportsmed.* 1996;24:89–95.

27. Kihlstrand M, Stenman B, Nilsson S, Axelsson O. Water-gymnastics reduced the intensity of back/low back pain in pregnant women. *Acta Obstet Gynecol Scand.* 1999;78:180–185.

28. Perkins J, Hammer RL, Loubert PV. Identification and management of pregnancy-related low back pain. *J Nurse-Midwifery.* 1998;43: 331–340.

29. Franklin ME, Conner-Kerr TC. An analysis of posture and back pain in the first and third trimesters of pregnancy. *J Sports Phys Ther.* 1998;28:133–138.

30. Kristiansson P, Svärdsudd K, vonSchoultz B. Serum relaxin, symphyseal pain, and back pain during pregnancy. *Am J Obstet Gynecol.* 1996;175:1342–1347.

31. Kristiansson P, Svärdsudd K, vonSchoultz B. Back pain during pregnancy: A prospective study. *Spine.* 1996;21:702–709.

32. Brynhildsen J, Hansson A, Persson A, Hammar M. Follow-up of patients with low back pain during pregnancy. *Obstet Gynecol.* 1998; 91.182–186.

33. MacEvilly M, Buggy D. Back pain and pregnancy: a review. *Pain.* 1996;64:405–414.

34. Dumas GA, Reid JG. Laxity of knee cruciate ligaments during pregnancy. *J Sports Phys Ther.* 1997;26:2–6.

35. Östgaard HC, Andersson GBJ, Karlsson K. Prevalence of back pain in pregnancy. *Spine.* 1991;16:549–552.

36. Fast A, Weiss L. Low back pain in pregnancy. Abdominal muscles, sit-up performance and back pain. *Spine.* 1990;15:28–30.

37. Östgaard HC. Assessment and treatment of low back pain in working pregnant women. *Semin Perinatol.* 1996;20:61–69.

38. McIntyre IN, Broadhurst NA. Effective treatment of low back pain in pregnancy. *Aust Fam Physician.* 1996;25:S65–S67.

39. Mens JM, Vleeming A, Stoeckart R, Stam H, Snijders CJ. Understanding peripartum pelvic pain; implications of a patient survey. *Spine.* 1996;21:1363–1370.

40. Wicks T. The sacroiliac joint: A major cause of backache in pregnancy. *Midwifery Today Childbirth Educ.* 1996;39:33–34.

41. Berg G, Hammar M, Moller-Nielsen J, et al. Low back pain during pregnancy. *Obstet Gynecol.* 1988;71:71–75.

42. Östgaard HC, Zetherström G, Roos-Hansson E, Svanberg B. Reduction of back and posterior pelvic pain in pregnancy. *Spine.* 1994;19:894–900.

43. Östgaard HC, Roos-Hanssen E, Zetherström G. Regression of back and posterior pelvic pain after pregnancy. *Spine.* 1996;21:2777–2780.

44. Hansen A, Jensen DV, Worslev M, et al Symptom-giving pelvic girdle relaxation in pregnancy II: Symptoms and clinical signs. *Acta Obstet Gynecol Scand.* 1999;78:111–115.

45. LeBan MM, Perrin JCS. Pregnancy and the herniated lumbar disc. *Arch Phys Med Rehabil.* 1983;64:319–321.

46. LeBan MM, Viola S, Williams DA, Wang AM. Magnetic resonance imaging of the lumbar herniated disc in pregnancy. *Am J Phys Med Rehabil.* 1995;74:59–61.

47. Garmel SH, Guzelian GA, D'Alton JG, D'Alton ME. Lumbar disk disease in pregnancy. *Obstet Gynecol.* 1997;89:821–822.

48. Fast A, Shapiro D, Ducommun EJ, et al. Low-back pain in pregnancy. *Spine.* 1987;12:368–371.

49. Topping J, Black AJ, Farquharson RG, Fraser WD. Osteoporosis in pregnancy: More than postural backache. *Prof Care Mother Child.* 1998,8.147–150.

50. Fokter SK, Vengust V. Displaced subcapital fracture of the hip in transient osteoporosis of pregnancy. *Int Orthop (SICOT).* 1997;21:201–203.

51. Bjorklund K, Naessen T, Nordstrom ML, Bergstrom S. Pregnancy-related back and pelvic pain and changes in bone density. *Acta Obstet Gynecol Scand.* 1999;78:681–685.

52. Nilsson-Wikmar LN, Harms-Ringdahl K, Pilo C, Pahlback M. Back pain in women post-partum is not a unitary concept. *Physiother Res Int.* 1999;4:201–213.

53. Turgut F, Turgut M, Cetinsahin M. A prospective study of persistent back pain after pregnancy. *Eur J Obstet Gynecol Reprod Biol.* 1998;80:45–48.

54. Macarthur A, Macarthur C, Weeks S. Epidural anaesthesia and low back pain after delivery: A prospective cohort study. *BMJ.* 1995;311:1336–1339.

55. Kofler M, Kronenberg MF. Bilateral femoral neuropathy during pregnancy. *Muscle Nerve.* 1998;21:1106.

56. Al-Hakim M, Katirji B. Femoral mononeuropathy induced by the lithotomy position: A report of 5 cases with a review of literature. *Muscle Nerve.* 1993;16:891–895.

57. Carter GT, McDonald CM, Chan TT, Margherita AJ. Isolated femoral mononeuropathy to the vastus lateralis: EMG and MRI findings. *Muscle Nerve.* 1995;18:341–344.

58. Lindner A, Schulte-Mattler W, Zierz S. Postpartum obturator nerve syndrome: Case report and review of the nerve compression syndrome during pregnancy and delivery. *Zentralbl Gynakol.* 1997;119:93–99.

59. Hagay Z, Weissman A. Management of diabetic pregnancy complicated by coronary artery disease and neuropathy. *Obstet Gynecol Clin North Am.* 1996;23:205–220.

60. Weiss AP, Akelman E. Carpal tunnel syndrome: A review. *RI Med.* 1992;75:303–306.

61. Graham RA. Carpal tunnel syndrome: A statistical analysis of 214 cases. *Orthopedics.* 1983;6:1283–1287.

62. Stolp-Smith KA, Pascoe MK, Ogburn PL. Carpal tunnel syndrome in pregnancy: Frequency, severity, and prognosis. *Arch Phys Med Rehabil.* 1998;79:1285–1287.

63. Courts RB. Splinting for symptoms of carpal tunnel syndrome during pregnancy. *J Hand Ther.* 1995;8:31–34.

64. Babayev M, Bodack M, Creatura C. Common peroneal neuropathy secondary to squatting during childbirth. *Obstet Gynecol.* 1998;91:830–832.

65. American College of Obstetricians and Gynecologists. *Exercise during Pregnancy and the Postnatal Period.* Washington, DC: American College of Obstetricians and Gynecologists; 1985.

66. American College of Obstetricians and Gynecologists. *Exercise during Pregnancy and the Postpartum Period.* Technical Bulletin No. 189. Washington, DC: American College of Obstetricians and Gynecologists; 1994.

67. Hale RW, Milne L. The elite athlete and exercise in pregnancy. *Semin Perinatol.* 1996;20(4):277–284.

68. Morgan WP. Anxiety reduction following acute physical activity. *Psychiatr Annals.* 1979;9:36–46.

69. Dishman RK. Medical psychology in exercise and sport. *Med Clin North Am.* 1985;69:123–143.

70. Pettruzello SJ, Landers DM, Hatfield BD, Kubitz KA, Salazar W. A meta-analysis on the anxiety-reducing effects of acute and chronic exercise. *Sports Med.* 1991;11(13):143–182.

71. Koltyn KF, Schultes SS. Psychological effects of an aerobic exercise session and a rest session following pregnancy. *J Sports Med Phys Fitness.* 1997;37:287–291.

72. Cohen GC, Prior JC, Vigna Y, Pride SM. Intense exercise during the first two trimesters of unapparent pregnancy. *Physician Sportsmed.* 1989;17:87–94.

73. Huch R. Physical activity at altitude in pregnancy. *Semin Perinatol.* 1996;20(4):303–314.

74. Artal R, Fortunato V, Welton A, et al. A comparison of cardiopulmonary adaptations to exercise in pregnancy at sea level and altitude. *Am J Obstet Gynecol.* 1985;172:1170–1180.

75. Kolasa KM, Weismiller DG. Nutrition during pregnancy. *American Fam Phys.* 1995;56:205–212.

76. Nielsen P, Nachtigall D. Iron supplementation in athletes: Current recommendations. *Sports Med.* 1998;26:207–216.

77. Rudd JS. *Nutrition and the Female Athlete.* New York: CRC Press; 1996.

78. Hamaoui E, Hamaoui M. Nutritional assessment and support during pregnancy. *Pregnancy and Gastrointestinal Disorders.* 1998;27:89–121.

79. Carpenter MW. Pregnancy. In: Shangold MM, Mirkin G. *Women and Exercise: Physiology and Sports Medicine.* 2nd ed. Philadelphia: FA Davis; 1994:172–186.

80. Stevenson L. Exercise in pregnancy: part 2: Recommendations for individuals. *Can Fam Physician.* 1997;43:107–111.

81. Artal R, Sherman C. Exercise during pregnancy: safe and beneficial for most. *Physician Sportsmed.* 1999;27:51–75.

82. Clapp JF. *Exercising Through Your Pregnancy.* Champaign, IL: Human Kinetics; 1998.

83. Bung P, Artal R, Khodiguian N, Kjos S. Exercise in gestational diabetes: An optional therapeutic approach? *Diabetes.* 1991;40:182–185.

84. Clapp JF. The course of labor after endurance exercise during pregnancy. *Am J Obstet Gynecol.* 1990;163:1799–1805.

85. Botkin C, Driscoll CE. Maternal aerobic exercise: Newborn effects. *Fam Pract Res J.* 1991;11:387–393.

86. Hall DC, Kaufmann DA. Effects of aerobic and strength conditioning on pregnancy outcomes. *Am J Obstet Gynecol.* 1987;157:1199–1203.

87. Wolfe LA, Walker RMC, Bonen A, McGrath MJ. Effects of pregnancy and chronic exercise on respiratory responses to graded exercises. *J Appl Physiol.* 1994;76:1928–1936.

88. Carey GB, Quinn TJ, Goodwin SE. Breast milk composition after exercise of different intensities. *J Hum Lact.* 1997;13:115–120.

89. Kulpa PJ, White BM, Visscher R. Aerobic exercise in pregnancy. *Am J Obstet Gynecol.* 1987;156:1395–1403.

CHAPTER 12

The Older Female Athlete

Stacy A. Harris and Ellen Coven

Aging is a process involving structural and physiological changes that create reduced functional reserves of all organ systems. This linear decline in functional reserves affects most body systems after the third decade of life.[1] Aging impairs the body's ability to respond appropriately to environmental stresses. The functional losses may be so gradual that they are undetectable during normal daily activities. These subtle changes may go unnoticed until the body is placed under significant stress, such as a physically demanding athletic event. The changes the older female athlete experiences include cardiovascular, pulmonary, muscular, nervous system, skeletal, thermoregulatory, flexibility, postural, connective tissue, cartilaginous, and integumentary. In addition, alterations in response to medications along with changes in the genitourinary system can significantly affect the older female athlete.

CARDIOVASCULAR CHANGES

After age 35, cardiac fitness gradually begins to decline. Maximal oxygen uptake (Vo_{2max}) decreases by approximately 8% to 10% every 10 years after the third decade of life.[2] Vo_{2max} is an indicator of cardiac fitness and is influenced by muscle function, as well as cardiovascular and pulmonary systems. The more physically fit one remains, however, the slower the rate of decline.[3]

Cardiac output, a product of stroke volume and heart rate, measures the amount of blood the heart can pump over a certain time period. With aging, stroke volume and heart rate are reduced at high workloads, which subsequently influences cardiac output.[4] The left ventricular hypertrophy commonly present in elderly persons is thought to be a result of prolonged increases in afterload and arterial stiffness.[5] In addition, reduced ventricular function contributes to the decline in stroke volume.[6]

Maximal attainable heart rate also decreases with aging, whereas resting heart rate remains unchanged. Return of heart rate to baseline after activity takes longer in elderly compared with younger persons. This slower return of heart rate to resting level requires longer recovery periods during interval training. Infiltration of cardiac tissues by collagen, elastin, reticulin, and fatty tissues alters the cardiac conduction system and makes the myocardium less compliant. The altered conduction system contributes to the reduced maximal heart rate, while the less compliant ventricle decreases cardiac output. In addition, the myocardium becomes less responsive to catecholamine stimulation.

Cardiovascular Changes in Aging

- Decreased Vo_{2max}
- Decreased ventricular function
- Decreased cardiac output
- Decreased stroke volume
- Decreased maximal heart rate
- Unchanged resting heart rate
- Decreased myocardial compliance
- Increased resting blood pressure
- Increased vascular resistance
- Increased exercising blood pressure

Clinical Guideline

Atherosclerosis narrows the lumens of blood vessels, which decreases vessel wall extensibility. These narrower blood vessels create increased blood flow resistance that results in higher resting blood pressure. Furthermore, the decreased microvascular supply to muscles, organs, and peripheral tissues[7] reduces the volume of blood delivered to working tissues. Overall, the decreased VO_{2max}, cardiac output, maximal heart rate, myocardial compliance, and increased vascular resistance of the aging cardiovascular system cause the heart to work harder to meet the metabolic demands of the body at any given workload.[8] In the older female athlete, cardiovascular loss manifests as progressive decline in aerobic performance.

PULMONARY CHANGES

In the aging female athlete, the pulmonary system becomes less efficient. Pulmonary changes related to aging include an increased sense of respiratory effort during exertion, breathlessness at minimal workloads, loss of pulmonary blood volume, decreased alveolar elastic recoil, and intercostal muscle weakness and stiffness.[8,9] In addition, inspiratory capacity, forced expiratory volume, tidal volume, vital capacity, and inspiratory airflow decrease, whereas residual volume and total lung capacity increase.[8] Furthermore, alveolar collagen deposition can create a diffusion barrier for oxygen and carbon dioxide gas exchange. Slowing of ventilation and gas exchange occurs during transition from rest to submaximal exercise.[10] Overall, these pulmonary changes increase the workload of both inspiration and expiration. The impaired ability to deliver oxygen to working tissues is especially apparent in the older female athlete during aerobic activity.

Clinical Guideline: Pulmonary Changes with Aging

- Respiratory muscle weakness
- Decreased tidal volume
- Respiratory muscle stiffness
- Decreased vital capacity
- Decreased alveolar elastic recoil
- Decreased inspiratory airflow
- Decreased inspiratory capacity
- Increased residual volume
- Decreased forced expiratory volume
- Increased total lung capacity

Clinical Guideline

MUSCULAR CHANGES

With aging, a number of alterations in skeletal muscle tissue occur. Fat and connective tissue replace skeletal muscle fibers, resulting in loss of muscle mass. The number of type I muscle fibers that are used for postural and low-intensity activities becomes more abundant compared with type II muscle fibers, which are used for short bursts of activity.[11] The motor unit includes the motor nerve and all muscle fibers it innervates. With aging, however, fewer muscle fibers are available in each motor unit. Younger athletes increase strength by muscular hypertrophy, whereas older athletes do so by increased motor recruitment. Due to possible delay in nerve impulse transmission at the motor end plate with aging, muscle contractile speed decreases. Because power is the maximal velocity of muscle contraction against a mass over time, the aging athlete experiences the greatest impairment during power events. In addition, muscle strength loss is greater in aging women than men. Overall, the aging process in the older female athlete results in loss of muscle strength, mass, and speed of contraction.

Muscular Changes with Aging

- Decreased muscle mass
- Decreased muscle fibers per motor unit
- Decreased contractile speed
- Increased type I fibers

Clinical Guideline

NERVOUS SYSTEM CHANGES

Decreased visual acuity and accommodation, along with impaired hearing, occur with aging. Visual and auditory deficits in the older female athlete cause loss of important cues during athletic events. In addition, slowed reaction time occurs as a result of delayed rate of muscle contraction, nerve impulse propagation, perceptual processing, sensory nerve conduction, and central processing time.[8] During highly competitive events, the ability to focus attention on a specific task decreases. This impaired attention leads to performance deficits and frustration. To improve performance and decrease frustration, exposing the older female athlete to stressful environments during training sessions may allow for adaptation of effective coping strategies. Furthermore, the older female athlete experiences an impaired ability to solve new complex problems; however, she does benefit from valuable knowledge gained through previous experience. Although the amount of sleep required with aging remains unchanged, the efficiency of sleep decreases, which interferes with the healing and recovery processes.

Nervous System Changes with Aging

- Decreased reaction time
- Delayed perceptual processing
- Decreased rate of muscle contraction
- Delayed sensory nerve conduction

- Delayed nerve impulse propagation
- Delayed central processing

Clinical Guideline

SKELETAL CHANGES

Bone tissue is a dynamic structure composed of a matrix of organic and inorganic materials that undergoes changes according to physical demands placed on it. The most frequent bone impairment in the aging female is osteoporosis. Because of the rate of bone resorption exceeds the rate of bone formation, bone mass loss occurs in osteoporosis. In women, bone mass decreases 20% by age 65 and 30% by age 80.[9] Type I osteoporosis affects only women and is related to the loss of estrogen associated with menopause. Type II osteoporosis, however, affects both men and women and is related to decline in osteoblastic activity associated with aging. In the older female athlete, a bone fracture occurring in response to minimal trauma may be the heralding sign of osteoporosis.

THERMOREGULATORY CHANGES

The change in the ability of the aging person to dissipate heat leads to decreased heat tolerance. Reduced and delayed sweat responses can be further aggravated by the relatively reduced body water state commonly present in aged persons.[12] The reduced thirst sensation associated with aging can cause the older female athlete to become dehydrated before her thirst sensation triggers drinking. Recommendations to avoid dehydration during activity include hydration before, during, and after the athletic event; drinking fluids before the occurrence of sense of thirst; training during the coolest part of the day; not restricting fluids during hot weather; staying in the shade; wearing light-colored clothing; monitoring urine for evidence of concentration; and recognizing the signs and symptoms of heat stress.[8] In addition, because of decreased subcutaneous tissue, altered cold perception,[4] and decreased blood flow to peripheral tissues caused by atherosclerosis, the older female athlete is at increased risk for localized cold injuries, such as frostbite.

Thermoregulatory Changes in Aging

- Decreased heat and cold tolerance
- Delayed sweat response
- Decreased subcutaneous tissue
- Decreased blood flow to tissues

Clinical Guideline

FLEXIBILITY CHANGES

Flexibility is the possible range of motion for one or multiple joints and depends on bony structures, muscle, fascia, ligaments, tendons, and joint capsules. Because connective tissue and joints become stiffer with age, the body loses flexibility. The decreased flexibility that occurs with aging increases the risk of tissue damage during physical activity. Warming up before activity, however, helps increase tissue compliance, which reduces the risk of injury.

POSTURAL CHANGES

Postural stability involves sensory, motor, and higher level systems, such as the basal ganglia, cerebellar, and perceptual. Because vestibular, visual, and somatosensory systems change with age, the feedback response to postural control is altered. Furthermore, muscle effectors are unable to respond appropriately to postural changes. In the older athletic female, postural stability impairments increase fall risk, especially during athletic events.

CONNECTIVE TISSUE AND CARTILAGINOUS CHANGES

Connective tissue constitutes fasciae, tendons, and ligaments while it provides both structure and support to body components. With aging, changes in collagen and elastin impair the ability of connective tissue structures to withstand stress. Both collagen and elastin become less compliant because of increased cross-linkage. In addition, collagen turnover rate, water content, thickness, and shock-absorbing capacity decrease. Because of these various changes, tendons, ligaments, and cartilaginous tissues become brittle.[8] As a result, the older female athlete is at increased risk for injury because of the impaired mechanical properties of these supporting structures.

Connective Tissue and Cartilaginous Changes with Aging

- Decreased collagen compliance
- Decreased collagen turnover rate
- Decreased elastin compliance
- Decreased collagen water content
- Increased collagen cross-linkage
- Decreased collagen thickness

Clinical Guideline

INTEGUMENTARY CHANGES

Some of the many functions of the integumentary system include protection against trauma, infection, environment and ultraviolet light, as well as thermoregulation and storage of energy. With aging, thinning of the epidermal, dermal, and subcutaneous skin layers occurs.[13] In addition, the rete pegs, or interdigitations between the epidermis and dermis, exhibit loosening. Alterations of these structures cause increased skin vulnerability to trauma, cold, blistering, and delayed healing. Also, more fragile vasculature leads to easy bruising, and less keen sensory function causes lack of early injury awareness. The skin exhibits decreased inflammatory response to sun damage and reduced protection from ultraviolet light. As a result, the older person can remain in the sun longer than the younger person before becoming sunburned yet can still experience ultraviolet damage. Recommendations for the older female athlete regarding age-associated skin changes include wearing a cap and light-colored clothing, exercising when the sun is least intense, using sunscreen, and having any suspicious skin lesion evaluated by a physician.[8]

Integumentary Changes with Aging

- Thinning of epidermal, dermal, and subcutaneous layers
- Loosening of rete pegs
- Increased vascular fragility
- Decreased sensory function
- Decreased inflammatory response
- Decreased ultraviolet light protection

Clinical Guideline

MEDICATIONS

Numerous pharmacokinetic changes occur in the aging body. These changes include decreased cell receptors and plasma-binding proteins, as well as altered medication absorption and distribution. Reduced renal and hepatic clearance acts to prolong the half-life of many medications. Nonsteroidal anti-inflammatory medications are widely used for osteoarthritis to control pain and inflammation; however, they increase the risk of gastrointestinal ulcer and renal impairment. Because nonsteroidal anti-inflammatory medications decrease the sensation of pain, the older female athlete may not identify when to stop activity to avoid injury. Thus, for those with osteoarthritis, administering a small medication dose or no dose before exercise and a full dose after exercise may be beneficial. In certain diseases, such as diabetes, medication schedule and dosage may require adjustment as a result of increased glucose use and insulin sensitivity during exercise. In addition, β-blockers can inhibit the normal physiological heart rate response to exercise. Recommendations regarding medication use in the older female athlete include using as few medications at the lowest dosages as possible, being aware of potential side effects and drug interactions, and stopping a medication if ineffective to try an alternative one.[8]

STRESS INCONTINENCE

Aging is associated with urinary dysfunction in females and involves small bladder capacity, increased residual urine, involuntary bladder contractions, and stress incontinence. Of all of these dysfunctions, stress incontinence is the most common, and its incidence increases with age. In stress incontinence, leakage of urine occurs when intravesical pressure exceeds intraurethral pressure and can become a source of distress and embarrassment. Running, jumping, and weight training increase abdominal pressure and can aggravate stress incontinence. Stress incontinence is usually associated with laxity of the pelvic floor muscles, bladder outlet weakness, or urethral sphincter weakness; however, it can occur in normal anatomy as well. If stress incontinence is mild and the anatomy is normal, reducing fluid intake 3 hours before and emptying bladder directly before exercise can help control symptoms. Replacing fluids immediately after exercise, however, is necessary to avoid dehydration. Also, Kegel exercises, which involve contracting the pubococcygeus muscle spontaneously or during urination to interrupt urine flow, aid in alleviating symptoms. In addition, wearing a mini-pad or panty liner can provide protection from bladder leakage. If anatomical deficits are present and symptoms persist despite Kegel exercises, then surgical intervention may become necessary. Exercise postoperatively, though, has an increased risk of causing stress incontinence recurrence. In addition to Kegel exercises and surgery, stress incontinence treatment may include medications, such as estrogen replacement therapy, which prevent urethral atrophy; α-adrenergic agonists, which increase urethral resistance; and anticholinergic agents, which relax the detrusor muscle.[14] Other alternatives in treatment include biofeedback and electrical stimulation.[15]

ASPECTS OF TRAINING THE OLDER FEMALE ATHLETE

Overview

Whether she is a master athlete or a weekly aerobic dance participant, the older female athlete must carefully consider the design of her training program. Her age-related functional declines and increased incidence of medical illnesses alter her ability to reach peak performance and increase her risk for injury. To safely achieve her goals and increase longevity in her sport, an effective training program must address any functional limitations or medical conditions.

Effective conditioning is the most critical component to training the older female athlete. Conditioning must encompass the needs of the whole athlete, including her aerobic capacity, muscular strength, joint mobility, and neuromuscular control. Balanced development, which includes flexibility, strength, and both standing and dynamic posture, is essential to every effective conditioning program. Optimal balance in opposing muscle groups along with adequate joint range of motion is necessary for correct body alignment. In addition, sufficient endurance is crucial for aerobic fitness. Lastly, an important characteristic of conditioning is awareness of the wide range of abilities not only between individuals of the same age but in the same person.[16]

Flexibility

Adequate joint mobility and range of motion are prerequisites for correct body alignment. Chronically tight muscles, in combination with weak stabilizers, result in faulty compensation patterns, inefficient body mechanics, and increased risk of injury. Muscles of the anterior shoulder girdle, such as the anterior deltoids and pectorals, are commonly problematic and manifest as rounded back and upper shoulders. A hyperextended back, which can contribute to low back pain, is frequently the result of impaired flexibility of the lumbar extensors, hip flexors, and hamstrings.[17,18]

Techniques to develop functional flexibility are best performed with a combination of static and active stretching exercises. Static stretches involve stretching the muscle to the end point of movement and then holding the position for an extended length of time. Active stretching is accomplished by contracting the opposing muscle group. Ballistic movements are contraindicated.

Guidelines for flexibility training have been prescribed by the American College of Sports Medicine (ACSM) and are widely followed by trainers and fitness professionals:

- Frequency: 2–3 days/per week[19]
- Intensity: To a position of mild discomfort
- Duration: 10–30 seconds for each stretch
- Repetitions: 3–5 for each stretch

Additional studies have suggested that flexibility work be done on a daily basis.[20]

The American Council on Exercise (ACE) and the American Senior Fitness Association (ASFA) add additional guidelines for older adults:[21,22]

- Always include an adequate warmup.
- Work a balanced combination of major muscle groups.
- Maintain proper body alignment.
- Maintain rhythmic breathing.
- Discontinue the move if the stretch position results in joint pain.

Strength

Strength conditioning should focus on the development of both muscular strength and endurance of the postural support muscles. Effective strength conditioning targets stabilizing the spine in neutral position known as "core stability." After the age of 50, women typically exhibit weak, overstretched spine extensors, abdominal muscles, pelvic stabilizers, hip extensors, and lower extremity antigravity muscles, such as the quadriceps and hamstrings. The following guidelines describe a compilation of guidelines for strength work, which has been researched and prescribed by a number of sources.[22-24]

Guidelines for Strength Training in Older Women

Frequency: 2–3 times weekly

One set of each exercise, 8–12 repetitions (to the point of volitional fatigue)

A safe and effective training load for the older female athlete is approximately 75% of maximum resistance. Studies have shown that this level is effective enough to produce good levels of strength development and light enough to reduce the risk of injury.

Progress gradually: The double progressive training approach is suggested. Begin with 8 good repetitions. When 12 receptions are successfully achieved, increase resistance by 5%.

Adherence to correct body alignment and form.

Perform every exercise through a full pain-free range of motion. Optimum functional strength development occurs when the muscle is worked from a fully stretched to a fully contracted position.

Perform both concentric (lifting) and eccentric (lowering) phase in a controlled manner. Research indicates that effective speed is a 6-second rep—that is 2 seconds on the up phase, 4 seconds on the down phase.

Maintain a continuous pattern: Breath holding, as well as isometric muscular contraction (holding the weight in a static position), can escalate blood pressure.

Use closed kinetic chain exercises whenever possible to integrate muscles needed for stabilization. For more balanced development, use free weights or elastic resistance instead of exercise machines (they externally stabilize the torso). For additional stabilizing development use exercise balls or foam rollers (Figure 12–1).

Vary position of exercises for a more balanced development.

Allow for sufficient rest and recovery; 2- to 3-minute rest periods between exercises and at least 48 hours between sessions are recommended.

Decrease speed for greater resistance.

Learn to read feedback: Avoid exercises that produce sharp or prolonged joint/muscle pain.

Clinical Guideline

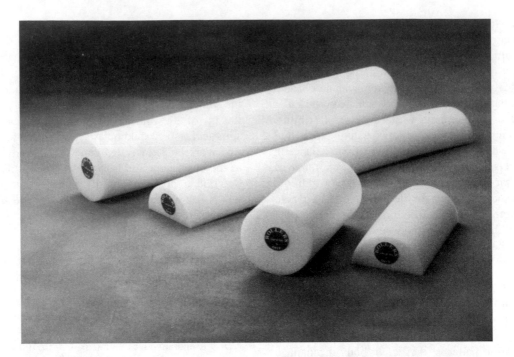

Figure 12–1 Foam Rollers.

Selected exercises promote core stability and balanced development of antigravity muscles. By adding hand-held weights, elastic resistance, or by using super slow technique, resistance progression can be achieved (see Appendix 12–B).

Static and Dynamic Balance

Once deficits in muscular balance are adequately restored, the athlete can then proceed to improve static and dynamic balance. Correct standing posture is necessary before effective training can progress. Standing posture should be checked, adjusted, and reinforced using a mirror and visualization cues to help the body learn and correct poor habits.

Because balance problems for older athletes are attributed to functional declines in the somatosensory and vestibular systems, any effective training strategy must strive to integrate and challenge these systems. Specific objectives involve increasing sensory input, improving kinesthetic awareness, and increasing reflex speed. An effective training design moves from stationary drills to increasingly more difficult tasks on unstable balance training equipment, such as balance boards (Figure 12–2).[25]

Balance drills are best performed with a partner or trainer. For the older female athlete who may have osteoporosis, it is especially important to ensure safety against the risk of a fall while performing balance exercises. Pool training is an effective and safe adjunct to land training. The buoyancy of water assists in developing balanced core strength and proprioception.

Balance Drills

- Single-leg stand with flexion/extension of the knee
- Same as above with eyes closed
- Single-leg stand with ball toss and catch
- Front walk over taped line
- Crossover walk over taped line (may not be appropriate for those with total hip replacement)
- Low beam walk
- T'ai chi exercises (controlled shift of weight)
- Standing 180 jump turns in water

Clinical Guideline

Building Endurance

Aerobic fitness is vital for optimal performance. Improved cardiopulmonary capacity builds endurance and positively affects balance ability. For the older female athlete who is at greater risk for cardiac and pulmonary disease or who may use medications, appropriate training intensity must be carefully determined. For those athletes with osteoporosis or arthritis, cross-training, such as pool training, helps to minimize stress in weight-bearing joints. In addition, cross-training helps to prevent overuse injuries, requires the body to recruit different muscle groups, and challenges stabilization tasks.[26,27]

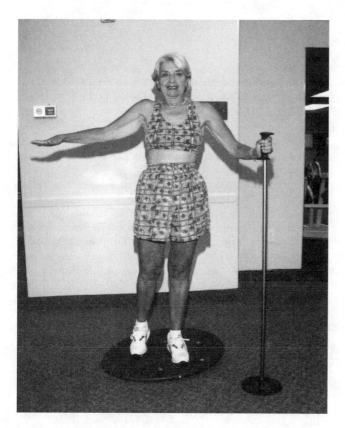

Figure 12–2 Balance Board.

SPORT-SPECIFIC TRAINING

The older female athlete armed with a strong conditioning program designed to target and correct functional deficits will enter any sports-specific program with a greater ability to achieve her athletic goals. With a solid foundation of strength, mobility, endurance, and balance, she can begin to develop the necessary skills for her specific sport. Integration of these elements promotes agility, coordination, and power. Whether to generate faster club-head speed, better racquet control, increased throwing power, or precision footwork, these elements ultimately lead to improved sports performance.

SPORT-SPECIFIC TRAINING MODEL FOR GOLF

Golf has become extremely popular among women and therefore serves as a useful example for the female athlete. Golf requires the athlete to integrate a complex series of rotary movements in most joints, good stabilizing function in the torso, and strength/power to generate effective club-head speed. A deficit in any of these areas can lead to poor or inconsistent performance and injury. Common sites of

injury in the amateur female golfer are the elbow, low back, shoulders, hands, and wrists. Improper technique, overuse, and poor upper body strength may be contributing factors to elbow injury, whereas low back injury is often the result of inadequate stabilizing strength in the torso.[28]

Strength training to help stabilize the spine during forceful rotational movements must be a top priority for injury prevention, especially in osteoporotic females. Many professionals would agree that an effective training design progresses from: flexibility → stability → strength → power → to specific skill mechanics. An overall plan for a golf-specific training program may include a program such as that outlined in the Clinical Guideline.

Sports-Specific Training Model—Golf

Focus: Warmup (can also include some cardio endurance work)
Exercise: Walking
Purpose: Preparation and endurance development

Focus: Flexibility
Exercise: Stretches/range of motion—neck, shoulders, wrists, torso/low back, hips, hamstrings, ankles
Purpose: Optimal joint mobility and injury risk reduction

Focus: Stability
Exercise: Mid back, abs/lower, abs/obliques, hip extensors, hip ab/adductors
Purpose: Power production and injury protection

Focus: Strength
Exercise: Deltoids, pectorals, arms, gluteals, and quadriceps
Purpose: Power production

Focus: Power
Exercise: Reverse wood chop (two-handed cable cross pull), weighted club swing
Purpose: To increase club-head speed

Focus: Skill refinement
Exercise: Video swing analysis
Purpose: Mechanical efficiency

Clinical Guideline

CONCLUSION

Clearly, the benefits of athletic activity in older women are multidimensional and invaluable. Despite aging challenges, physical activity maintains youthfulness. Future research will provide answers to theories and questions in active women with more acceptance, understanding, and increased participation.

REFERENCES

1. Siegel AJ, Warhol MJ, Lang E. Muscle injury and repair in ultra long distance runners. In: Sutton JR, Brock RM, eds. *Sports Medicine for the Mature Athlete.* Indianapolis: Benchmark Press; 1986:35–43.

2. Rogers MA, Hagberg JM, Martin WH, et al. Decline in Vo_{2max} with aging in master athletes and sedentary men. *J Appl Physiol.* 1990;68: 2195–2199.

3. Jackson AS, Beard EF, Weir LT, et al. Changes in aerobic power of men ages 25–70. *Med Sci Sports Exerc.* 1995;27:113–120.

4. Berman R, Haxby JV, Pomerantz RS. Physiology of ageing. Part I: Normal changes. *Patient Care.* 1988;22:20–36.

5. Folkow B, Svanborg A. Physiology of cardiovascular aging. *Physiol Rev.* 1993;73(4):725–764.

6. Lakatta EG. Cardiovascular regulatory mechanisms in advanced age. *Physiol Rev.* 1993;73:413.

7. Goldman R. Speculations on vascular changes with age. *J Am Geriatr Soc.* 1970;18:765–769.

8. Menard D. The ageing athlete. In: Harries M, Williams C, Stanish WD, et al, eds. *Oxford Textbook of Sports Medicine.* 2nd ed. Oxford: Oxford University Press; 1998:787–813.

9. Roberts RA, Roberts SO. Exercise and aging. In: Roberts RA, Roberts SO, eds. *Exercise Physiology: Exercise, Performance, and Clinical Applications.* St. Louis: Mosby; 1997:578–599.

10. Babcock MA. Exercise on transient gas kinetics are slowed as a function of age. *Med Sci Sports Exerc.* 1994;26:440.

11. McArdle WD, Katch FI, Katch VL. Physical activity, health, and aging. In: McArdle WD, Katch FI, Katch VL, eds. Philadelphia: Williams & Wilkins; 1991:635–668.

12. Astrand PO, Rodahl K. *Textbook of Work Physiology.* Singapore: McGraw-Hill; 1986:617.

13. Frenske NA, Lober CW. Skin changes of ageing: Pathological implications. *Geriatrics.* 1990;45:27–32.

14. Cardenas DD, Mayo ME, King JC. Urinary tract and bowel management in the rehabilitation setting. In: Braddom RL, ed. *Physical Medicine and Rehabilitation.* Philadelphia: WB Saunders; 1996:555–579.

15. Cobbs EL, Ralapati AN. Health of older women. *Med Clin North Am.* 1998;82(1):127–144.

16. Spirduso W. *Physical Dimensions of Aging.* Champaign, IL: Human Kinetics; 1995.

17. Kendall FP, McCreary EK, Provance PG. *Muscles, Testing and Function.* Baltimore: Williams & Wilkins; 1993.

18. Baxter RE. *Pocket Guide to Musculoskeletal Assessment.* Philadelphia: WB Saunders; 1998.

19. American College of Sports Medicine (ACSM) Position Stand. The recommended quantity and quality of exercise for developing and maintaining cardiorespiratory and muscular fitness in healthy adults. *Med Sci Sports Exerc.* 1998;30(6):975–991.

20. Alter MJ. *Science of Flexibility.* 2nd ed. Champaign, IL: Human Kinetics; 1996.

21. American Council on Exercise. *Personal Trainer Manual.* San Diego CA: The Council; 1991.

22. Clark J. *Senior Fitness Instructor Training Manual.* New Smyrna Beach, FL: American Senior Fitness Association; 1994.

23. Wescott WL, Baechle TR. *Strength Training Past 50.* Champaign, IL: Human Kinetics; 1998.

24. Peterson JA, Bryant CX. *Strength Training for Women.* Champaign, IL: Human Kinetics; 1995.

25. Ellison D. A Balancing act. *IDEA Health Fitness Source* 1998;3:48–56.

26. Pollack ML, Wilmore JH. *Exercise in Health and Disease: Evaluation and Prescription for Prevention and Rehabilitation.* 2nd ed. Philadelphia: WB Saunders; 1990.

27. ACSM. *Exercise Management for Persons with Chronic Diseases and Disabilities.* Champaign, IL: Human Kinetics; 1997.

28. Metz JP. Managing golf injuries. *Physician Sportsmed.* 1999;7:41–56.

APPENDIX 12–A

Selected Stretches for Chronically Tight Areas That Contribute to Poor Alignment and Posture

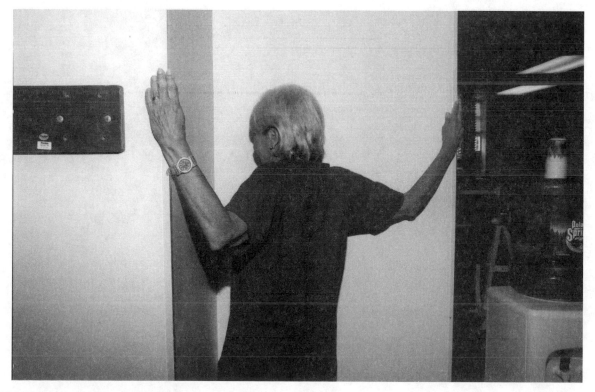

Figure 12–A1 Corner Stretch: *Anterior Deltoids and Pectorals.*

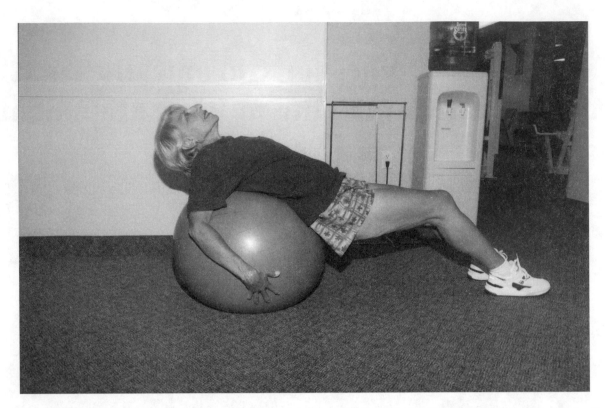

Figure 12–A2 Extended Upper Body Stretch (Can Be Done Supine with Pillow Instead of Ball or Seated): *Pectorals, Anterior Traps and Cervical Muscles, Abdominal Muscles.*

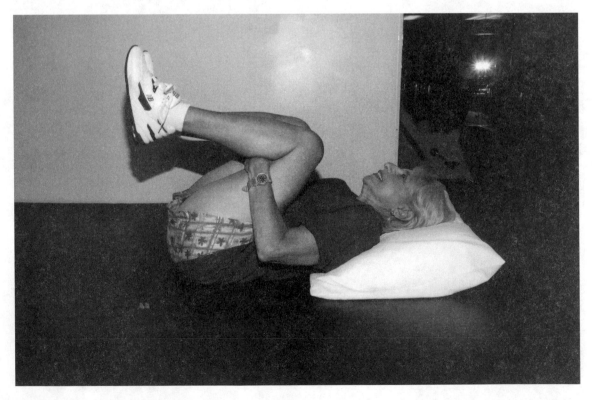

Figure 12–A3 Knees to Chest Curl: *Paraspinals, Gluts, Lower Paraspinals.*

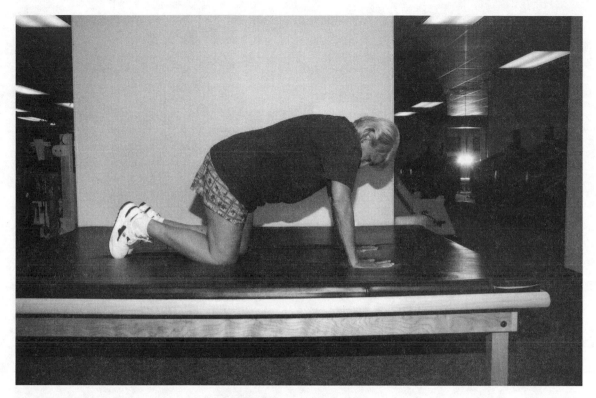

Figure 12–A4 Cat Stretch-Flexion; On Hands and Knees, Trunk Flexion: *Paraspinals.*

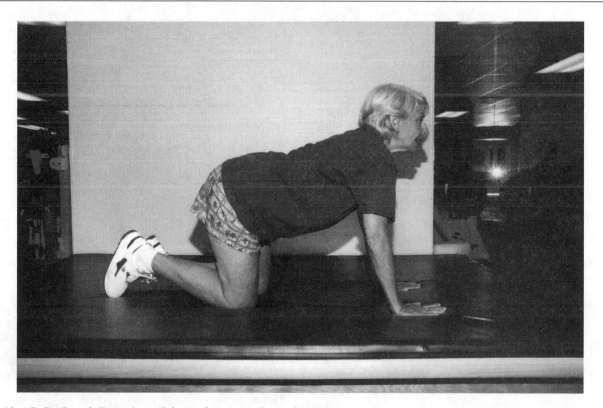

Figure 12–A5 Cat Stretch-Extension: *Abdominal, Anterior Cervical Muscles.*

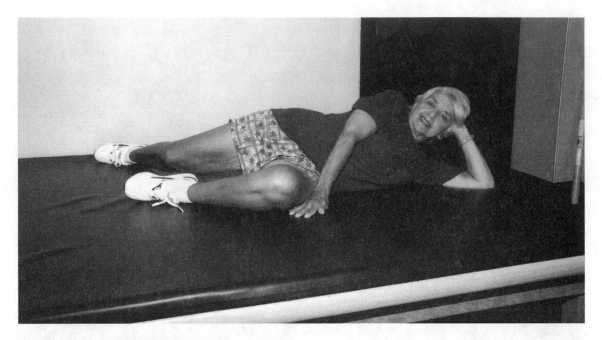

Figure 12–A6 Seated Hip Flexor Stretch: *Hip Flexors, Quads, Obliques.*

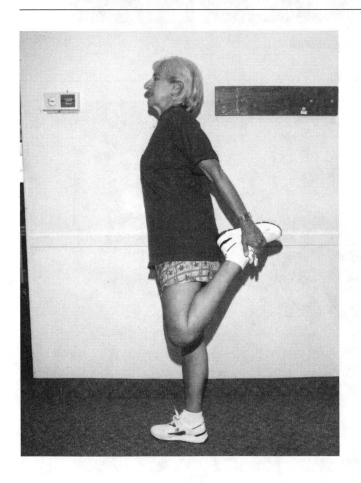

Figure 12–A7 Standing Hip Flexor Stretch: *Iliopsoas, Quads.*

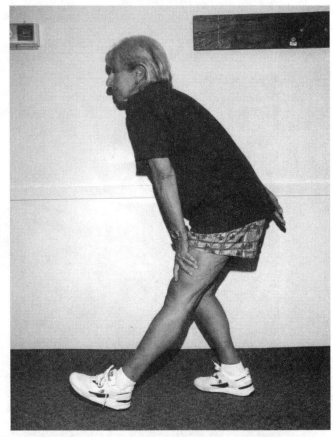

Figure 12–A8 Standing Hamstring Stretches; Can Be Done Seated and with Active Contraction of Quads: *Hamstrings, Gastrocs.*

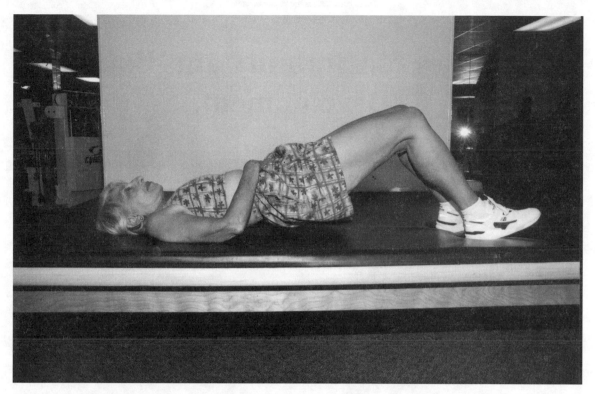

Figure 12–A9 Pelvic Tilts; Can Be Done Standing; Incorporate Lateral, Front, and Circular Motions: *Lower Lumbar Paraspinals.*

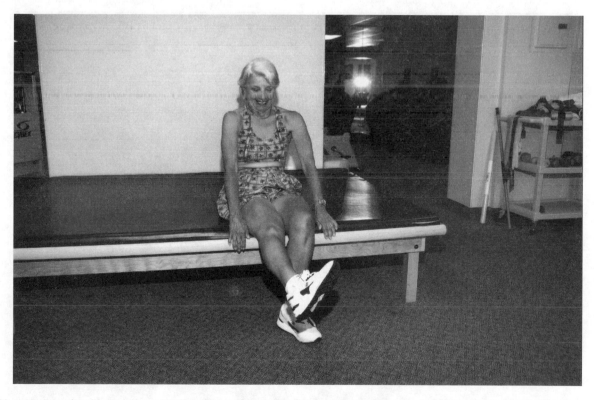

Figure 12–A10 Seated Ankle Rotation: *Achilles, Peroneals, Tibialis, Plantar Fascia, Gastrocs (with Knee Straight), Soleus (Knee Bent).*

APPENDIX 12–B

Exercises for Stability and Balance Development

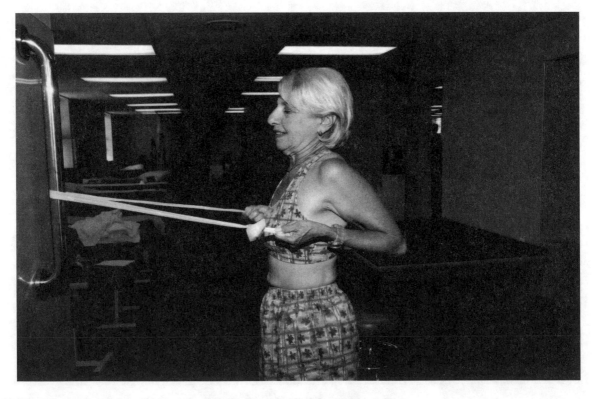

Figure 12–B1 Scapular Retraction with Resistance Band: *Scapular Stabilizers, Upper Traps.*

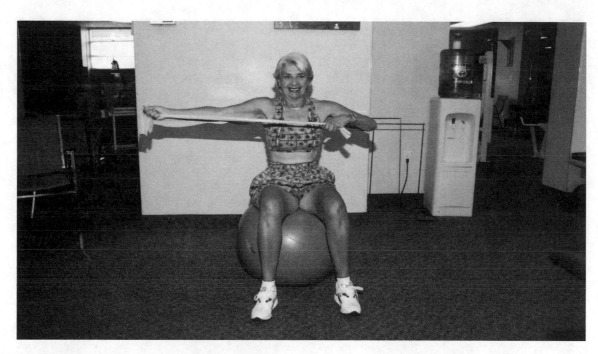

Figure 12–B2 Bow and Arrow Seated on a Ball for Additional Core Stability Challenge: *Scapular Stabilizers, Middle Traps, Triceps, Deltoids.*

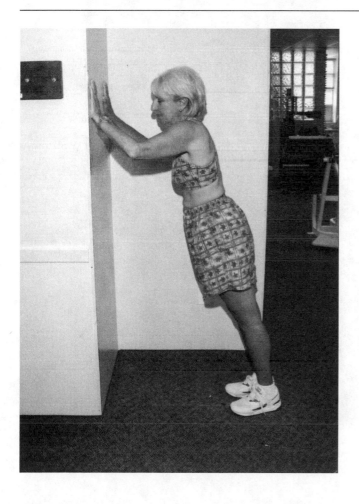

Figure 12–B3 Standing Push Up: *Multisite Torso Stabilization, Triceps, Pecs, Scapular Stabilizers (Caution with Hand and Wrist or Carpal Tunnel Syndrome).*

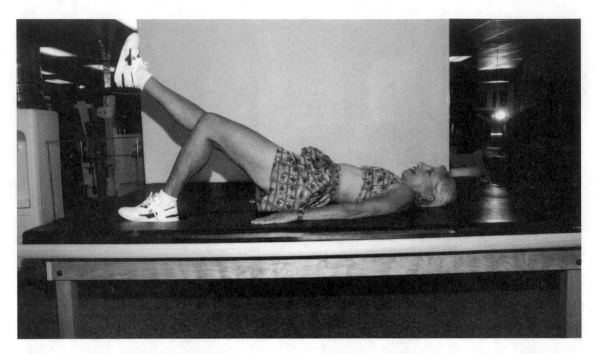

Figure 12–B4 Bridge with Leg Extension: *Multisite Torso/Hip Stabilization, Rectus Abdominis, Quads.*

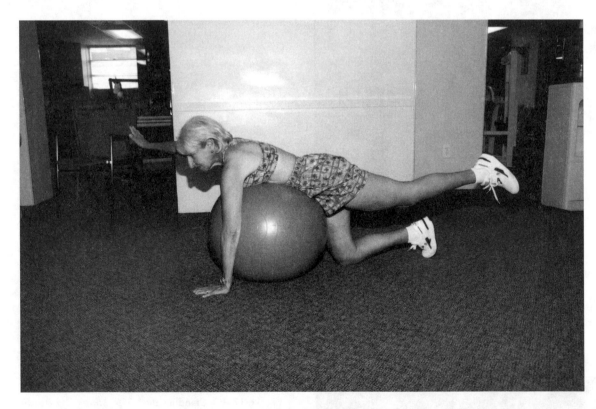

Figure 12–B5 All Fours Alternating Leg/Arm Extension using Stability Ball: *Multisite Torso Stabilization, Leg Extensors, Deltoids, Triceps, Scapular Stabilizers.*

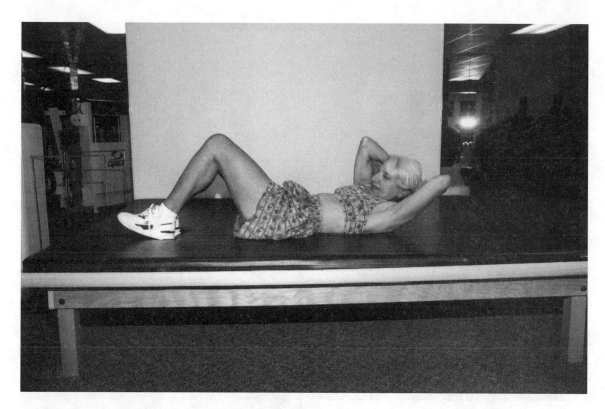

Figure 12–B6 Diagonal Crunch: *Obliques, Rectus Abdominis, Paraspinals.*

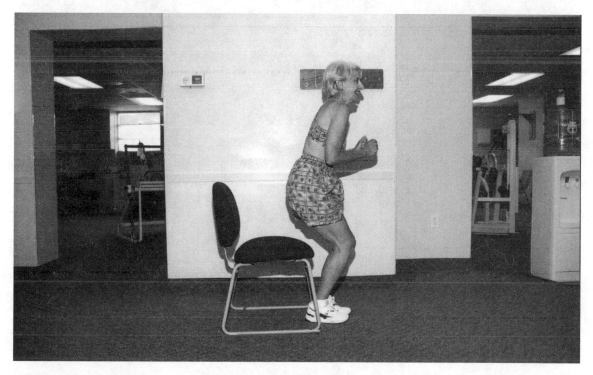

Figure 12–B7 Squat from Chair: *Extensors, Quads, Hamstrings, Paraspinals, Glutes.*

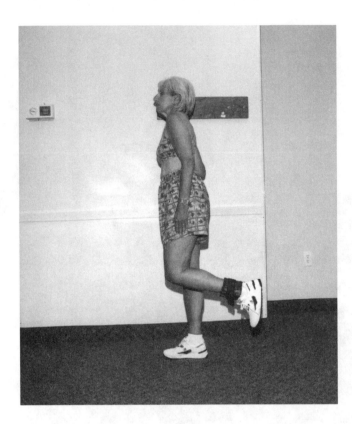

Figure 12–B8 Standing Curl with Ankle Weight: *Hamstrings, Paraspinals*.

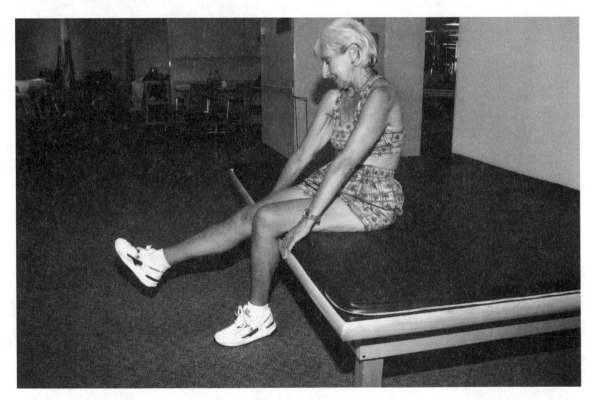

Figure 12–B9 Seated Leg Extension: *Quads (Can Add Ankle Weights)*.

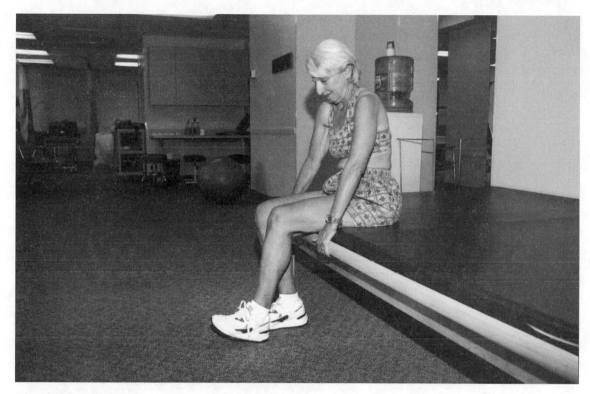

Figure 12–B10 Toe Taps: *Anterior Tibialis, Peroneals, Extensor Hallucis.*

PART III

Medical Issues

Medical Challenges

Sandra J. Hoffmann

INTRODUCTION

The primary focus of many clinicians in the fields of exercise science and sports medicine has been on orthopaedic issues of women. This chapter will focus on many of the common medical issues that athletes and active women face that can have an impact on healthy participation.

ACUTE ILLNESSES

Upper Respiratory Tract Infection

Upper respiratory infections (URIs) are ubiquitous in exercising and athletic women and are one of the most common reasons for women to seek medical attention. Most URIs are viral in nature. Symptoms include fever, chills, myalgias, cough, nasal congestion, sore throat, and fatigue. These symptoms can be exacerbated in an overtrained or immunocompromised athlete. Women should be carefully evaluated for the presence of secondary bacterial infections such as otitis media, bacterial sinusitis, pharyngitis, pneumonia, and, rarely, bacterial meningitis. Treatment consists primarily of supportive care with fluids. Antipyretics, decongestants, topical nasal anticholinergics, antihistamines, cough suppressants, and throat lozenges (antiseptic, vitamin C, or zinc) can be used for symptomatic relief.[1] Antibiotics are indicated for acute bacterial infections. No evidence exists that popular herbal supplements such as Echinacea prevent or cure viral syndromes. Elite athletes should be warned that production of herbals is unregulated in the United States, and herbals may contain substances banned by their governing bodies. Athletes may continue or return to participation

when their fevers are less than 100.5° and cough and myalgias have resolved.

Common Bacterial Infections Associated with URIs

- Otitis media
- Sinusitis
- Pharyngitis
- Pneumonia
- Meningitis

Clinical Guideline

Infectious Mononucleosis

Infectious mononucleosis is a viral infection caused by the Epstein-Barr virus. In the United States, more than 90% of the population have developed antibodies by age 30.[2] Many cases are transient and mild and mistaken by women and clinicians as URIs. The virus is excreted in saliva and has an incubation period of 30 to 50 days. Prodromal signs and symptoms, which are indistinguishable from other viral illnesses, occur during the first 3 to 5 days of the acute illness and include headache, malaise, anorexia, fevers, fatigue, and myalgias. Beginning on days 7 to 21, more specific symptoms such as exudative pharyngitis (can be concurrently infected with group A streptococci), tender lymphadenopathy, jaundice, rash, and splenomegaly may occur. Diagnosis is made by a positive heterophil antibody absorption test and elevated white blood cell count with lymphocytosis and atypical lymphocytes. Liver transaminases will be elevated in 90% of cases.

Treatment is primarily supportive with relative rest, fluids, and mild analgesics and antipyretics. Women should be monitored closely for complications. Documented streptococcal pharyngitis should be treated with appropriate antibiotics. Use of ampicillin can induce a rash and should be avoided. Severe tonsillar enlargement can lead to pharyngeal edema and should be treated with high-dose parenteral corticosteroids and close observation for airway obstruction. Other indications for corticosteroid use include the development of severe cytopenias, hepatitis, encephalitis, or myocarditis. Splenic rupture, although rare, can be life threatening, and immediate hospitalization and surgical consultation are warranted.[3]

Athletes should be restricted from practice and competition for a minimum of 3 weeks. After that period, noncontact activities may be allowed if there has been clinical and laboratory resolution of signs and symptoms and no evidence of splenomegaly. Contact sports are allowed 4 weeks after onset of symptoms if the spleen has returned to normal size. Some authors advocate use of ultrasonography measurement of spleen size before returning to contact activities, but this is not widely practiced.[4]

Vaccinations

Several common infectious diseases that can result in lost playing and practice time for competitive athletes can be prevented with the use of vaccines. Athletes should be counseled that despite being physically fit, they are not at lower risk than the general population for certain contagious diseases. Collegiate athletes, especially those that participate in winter sports, are a relatively high risk for exposure to influenza, and athletes should consider receiving a yearly influenza vaccine. Measles, mumps, rubella, varicella, and hepatitis B vaccines should be offered to adolescent women if they have not developed childhood immunity or previously been vaccinated. Clinicians should ensure that athletes have received the appropriate childhood vaccinations and receive a tetanus and diphtheria toxoid booster at appropriate intervals. Meningococcus vaccine should be considered in college students, especially those living in group housing. Hepatitis A vaccination is recommended for athletes traveling to endemic areas.[5] All women receiving vaccines should be counseled on pregnancy prevention immediately before and after being vaccinated.

Exercise-Induced Anaphylaxis and Cholinergic Urticaria

Exercise-induced anaphylaxis is an immunoglobulin E (IgE)–mediated allergic reaction to exercise that affects women two times more commonly than men.[6] Co-precipitants such as food, drugs, environmental pollens, ambient temperature extremes, or hormones can contribute to the reaction, but only in conjunction with exercise. Signs and symptoms include flushing, pruritus, nausea, vomiting, throat tightening, and large (10–25 mm) skin wheals. Development of angioedema, bronchospasm, laryngospasm, and hypotension can lead to anaphylactic shock and death. Basic life support should be ensured, and the patient should be immediately transported to a medical facility. Epinephrine and inhaled beta-agonists are the primary treatment of acute attacks. Prevention by avoidance of co-precipitants before exercise should be stressed. All women who have experienced an acute attack should carry a prefilled epinephrine syringe with them when exercising, wear a medical alert bracelet identifying the disorder, and be cautioned about exercising alone.

Cholinergic urticaria is also a physical IgE-mediated allergic reaction to raising of core body temperature 0.5 to 1.5°C either through passive or active warming.[6] Signs and symptoms of cholinergic urticaria include development of small (2mm) pruritic papules, sweating, flushing, headache, abdominal cramping, and diarrhea. Respiratory symptoms of bronchospasm such as dyspnea and wheezing are seen more commonly than in exercise-induced anaphylaxis. Angioedema often occurs. Treatment is with antihistamines both prophylactically and during an acute flare.

PULMONARY DISORDERS

Lung function is essential for oxygen exchange and eventual delivery to exercising muscles. Many pulmonary conditions can limit this exchange, and thus have a negative impact on the ability to exercise and participate in sports. Several of these chronic conditions, a few which are more prevalent in women, can also affect quality of life and life expectancy.

Asthma and Exercise-Induced Asthma

Asthma is a chronic, episodic medical condition that is characterized by increased airway responsiveness to a variety of stimuli. In childhood, males are more commonly affected, but this gender prevalence equalizes by age 30. More than 30% of women self-report premenstrual or perimenstrual exacerbation of their asthma symptoms.[7] Women who have perimenstrual asthma (PMA) tend to be older, have a longer duration of their chronic symptoms, and have increased severity of symptoms compared with women without cyclic exacerbations.[7] The purported mechanism of the cyclic changes is a decrease in progesterone level at the time of menses, and thus less hormonal-mediated relaxation of bronchial smooth muscle.[8]

A few uncontrolled studies have looked at treating PMA with hormonal manipulation, diuretics, and nonsteroidal anti-inflammatory medications, but none have been found to be effective.[7] Standard treatment of PMA exacerbations is determined by the extent of symptoms, which are no different than those not related to menses. Detailed treatment of chronic asthma and PMA is beyond the scope of this chapter but involves objective measures of lung function, pharmacological therapy, environmental measures, and patient education.[9]

Exercise is one of the most common precipitants that triggers acute asthma.[10,11] Exercise-induced asthma (EIA) is defined as reversible airway obstruction that leads to a fall in peak expiratory flow rate or FEV_1 of at least 15% after an exercise challenge that resolves after completion of activity.[11] There is a 70% to 90% prevalence of EIA in people with chronic asthma and a 40% prevalence in people with allergic rhinitis.[2]

Environmental Triggers of EIA

- Cold air
- Dry air
- Allergens
- Pollution
- Dust
- Respiratory infections
- Pool chemicals

Clinical Guideline

Signs and symptoms of EIA include dyspnea, wheezing, chest tightness, and cough with or after exercise. Some women will also complain of "feeling out of shape."[12,13] Exercising in cold and dry air makes symptoms worse, as does concurrent URIs and exposure to pollution, dust, and allergens.[2]

The differential diagnosis of EIA includes other causes of dyspnea during exercise such as general deconditioning, airway obstruction, glottic dysfunction, tracheal narrowing, occult cardiac or pulmonary disease, and disorders of muscle metabolism.[11,14,15] Diagnosis, however, is often based on clinical signs and symptoms and response to standard treatments. If the diagnosis is questionable, it can be confirmed with an exercise challenge test (ECT). An ECT is performed most often in a laboratory setting under controlled conditions that sometimes do not evoke a particular athlete's symptoms. If this occurs, performance of the test in the field or environment under conditions closest to those of that woman's particular sport is warranted.[11,16]

Treatment of EIA is primarily aimed at preventing attacks. This can be accomplished by adequate, slow warmup; breathing through nasal passages; breathing warm, humidified air; and appropriate conditioning. More effective control can be achieved with pharmacological treatment.[2,11–13,15,17]

Common Pharmacological Treatment of EIA

- Short-acting inhaled beta-adrenergic agonists
- Long-acting inhaled beta-adrenergic agonists
- Mast cell inhibitors
- Leukotriene antagonists
- Inhaled corticosteroids
- Antihistamines

Clinical Guideline

Exercise and Obstructive Pulmonary Diseases

As the general population ages, more women with chronic pulmonary diseases will seek advice from clinicians about exercise as an adjunct treatment for their chronic conditions or as part of initiating or maintaining a healthy lifestyle. Research has shown exercise training in patients with chronic obstructive pulmonary disease (COPD) can reduce disability and deconditioning, increase exercise tolerance, delay the appearance of dyspnea, and improve quality of life despite permanent and severe structural damage to the lungs.[18] No particular mode of exercise has been found to be better than others, but clinicians must remember that in these women progress may be slow. Women with severe COPD should initially be referred to a supervised rehabilitation program. Those with mild-to-moderate disease and graduates of supervised programs can be given exercise prescriptions for home programs using arm ergometers, stationary bicycles, treadmills, walking, or stair climbing.[18] Aggressive pharmacological therapy and pulmonary hygiene should accompany all exercise programs.

Because the median survival rate for women with cystic fibrosis (CF) has increased, exercise and sports participation have become important issues, from both a medical and psychosocial perspective. Exercise has been shown to improve quality of life and survival in women with CF,[19] and all women with this condition should be encouraged to remain as physically active as possible. Little research has been published on exercise as an adjunct treatment for other forms of obstructive lung disease such as bronchopulmonary dysplasia. Specialists in physical medicine and rehabilitation, sports medicine, and pulmonary medicine are encouraged to develop multidisciplinary programs to help women with pulmonary disabilities enjoy and safely participate in physical activity.

Exercise and Restrictive Lung Diseases

Women with restrictive lung disorders caused by neuromuscular diseases or thoracic deformities should be encouraged by clinicians to participate in sports and exercise to the fullest extent possible. In particular, water sports and horseback riding have been found to increase quality of life for cerebral palsy patients.[19] Again, a multidisciplinary approach to helping these women maintain physical fitness is encouraged.

Pulmonary Disorders Associated with Menses

The most common pulmonary disorder associated with menses is asthma exacerbations.[8] Management is with standard pharmacological therapy. Athlete education and awareness of cyclic exacerbations may allow better environmental control and possible prevention.

Catamenial pneumothorax is a rare condition in which recurrent episodes of a spontaneous pneumothorax occur at menses.[8] The diagnosis should be considered in athletes who sustain a pneumothorax with minimal trauma or have recurrent episodes of a pneumothorax. Thought to possibly be related to endometriosis of the pleura or diaphragm, this condition has been successfully treated with gonadotropin-releasing hormone agonists.[8]

Pulmonary Trauma and Emergencies

Pulmonary trauma and emergencies can be life threatening and require quick response by clinicians. Treatment with basic life support measures while awaiting transport to a medical facility can be life saving. Common pulmonary trauma and emergencies include pneumothorax, diaphragm paralysis, chest wall trauma, and sternoclavicular dislocation. Although spontaneous pneumothoraces are more commonly seen in men, smoking increases a woman's risk ninefold.[20] Women may also experience catamenial pneumothoraces or a pneumothorax related to a rib fracture sustained in a sport such as soccer. In sports such as gymnastics, diving, and ice hockey, diaphragmatic paralysis can accompany a neck or cervical spine injury.[20] Athletes should be evaluated for rib fractures and pulmonary contusions whenever there is blunt trauma to the chest wall. Last, posterior dislocation of the sternoclavicular joint may compress the trachea and great vessels, leading to cardiopulmonary compromise and the need for urgent reduction.[20]

GASTROINTESTINAL DISORDERS

Exercise can be thought of as the "graded stress test" for the colon.[21] Common gastrointestinal (GI) symptoms seen with exercise and sports include heartburn/acid reflux, bloating, diarrhea, GI bleeding, abdominal pain, and trauma. Although irritable or functional bowel syndrome (IBS) is markedly more common in women than men, there are little data on gender differences in reporting of other GI symptoms or syndromes during exercise or athletic competition.[22,23] GI symptoms are thought of as occurring primarily in runners,

but studies have shown a high incidence in sports such as swimming and gymnastics.[24] In addition, surveys show that both upper and lower GI symptoms are experienced equally by athletes.

Gastrointestinal Bleeding

Many studies on the association between exercise and GI bleeding have been done, but most have had a predominance of male subjects. One study on marathon runners, in which 46% of the subjects were women, reported a significant increase in prerace and postrace hemoccult positive results.[22] The underlying mechanism causing bleeding is postulated to be ischemia to the GI tract. During activity, approximately 40% to 80% of normal blood flow to the GI tract is shunted to other organs such as the heart and skeletal muscles. Increasing the intensity of exercise or relative dehydration decreases blood flow to GI structures and increases the risk of mucosal bleeding from both the upper and lower tracts. Other proposed factors that contribute to gut ischemia and possible bleeding include mechanical trauma from repetitive motion and alteration of GI hormones.

Heartburn and Acid Reflux

Heartburn and acid reflux are common exercise-associated symptoms. Treatment is centered around lifestyle changes such as tobacco, alcohol, and caffeine cessation; avoidance of large or fatty meals; not eating before lying down; and avoidance of medications that decrease lower esophageal sphincter (LES) pressure. It should be noted that exercise itself has been shown to cause a decrease in LES tone that can be exacerbated by any of the previously mentioned factors. Medical therapy includes antacids, histamine blockers, and proton pump inhibitors. If symptoms persist for longer than 2 weeks of medical therapy or are associated with weight loss or anemia, referral to a specialist is warranted, because chronic reflux can lead to esophageal strictures and cancer.

Common Causes of Acid Reflux in Female Athletes

- Exercise
- Medications (estrogens, theophylline)
- Tobacco
- Alcohol
- Caffeine
- Eating large or fatty meals
- Eating before sleeping
- Certain foods (chocolate, peppermint)

Clinical Guideline

Bloating and Gas

Gas and abdominal bloating are primarily caused from gas-forming foods, especially cruciferous vegetables and legumes. Diets that include protein powder, high fiber, and protein food bar supplements are also contributors. Questioning patients about a personal or family history of lactose intolerance can be helpful. Bloating can be successfully treated in most cases by diet modifications, enzyme supplementation, or over-the-counter products that contain simethicone or activated charcoal.

Diarrhea

Diarrhea that occurs during exercise is commonly called "runner's trots" but can be caused by a variety of etiological agents. Runner's diarrhea is actually a diagnosis of exclusion and should be considered only after a thorough history and physical examination precludes an underlying medical illness. Because of the high incidence in women with IBS, inflammatory bowel disease, and rheumatological conditions, diarrhea associated with weight loss, anemia, or evidence of GI bleeding deserves a full medical evaluation. Persistent diarrhea without evidence of blood loss can be evaluated by a few tests, including stool sample for fecal leukocytes and *Clostridium difficile* toxin, stool culture, and thyroid-stimulating hormone level. Diarrhea can be a manifestation of laxative abuse in bulimic women, and a careful screening for an eating disorder should be undertaken.

Treatment of runner's diarrhea includes maintenance of adequate hydration and avoidance of caffeine, nonsteroidal anti-inflammatory medications, and high-carbohydrate sports drinks. Reducing lactose, sorbitol, and high glycemic foods before exercise and avoidance of exercise immediately after meals can be helpful adjuncts. Use of antimotility agents can be considered, but these medications often have side effects that can impair performance. Treatment of other causes of diarrhea depends on the specific cause and is beyond the scope of this chapter.

Common Causes of Diarrhea in Female Athletes

- Runner's diarrhea
- Irritable bowel syndrome
- Viral gastroenteritis
- Bacterial toxins
- Systemic lupus erythematosus
- Inflammatory bowel disease
- Endocrine disorders (hyperthyroidism, Addison's disease)
- Laxative abuse
- Sorbitol (chewing gum)
- Lactose intolerance

Clinical Guideline

Abdominal Pain

Abdominal pain is a common complaint in primary care practice and one of the most common reasons for emergency department visits. Diagnosis of the cause of abdominal pain is often challenging, even for experienced clinicians. It can be much more difficult to determine the cause of abdominal pain in women, because inflammation of the pelvic reproductive organs needs to be included in a differential diagnosis. Despite the difficulty, the role of the clinician evaluating abdominal pain in active women centers on whether the woman needs an immediate referral for surgical intervention. In addition, decisions regarding the ability of the women to continue exercising or participating in competition need to be made in a timely fashion. Women in whom the pain is acute in onset, severe or progressive, lasts more than 6 hours, occurs during inactivity, or in which emesis or anorexia develops after the onset of pain should be referred immediately to a surgeon for evaluation.

Abdominal Trauma

Severe abdominal trauma is rare in athletes but accounts for about 10% of emergency department visits for abdominal trauma.[25] Of particular and immediate concern in blunt abdominal trauma is the determination of rupture or damage to the liver, spleen, kidney, or bowel. All abdominal trauma needs immediate evaluation by a qualified clinician. If one is not readily available at the site of injury, prompt transport to an emergency facility is warranted.

GENITOURINARY ISSUES

Dysuria

Irritable voiding symptoms are a common complaint in women and can be from a number of causes including urinary tract infections (UTIs), vaginitis, sexually transmitted diseases, and interstitial cystitis. Urinalysis should be performed in all women with irritable voiding symptoms. Microscopic examination of vaginal secretions and cultures or nucleic acid amplification tests for chlamydia and gonorrhea should be performed when directed by the history or physical examination, and appropriate treatment prescribed.[26–28] In women who have a history of IBS, fibromyalgia, systemic lupus erythematosus, or frequent "culture-negative" UTIs, the diagnosis of interstitial cystitis should be considered. In these women, avoidance of caffeine, alcoholic beverages, citrus fruits, and high doses of vitamin C can be helpful. A therapeutic trial of nonsteroidal anti-inflammatory medications, antihistamines, or low doses of amitriptyline can be considered.[29] Referral to a urologist is needed for definitive diagnosis.

Urinary tract infections are ubiquitous in women and a common cause of dysuria. They are usually classified as complicated or uncomplicated. Complicated UTIs are those in which the woman has an underlying chronic medical condition; those that occur more than three times in 6 months; or those that are associated with severe systemic symptoms such as nausea, vomiting, or rigors.[30] Treatment of complicated UTIs often requires hospitalization and administration of intravenous antibiotics. Uncomplicated UTIs are more commonly seen in younger women and are often associated with sexual intercourse. Symptoms include frequency, urgency, dysuria, and suprapubic pain. Diagnosis can be made in the office with a urine dipstick that is positive for leukocytes. Treatment is with antibiotics directed at enteric gram-negative bacteria, the most common etiological organisms. Choice of antibiotic therapy depends on patient allergies, cost, and community sensitivity patterns.[30] There is no need for routine urine cultures for uncomplicated UTIs.

Proteinuria

During exercise, renal blood flow decreases as blood is shunted to the heart and skeletal muscles and away from visceral organs. The drop in renal blood flow is proportional to the intensity of exercise. Other physiological responses of the kidney to exercise include a decrease in glomerular filtration rate, increase in sodium reabsorption, and decrease in free water clearance. Despite these attempted compensatory mechanisms of the kidney to maintain equilibrium, the net result is a deficit of total body water and plasma volume. Decreases in plasma volume stimulate the renin-angiotensin system to increase the glomerular filtration fraction. These mechanisms increase the concentration of plasma proteins in glomerular capillaries, increase glomerular permeability to these proteins, and thus increase protein excretion in the urine.[31]

Transient proteinuria is commonly seen in women who are athletes and who participate in regular exercise. Dipstick readings of 2+ can be considered normal after a bout of intense exercise. Maximal protein excretion is seen within 30 minutes of cessation of activity. Proteinuria in athletic women has many causes. Initial evaluation of proteinuria should begin with a thorough history and physical examination and a urine dipstick. Positive dipstick results should be repeated after 48 hours of relative rest. If the dipstick test remains positive, a supine (first morning void) sample should be taken. Proteinuria that resolves with rest is likely to be the result of physiological changes associated with exercise described previously. Athletes who continue to excrete protein or have abnormal findings on physical examination should undergo a complete medical evaluation, including a 24-hour urine collection for protein and creatinine, urine protein electrophoresis, and serum measurements of creatinine and blood urea nitrogen (BUN). An imaging study such as renal ultrasonography or intravenous pyelography (IVP) should also be performed. Any woman who has more than 3 g of protein in a 24-hour urine collection should be referred to a specialist for further evaluation.

Hematuria

Hematuria can be caused by inflammation or infection anywhere in the genitourinary (GU) tract or from any condition that causes red blood cell hemolysis. There are many causes of hematuria in female athletes, including "sports" or exercise-induced hematuria. Other common causes include GU trauma, medications, infections, GU tract stones, cancer, glomerulonephritis, or coagulation disorders.

- Stones
- Cancers
- Glomerulonephritis
- Bleeding disorders
- Medications
- Rifampin
- Sulfamethoxazole
- Macrodantin
- Ibuprofen

Clinical Guideline

Exercise-induced hematuria is seen equally in women and men. Exercise-induced hematuria is more common after intense exercise in asymptomatic women and resolves with rest.[32,33]

Evaluation of hematuria begins with a thorough history and physical examination. Hematuria associated with fever, flank pain, dysuria, joint swelling, skin lesions, or any other symptoms should have a symptom-focused evaluation. Evaluation of asymptomatic hematuria should begin with a repeat urinalysis after 48 to 72 hours of relative rest. If the hematuria has resolved, a diagnosis of exercise-induced hematuria can be made.[31] Hematuria that persists requires further evaluation.[32] All possible medications should be discontinued. If the hematuria is associated with leukocytes on the urine dipstick, empiric antibiotic treatment is warranted. Causes of myoglobinuria should be sought if there is evidence of hematuria but no red blood cells on urine dipstick. Hematuria associated with proteinuria or red blood cell casts requires extensive evaluation for causes of glomerulonephritis. Laboratory studies should include measurements of serum creatinine, BUN, protein electrophoresis, rapid plasma reagent, cryoglobulins, antinuclear antibody, complement levels, antistreptolysin O titer, and antiglomerular basement membrane (anti-GBM) antibody. If the history or physical examination is suggestive, testing for sickle cell disease or a coagulation disorder should be considered. Further evaluation to a specialist may be warranted for diagnostic testing such as cystoscopy or renal biopsy.

Treatment of exercise-induced hematuria includes increasing hydration during activity, decreasing the intensity of workouts, and exercising with a small amount of urine in the bladder.[32] Treatment of other causes of hematuria is directed toward the underlying cause.

Acute Renal Failure

Exercise is a rare cause of acute renal failure (ARF). The mechanism is likely multifactorial, with volume depletion being a significant trigger. Risk factors such as sickle-cell trait, nonsteroidal anti-inflammatory use, or rhabdomyolysis can contribute to the insult to the kidneys. Unless treated promptly, primarily with aggressive fluid hydration, ARF can lead to permanent loss of function or death.[31]

GU Trauma

Trauma to the kidney during sports is due to a direct blow to the flank or abdominal area. Typically, this occurs during contact or collision sports. Hematuria from kidney trauma is seen less often in women than men, possibly because women have more perirenal fat. Presentation can range from mild hematuria and pain to an acute condition of the abdomen. Contusions are treated symptomatically with relative rest, mild analgesics, and protective padding to prevent further trauma. More severe injuries such as a renal fracture or vascular injury require immediate surgical repair.

Bladder contusions are more commonly seen in men than women, particularly in runners who exercise with completely empty bladders. The mechanism is postulated to be due to the repetitive trauma of the loose, empty bladder "slapping" against the pelvic wall. Symptoms can be alleviated by running with a partially full bladder.

Direct trauma to the bladder can occur during sports such as martial arts or gymnastics. Athletes at risk of bladder trauma should be advised against competing and practicing with an empty bladder to decrease the chance of injury. In female cyclists and equestrians, perineal numbness or trauma may occur.[34]

HEMATOLOGICAL ISSUES

Anemia

Anemia affects approximately 6% of women aged 15 to 44.[35] It is more commonly seen in women as a result of menstrual blood loss, which can lead to iron-deficiency anemia (IDA). The causes of anemia in athletic women are numerous, including nutritional deficiencies, sports (dilutional) pseudoanemia, footstrike hemolysis, bone marrow disorders, and factors that cause increased red blood cell destruction.

Common Causes of Anemia in Female Athletes

- Sports anemia
- Footstrike hemolytic anemia
- Nutritional/precursor deficiencies:
  Iron
  Vitamin B_{12}
  Folate
  Erythropoietin
- Anemia of chronic disease

- Bone marrow disorders:
  Infiltrative diseases (cancer)
  Suppression (sepsis)
  Primary marrow failure (aplastic anemia, leukemia)
- Other causes of RBC destruction:
  Hemoglobinopathies (sickle cell disease)
  Deficiencies of RBC enzymes (glucose-6-phosphate dehydrogenase deficiency)
  Inherited RBC membrane defects (hereditary spherocytosis)
  Extrinsic factors (ie, hypersplenism, antibody production)

Clinical Guideline

Signs and symptoms of anemia include exertional fatigue, dyspnea, presyncope (especially in hot weather), pica (craving for ice), heaviness or burning in muscles with activity, and decreased performance.[36] Physical examination may show pallor, pulmonary flow murmur, or mild cognitive deficits. Jaundice, scleral icterus, bruising, or splenomegaly may be present, depending on the underlying cause of the anemia.

Sports or "dilutional" anemia is common in highly trained female athletes. During and immediately after intense exercise, the physiological response of the body to hemoconcentration is an increase in hormones such as renin, aldosterone, and vasopressin to stimulate sodium and water retention. The result is a reduction in hemoglobin concentration caused by an expansion of plasma volume.[2] The lower limits of hemoglobin measurement seen in women with dilutional anemia depend on the intensity of exercise. An elite aerobic athlete may have hemoglobin levels as low as 11 g/dL, whereas in a sedentary women a level less than 12 g/dL would warrant an evaluation.[37] Despite a low hemoglobin and hematocrit level, measurements of ferritin, serum iron, total iron-binding capacity (TIBC) and mean corpuscular volume (MCV) are normal in sports anemia. Because this is an acute response to exercise, hemoglobin levels should return to normal values 3 to 5 days after cessation of activity.[2]

Footstrike or "water-slap" anemia is an entity seen in endurance runners and swimmers. The pathogenesis is thought to be related to hemolysis of red blood cells (RBCs) caused by repetitive trauma of the heel against a hard surface during running or the arm continuously "slapping" the water in endurance swimming. Laboratory evidence of footstrike hemolytic anemia is similar to other pathological processes that cause hemolysis and includes decreased haptoglobin, mild macrocytosis, mild reticulocytosis, and free hemoglobin in the urine.[37] Treatment of this entity primarily involves decreasing running or swimming mileage. In runners, better shoe cushioning and running on softer surfaces may also be helpful.

Iron-deficiency results from an imbalance of dietary iron intake and iron losses through menses, sweat, urine, and feces. In sedentary women, there are three distinct stages of iron deficiency. The first stage is depletion of iron stores, measured as low serum ferritin levels. The next stage is iron-deficient erythropoiesis, which is marked by a decrease in both serum ferritin and transferrin saturation. Finally, if sufficient iron is not supplied to keep up with demand, IDA results.[38] Laboratory markers of IDA include decreased hemoglobin and hematocrit levels, decreased serum ferritin, decreased serum iron, decreased transferrin saturation, and increased total iron-binding capacity. MCV of RBCs is also markedly reduced. Unlike sedentary women, it is unclear in female athletes whether measures of serum ferritin alone can be used as a marker of depletion of iron stores, because serum ferritin values decline as a response to intensive training.[39–41]

IDA is more common in women than men primarily because of menstrual losses. IDA may be more common in active women than women who lead a more sedentary lifestyle because of increased losses from sweat and occult fecal loss from gut ischemia during intense exercise. Active premenopausal women are particularly at risk of developing IDA because of their lower iron stores from recurrent menses. Athletes who are at high risk of IDA developing include vegetarians, those with eating disorders, or women who have menorrhagia. Signs and symptoms of IDA are indistinct from other causes of anemia, but laboratory studies are diagnostic. The most accurate test for diagnosing IDA is bone marrow staining for hemosiderin; however, this invasive and expensive test is rarely indicated. A low hemoglobin and hematocrit associated with low serum ferritin, low serum iron, and elevated TIBC indicates IDA.

Treatment of IDA should not be undertaken without identifying and correcting the underlying cause. Women who have guaiac-positive stools should be referred for further diagnostic testing. Dietary habits should be examined, and women should be encouraged to eat foods high in iron such as poultry, fish, lean red meat, beans, and peas. Supplementation with ferrous salts, 325 mg orally three times daily, should be prescribed. Increased absorption of iron by means of the diet or oral supplement occurs when taken with vitamin C. Caffeine use decreases absorption and should be discouraged. Side effects of supplements include bloating, gas, and constipation. Ferrous gluconate or polysaccharide-iron complexes are associated with less constipation and bloating than ferrous sulfate by many women. The addition of a stool softener that contains docusate sodium is also helpful. Supplementation should be continued for 3 to 6 months after normalization of laboratory values to help build iron stores. Use of iron supplementation by athletes for low serum ferritin levels without associated anemia has not been shown to enhance performance.[40] Supplementation without medical supervision should be discouraged because of the high prevalence of hemochromatosis in the population, particularly in Caucasian women.

Sickle Cell Disease

Sickle cell disease is a multisyndrome disorder caused by an inherited mutant sickle cell hemoglobin, HbS. HbS causes erythrocytes to lose solubility and polymerize when deprived of oxygen. Different inheritance patterns of the sickle cell gene cause the various clinical syndromes of sickle cell disease or sickle cell trait. Sickle cell disease is clinically manifested by chronic anemia and recurrent pain crises. It is associated with homozygosity for the sickle cell gene or heterozygosity of another mutant beta globin gene with the sickle cell gene.[42] Women with sickle cell disease have an average life expectancy of 48 years; however, in many women these years are also associated with major morbidity.[42] Delayed skeletal maturation, growth retardation, and delayed menarche in young women can affect sports participation. Sickle cell disease is not an absolute contraindication to athletics, and young women should be encouraged to participate in any activities except those that involve extreme exertion or contact sports.[43] Acute complications such as infections, bone infarctions, pain crises, or worsening anemia are contraindications to exercise.

Sickle cell trait is inherited heterozygosity of the sickle cell gene with a normal beta globin gene. The prevalence of sickle cell trait in African-Americans is approximately 9%. Sickle cell trait is not associated with any hematological manifestations but can be associated with splenic infarctions, hematuria, and impaired urine-concentrating ability.[42] In male military recruits there is a 30-fold increase of sudden death associated with exercise. Risk factors include dehydration, increased environmental temperature, altitude, poor conditioning, and increased exercise intensity. Dehydration and hypoxia cause hemoglobin sickling, which in turn causes infarction of major organs such as the kidneys, spleen, heart, and skeletal muscle. Cardiac ischemia can lead to dysrhythmias and sudden death. Resultant skeletal muscle necrosis from infarction can lead to rhabdomyolysis, acute renal failure, and death.[44] Aggressive rehydration and supportive care are the cornerstones of therapy.

No cases of sudden death in women with sickle cell trait have been reported in the literature. It is not known whether this is due to protective hormonal influences, more attention to hydration, better conditioning, less strenuous exertion, or underreporting of cases by health care professionals. Women with sickle cell trait should be encouraged to stay well-hydrated during exercise, decrease exercise intensity in hot weather, not exercise at altitude, and remain well-conditioned.

DERMATOLOGICAL ISSUES

Promotion of Healthy Skin

Promotion of healthy skin should be a goal of every active woman. Daily physical activity, balanced nutrition, and adequate hydration are essential. Every woman who participates in outdoor sports should always wear sunscreen on all areas of exposed skin. Sunscreens with an SPF-15 or higher should be applied 30 minutes before going outdoors and reapplied frequently. Sunscreen should be used regardless of time of day or season. Abstinence from cigarettes, other tobacco products, and alcohol can help maintain skin health. Rapid weight fluctuations can be harmful, because of stressing the elastic components of skin, and should be discouraged.

Promotion of Healthy Skin in Active Females

- Sun protection
- Balanced nutrition
- Adequate hydration
- Regular exercise
- Avoidance of alcohol and tobacco
- Avoidance of rapid weight changes

Clinical Guideline

Environmental Skin Disorders

Sun

Climate-related skin disorders are likely to be seen in women who participate in outdoor activities. Sun-related disorders include acute sunburn, premature aging, and skin cancers. Acute sunburn can be prevented by use of appropriate clothing and sunscreens. Treatment consists of tepid baths and mild analgesics. Premature aging is primarily due to chronic sun damage. Prevention is by use of sunscreen and appropriate clothing. Treatment of sun-damaged skin with alpha hydroxy acids and tretinoin (Retin-A) may be indicated in some women. Chronic sun exposure in women increases the likelihood of certain types of skin cancers developing. Clinicians caring for active and athletic women should be able to recognize abnormal skin lesions and either have the skills to appropriately treat these lesions or refer to a specialist when warranted.

Heat

Heat and sweating are common causes of skin disorders in active women. Moisture provides an excellent growth medium for infectious organisms, and efforts to control moisture may help control secondary infections. Wet exercise clothing, including footwear, should be removed immediately after exercise. Bathing as soon as possible after a workout can reduce the risk of bacterial folliculitis, impetigo, and fungal skin infections.

Cold

Athletes who exercise outdoors during winter months are at risk for cold-induced skin disorders. Chafing and dry skin can be treated with clothing protection and moisturizers. Severe environmental cold exposure can lead to frostbite. Frostbite can occur with or without hypothermia, which is a medical emergency. Localized freezing of tissue can lead to permanent loss of function, sepsis, and gangrene. As with most environmental skin injuries, prevention is the optimal treatment.

Raynaud's phenomenon is five to eight times more common in women than men. In women who have Raynaud's phenomenon, cold exposure precipitates intense vasoconstriction of digital arteries of the fingers and toes. If untreated, pain and digital infarction with subsequent necrosis can develop. Athletes with Raynaud's phenomenon should have a thorough evaluation to look for secondary causes such as connective tissue diseases or blood dyscrasias. Prevention, by keeping the body and extremities warm, is essential. Use of gloves even while indoors can be helpful. Severe cases often require medical therapy with small doses of topical nitroglycerin paste or systemic vasodilators, but their use is often limited by headache, hypotension, and syncope. Women with Raynaud's phenomenon should be cautioned to warm their hands frequently if participating in cold weather activities.

Insect Bites and Stings

Insect bites and stings are common consequences of outdoor activity. As for most climate-related skin disorders, prevention is the most important therapy. Liberal use of insect repellants before outdoor activity can be helpful. If bites or stings do occur, treatment with cold compresses can be soothing. Use of systemic antihistamines or judicious use of low-potency topical corticosteroids is indicated for pruritus. Systemic steroids should be reserved for cases with severe pruritus, multiple diffuse lesions, or associated angioedema of the respiratory system.

Common Skin Disorders Related to Environmental Conditions in Female Athletes

- Sun:
  Sunburn
  Premature aging
  Skin cancer
- Heat:
  Folliculitis
- Cold:
  Frostbite
  Raynaud's phenomenon
- Insect bites and stings
  Urticaria
  Abscesses/infections

Clinical Guideline

Skin Disorders Related to Injury

Chafing and Blisters

Chafing occurs from unprotected skin rubbing against other skin or clothing. Chafing is prevented by wearing of loose, seamless, dry clothing, or use of petroleum jelly over areas of contact.[45] Blisters occur from friction between skin and another surface, most commonly shoes. Moisture increases friction, so keeping skin dry, especially feet, can be preventive. Wearing a thin pair of socks next to the skin with a thicker, absorbent outer pair can decrease friction. Use of petroleum jelly or moleskin donuts may also be helpful for prevention.[46] Soaking feet in tannic acid promotes hyperplasia and toughening of skin. If blisters develop, needle drainage with preservation of the top epithelial layer is the optimal treatment. If blisters are severe, use of a hydrocolloid occlusive dressing can promote epithelialization.

Corns and Calluses

Corns and calluses are areas of hyperkeratosis caused by excessive friction, usually over areas of bony prominences. Proper footwear and biomechanics during activity can prevent corn and callus formation. Treatment consists of thinning the area of hyperkeratosis. This is typically accomplished by soaking in warm water and then removing epidermis by scalpel, pumice stone, or salicylic acid.[47]

Infectious Skin and Nail Disorders

Bacterial

Moist warm skin, particularly areas that are irritated or chaffed, provides an excellent growth medium for bacterial and fungal skin infections. Keeping skin dry through use of "wick-away" clothing, including socks, and showering soon after activity are helpful in preventing skin infections in active women.

Impetigo is a bacterial skin infection that is spread by contaminated skin, athletic equipment, or by surfaces in showering areas. Skin that has areas of breakdown or dermatitis is predisposed to this infection developing. *Streptococcus pyogenes* and *Staphylococcus aureus* are the most common etiological organisms.[5,47] Empiric treatment is with systemic antibiotics with good skin penetration such as erythromycin, cephalexin, dicloxacillin, or amoxicillin-clavulanic acid. Athletes with active lesions should be discouraged from participating in water or contact sports and sharing towels or other equipment.

Folliculitis is a bacterial infection of hair follicles that develops in areas of excessive moisture. In addition to moisture control, folliculitis can be treated by daily washing of the affected area with antibacterial soap. Thorough cleansing of contaminated equipment is helpful in preventing recurrences.[5,47] If the athlete has furuncles or carbuncles, incision and drainage of lesions should be performed. Antibiotic therapy is similar to that for impetigo, unless the athlete has "hot tub" folliculitis, which requires antipseudomonal antibiotic therapy. An athlete with folliculitis can participate in sports if the lesions are covered. Furuncles should be healed before participating in swimming or contact sports.[5,47]

Viral

Warts are caused by human papillomavirus and can impair activity and athletic performance if they occur on pressure points and cause pain. There is no gender affinity for development of warts. Warts are distinguished from talon noir (black heel) by the soft keratinized skin with punctate black dots seen after scraping off the overlying dead skin and the anatomical location in which they occur. Plantar warts, which frequently occur on the metatarsal heads or heel of the foot, are the most problematic because of pressure and pain. Transmission of warts is from autoinoculation, skin-to-skin contact, or through contaminated equipment and athletic surfaces.[5,47,48] Warts may resolve spontaneously or can be treated with agents that will increase local immune activity. A variety of destructive techniques can be used. Paring and daily use of salicylic acid can be done by athletes themselves. Clinicians can use liquid nitrogen on a biweekly or monthly basis as an adjunct. Curettage, topical podofilox or imiquimod, lasers, cauterizations, and injections with interferon or bleomycin are alternative modalities.[5,46]

Treatments for Warts in Athletic Women

- Paring
- Curettage
- Cauterization
- Laser therapy
- Salicylic acid
- Liquid nitrogen
- Topical podofilox

- Topical imiquimod
- Interferon injection
- Bleomycin injection

Clinical Guideline

Herpes simplex virus type I infection is a highly contagious viral skin infection spread by direct contact between athletes. Commonly seen in contact sports such as wrestling, this infection is also spread by skin-to-skin contact in sports such as basketball, synchronized skating, or cheerleading in female athletes. Treatment, if initiated at the onset of symptoms, is with one of the systemic antivirals, acyclovir, famciclovir, or valacyclovir, for 10 days. Severe, recurrent cases may require suppressive therapy throughout the competitive season.

Fungal

Fungal skin infections in athletes occur often because of exposure to moisture and humidity, especially of intertriginous areas. Dermatophytes and *Candida* species are normal inhabitants of the skin and can cause clinical disease when there is excessive moisture and areas of skin breakdown or immunosuppression. Common areas where fungal infections occur in women are the feet (tinea pedis), gluteal and inguinal folds, under the breast, and on the scalp (tinea capitis). Drying of the skin is the cornerstone to prevention of fungal skin infections. Drying between the toes, applying absorbent foot powder, and frequent changing of socks can prevent development of tinea pedis. Treatment of tinea pedis is prolonged (1 month) once or twice daily application of antifungal creams.[5,46,47] Athletes in contact sports must completely cover all lesions before participation.

Clinical Guideline: Common Antifungal Creams Used To Treat Tinea Pedis

- Nonprescription:
  Tolnaftate
  Undecylenic acid
- Prescription:
  Terbinafine
  Naftifine
  Miconazole
  Clotrimazole
  Econazole

Clinical Guideline

Onychomycosis occurs in active women because of sweat in footwear or frequent exposure to warm water on the hands. Onychomycosis occurs in both the hands and feet but is more common in the toenails in active women because of athletic shoes and walking in locker rooms. Risk factors that predispose women to onychomycosis are chronic tinea pedis, hyperhidrosis, older age, decreased immunity (including diabetes), and repetitive trauma. Onychomycosis increases the risk of lower extremity cellulitis by providing an entry port for bacteria through damaged skin and nails. Athletes can also experience pain or altered biomechanics with activity if the nail becomes distorted.

Risk Factors for Development of Onychomycosis

- Chronic tinea pedis
- Hyperhidrosis
- Age >50
- Altered immunity
- Repetitive trauma

Clinical Guideline

Diagnosis is made by scraping the under portion of the nail and placing the scrapings on a heated slide with potassium hydroxide (KOH). Hyphae seen under microscopic examination confirm the diagnosis. If the KOH scraping is negative, nail culture or biopsy of the nail plate is usually diagnostic.[49] The oral antifungals itraconazole, terbinafine, and fluconazole are used for treatment of onychomycosis.[49] Liver enzymes should be routinely monitored during the treatment period. If taken as directed, treatment is typically successful, but expensive ($500–$1,000).

NEUROLOGICAL DISORDERS

Seizure Disorders

Seizures occurring during sports or exercise are rare. They most often occur within 3 hours of intense exercise, likely as a result of mild acidosis.[50] Overall, seizure disorders may actually improve in women who exercise regularly because of improved psychological factors such as increased sense of well-being.[50,51] Clinicians caring for physically active women who have seizure disorders need to be careful which antiepileptic drug (AED) they prescribe. Potential side effects such as diplopia, impaired coordination, and reduced concentration can limit performance and actually place athletes at risk for injury in certain sports. Exercise can also affect the metabolism of AED, so careful monitoring of drug levels should be done when beginning or altering the intensity or duration of an established activity program.[50,52]

Athletes with seizure disorders should be counseled on maintaining adequate hydration, nutrition, sleep hygiene, and avoidance of exercising at high environmental tempera-

tures, altitude, or when fatigued. Participation in specific sports depends on the degree of seizure control, side effects of AED, and overall risk for injury. In general, sports such as archery, riflery, weight lifting, swimming, car racing, or those involving heights should be avoided.[43,50,52]

Catamenial epilepsy occurs in 12% of women who have a seizure disorder. Contributing factors include cyclic alterations of hormone levels and drug metabolism. Treatment of catamenial epilepsy includes progesterone contraceptives such as medroxyprogesterone, levonorgestrel implants, or a daily pill containing norgestrel or norethindrone.[8] Natural progesterone delivered transdermally by mouth or as rectal suppositories 2 to 3 days before menses is used by some clinicians.[53]

There is no published literature on the relationship between exercise and catamenial seizures. Overall, it is prudent to recommend the same precautions for participation as for women who do not have perimenstrual seizure exacerbations, with particular attention to adequate sleep, nutrition, and hydration.

ENDOCRINE DISORDERS

Thyroid

Hyperthyroidism is caused by an excess of thyroid hormone, which leads to the clinical syndrome of thyrotoxicosis. This clinical disorder that affects primarily women has several causes, including Graves' disease, toxic nodular goiter, exogenous hyperthyroidism, and thyroiditis. Graves' disease, which has a 7:1 predilection for women, causes 60% to 90% of thyrotoxicosis.[54] Seen mostly in women in their third and fourth decades, Graves' disease is caused by an autoantibody to thyroid-stimulating hormone (TSH) receptors signaling the thyroid gland to produce excess thyroxine.

Causes of Thyrotoxicosis in Women

- Graves' disease
- Toxic adenoma
- Toxic multinodular goiter
- Subacute thyroiditis:
  Lymphocytic (painless)
  Granulomatous (painful)
- Factitious hyperthyroidism
- Carcinomas:
  Choriocarcinoma
  TSH-producing pituitary tumor
  Ovarian teratoma
  Hydatiform mole
  Metastatic disease from follicular thyroid carcinoma

Clinical Guideline

Clinical features of thyrotoxicosis include proximal muscle weakness, anxiety, depression, insomnia, diarrhea, palpitations, weight loss, heat intolerance, sweating, or menstrual abnormalities. Many of these signs and symptoms can be confused in athletic women with overtraining, chronic fatigue, depression, or performance anxiety and therefore warrant a thorough physical examination and laboratory evaluation. Examination may reveal ophthalmoplegia, elevated blood pressure, tachycardia, atrial fibrillation, hyperreflexia, or tremors. Thyromegaly and infiltrative dermopathy are present in Graves' disease. Thyroid nodules are prominent with toxic adenomas or toxic multinodular goiter.

Signs and Symptoms of Thyrotoxicosis in Active Women

- Muscle atrophy
- Proximal muscle weakness
- Hyperreflexia
- Emotional lability
- Tremor
- Palpitations
- Tachycardia
- Atrial fibrillation
- Diarrhea
- Oligomenorrhea
- Amenorrhea
- Weight loss
- Hair loss
- Warm skin
- Heat intolerance

Clinical Guideline

Diagnosis of hyperthyroidism is made by measuring serum TSH levels, which are markedly decreased along with elevations of T_3 and T_4 levels. In Graves' disease there are also elevations of thyroid-stimulating antibody, antithyroid peroxidase antibody, and antithyroglobulin antibody.

Radionuclide scanning is helpful in determining the cause of hyperthyroidism. Thyroid scanning in Graves' disease demonstrates normal or diffusely increased uptake. Nodular disease will appear as focal areas of increased uptake, whereas thyroiditis or use of exogenous thyroxine appears as low uptake on scans.

General therapy of thyrotoxicosis consists of use of beta-adrenergic blockers to control adrenergic symptoms and specific treatment directed to the underlying cause. For women with Graves' disease, the antithyroid medications propylthiouracil or methimazole can control the disease until the woman becomes euthyroid.[54,55] Thyroid ablation by radioactive iodine therapy or surgery is an option. Cessation or decreased use of exogenous thyroxine will be curative in factitious hyperthyroidism. Thyroiditis and toxic nodules

typically "burn out," and the hyperthyroidism spontaneously resolves.[55,56]

Hypothyroidism is caused by thyroid hormone deficiency. In active women it can initially be seen as fatigue, or symptoms of fibromyalgia, overtraining, or multiple overuse injuries.[54,57] Hypothyroidism can be due to disease of the gland itself (primary) or dysfunction of the hypothalamic-pituitary axis (secondary). Primary hypothyroidism is markedly more common in women and is usually caused by gland ablation for hyperthyroidism or idiopathic loss of gland function.[57]

Typical clinical signs and symptoms of hypothyroidism are fatigue, cold intolerance, weight gain, dry skin, depression, dementia, and menorrhagia. Musculoskeletal manifestations include muscle weakness, myalgias, arthralgias, joint effusions, and nerve entrapment syndromes.[57] Physical examination reveals decreased deep tendon reflexes, doughy skin, and enlarged thyroid gland.

Signs and Symptoms of Hypothyroidism in Active Women

- Muscle weakness
- Myalgias
- Arthralgias
- Joint effusions
- Tendinitis
- Nerve entrapment syndromes
- Fatigue
- Weight gain
- Dry skin
- Cold intolerance
- Menorrhagia
- Depression

Clinical Guideline

An elevated serum TSH is diagnostic in primary hypothyroidism. If secondary hypothyroidism is suspected, a full workup for pituitary insufficiency is indicated.[54,57] Treatment is with levothyroxine started at doses of 0.025 to 0.05 mg daily in women older than age 50, and .005 to 0.1 mg daily in younger patients, with incremental adjustments every 4 to 8 weeks as needed. The typical replacement dosage for adults is 1–2 µg/kg/day.[54]

Diabetes Mellitus

Diabetes mellitus is a chronic disease characterized by relative or absolute insulin deficiency. Type 1 diabetes affects 0.3% of the population of the United States, with type 2 diabetes affecting 10% to 15% of the US population older than the age of 50.[58] Although there is not a gender predilection, diabetes causes premature morbidity and mortality for many women, including end-stage renal disease, blindness, limb amputations, coronary artery disease, and peripheral and cerebrovascular disease.[58] Major clinical trials have shown for both types of diabetes that diabetic complications decrease as glucose control improves.[59,60]

Exercise is one nonpharmacological method that has been shown to improve glucose tolerance,[61–67] diabetic control,[68–71] and reduce cardiovascular risk factors[61–62,65,67,72] in adults with type 2 diabetes. In individuals with type 1 diabetes, exercise is important to overall health and prevention of cardiovascular risk factors but has not been shown to improve glycemic control.[58,67] The American Diabetes Association thus encourages regular exercise for all women with diabetes.[73]

Women with both type 1 and type 2 diabetes should have a thorough history and physical examination and a written exercise prescription before starting an exercise program.[74] A graded exercise stress test should be performed if the patient is embarking on a vigorous program, has been diagnosed with diabetes for a long period of time, is older, has coronary artery disease, or has any microvascular or macrovascular complications of diabetes.[73] Care should be taken in developing safe exercise prescriptions for patients with diabetic complications, especially retinopathy, autonomic dysfunction, neuropathy, and peripheral vascular disease.[67,75] All individuals with diabetes should be instructed on use of proper footwear and daily foot examinations.

Blood glucose should be measured before, immediately after, and during prolonged (>1 hour) activity and insulin dosing and carbohydrate intake adjusted accordingly. Women with blood glucose measurements greater than 300 mg/dL should not begin activity until they achieve better glucose control.[73] Although not supported by research, use of lispro insulin may help glucose control during and immediately after exercise, because it is fast acting and has a short half-life.[67,75–77]

A general exercise program for diabetic patients should include 5-minute warm-up and cool-down periods with a 20- to 60-minute period of aerobic activity between.[67] Stretching to increase and maintain flexibility is important, as is resistance training with light weights and frequent repetitions.[50,78–79] Women should begin a program even if they cannot participate in a full 20 to 60 minutes of aerobic conditioning. Participating in activities that a woman is interested in and perceives as fun may help compliance.[74] Proper hydration should be judiciously maintained throughout and after all activity.

RESEARCH

There continues to be a scarcity of research on gender differences in the risk factors, clinical presentation, and treatment of medical illnesses despite a mandate by the National Institutes of Health (NIH) that women be enrolled as subjects in all clinical trials that receive NIH funding. There is also little research on how exercise and sports participation has an impact on women's overall health or affects the progression of chronic medical conditions. Sports health professionals are particularly encouraged to develop or participate in research trials involving women of all ages and ethnicity, which not only address the effects of exercise on musculoskeletal health but also focus on prevention and treatment of both acute and chronic medical illnesses.

REFERENCES

1. Swain RA, Kaplan B. Upper respiratory infections. Treatment selection for active patients. *Phys Sportsmed.* 1998;26(2):85–96.

2. Nichols A. Nonorthopaedic problems in the aquatic athlete. *Clin Sports Med.* 1999;18(2):395–411.

3. Sevier TL. Infectious disease in athletes. *Med Clin North Am.* 1994;78(2):389–412.

4. Eichner ER. Infectious mononucleosis. Recognizing the condition, "reactivating" the patient. *Phys Sportsmed.* 1996;24(4):49–54.

5. Patel D, Gordon RC. Contagious diseases in athletes. *Contemp Pediatr.* 1999;16(9):139–164.

6. Terrell T, Hough D, Alexander R. Identifying exercise allergies. Exercise-induced anaphylaxis and cholinergic urticaria. *Phys Sportsmed.* 1996;24(11):76–89.

7. Shames R, Heilbron D, Janson S, et al. Clinical differences among women with and without self-reported perimenstrual asthma. *Ann Allergy Asthma Immunol.* 1998;81:65–71.

8. Case A, Reid R. Effects of the menstrual cycle on medical disorders. *Arch Intern Med.* 1998;158:1405–1412.

9. Highlights of the Expert Panel Report 2. Guidelines for the Diagnosis and Management of Asthma. *National Institutes of Health Publication.* No 97–4051A. Bethesda MD: National Institutes of Health, National Heart, Lung and Blood Institute; 1997.

10. Disabella V, Sherman C, DiNubile N. Exercise for asthma patients. Little risk, big rewards. *Phys Sportsmed.* 1998;26(6):75–84.

11. McFadden ER, Gilbert IA. Exercise-induced asthma. *N Engl J Med.* 1994;330(19):1362–1367.

12. Lacroix V. Exercise-induced asthma. *Phys Sportsmed.* 1999;27(12):75–92.

13. Storms W. Exercise-induced asthma: Diagnosis and treatment for the recreational or elite athlete. *Med Sci Sports Exerc.* 1999;31(1S):33–38.

14. Brugman S, Simons S. Vocal cord dysfunction. Don't mistake it for asthma. *Phys Sportsmed.* 1998;26(5):63–85.

15. Leff JA, Busse WW, Pearlman D, et al. Montelukast, A leukotriene-receptor antagonist for the treatment of mild asthma and exercise-induced bronchoconstriction. *N Engl J Med.* 1998;339(3):147–152.

16. Mannix ET et al. A comparison of two challenge tests for identifying exercise-induced bronchospasm in figure skaters. *Chest.* 1999;115(3):649–653.

17. Smith B, LaBotz M. Pharmacologic treatment of exercise-induced asthma. *Clin Sports Med.* 1998;17(2):343–363.

18. Mink BD. Exercise and chronic obstructive pulmonary disease. *Phys Sportsmed.* 1997;25(11):43–52.

19. Homnick DN, Marks JH. Exercise and sports in the adolescent with chronic pulmonary disease. *Adolesc Med State Art Rev.* 1998;9(3):467–481.

20. Erickson SM, Rich BSE. Pulmonary and chest wall emergencies. *Phys Sportsmed.* 1995;23(11):95–104.

21. Eichner ER, Scott W. Exercise as disease detector. *Phys Sportsmed.* 1998;26(3):41–52.

22. McCabe ME et al. Gastrointestinal blood loss associated with running a marathon. *Dig Dis Sci.* 1986;31:1299–1232.

23. Wald A et al. Gastrointestinal transit: The effect of the menstrual cycle. *Gastroenterology.* 1981;80:1497–1500.

24. Putukian M, Potera C. Don't miss gastrointestinal disorders in athletes. *Phys Sportsmed.* 1997;25(11):80–94.

25. Bergman RT. Assessing acute abdominal pain. *Phys Sportsmed.* 1996;24(4):72–82.

26. Centers for Disease Control and Prevention. 1998 guidelines for treatment of sexually transmitted diseases. *MMWR.* 1998;47 (RR-1):1–116.

27. Clark J. Sexually transmitted diseases. Detection, differentiation, and treatment. *Phys Sportsmed.* 1997;25(1):76–91.

28. Sobel JD. Vaginitis. *N Engl J Med.* 1997;337(26):1896–1903.

29. Gormley EA. Irritative voiding symptoms: Identifying the cause. *Hosp Pract.* 1999;Dec 15:91–196.

30. Ryan S. Managing urinary tract and vaginal infections. *Phys Sportsmed.* 1996;24(7):101–106.

31. Fishbane S. Exercise-induced renal and electrolyte changes. Minimizing the risks. *Phys Sportsmed.* 1995;23(8):39–46.

32. Gambrell RC, Blount BW. Exercise-induced hematuria. *Am Fam Phys.* 1996;53(3):905–911.

33. Jones GR, Newhouse I. Sport-related hematuria: A review. *Clin J Sports Med.* 1997;7:119–125.

34. LaSalle MD, Salimpour P, Adelstein M, et al. Sexual and urinary tract dysfunction in female bicyclists. Presented at the 94th Annual Meeting of the American Urological Association; May 4, 1999. Dallas, TX.

35. Dallman PR, Yip R, Johnson C. Prevalence and causes of anemia in the United States, 1976–1980. *Am J Clin Nutr.* 1984;39:437.

36. Andrews N. Disorders of iron metabolism. *N Engl J Med.* 1999;341(26):1986–1995.

37. Eichner ER. The anemia of athletes. *Phys Sportsmed.* 1986;14:122–130.

38. Chatard JC, Mujika I, Guy C, Lacour JR. Anaemia and iron deficiency in athletes. *Sports Med.* 1999;27(4):229–240.

39. Ashenden M, Martin D, Dobson G, et al. Serum ferritin and anemia in trained female athletes. *Int J Sport Nutr.* 1998;8:223–229.

40. Cook JD. The effect of endurance training on iron metabolism. *Semin Hematol.* 1994;31:146–154.

41. Garza DI, Shrier HW, et al. The clinical value of serum ferritin tests in endurance athletes. *Clin J Sports Med.* 1997;7:46–53.

42. Enbury SH. Sickle cell anemia and associated hemoglobinopathies. In: Goldman L, Bennet JCL, eds. *Cecil Textbook of Medicine.* Philadelphia: WB Saunders: 2000:893–905.

43. American Academy of Family Physicians. Preparticipation physical evaluation. 2nd ed. Minneapolis, MN: The Physician and Sports Medicine Division of McGraw-Hill; 1997.

44. Kerle KK, Nishimura KD. Exertional collapse and sudden death associated with sickle cell. *Am Fam Phys.* 1996;54(1):237–240.

45. Ramsey ML. Skin care for active people. *Phys Sportsmed.* 1997;25(3):131–132.

46. Burkhart CG. Skin disorders of the foot in active patients. *Phys Sportsmed.* 1999;27(2):88–101.

47. Knopp WD. Dermatology. In: Sallis RE, Massimino F, eds. *ACSM's Essentials of Sports Medicine.* St. Louis, MO: Mosby; 1997:110–117.

48. Lillegard WA, Butcher J. Dermatologic conditions in athletes. In: Kibler WB, ed. *ACSM's HandBook for the Team Physician.* Baltimore: Williams & Wilkins; 1996:115–140.

49. Seraly MP, Fuerst ML. Diagnosing and treating onychomycosis. *Phys Sportsmed.* 1998;26(8):59–67.

50. Sirven JI, Varrato J. Physical activity and epilepsy. *Phys Sportsmed.* 1999;27(3):63–70.

51. Nakken KO. Physical exercise in outpatients with epilepsy. *Epilepsia.* 1999;40(5):643–651.

52. Cantu RV. Epilepsy and athletics. *Clin Sports Med.* 1998;17(1):61–69.

53. Herzog AG, Klein P, Ransil BJ. Three patterns of catamenial epilepsy. *Epilepsia.* 1997;38:1082–1088.

54. Dillmann WH. The thyroid. In: Goldman L, Bennett JC, eds. *Cecil Textbook of Medicine.* Philadelphia: WB Saunders; 2000:1231–1250.

55. Wang DH, Koehler SM, Mariash CN. Detecting Graves' disease. *Phys Sportsmed.* 1996;24(12):35–40.

56. Daniels GH. Hyperthyroidism: Multiple possibilities in the female patient. *Int J Fertil.* 1999;44(1):6–11.

57. Knopp WD, Bohm ME, McCoy JC. Hypothyroidism presenting as tendinitis. *Phys Sportsmed.* 1997;25(1):47–55.

58. Sherwin RS. Diabetes mellitus. In: Goldman L, Bennett JC, eds. *Cecil Textbook of Medicine.* Philadelphia: WB Saunders; 2000:1263–1285.

59. Diabetes Control and Complications Trial Research Group. The effects of intensive treatment of diabetes on the development and progression of long-term complications in insulin-dependent diabetes mellitus. *N Engl J Med.* 1993;329:977.

60. Turner RC, Holman RR, Cull CA, et al. Intensive blood-glucose control with sulfonureas or insulin compared with conventional treatment and risk of complications in patients with type 2 diabetes (UKPDS 33). *Lancet.* 1998.352–837.

61. Clark DO. Physical activity efficiency and effectiveness among older adults and minorities. *Diabetes Care.* 1997;20(7):1176–1182.

62. Dunstan DW, Mori TA, Puddey IB, et al. The independent and combined effects of aerobic exercise and dietary fish intake on serum lipids and glycemic control in NIDDM. *Diabetes Care.* 1997;20:913–921.

63. Goodyear LJ, Kahn BB. Exercise, glucose transport, and insulin sensitivity. *Annu Rev Med.* 1998;49:235–261.

64. Helmrich SP, Ragland DR, Leung RW, et al. Physical activity and reduced occurrence of non-insulin-dependent diabetes mellitus. *N Engl J Med.* 1991;325:147–152.

65. Lehmann R, Vokac A, Niedermann K, et al. Loss of abdominal fat and improvement of the cardiovascular risk profile by regular moderate exercise training in patients with NIDDM. *Diabetologia.* 1995;38:1313–1319.

66. Manson JE, Rimm EB, Stampfer MJ, et al. Physical activity and incidence of non-insulin-dependent diabetes mellitus in women. *Lancet.* 1991;338:774–778.

67. Peirce NS. Diabetes and exercise. *Br J Sports Med.* 1999;33:161–173.

68. Bourn DM, Mann JI, McSkimming BJ, et al. Impaired glucose tolerance and NIDDM: Does a lifestyle intervention program have an effect? *Diabetes Care.* 1994;17:1311–1319.

69. Ericksson JG. Exercise and the treatment of type 2 diabetes mellitus. *Sports Med.* 1999;27(6):381–391.

70. Ligtenberg PC, Hoekstra JBL, Bol E, et al. Effect of physical training on metabolic control in elderly type diabetes mellitus patients. *Clin Sci.* 1997;93:127–135.

71. Schneider SH, Khachadurian AV, Amorosa LF, et al. Ten-year experience with an exercise-based outpatient life-style modification program in the treatment of diabetes mellitus. *Diabetes Care.* 1992;15(Suppl 4):1800–1810.

72. NIH Consensus development panel on physical activity and cardiovascular health. *JAMA.* 1996;276:241–246.

73. American Diabetes Association. Diabetes Mellitus and Exercise. *Diabetes Care.* 1999;22(Suppl 1):S49–53.

74. Walberg-Henriksson H, Rincon J, Zierath JR. Exercise in the management of non-insulin-dependent diabetes mellitus. *Sports Med.* 1998;25(1):25–35.

75. White RD, Sherman C. Exercise in diabetes management. *Phys Sportsmed.* 1999;27(4):63–76.

76. Kappel C, Dills DG. Type 2 diabetes: Update on therapy. *Comp Ther.* 1998;24(6/7):319–326.

77. Petrella RJ. Exercise for older patients with chronic disease. *Phys Sportsmed.* 1999;27(11):79–104.

78. Eriksson J, Taimela S, Eriksson K, et al. Resistance training in the treatment of non-insulin-dependent diabetes mellitus. *Int. J Sports Med.* 1997;18(4):242–246.

79. Smutok MA, Reece C, Kokkinos PF, et al. Effects of exercise training modality on glucose tolerance in men with abnormal glucose regulation. *Int J Sports Med.* 1994;6:283–289.

CHAPTER 14

Cardiac Issues in the Female Athlete

Holly S. Andersen

Cardiovascular disease is the leading cause of death among women in this country, accounting for more deaths each year than from all cancers combined. However, the most recent population survey data show us that even today US women do not perceive heart disease as a priority health problem. Once a woman is diagnosed with coronary heart disease, she has increased morbidity and mortality compared to a man. Fortunately, there is a tremendous amount that can be done to prevent heart disease, and being physically active is an extraordinarily important part of maintaining a healthy heart.

EXERCISE PHYSIOLOGY

The cardiovascular response to exercise is similar in women and men; however, it is important to be aware of the definite physiological differences that exist when evaluating and treating women. Women normally have smaller hearts (even when corrected for body size), smaller stroke volumes, and higher heart rates. They normally have a lower blood volume and hematocrit, making their total oxygen carrying capacity less than a man's. In addition, their body fat percentage is normally higher. Combined, these differences account for their generally lower maximal aerobic capacity.[1,2] Highly trained female athletes can, however, achieve maximal oxygen uptakes equal to similarly trained males.[3] Nonetheless, when evaluating exercise performance in women, sex-specific standards for maximal aerobic capacity and nomograms for the calculation of maximal capacity from submaximal heart rates and oxygen consumption should be used.

The hearts of both men and women adapt similarly to exercise, although to slightly different degrees. Highly trained athletes frequently demonstrate cardiac dimensional changes as an adaptation to physical training. Left ventricular cavity size exceeding normal limits can occur in a minority of elite female athletes, but it is rarely in the range of a dilated cardiomyopathy.[4] Endurance sports such as cycling (Figure 14–1), Nordic skiing, and rowing have the greatest effect on cavity dimension. Unlike men, substantial increases in left ventricular wall thickness do not appear to occur in high-performance female athletes, making the diagnostic distinction of hypertrophic cardiomyopathy a dilemma restricted to the elite male athlete.[4]

CORONARY RISK REDUCTION

A sedentary lifestyle is now recognized as an independent risk factor for coronary heart disease, and more than 75% of the US population is sedentary or nearly so. It has been clearly established that all-cause mortality is lower among more fit women. Women with the lowest level of fitness have been found to have higher blood glucose levels with less favorable lipid profiles and anthropometric indexes than those with moderate and high levels of fitness. Exercise has been shown to prospectively increase high density lipoprotein (HDL) levels in women.[5] In postmenopausal women, higher levels of cardiorespiratory fitness are associated with significantly lower total cholesterol, low density lipoprotein (LDL), triglyceride, and fibrinogen levels.[6] Exercise helps prevent coronary artery disease; even modest amounts of physical activity can have a profound impact. A strong

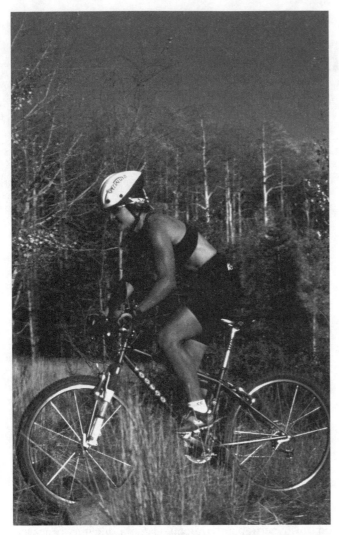

Figure 14–1 Endurance Sports Such As Cycling Have the Greatest Effect on Cardiac Intracavitary Dimension.

graded inverse association has been found between physical activity and coronary event risk. Walking is an excellent form of activity, and because elderly women, who are at particular risk for cardiovascular disease, are unlikely to take up new sports, the importance of walking should be emphasized to them. Women who walk ≥3 hours per week at a brisk pace have similar coronary risk reductions (30%–40%) as women who participate in regular vigorous exercise.[7] It is never too late to start; sedentary women who become active later in adulthood can significantly reduce their risk of coronary heart disease compared with women who remain sedentary.[6] Study after study has shown that the greatest magnitude of risk reduction is achieved in going from a sedentary lifestyle to a moderate level of activity. Gradual increases in the intensity and duration of physical activity should be made, and pre-exercise cardiac stress testing should be strongly considered for those women at particular risk.

Physiologic Parameters Improved with Exercise

- Blood pressure
- Glucose tolerance
- Total cholesterol
- HDL
- Triglycerides
- Fibrinogen
- Overall coronary artery disease risk

Clinical Guideline

CARDIAC STRESS TESTING

All noninvasive modalities of stress testing are disadvantaged by the lower prevalence of coronary artery disease in women, as Bayesian theory predicts (lower prevalence of disease in a population will increase the false-positive rate). Numerous studies have examined the results of the standard electrocardiogram (ECG) treadmill test and have emphasized the high false-positive rate in the female population. The largest series comes from the Coronary Artery Surgery Study,[8] which reported the false-positive rate to be 12% in men and 54% in women. On subgroup analysis, which matched for age and extent of coronary artery disease, however, there was no longer a significant difference with respect to false positives. Therefore, these investigators concluded that the initial difference was due solely to disease prevalence. These conclusions have been challenged by subsequent studies; Barolsky evaluated men and women with similar disease prevalence, and among these patients, a striking difference in the false-positive rate remained—23% for men and 53% for women[9]—strongly implicating a non-Bayesian factor. Premenopausal women have the highest false-positive rates with the ECG treadmill test. Estrogen has a molecular structure similar to digoxin and may cause a digitalis-like false-positive ECG response. ECG responses have been shown to vary during the menstrual cycle and in response to estrogen therapy, but to date studies investigating hormonal influences have been somewhat conflicting.

Stress testing with radionuclide cineangiography (RNCA) is also fraught with significantly higher false-positive rates in women. RNCA looks at the change in ejection fraction with exercise. A normal response has been defined as a 5% increase.[10] In men, stroke volume increases with exercise primarily because of an increase in the ejection fraction. In women, however, stroke volume is increased primarily by an increase in the left ventricular end diastolic volume. It has been reported that as many as 50% of women with normal coronary arteries will fail to increase their ejection fraction (whereas this phenomenon occurs in only 10% of normal men).[11] In this test as with the ECG treadmill test, a totally normal response to exercise is a good indicator that significant coronary artery disease is unlikely to be present (good negative predictive value), but an abnormal response in a woman is often not clinically helpful.

Higher false-positive rates in women also occur with stress thallium imaging. Breast tissue can attenuate radioactivity and produce artifactual defects in the septum and anterior wall, rendering it a less accurate test in women. The use of technetium-99m sestamibi single photon emission computed tomographic stress imaging has been demonstrated to be as sensitive as thallium imaging, but because this study enables visualization of wall motion, it has greater specificity, decreasing the number of false-positive readings of the anterior wall.[12]

Stress echocardiography has been proposed as the most efficient, cost-effective screening test for women, particularly for premenopausal women. According to a study by the Cleveland Clinic, it was found to be more specific and accurate than the standard exercise ECG, and therefore many inappropriate, follow-up studies, including more expensive stress tests and angiograms, were avoided.[13] Furthermore, the psychological burden of undergoing further testing for patients considered to have a diagnosis of heart disease should not be underestimated.

CARDIAC REHABILITATION

For those who are recovering from a cardiac event or procedure, multiple studies have now shown that rehabilitation can improve exercise capacity and decrease morbidity and possibly mortality. Still, only a great minority enroll in these programs, and women are consistently less likely to enroll than men.[14] Women are referred less often than men; and even when they do enroll, they have significantly higher dropout rates.[15] This is especially important in view of much evidence to suggest that women may actually benefit more from their rehabilitation. It may be that women often have more room for improvement at the beginning than men. We know that women at any age are more likely to die from their coronary heart disease. In addition, women at entry into cardiac rehabilitation programs have reported higher degrees of psychosocial impairment and lower levels of physical functioning than men.[16] Not unlike men, depression is prevalent in women after major coronary events and this increases their morbidity and mortality. Formal outpatient cardiac rehabilitation and exercise training programs have been shown to have marked benefits in exercise capacity, weight loss, and quality of life for these patients.[17] It also appears that women are better able to achieve greater and more lasting improvements in their lipid profiles with cardiac rehabilitation than are men. Clearly, formal cardiac rehabilitation is an underused important treatment for coronary heart disease in women. We need to routinely recruit women to engage in these programs, and we need to better adapt our programs to the needs of women so that they are more likely to successfully complete them.

EVALUATION OF PALPITATIONS, CHEST PAIN, AND SYNCOPE

Palpitations

"Palpitations" are a subjective term used to describe a plethora of symptoms. A careful history to discern what a patient means by palpitations is essential. Quite often, especially in younger athletic individuals, simple benign atrial premature contractions can cause profound symptoms. After an atrial premature contraction, there is normally a compensatory pause in the heart rate. This allows the ventricle to fill with more blood than usual, and when it contracts again, it does so more forcibly. The extrasystole, the pause, and the postextrasystole hypercontracted beat are completely asymptomatic in most individuals, but in others the symptoms can be so disconcerting that they seek out emergency department treatment. If they are not appropriately convinced of the benign nature of these extra beats, they will often go from doctor to doctor undergoing expensive and repeated testing. Taking the time to completely reassure this patient will most often prove to be adequate therapy; infrequently, a ß-blocker can be successfully used to lessen the frequency of the atrial premature contractions and lessen the patient's perception of them.

Patients who describe "skipped" beats or "extra" beats may also be experiencing *ventricular* premature contractions. When these are found on an ECG, a Holter monitor, or an event monitor, a thorough workup is required to rule out underlying cardiac pathology. Careful questioning to uncover a history of syncope, chest pain, or dyspnea is important. Questions as to medications, both prescribed and over-the-counter, are essential, because many drugs are arrhythmogenic. A recent viral (particularly an upper respiratory) infection might raise suspicion for myocarditis, which can provoke arrhythmias. Caffeine, alcohol, dehydration, and thyroid disorders can all provoke arrhythmias and should be considered when evaluating these patients.

If a patient describes palpitations as a sudden onset of heart "racing," this may suggest a paroxysmal supraventricular tachycardia, atrial fibrillation, or, less likely, ventricular tachycardia. Associated symptoms of chest pain, light-headedness, dyspnea, or diaphoresis must be explored to determine whether there is associated ischemia or hemodynamic compromise. Again, Holter or event monitoring is crucial to document the arrhythmia. Once documented, medical therapy can often successfully suppress the arrhythmias. Some arrhythmias can be cured by the electrophysiological intervention of radiofrequency ablation. Automatic implantable cardiac defibrillators are now commonplace in the treatment of ventricular tachycardia.

Endurance athletes experience a significantly greater degree of bradyarrhythmias than age-matched controls. Physical activity increases the body's sympathetic drive, which increases the blood pressure, heart rate, and stroke volume. Chronic exposure to habitual exercise causes adaptive changes that gradually down-regulate the sympathetic nervous system and up-regulate the parasympathetic system (increased vagal tone). As a result, automaticity of the heart decreases, producing a slower resting sinus rhythm and occasionally even a junctional rhythm. Conductivity also decreases and can produce brief delays in sinoatrial (first-degree heart block) and atrioventricular (AV) nodal conduction (Mobitz type 1 second-degree heart block). In one study, profound bradycardia (<35 beats per minute) was found in 40% of the athletes compared with 5% of the controls, and transient periods of first- or second-degree AV block were noted in 50% of the athletes and in none of the controls.[18] These atrial arrhythmias are usually completely asymptomatic and benign. Prolonged sinus pauses, profound bradyarrhythmias, and higher degrees of heart block, all of which can produce symptoms, are not considered normal adaptive changes to exercise and need to be investigated and treated accordingly.

Possible Causes of Palpitations

Patient's complaint: skipped beats or extra beats
Consider: atrial premature contractions or ventricular premature contractions
Recommendations: reassurance; avoid alcohol, caffeine, dehydration; possibly ß-blockers; or full evaluation
Patient's complaint: Heart racing
Consider: supraventricular tachycardia, atrial fibrillation, atrial flutter, ventricular tachycardia
Recommendations: full evaluation

Clinical Guideline

Chest Pain

Chest pain is an important symptom that requires prompt evaluation. It is a frequent complaint of athletes and non-athletes alike and can have myriad causes. Chest pain that predictably occurs with a certain amount of physical stress, which is relieved by rest, is of significant concern. With stress, myocardial oxygen demand increases. If there is an arterial blockage impairing blood delivery to a part of the heart, it will become ischemic. Ischemia usually produces pain, and the pain of the heart is most often referred to the chest substernally (angina). Women are more likely to have pain referred to their arm (left > right), back, stomach, and neck than are men. Women are also more likely to experience "silent" ischemia. Chest pain that is provoked by physical or emotional stress should, in most cases, be evaluated by a stress test. Sometimes the presentation is so classic for angina that proceeding directly to an angiogram is warranted.

A patient experiencing a myocardial infarction will most likely present with sudden onset of chest pain. It is not uncommon for the pain to radiate to the left shoulder or arm, and it is often associated with diaphoresis. Chest pain (signaling myocardial ischemia) usually needs to last for >30 minutes to produce a myocardial infarction. Men are more likely to have a myocardial infarction as their initial presentation of coronary heart disease, whereas women are more likely to have angina. Unremitting chest pain should be considered a medical emergency and dealt with as such.

Chest pain that is "pleuritic" (worsens with a deep breath) can signify inflammation of the heart lining (pericarditis) or muscle (myocarditis). The pain from these conditions is usually exacerbated by lying flat and relieved by leaning forward. Cardiac auscultation of a pericardial friction rub; blood analysis including a complete blood count, erythrocyte sedimentation rate, and myocardial enzymes; and an echocardiogram can help confirm the diagnosis. Pulmonary pleurisy and some types of musculoskeletal pain can also produce pleuritic chest pain.

Esophageal reflux, gastritis, or ulcer pain can mimic cardiac ischemic pain. Gastric pain, however, usually is not provoked by physical stress. It is more likely to occur 30 to 90 minutes postprandially or at night when the patient is recumbent. It is oftentimes transiently relieved by food or antacids. Musculoskeletal pain is a frequent complaint of athletes, especially when they begin a new upper body exercise. This pain is usually not provoked by physical stress, unless it is the activity that provoked the injury. It is usually positional and can wax and wane in intensity over several hours. It is oftentimes relieved by anti-inflammatory medications. Quite often, it is difficult to distinguish cardiac from noncardiac pain, and further diagnostic evaluation, particularly stress testing, is required.

Coronary Artery Disease in Women

- Women are more likely to have atypical angina (arm, back, neck, or epigastric pain, fatigue, dyspnea).
- Women are more likely to experience "silent" ischemia.
- Women are more likely to have angina as their initial presentation of coronary heart disease, whereas men are more likely to have myocardial infarction.

- Women are more likely to be diagnosed at a later stage with their heart disease.
- Women are more likely to have comorbidities of hypertension and diabetes.
- Women are more likely to die from their heart attacks.

Clinical Guideline

Syncope

Syncope is a brief sudden loss of consciousness and muscle tone as a result of cerebral hypoperfusion. Exercise-induced syncope can be a harbinger of underlying significant cardiac disease. It may be the presenting symptom of a cardiomyopathy, the long-QT syndrome, other arrhythmias (including the Wolff-Parkinson-White syndrome, arrhythmogenic right ventricular dysplasia, and right ventricular outflow tract tachycardia) or coronary artery anomalies, all of which may put a patient at risk for sudden cardiac death. Therefore, a patient who is initially seen with exercise-induced syncope should have a careful cardiac evaluation, including a detailed clinical and family history, a physical examination, and an ECG. An echocardiogram should be considered for all and performed in those patients with an abnormal cardiac examination or ECG. Stress testing and Holter or event monitoring may be additionally needed to evaluate for ischemia and arrhythmias.

Most often, especially in otherwise healthy appearing athletes, the diagnosis is a benign one such as orthostatic hypotension or "vasodepressor," or more accurately, "neurocardiogenic" syncope. Neurocardiogenic syncope occurs as a result of an abnormal hyper-reflexic increase in vagal tone in response to an adrenergic stimulus. Paradoxically, instead of the heart rate and blood pressure increasing in response to a stressor, the heart rate and blood pressure drop. This is in contrast to orthostatic hypotension, in which the blood pressure drops, but the heart rate increases. Dehydration associated with exercise can exacerbate both conditions, so these athletes should be encouraged to remain well hydrated. The head-up tilt table test is an important diagnostic tool for the evaluation and management of neurocardiogenic syncope. ß-blockers and low-dose panoxetine have been particularly successful in eliminating or lessening the associated symptoms. Most patients with neurocardiogenic syncope can be managed successfully and can safely continue to participate in athletics.[19] Exercise itself may increase orthostatic tolerance and improve symptoms for these patients.[20]

Cardiac Causes of Exercise-induced Syncope

- Hypertrophic cardiomyopathy
- Long QT syndrome

- Wolff-Parkinson-White syndrome
- Arrhythmogenic right ventricular dysplasia
- Right ventricular outflow tract tachycardia
- Coronary artery anomalies

Clinical Guideline

HYPERTENSION

Hypertension is a powerful risk factor for cardiovascular disease. Prospective studies of both men and women confirm the strong association between hypertension and heart disease. A normal blood pressure is now considered to be a systolic pressure of ≤ 140 mm Hg and a diastolic pressure of ≤ 85 mm Hg. Isolated systolic hypertension is more prevalent among women, particularly among those of African-American descent. It increases with age, estimated to occur in 30% of women older than 65 years. Lowering blood pressure in hypertensive individuals is crucial. In a landmark study of systolic hypertension in the elderly, antihypertensive therapy resulted in a 36% and a 27% decrease in the incidence of stroke and coronary heart disease, respectively.[21] The treatment of diastolic hypertension is also extremely important. A decrease in the diastolic blood pressure by six has been shown to significantly decrease the occurrence of stroke and myocardial infarction.[22] Hypertensive individuals have also been shown to have reduced cardiopulmonary function during exercise. This is believed to be related to impaired peripheral vascular autoregulation.[23] Another important reason to aggressively treat hypertension is that some patients, as a consequence, will develop left ventricular hypertrophy, which is itself a strong independent risk factor for cardiovascular death, in particular, sudden cardiac death.

Athletes of any age with hypertension should be evaluated if the blood pressure is >125/75 mm Hg in those less than 10 years or >135/85 mm Hg in those older than 10 years.

Clinical Guideline

Athletes of any age with hypertension should be evaluated if the blood pressure is >125/75 mm Hg in those less than 10 years, or >135/85 mm Hg in those older than 10 years.[24] Exercise testing is an important diagnostic and prognostic procedure in the assessment of patients with hypertension. In both women and men, an exaggerated blood pressure response to exercise, particularly the diastolic blood pressure,[25] has been found to be one of the best predictors of future hypertension. These athletes should be checked regularly for the development of hypertension.

A nonpharmacological approach to the treatment of hypertensive individuals is a critical first step in management, regardless of whether antihypertensive medications are additionally needed. The nonpharmacological modalities include a diet low in salt and saturated fat, exercise, weight loss, alcohol restriction to less than 2 ounces daily, and smoking cessation. Aerobic exercise is effective in lowering blood pressure, but only if performed regularly. Isometric exercise is not an effective alternative to aerobic exercise with respect to blood pressure lowering. Isometric exercise, however, can be performed safely once a patient's blood pressure is well controlled. Excitingly, aerobic exercise has been shown to have a favorable impact on the cardiorespiratory fitness and blood pressures of high-risk adolescent girls.[26]

MITRAL VALVE PROLAPSE

Mitral valve prolapse (MVP) is the most common cardiac valvular abnormality in industrialized nations, affecting 2% to 3% of men and 4% of women. It describes the superior and posterior displacement of the mitral valve leaflets into the left atrium from their normal position in the left ventricle during systole. MVP most often occurs as a primary condition with an autosomal dominant pattern of inheritance with incomplete penetrance in male subjects but nearly 100% penetrance in female subjects aged 16 to 50 years.[27] MVP may also be found as a secondary condition in Marfan syndrome, Ehlers-Danlos syndrome, and heritable polycystic kidney disease. It is important to note that MVP may also be acquired in conditions that cause the left ventricle to be abnormally small, such as anorexia nervosa, or in the presence of an atrial septal defect. This acquired form disappears when the underlying cause is resolved. Conversely, MVP may be masked in conditions in which the left ventricle is transiently dilated such as in the normal volume overload of pregnancy.

Secondary Conditions Associated with Mitral Valve Prolapse

- Marfan syndrome
- Ehlers-Danlos syndrome
- Heritable polycystic kidney disease

Clinical Guideline

MVP is usually first diagnosed during routine examination of the heart. Auscultatory and echocardiographic findings usually do not appear until late childhood or adolescence. The two classic auscultatory features of MVP are a midsystolic click and a late systolic murmur heard best directly over or just medial to the left ventricular impulse. It is important to remember that the auscultatory manifestations of MVP can vary greatly within the same patient from office visit to office visit. ECGs with Doppler should be used

to confirm the diagnosis of MVP and to grade any associated mitral regurgitation and structural valvular abnormality.

Past literature and unfortunately traditional teaching have propagated the existence of an MVP "syndrome," which reportedly includes chest pain, dyspnea, palpitations, anxiety, hysteria, and even panic attacks. The early studies that reported these associations were weakened by selection bias. More recently, case-controlled studies have demonstrated no significant associations between MVP and these symptoms, the one exception being palpitations.[28] Patients with MVP have a slightly higher prevalence of atrial tachycardias. In addition, there is an excess of orthostatic hypotension in patients with MVP, which can lead to presyncope and syncope. This is believed to be due to a low blood volume, which is often exacerbated by a low-salt diet, physical activity, and menstruation, all of which can contribute to dehydration.[29]

There are extracardiac manifestations of primary MVP that include a tendency toward leaner bodies[30] with lower body weights and lower blood pressures.[31] Other studies have found that women with MVP were taller, thinner, had longer arm spans, and had narrower anteroposterior chest diameters than women without MVP.[32] These desirable characteristics are likely responsible for the "selection advantage" that accounts for the high prevalence of this genetic condition in our population. One study even found that the age at death in patients with MVP tended to be greater than in patients without this condition.[33] Finally, a small proportion of MVP patients will demonstrate increased joint mobility, a feature dramatically demonstrated in the Marfan and Ehlers-Danlos syndromes, but they are no more likely to have joint displacement, injury, or arthritis.

Extracardiac Manifestations of Primary MVP

- Leaner bodies
- Lower body weights
- Lower blood pressures
- Taller
- Thinner
- Longer arm spans
- Narrower anteroposterior chest diameters
- Increased joint mobility

Clinical Guideline

The prognosis for most patients with MVP is benign. Serious complications will occur, however, in a minority. Male gender, age greater than 45, and the presence of mitral regurgitation are independent predictors of increased risk. Traditionally, severe mitral regurgitation, infectious endocarditis, stroke, and sudden death were believed to be the possible major complications of MVP; recent data, however, have found no increased risk of neurological ischemic events,[34] and only older forensic studies have demonstrated an extremely rare association between sudden death and MVP. It is clear that patients with MVP and hemodynamically significant mitral regurgitation have an increased risk of sudden death, just as those with hemodynamically significant mitral regurgitation from other causes, but it is uncertain that patients without associated significant regurgitation are at an increased risk.

Severe mitral regurgitation is the most common major complication of MVP. Five and a half percent of men and 1.5% of women with MVP will require mitral valve repair or replacement by age 75.[35] Mild mitral regurgitation can progress significantly during long-term follow-up; therefore, appropriated monitoring is crucial.

Infectious endocarditis occurs in patients with MVP at a relative risk of three to eight times the general population[36]; however, the cumulative risk for contracting it by age 75 is less than 1%. Dental procedures have been shown to be responsible for the inciting bacteremia in approximately one-third of the cases.

Management of patients with MVP varies depending on their risk. Younger women (<45 years) without mitral regurgitation should be reassured that their condition is benign, and the associated low blood pressure and body weight are desirable. Endocarditis prophylaxis does not clearly benefit this low-risk group.[37] They should be re-evaluated every 5 years to ensure that they have not progressed into a higher risk group.

Patients with MVP who have mild mitral regurgitation are a group with a slightly increased risk of endocarditis and the development of mitral regurgitation. Antibiotic prophylaxis (2 g amoxicillin 1 hour before procedure; clindamycin in penicillin-allergic patients) is recommended before dental work that may cause gum bleeding.[22,38]

Management of MVP Relative to Risk of Complications

- Low risk—No mitral regurgitation (especially in women younger than 45 years).
  Management: Reassurance
  No absolute indication for antibiotics
  Re-evaluate clinically and with echocardiography every 5 years
- Moderate risk—Mild mitral regurgitation on Doppler
  Management: Antibiotic prophylaxis before dental work
  (2 g amoxicillin, 1 hour before procedure; clindamycin if penicillin allergy).
  Treat even mild hypertension.
  Re-evaluate clinically and with echocardiography every 2–3 years.
- High risk—Moderate or severe mitral regurgitation.
  Management: Antibiotic prophylaxis before dental work.
  (2 g amoxicillin, 1 hour before procedure; clindamycin if penicillin allergy).

Treat even mild hypertension.
Re-evaluate clinically and with echocardiography annually.
Mitral valve repair/replacement needs to be considered if exertional dyspnea or left ventricular impairment is present.

Clinical Guideline

MVP patients with recurrent syncope or presyncope may be symptomatic from orthostatic hypotension resulting from a relatively reduced blood volume, and, as mentioned earlier, this is oftentimes exacerbated by factors that can contribute to dehydration. This can be relieved by fluid intake and salt supplementation. Refractory symptoms can be treated with fludrocortisone (Florinef), 0.05 to 0.10 mg/day.

SUDDEN CARDIAC DEATH

Occurrences of sudden death in athletes are of intense concern and interest to both the medical and lay communities. However, sudden cardiac death in competitive athletes is an extremely rare event. Between 10 and 25 sports-related sudden cardiac deaths occur annually in the United States.[39] Exercise does acutely and transiently increase the risk of cardiac events; however, the absolute instances of exercise deaths are quite low. Only approximately 0.75 and 0.13 per 100,000 young male and female athletes, respectively, and 6 per 100,000 middle aged men die during exertion per year.[40] Collapse usually occurs during or shortly after exercise, either in training or competition. Age is the most useful variable in predicting the underlying pathological condition. Most sudden cardiac deaths are due to congenital abnormalities in athletes less than 35 years, whereas atherosclerotic coronary artery disease is the most common cause in those older than 35. The most common congenital causes are hypertrophic obstructive cardiomyopathy, coronary artery anomalies, and aortic dissection associated with Marfan syndrome. Atherosclerotic heart disease is found in only 10% of this younger group compared with 80% in those older than 35 years.[41]

Overall, sudden cardiac death accounts for approximately 300,000 to 400,000 deaths each year in this country. Women have a significantly lower incidence of sudden cardiac death compared with men who make up 70% to 89% of all sudden cardiac death victims.[42-44] A higher percentage of sudden cardiac deaths in women occurs in patients without a previous diagnosis of heart disease (64% vs 50%).[45] Among survivors of sudden cardiac death, only 45% of women compared with 80% of men have underlying coronary artery disease. Women are more likely to have valvular heart disease (13% vs 5%), idiopathic dilated cardiomyopathy (19% vs 10%), or a "normal" heart (10% vs 3%).[44]

Sudden Cardiac Death

- More common in men.
- Women are less likely to have a previous diagnosis of heart disease.
- Women survivors are less likely to have underlying coronary artery disease.

Clinical Guideline

Structural abnormalities can be identified in greater than 90% of young victims of sudden cardiac death.[46–48] In the pediatric population, about 40% of sudden cardiac deaths occur in patients with surgically corrected congenital cardiac abnormalities, tetralogy of Fallot and transposition of the great vessels being the most common.[49] In otherwise healthy appearing young individuals, however, sudden cardiac death is often the first manifestation of underlying cardiac disease. Hypertrophic obstructive cardiomyopathy is a relatively uncommon cardiac malformation (0.1%–0.2% of the general population); however, it is of great importance because it is probably the most common cause of unexpected cardiac death in young people, including competitive athletes. The incidence of sudden death in patients with hypertrophic cardiomyopathy is 2% to 4% per year in adults and 4% to 6% per year in children and adolescents.[50]

It is a condition characterized by an asymmetrically hypertrophied and nondilated left ventricle in the absence of another cardiac or systemic disease associated with left ventricular hypertrophy. It produces a systolic murmur distinguished by accentuating with the Valsalva maneuver. It is genetically heterogeneous, having been found to be attributed to several distinct genetic defects involving myocardial contractile proteins and the ß-myosin heavy chain. Its morphological and clinical expression is particularly diverse. Recent guidelines to help delineate risk for sudden death have been described by Barry Maron.[51]

Hypertrophic Obstructive Cardiomyopathy— Prognostic Indicators of Risk for Sudden Death

High risk
History of:
Cardiac arrest
Sustained ventricular tachycardia
Multiple familial sudden deaths
Repetitive nonsustained ventricular tachycardia
Presence of:
Massive left ventricular hypertrophy (>35 mm)
Adverse genotype
Low risk
Absence of:
Symptoms

Massive left ventricular hypertrophy (<35 mm)
Ventricular tachycardia on Holter monitoring
Hypotensive blood pressure response to exercise

Clinical Guideline

Major Causes of Sudden Death in Young Athletes

- Coronary artery anomalies
- Aortic dissection from the Marfan syndrome
- Wolff-Parkinson-White syndrome
- Long QT syndrome
- Arrhythmogenic right ventricular dysplasia
- Right ventricular outflow tract tachycardia
- Myocarditis
- Dilated cardiomyopathy
- Cocaine use
- Electrolyte abnormalities, particularly hypokalemia and hypomagnesemia

Clinical Guideline

PREPARTICIPATION SCREENING

The cardiovascular evaluation is an extremely important component of the preparticipation examination of the athlete. Screening programs for identifying the relatively rare cardiac abnormalities that may cause sudden cardiac death in large populations of asymptomatic athletes have been found to be costly and inefficient.[52] General screening for participation in sports should always include a detailed personal and family medical history. The athlete should be questioned about chest pain, dyspnea, palpitations, lightheadedness, and frank syncope. The family history should focus on premature or sudden death, syncope, arrhythmias, hypertension, and coronary heart disease. Blood pressure should be measured in all children 3 years of age or older. A careful cardiac examination needs to be performed with auscultation of the heart and examination of extremity pulses. The American Heart Association Science Advisory and Coordinating Committee appointed a panel to compose a consensus statement regarding the preparticipation screening of athletes. Those recommendations are found in the Clinical Guideline below.[53] The American Heart Association Statement recommends that a history and physical examination be performed before participation in organized high school and college sports and be repeated every 2 years. In intervening years, a repeat history should be obtained. Cholesterol levels should be measured in anyone older than 25 years of age, in obese or hypertensive children, and in children with a family history of hypercholesterolemia or premature coronary artery disease.[54] Electrocardiograms, echocardiograms, and other noninvasive tests are generally reserved for those with any abnormalities on the initial evaluation.[55]

The American Heart Association's Recommendations for Cardiovascular Preparticipation Screening of Competitive Athletes

*History**

Personal history of
  Exertional chest pain
  Syncope and presyncope
  Excessive exertional dyspnea or fatigue
Past detection of
  Heart murmur
  Hypertension
Family history of
  Premature death
  Sudden death
  Significant coronary artery disease in close relatives <50 years
  Hypertrophic cardiomyopathy
  Dilated cardiomyopathy
  Long QT syndrome
  Marfan syndrome
  Clinically important arrhythmias

Physical examination

Precordial auscultation in supine and standing positions, specifically attempting to identify a murmur of left ventricular outflow obstruction
Assessment of femoral artery pulses to exclude coarctation of aorta
Recognition of physical stigmata of Marfan syndrome (tall stature, joint hypermobility, pectus excavatum, reduced thoracic kyphosis, scoliosis, arachnodactyly, myopia)
Brachial blood pressure measurement in sitting position

*Parents should be involved with completing the history for a minor athlete.

Clinical Guideline

RECOMMENDATIONS FOR PARTICIPATION IN SPORTS FOR PATIENTS WITH HEART DISEASE

Physicians and other health care providers make recommendations to patient athletes. Recent controversies involving high-profile athletes as to whether they should be allowed to compete have undermined the trust of the medical community by the lay public. Medical experts were sharply divergent with regard to their diagnosis and evaluation of the risks associated with Reggie Lewis, the Boston Celtic's basketball player. One team of doctors advised him not to play, whereas others thought he could. Lewis died during a medically unsupervised workout, and an autopsy showed his heart to be abnormal, with ventricular cavity enlargement and scarring, findings consistent with a healed myocarditis.

Anthony Penny was a promising basketball player at Central Connecticut State University. In 1989 he filed a malpractice suit against a cardiologist who diagnosed him with hypertrophic cardiomyopathy and recommended against his continued participation in college basketball. After two other cardiologists concurred with his opinion, the university refused to allow him to play for two seasons. He ultimately obtained medical clearance from two other cardiologists. *Penny v Sands* claimed economic harm to Penny's anticipated professional basketball career by his forced exclusion from intercollegiate competition. Penny subsequently collapsed and died suddenly in 1990 while playing in a professional basketball game in England. Although the suit had been voluntarily dismissed before his death, his story points out the high stakes involved when making such recommendations.

The cardiology community has established a consensus statement for athletic participation for patients with a diagnosis of a cardiovascular disorder. The reader is referred to this most recent Task Force on Cardiovascular Abnormalities in the Athlete and its recommendations regarding eligibility of patients for competition. This is the most comprehensive consensus statement available. Its purpose is to provide guidelines. There are no gender-specific recommendations, because currently no evidence exists to warrant them.[52]

REFERENCES

1. Astrand PO. Human physical fitness with special reference to sex and age. *Physiol Rev.* 1956;36:307–316.
2. Astrand I. Aerobic work capacity in men and women with special reference to age. *Acta Physiol Scand.* 1960;49:169–180.
3. O'Toole ML, Hiller WDB, Douglas PS, et al. Cardiovascular responses to prolonged cycling and running. *Med Sci Sports Exerc.* 1985;17:219–224.
4. Pelliccia A, Maron BJ, Culasso F, et al. Athlete's heart in women. Echocardiographic characterization of highly trained elite female athletes. *JAMA.* 1996;276:211–215.
5. Williams PT. High-density lipoprotein cholesterol and other risk factors for coronary heart disease in female runners. *N Engl J Med.* 1996;330:1325–1327.
6. Haddock BL, Hopp HP, Mason JJ, et al. Cardiorespiratory fitness and cardiovascular disease risk factors in postmenopausal women. *Med Sci Sport Exerc.* 1998;30:893–898.

7. Manson JE, Hu FB, Rich-Edwards JW, et al. A prospective study of walking as compared with vigorous exercise in the prevention of coronary heart disease in women. *N Engl J Med.* 1999;341:650–658.

8. The CASS Investigators. Myocardial infarction and mortality in the Coronary Artery Surgery Study (CASS) randomized trial. *N Engl J Med.* 1984;310:750–758.

9. Barolsky SM, Gilbert CA, Faruqui A, et al. Differences in electrocardiographic response to exercise in women and men: A non-Bayesian factor. *Circulation.* 1979;60:1021–1024.

10. Borer JS, Bacharach SL, Green MV, et al. Real-time radionuclide cineangiography in the non-invasive evaluation of global and regional left ventricular function at rest and during exercise in patients with coronary artery disease. *N Engl J Med.* 1977;296:839–843.

11. Higginbotham MB, Morris KG, Coleman E, et al. Sex-related differences in the normal cardiac response to upright exercise. *Circulation.* 1984;70:357–362.

12. Taillefer R, De Puey EG, Udelson JE, et al. Comparative diagnostic accuracy of Tl-201 and Tc-99m sestamibi SPECT imaging (perfusion and ECG-gated SPECT) in detecting coronary artery disease in women. *J Am Coll Cardiol.* 1997;29:69–77.

13. Marwick TH, Anderson T, Williams MJ, et al. Exercise echocardiography is an accurate and cost-efficient technique for detection of coronary artery disease in women. *J Am Coll Cardiol.* 1995;26:335–341.

14. Harlan WR, Sandler SA, Lee KL, et al. Importance of baseline functional and socioeconomic factors for participation in cardiac rehabilitation. *Am J Cardiol.* 1995;76:36–39.

15. Halm M, Penque S, Doll N, et al. Women and cardiac rehabilitation: Referral and compliance patterns. *J Cardiovasc Nurs.* 1999;13:83–92.

16. Brezinka V, Dusseldorp E, Maes S. Gender differences in psychosocial profile at entry into cardiac rehabilitation. *J Cardiopulm Rehabil.* 1998;18:445–449.

17. Lavie CJ, Milani RV, Cassidy MM, et al. Effects of cardiac rehabilitation and exercise training programs in women with depression. *Am J Cardiol.* 1999;83:1480–1483.

18. Northcote RJ, Canning GP, Ballantyne D. Electrocardiographic findings in male veteran endurance athletes. *Br Heart J.* 1989;61:155–160.

19. Calkins H, Seifert M, Morady F. Clinical presentation and long-term follow-up of athletes with exercise-induced vasodepressor syncope. *Am Heart J.* 1995;129:1159–1164.

20. Mtinangi BL, Hainsworth R. Increased orthostatic tolerance following moderate exercise training in patients with unexplained syncope. *Sports Med.* 1995;19:223–234.

21. Systolic Hypertension in the Elderly Program (SHEP) Cooperative Research Group. Prevention of stroke by antihypertensive drug treatment in older persons with isolated systolic hypertension. *JAMA.* 1991;265:3255–3264.

22. Shahi M, Thom S, Poulter N, et al. Regression of hypertensive left ventricular hypertrophy and left ventricular diastolic function. *Lancet.* 1990;336:458–461.

23. Modesti PA, Olivo G, Pestelli F, et al. Peripheral vascular resistance limits exercise functional capacity of mild hypertensives. *Angiology.* 1999;50:473–478.

24. Feinstein RA, Soileau EJ, Daniel WA Jr. A national survey of pre-participation physical examination requirements. *Phys Sportsmed.* 1988;16:51–59.

25. Singh JP, Larson MG, Manolio TA, et al. Blood pressure response during treadmill testing as a risk factor for new-onset hypertension. The Framingham heart study. *Circulation.* 1999;99:1831–1836.

26. Ewart CK, Young DR, Hagberg JM. Effects of school-based aerobic exercise on blood pressure in adolescent girls at risk for hypertension. *Am J Public Health.* 1998;88:949–951.

27. Devereux RB, Kramer-Fox R, et al. Inheritance of mitral valve prolapse: Effect of age and sex on gene expression. *Ann Intern Med.* 1982;97:826–832.

28. Devereux RB, Kramer-Fox R, Brown WT, et al. Relation between clinical features of mitral valve prolapse syndrome and echocardiographically documented mitral valve prolapse. *J Am Coll Cardiol.* 1986;8:763–772.

29. Santos AD, Mathew PK, Hilal A, et al. Orthostatic hypotension: A commonly unrecognized cause of symptoms of mitral valve prolapse. *Am J Med.* 1981;71:746–750.

30. Savage DD, Garrison RJ, Devereux RB, et al. Mitral valve prolapse in the general population. 1. Epidemiologic features: The Framingham Study. *Am Heart J.* 1983,106:571–576.

31. Devereux RB, Brown WT, Lutas EM, et al. Association of mitral valve prolapse with low body weight and low blood pressure. *Lancet.* 1982;2:792–795.

32. Schutte JE, Gaffney FA, Blend L, et al. Distinctive anthropometric characteristics of women with mitral valve prolapse. *Am Med J.* 1981;71:533–538.

33. Davies MJ, Moore BP, Baimbridge MV. The floppy mitral valve. Study of incidence, pathology, and complications in surgical necroscopy, and forensic material. *Br Heart J.* 1978;40:468–481.

34. Gilon D, Buonanno FS, Jaffe MM, et al. Lack of evidence of an association between mitral valve prolapse and stroke in young patients. *N Engl J Med.* 1999;341:8–13.

35. Zuppirolia A, Rinaldi M, Kramer-Fox R, et al. Natural histories of mitral valve prolapse. *J Am Coll Cardiol.* 1997;29:506A.

36. MacMahon S, Roberts JK, Kramer-Fox R, et al. Mitral valve prolapse and infective endocarditis. *Am Heart J.* 1987;113:1291–1298.

37. Devereux RB, Frary CJ, Kramer-Fox R, et al. Cost-effectiveness of infective endocarditis prophylaxis for mitral valve prolapse with or without a mitral regurgitant murmur. *Am J Cardiol.* 1994;74:1024–1029.

38. Dajani AS, Taubert KA, Wilson W, et al. Prevention of bacterial endocarditis. Recommendations by the American Heart Association. *JAMA.* 1997;277:1794–1801.

39. Liberthson RR. Sudden death from cardiac causes in children and young adults. *N Engl J Med.* 1996;334:1039–1044.

40. Thompson PD. The cardiovascular complications of vigorous physical activity. *Arch Intern Med.* 1996;156:2297–2302.

41. Maron BJ, Epstein SE, Roberts WC. Causes of sudden death in competitive athletes. *J Am Coll Cardiol.* 1986;7:204–214.

42. Kannel WB, Thomas HE Jr. Sudden coronary death: The Framingham Study. *Ann NY Acad Sci.* 1982;382:3–20.

43. Kannel WB, Schatzkin A. Sudden death: Lessons from subsets in population studies. *J Am Coll Card.* 1985;5(Suppl);141B–149B.

44. Albert CM, McGovern BA, Newell JB, et al. Sex differences in cardiac arrest survivors. *Circulation.* 1996;93:1170–1176.

45. Kannel WB, Cupples LA, D'Agostino RB. Sudden death risk in overt coronary heart disease: The Framingham study. *Am Heart J.* 1987;113:799–804.

46. Driscoll DJ, Edwards WD. Sudden unexpected death in children and adolescents. *J Am Coll Cardiol.* 1985;5(Suppl):118B–121B.

47. Liberthson RR. Sudden death from cardiac causes in children and young adults. *N Engl J Med.* 1996;334:1039–1044.

48. Topaz O, Edwards JE. Pathological features of sudden death in children, adolescents and young adults. *Chest.* 1985;87:476–482.

49. Garson CA Jr, McNamara DG. Sudden death in a pediatric cardiology population, 1958–1983: Relation to prior arrhythmias. *J Am Coll Cardiol.* 1985;5(Suppl):134B–137B.

50. McKenna WJ, Camm AJ. Sudden death in hypertrophic cardiomyopathy: A profile of 78 patients. *Circulation.* 1989;80:1489–1492.

51. Maron BJ. Hypertrophic cardiomyopathy. *Lancet.* 1997;350:127–133.

52. Maron BJ, Bodison S, Wesley Y, et al. Results of screening a large population of intercollegiate athletes for cardiovascular disease. *J Am Coll Cardiol.* 1987;10:1214–1222.

53. McGrew CA. Insights into the AHA scientific statement concerning cardiovascular preparticipation screening of competitive athletes. *Med Sc. Sports Exerc.* 1998;30:351–353.

54. Gutgesell HP, Atkins DL, Day RW. Common cardiovascular problems in the young: Part II. Hypertension, hypercholesterolemia and preparticipation screening of athletes. *Am Fam Physician.* 1997;56:1993–1998.

55. Maron BJ, Mitchell JH. 26th Bethesda Conference: Recommendations for determining eligibility for competition in athletes with cardiovascular abnormalities. *J Am Coll Cardiol.* 1994;24:845–899.

CHAPTER 15

Exercise and the Female with Cancer

Stacy A. Harris

INTRODUCTION

Cancer continues to be one of the leading causes of morbidity and mortality in women in the United States. Breast cancer constitutes 30% of all new cancer cases in women; whereas lung and colorectal cancers account for 13% and 11%, respectively.[1] Current statistics estimate that one in eight women will develop breast cancer during her lifetime.[2] Fortunately, recent major advances in medical treatments have drastically increased the rates of cancer survival and cure.

Today, compared with several decades ago, more women participate in regular exercise. As a result, cancer frequently strikes women who are physically active. Unfortunately, limited information exists regarding exercise during cancer therapy and after medical treatment ends. Because of the traditional belief that vigorous exertion is potentially harmful for cancer patients, many physicians are cautious when advising their cancer patients about return to exercise. This chapter examines the present knowledge of the benefits of exercise in cancer, reviews the impact of cancer and its treatments on exercise ability, presents recommended guidelines and precautions, and suggests areas for future research.

ETIOLOGY

The literature well documents the role of exercise in the prevention of many chronic diseases.[3,4] Evidence that physical activity is associated with a reduced risk of cancer,

however, has been less clear. Some studies have suggested that physical activity influences cancer risk through various mechanisms, whereas other studies have failed to demonstrate this association. Researchers have hypothesized that exercise may protect against breast cancer by altering ovulatory cycles, changing body fat composition, or by promoting natural immunity.[5–8]

Common reproductive patterns and obesity in women who develop breast cancer suggest that female hormones and metabolism contribute to the cause of the disease.[5] Strenuous exercise during adolescence may reduce breast cancer risk by causing increased age at menarche, anovulation, and longer cycle lengths, which all decrease total exposure to cyclic estrogen and progesterone.[7] Frisch[9] observed delayed menarche and amenorrhea in young female ballet dancers. In another study, Frisch et al[10] demonstrated that women who participated in college athletics regularly were less likely to develop breast and reproductive system cancers. A study by Paffenbarger et al,[11] however, failed to show an association between college athletes and breast cancer. Furthermore, data collected by Dorgan et al[12] did not support a protective effect of moderate to heavy physical activity during adulthood from breast cancer. In a prospective study of 25,624 women, Thune et al[13] found a 37% reduction in the risk of breast cancer among women who participated in regular exercise. The greatest risk reduction, however, occurred in lean women of all ages. Although the exact mechanism of how obesity is associated with breast cancer is unknown, it is thought to possibly result from alterations in the production and metabolism of estrogen by adipose tissue. By reducing body fat stores, exercise decreases the conversion of androgens and estrogens to potent carcinogenic agents.[14,15]

The author gratefully acknowledges Henry Jones, PhD, for assistance in preparation of this chapter.

The long-term effects of endurance training on the immune system include increased number and activity of macrophages, natural killer cells, and lymphokine-activated killer cells and their regulatory cytokines. In a randomized controlled study, Nieman and Henson[8] found that moderate exercise training is associated with reduced upper respiratory tract infections. A review by Shephard et al[16] suggested that moderate endurance exercise has a beneficial effect on the immune system, whereas intense exhausting exercise tends to produce an adverse effect on the immune response. Thus, the intensity of exercise appears to determine whether the immune system responds favorably or negatively. Despite the lack of clear evidence that exercise reduces the risk of breast cancer, physicians should encourage patients to keep physically active because of the proven role of exercise in reducing the risk of other forms of cancer and chronic diseases.[17,19]

THE GOALS OF EXERCISE IN CANCER PATIENTS

Exercise is a specific physical activity performed to obtain a therapeutic response. Most cancer patients experience deficits in strength, range of motion, and endurance as a result of the effects of chemotherapy, radiation therapy, and surgery. These deficits can be minimized or corrected through exercise. The goals of exercise depend on the type of cancer, stage of disease, required treatment, and premorbid physical condition. The purpose of exercise in cancer patients may be preventative during early stages to avoid deconditioning and contractures. During remissions or after cure, exercise may be restorative to combat the effects of illness and treatments. Those cancer patients who were mild to moderate exercisers before diagnosis may merely wish to resume their premorbid exercise program. On the other hand, those who were competitive athletes may desire to return to a vigorous exercise program necessary for training.

CANCER-RELATED FATIGUE

Fatigue is the most common and debilitating problem among cancer patients. Fatigue and impaired physical performance affect up to 70% of cancer patients during chemotherapy or radiation therapy.[20] Potential causes of fatigue include sleep disturbances,[21] impaired nutrition, decreased level of activity, psychosocial factors, and biochemical changes resulting from disease and treatment.[22] Return of energy to premorbid level is inversely proportional to age, stage of disease, and intensity of treatment and may take months to years.[23] Most patients undergoing chemotherapy treatment experience tiredness,[24,25] and women receiving intracavitary radiation for gynecologic cancer report increased physical fatigue.[26] Postchemotherapy treatment fatigue occurs during the first several days, peaks at approximately 10 days, and decreases until the next treatment.[27] In addition, cancer patients describe decreased symptoms of fatigue on weekends when not undergoing radiation therapy[28] and a gradual decline of these symptoms 3 months after completion of radiation therapy.[29] Fatigue can become severe enough to interfere with daily activities, limit treatment doses, and impair quality of life.

DECONDITIONING

Inevitably, physiological body changes occur in cancer patients that cause them to decrease their activity levels. Prolonged sedentariness leads to deconditioning, which affects every major body system. For instance, cardiorespiratory insufficiency, orthostatic hypotension, joint contractures, skin breakdown, urinary calculi, osteoporosis, phlebothrombosis, and psychological deterioration can occur during prolonged bedrest. During the first week of bedrest, muscular atrophy occurs with 3% loss of muscle strength per day.[30] To diminish fatigue, physicians often prescribe bedrest and reduced activity level. Unfortunately, the syndrome of deconditioning can further exacerbate cancer-related fatigue.

THE BENEFITS OF EXERCISE IN CANCER

Several studies of cancer patients have demonstrated numerous benefits from an exercise program. These benefits include a decrease in pain and other treatment side effects as well as improvement in emotional status, functional capacity, and quality of life. By enhancing levels of endorphins,[31] physical exercise has been shown to raise the pain threshold.[32,33] In a randomized study by Dimeo et al[34] of 33 cancer patients receiving high-dose chemotherapy followed by autologous peripheral blood stem cell transplantation, the training group, which participated in a supine bicycle ergometry progressive exercise program, required less analgesics compared with the control group. This study also demonstrated a shorter duration of neutropenia and length of hospital stay in the training group. In a randomized study of 42 women with breast cancer, Winningham and MacVicar[35] showed moderate activity with supine bicycle ergometry to be beneficial in managing chemotherapy-induced nausea. In a study of 46 women with breast cancer, Mock et al[36] demonstrated that a self-paced, home-based walking exercise program improved physical functioning, managed anxiety, decreased insomnia, and reduced fatigue during radiation treatment. Another study by Dimeo et al[37] has also shown that an exercise training program consisting of 6 weeks of daily treadmill walking is effective in decreasing fatigue, improving emotional stability, and increasing confidence and independence. Although symptoms of fatigue and side effects of treatment may alter a cancer patient's ability to exercise, MacVicar et al[38] demonstrated that aerobic training can still induce physiological adaptation sufficient to improve functional capacity. Because cancer treatments can deplete the body of natural and exogenous estrogens, cancer patients have an increased risk of coronary artery disease and osteoporosis developing. Aerobic exercise reduces the risk of coronary artery disease and osteoporosis. In addition, aerobic exercise can decrease weight gain that often accompanies adjuvant chemotherapy.[39] Furthermore, women with breast cancer who exercise experience a higher quality of life compared with those with breast cancer who do not exercise.[40]

The Benefits of Exercise in Cancer

- Decreased pain
- Decreased chemotherapy-induced nausea
- Improved emotional status
- Decreased fatigue
- Increased functional capacity
- Decreased insomnia
- Improved quality of life
- Improved anxiety
- Decreased duration of neutropenia
- Increased confidence
- Decreased length of hospitalization
- Increased independence
- Decreased coronary artery disease
- Decreased osteoporosis

Clinical Guideline

THE IMPACT OF CANCER ON EXERCISE

Many physically active women who are diagnosed with cancer desire to continue exercising both during and after treatment. They are often unaware, however, of the consequences of cancer and treatment side effects on exercise ability. Treatment typically consists of chemotherapy, radiation therapy, or surgery, either alone or in combination. Potential side effects of cancer treatments include nausea, vomiting, diarrhea, anorexia, nutritional deficiencies, metabolic disturbances, and electrolyte imbalances. These side effects along with hematopoietic abnormalities such as leukopenia, thrombocytopenia, and anemia can impair exercise ability. In addition, cancer treatment often includes the use of corticosteroids, which, if used long term, can cause hyperglycemia and osteoporosis. The side effects of cancer treatments can occur weeks, months, to even years after completion of therapy. Furthermore, the antineoplastic mechanisms of chemotherapy and radiation therapy that involve inhibition of protein synthesis may alter the biochemical adaptation process necessary for a training effect.

Cancer Treatment Side Effects That Impair Exercise Ability

- Nausea
- Nutritional deficiencies
- Vomiting
- Metabolic disturbances
- Diarrhea
- Electrolyte imbalances
- Pain
- Leukopenia
- Fatigue
- Thrombocytopenia
- Anorexia
- Anemia

Clinical Guideline

Treatments

Chemotherapy

Chemotherapeutic agents target and destroy rapidly dividing cancer cells. Unfortunately, actively dividing normal cells are also susceptible to the deleterious effects of these agents. The action of chemotherapeutic drugs on the rapidly dividing cells of the gastrointestinal lining can lead to nausea, vomiting, anorexia, stomatitis, and mucosal ulcerations. Furthermore, chemotherapeutic agents can alter taste sensation, which along with the consequences of the compromised gastrointestinal tract can impair nutritional status.[41] Some chemotherapeutic agents can cause hepatic and renal impairment, whereas others can alter the function of hormone-producing organs. Dysfunction of the ovaries caused by chemotherapeutic drugs can lead to early menopause.[42] Because of the effects of chemotherapeutic drugs on the bone marrow cells and blood, hematopoietic abnormalities frequently occur, such as anemia, leukopenia, and thrombocytopenia.[41] A below normal white blood count can increase the risk of infection, whereas low platelets can increase the risk of bruising and intra-articular bleeding. Anemia may cause fatigue; however, research has failed to show a correlation between the amount of fatigue and the severity of anemia,[43] except when hemoglobin levels are extremely low.[44] Fluorouracil can lead to cerebellar dysfunction, whereas intrathecal methotrexate can produce delayed encephalopathy. In addition to fatigue, some chemotherapeutic agents can cause cognitive deficits such as visual-perceptive, verbal, memory, and judgment impairments.[45] Doxorubicin hydrochloride can cause cardiac dysfunction, whereas bleomycin sulfate can lead to pulmonary fibrosis. In addition, cisplatin, mitomycin, carmustine, and cyclophosphamide can cause hearing loss, while vincristine and cytarabine may lead to peripheral neuropathy. Finally, another effect of chemotherapeutic agents involves increasing treated patients' risk of developing secondary cancers, such as leukemia or solid tumors.[42]

Although each chemotherapeutic agent typically causes characteristic side effects, each patient's experience with treatment is different. This variability in manifestation of side effects is due to the kind of chemotherapy administered, total dose of medication received, duration of treatment, previous or concurrent treatments, such as radiation therapy, and route of therapy, such as oral, intravenous, or intrathecal.[42]

Chemotherapy Side Effects

- Nausea
- Leukopenia
- Hearing loss
- Vomiting
- Thrombocytopenia
- Cardiac dysfunction
- Fatigue
- Peripheral neuropathy
- Pulmonary fibrosis
- Anorexia
- Encephalopathy
- Nephrotoxicity
- Mucosal ulceration
- Cognitive deficits
- Hepatotoxicity
- Stomatitis
- Cerebellar dysfunction
- Metabolic disturbances
- Anemia
- Early menopause
- Electrolyte imbalances
- Secondary malignancy

Clinical Guideline

Radiation Therapy

The effects of radiation therapy depend on the region of the body treated. Like chemotherapy, radiation therapy causes damage to rapidly dividing cells. Exposure of the actively dividing normal cells of the linings of the respiratory and gastrointestinal tracts to radiation can cause dry mouth, sore throat, altered taste, difficulty swallowing, and diarrhea. Late effects of radiation to the bowel can lead to bowel obstruction as a result of scarring. In addition, cancers that require radiation to the chest, such as breast and lung cancers, may cause pneumonitis and pulmonary fibrosis with resultant restrictive lung disease. Exposure of the thyroid and ovaries to radiation can lead to metabolic abnormalities, early menopause, and infertility. Acutely, ra-

diation to the head can cause headaches and nausea. Delayed effects of radiation to the head, however, can lead to focal necrosis of white matter, cognitive deficits, calcification, necrotizing leukoencephalopathy, and aneurysms. Like chemotherapy, radiation therapy can cause thrombocytopenia and increase the risk of secondary cancers. Finally, radiation to the spinal cord and peripheral nervous system can cause myelopathy and plexopathy.[41]

Radiation Therapy Side Effects

- Nausea
- White matter necrosis
- Infertility
- Vomiting
- Brain calcification
- Bowel obstruction
- Diarrhea
- Necrotizing leukoencephalopathy
- Aneurysm
- Headache
- Pneumonitis
- Plexopathy
- Altered taste
- Pulmonary fibrosis
- Myelopathy
- Swallowing difficulties
- Cognitive deficits
- Thrombocytopenia
- Demyelination
- Metabolic disturbances
- Early menopause
- Secondary malignancy

Clinical Guideline

Surgery

The effects of surgical treatment for cancer usually manifest immediately after surgery. Some of these effects resolve within weeks, whereas others may exhibit a protracted course. Initially, surgical procedures increase energy demands of the body for healing of the surgical incision, reduce activity level, cause pain, and require pain medications for comfort. Hormonal and metabolic changes, however, because of loss of organ function, may have long-term side effects. In addition, altered body image or function as a result of mastectomy or amputation may require significant adaptations and have long-lasting implications.[42]

Exercise and the Premorbidly Active Cancer Patient

Prior research has focused on sedentary subjects with cancer who exercise, but several recent studies have addressed exercise in the premorbidly physically active cancer patient. In a preliminary report of 55 physically active women with breast cancer who were primarily cyclists or runners, Schwartz and Winningham[46] reported fatigue, generalized weakness, muscular weakness, and irritability as the most frequently experienced symptoms. In a study by Wiley et al[47] that evaluated exercise tolerance before and after breast cancer therapy, data showed that subjects treated with chemotherapy experienced reduced cardiorespiratory fitness and loss of functional capacity. In a survey by MacVicar and Winningham[48] of 254 cancer patients who identified themselves as regular exercisers, 40% of the respondents reported problems maintaining an exercise program. Although fatigue was reported as the major limiting factor in half of these respondents, more than half were able to continue an exercise program throughout the treatment period. In a survey of 219 premorbidly active male and female cancer patients who were an average of 43 months after treatment, Schwartz[49] studied the effects of cancer-related fatigue on exercise. Most respondents were recreational or national class athletes in a variety of sports who trained an average of 9 hours per week. Those that received chemotherapy, radiation therapy, and surgery experienced the most intense cancer-related fatigue. Although cancer-related fatigue significantly limited the subjects' abilities to maintain a high-intensity exercise program, most used moderate-intensity exercise as an effective strategy to reduce fatigue. Those subjects with non-Hodgkin's lymphoma, however, experienced different cancer-related fatigue and reported less benefits from exercise than breast cancer subjects.

The Most Frequent Complaints of Athletes with Breast Cancer

- Fatigue
- Generalized weakness
- Muscular weakness
- Irritability

Clinical Guideline

GUIDELINES AND PRECAUTIONS

The type of cancer, stage of disease, and treatment impose certain limitations on exercise. The sequela of the disease and the potentially harmful side effects of cancer treatment make exercise guidelines and precautions crucial. The literature outlines concerns and suggestions for optimal and safe exercise programs in cancer patients.

Screening

Before the initiation of an exercise program, all cancer patients should undergo medical screening.[50] This screening should include laboratory tests to assess platelets, hemoglobin, osmolality, glucose, and electrolytes, especially sodium and potassium. Because of the possible negative effects of cancer treatments on the heart and lung, cardiopulmonary status should be evaluated with pulmonary function tests, chest X-ray examination, electrocardiogram, and ejection fraction. Bone series X-ray studies and bone scans are necessary to rule out bony metastases. In addition, careful review of all medicines allows for identification of any side effects that may alter exercise response. Beta blockers, for example, interfere with the normal heart rate response to exercise.[51]

The Exercise Prescription

The exercise prescription must specify the type, frequency, intensity, and duration of exercise. For conditioning healthy persons, the American College of Sports Medicine recommends aerobic exercise, at a frequency of 3 to 7 days per week, at an intensity of 70% to 90% of maximal heart rate for 20 to 30 minutes' total duration.[50] Aerobic exercise involves rhythmic, repetitive movement of large muscle groups, such as walking, swimming, and bicycling. To stimulate the body to increase cardiopulmonary endurance or fitness, each body system must be challenged by aerobic exercise. Aerobic exercise improves the oxidative capacity of skeletal muscles and promotes adaptation of the aerobic biochemical system. This adaptation to exercise stimuli is the training effect.

The highest metabolic rate an individual can achieve on exertion is maximal oxygen uptake. Maximal oxygen uptake is an effective measure of functional capacity.[52] To maintain functional capacity, one must perform aerobic exercises. To obtain maximal benefits from exercise, a target heart rate based on a maximal heart rate must be reached during exercise. Generally, maximal heart rate can be identified by calculating 220 minus the age.[50] Setting the intensity of exercise based on rate of perceived exertion, such as the Borg scale, rather than on target heart rate may be necessary in some cancer patients because of treatment-related abnormal and variable physiological responses to exercise.[53] In the cancer patient undergoing treatment, however, a target of 40% to 65% of maximal heart rate is recommended when performing continuous exercise, such as walking.[50] If the target heart rate is greater than this, exercise in a supervised environment is advised.[54] Because heart rate is an indicator of exercise intensity, cancer patients should learn to monitor pulse during exercise.

The duration of exercise is determined by the premorbid activity level. A cancer patient who is very deconditioned because of surgery or other treatments should start with short exercise periods of 5 to 10 minutes and gradually progress as tolerated.[39] The important factor is the total duration of exercise, whether it is performed in many brief sessions or in one single session. The exercise prescription must include warm-up and cool-down periods and provide flexibility to accommodate fluctuations in the physical condition of cancer patients. In designing the exercise program, the team approach is most efficient with the team members, including the patient, exercise physiologist, oncology nurse, physical therapist, dietitian, and physician. The exercise program must be tailored to the individual needs and limitations of each cancer patient. Changes in the exercise program may include cross-training or modifying sport to accommodate any restrictions caused by the disease or treatment.

Other recommendations for cancer patients who exercise include wearing proper shoes and comfortable nonrestrictive clothing, carrying identification with medical and physician information, and exercising with a partner. They should schedule exercise during a time of the day when energy level is high and drink plenty of fluids before, during, and after exercise to avoid dehydration. They must make sure calorie and nutrient intakes are sufficient to meet the high nutritional demands of disease and increased physical activity. In addition, an exercise diary maintained by the patient helps to monitor response to exercise and to adjust the prescription accordingly.[54]

Contraindications to Exercise

At times, the effects of cancer and its treatment necessitate temporary restriction of exercise. Contraindications to exercise include unusual fatigability, unusual muscular weakness, fever, bleeding, development of irregular pulse, leg pain or cramps, chest pain, acute onset of nausea during exercise, vomiting or severe diarrhea within the previous 24 to 36 hours, disorientation, confusion, dizziness, blurred vision, faintness, pallor, cyanosis, sudden onset dyspnea, decrease in heart rate and/or blood pressure with increased workload, and intravenous chemotherapy within 24 hours.[55] Because one study has shown an increase in cardiac dysrhythmias within the first several hours after chemotherapy administration, exercise is discouraged on the same day of treatment.[56] Strenuous activity can cause a false elevation of white blood cell count and a nonspecific rise in liver enzymes. Because these laboratory results frequently serve to evaluate response to treatment and determine future therapy, cancer patients should avoid exercise on the day of blood tests. Leukopenia resulting from chemotherapy and radiation therapy leads to increased susceptibility to infection.

To reduce contact with potential pathogens during this vulnerable period, cancer patients should avoid crowded exercise facilities and swimming pools.[54] Chemotherapy treatment and disease recurrence preclude high-impact aerobic exercise.[39]

To avoid complications of bleeding, patients should not exercise if platelets fall below 20,000 to 25,000 mm. When platelets are between 25,000 and 50,000 mm, isometric and isotonic exercises using light weights are permitted; however, prolonged stretching, heavy resistive, and isokinetic exercises are contraindicated. If platelets are greater than 50,000 mm, most exercise programs are tolerated.[51] When the hemoglobin level drops to less than 10 g/dL, isometric and range of motion exercises are encouraged, whereas aerobic and isotonic exercises are discouraged. Light aerobic and isotonic exercises are allowed when hemoglobin level is between 10 and 12 g/dL. Most exercise programs are tolerated when the hemoglobin level is greater than 12 g/dL. Exercise is contraindicated in the presence of hyponatremia, hypokalemia, and low serum osmolality. Sodium and potassium levels less than 130 and 3.0, respectively, warrant medical evaluation and treatment. In addition, arrhythmias or any other abnormalities on electrocardiogram preclude exercise and should be investigated.[51]

Contraindications to Exercise

- Unusual fatigability
- Disorientation
- Unusual muscular weakness
- Confusion
- Fever
- Dizziness
- Bleeding
- Blurred vision
- Development of irregular pulse
- Faintness
- Leg pain or cramps
- Pallor
- Acute nausea
- Cyanosis
- Vomiting
- Sudden dyspnea
- Platelets <20,000–25,000 mm
- Chest pain
- Severe diarrhea within previous 24–36 hours
- Hyponatremia
- Intravenous chemotherapy within previous 24 hours
- Hypokalemia
- Decrease in heart rate or blood pressure with increased workload
- Low osmolality

Clinical Guideline

Chemotherapy Precautions

- Do not exercise on day of treatment.
- Avoid crowded exercise settings.
- Avoid exercising on day of blood tests.

Clinical Guideline

Hematopoietic Precautions

Platelets <20,000–25,000 mm: Do not exercise

Platelets 25,000–50,000 mm: Isometric and isotonic exercises with light weights only

Platelets >50,000 mm: Most exercises tolerated

Hemoglobin <10 g/dL: Isometric and range of motion exercises only

Hemoglobin 10–12 g/dL: Light aerobic and isotonic exercises

Hemoglobin >12 g/dL: Most exercises tolerated

Clinical Guideline

Monitoring

Treatments for specific types of cancer are standard; however, responses of patients to treatments widely vary. One cancer patient may have debilitating side effects from a treatment protocol, whereas another patient may experience minimal side effects. Because of this variability, any exercise program must be carefully monitored and routinely reevaluated. Frequent follow-up with the physician is imperative to evaluate for signs of decreased tolerance to exercise to modify the exercise program accordingly. In addition, cancer patients have an increased risk of a second cancer developing because of late effects of treatment.[57] Close monitoring allows for early identification and treatment of any secondary malignancy.

EXERCISE IN SPECIFIC TYPES OF CANCER

Breast Cancer

For decades, women with breast cancer who were treated with mastectomy have avoided vigorous exercise of the affected upper extremity because of fear of lymphedema. According to literature, the rates of breast cancer patients who experience lymphedema vary from 25.5% in those treated with radical mastectomy to 38.3% in those who underwent axillary node dissection.[58] Although the exact cause of lymphedema is unclear, it can be unpredictable and irreversible. Manifestations of lymphedema range from transient acute upper extremity swelling that occurs 6 weeks after surgery to a more gradual swelling that develops weeks to years later. Although a correlation exists between the number of lymph nodes surgically removed and the amount of lymphedema,[58] the incidence is higher in those postmastectomy patients who received radiation therapy and experienced delayed surgical wound healing.[59] Treatment for lymphedema generally includes upper-extremity elevation, exercise, gentle massage, elastic support garments, and intermittent compression pump.

Postmastectomy shoulder and upper extremity exercise programs vary according to the specific surgical procedure performed. Some researchers advocate immediate mobilization,[60] whereas others recommend avoiding full mobilization during the first several days postoperatively to allow the inflammatory reaction to decrease.[61] If mastectomy and reconstruction procedures were performed simultaneously, certain restrictions could last even longer. Generally, the exercise program begins during hospitalization and includes active hand and elbow range of motion exercises followed by hand and forearm isometric exercises. Next, active assisted shoulder range of motion exercises begin with gentle resistive exercises added after drain removal. Progressive resistance exercises begin several weeks postoperatively.[62] As a result of axillary node dissection,[63] serratus anterior palsy can cause latissimus dorsi and deltoid weakness. Often, tightening of the shoulder soft tissue occurs after radiation therapy. To prevent impaired shoulder function, a range of motion exercise program should be participated in indefinitely. Exercises that require prolonged dependent positions or intense exercise with heavy weights are contraindicated.[62] Within a few months, however, postmastectomy patients can resume activities such as swimming, golfing, and tennis,[64] as long as they are careful to avoid cuts, abrasions, or sunburns to the affected extremity. An article by McKenzie[65] reviewed the experience of 24 women breast cancer survivors who trained for and participated in dragon boat racing. In this group, McKenzie described anecdotal findings of no new cases of lymphedema.

Primary Bone Tumors and Bone Metastasis

Like renal cell, thyroid, lung, and prostate cancers, breast cancer has a high propensity to metastasize to bones with the proximal femur being the most commonly affected long bone site.[66] Pathological fractures occur in 10% to 30% of patients with metastatic lesions.[67] When painful bone lesions are greater than 2.5 cm in diameter, occupy 50% or greater of cortical diameter, or involve more than 50% of medullary cross-sectional or cortical areas, the risk of fracture is high.[66] Cortical involvement greater than 50% requires non-weight-bearing precaution and precludes exercise. Cortical involvement between 25% and 50% allows for partial weight bearing and range of motion exercises only.[48] Both isokinetic and progressive resistive exercises should be avoided in bony metastasis because of placing excessive stress on bones.[51] Whether the bone lesion is due to metastasis or primary bone tumor, treatment may involve surgical repair in the form of limb salvage or amputation procedures. Both of these procedures may necessitate casting, specific exercises, and weight-bearing precautions. Designing the optimal and safest exercise program requires consultation with the surgeon.

Exercise programs for patients after a limb-salvage procedure depend on the type of surgery performed. In general, the program should initially include range of motion and isometric exercises distal to the operated area with non-weight-bearing restrictions. As healing occurs, with permission of the surgeon, passive range of motion and isometric exercises of the affected joint begin with partial weight-bearing precautions. Later active range of motion, isometric, and light isotonic exercises of the affected joint follow with full weight-bearing. In addition, atrophied and partially resected muscles require strengthening and re-education.[51]

In the treatment of primary bone tumors, limb salvage procedures require less energy consumption with ambulation compared with above-the-knee amputations.[68] Amputations for primary tumors are performed at a higher anatomical level compared with those done for traumatic injuries or vascular disease. Frequent procedures include short above-the-knee amputation, short above-the-elbow amputation, forequarter, hip disarticulation, and hemipelvectomy. Patients who have undergone hemipelvectomies require 125% more energy to ambulate with prostheses compared with normal persons.[69] Because of the great energy expenditure required, cardiopulmonary status and limitations must be considered when planning an exercise program. The exercise program for amputations should include preoperative isometric and range of motion exercises and postoperative isometric and isotonic exercises. In addition, aerobic exercises are executed to prevent contractures, increase strength, and improve endurance.[51] Exercises in both patients with limb-savage procedures and amputations aid in preparation for and successful use of braces or limb prostheses.

Lung Cancer

Often, the treatment of primary lung tumors or pulmonary metastasis includes chemotherapy, radiation therapy, and surgical resection. The side effects of treatment, however, can cause impaired pulmonary function and altered breathing mechanics. Pulmonary function tests are helpful in accurately assessing lung status. During and after lung cancer treatment, exercises should focus on improving diaphragm excursion, teaching breathing techniques, incorporating energy-conservation strategies, and increasing endurance. Symptoms and oxygen saturation levels during exercise determine any necessary supplemental oxygen requirements.

Colorectal Cancer

Many patients who are diagnosed with colorectal cancer undergo ileostomy or colostomy surgeries. Exercise not only firms and strengthens the abdominal muscles that may be weakened as a result of surgery but also maintains regular gastric motility that aids in ostomy management. Ostomies do not prohibit patients from exercise and sports activities. Postostomy patients can participate in running, cycling, tennis, skiing, golfing, and even swimming with a nonwater-soluble pouch seal. If participating in contact sports, however, belts, girdles, and other protective equipment may be helpful. In addition, excessive sweating may make more frequent pouch changes necessary and require increased oral fluid intake to replace fluid losses.[70]

Cancers Requiring Bone Marrow Transplantation

Patients who are diagnosed with leukemia and some other forms of cancer frequently undergo bone marrow transplantation. This type of treatment requires significantly prolonged hospitalizations that lead to severe deconditioning. Exercise after bone marrow transplantation should focus on reducing and preventing muscle atrophy while maintaining joint range of motion, endurance, balance, and coordination. The exercise program should start slowly with range of motion, stretching, and isometric stretching exercises followed by light isotonic strengthening and submaximal aerobic exercises. To reduce the risk of bleeding or infection, hematological precautions should be carefully followed.[51] One recent study by Dimeo et al[71] has shown that cancer patients can participate in an aerobic exercise program after bone marrow transplantation without dangerous consequences.

Primary Brain Tumors and Brain Metastasis

The treatment of primary brain tumors and brain metastasis depends on the type of tumor, location, and number of lesions. Frequently, brain lesions and subsequent treatments cause neurological deficits such as hemiparesis and altered sensation, as well as impaired cognition, balance, and coordination. Because of cognitive deficits, patients may lose awareness of their limitations. Each of these sequela can adversely affect the ability to exercise. Some clinicians suggest that patients with severe cerebellar dysfunction should avoid aerobic exercise.[51]

Head and Neck Cancers

Surgeries for head and neck tumors often result in neck and shoulder dysfunction. Radical neck dissection involves removal of the sternocleidomastoid, mylohyoid, anterior digastric, and platysma muscles with excision of the spinal accessory nerve. The absence or alteration of these structures can cause asymmetrical neck mechanics, shoulder limitations in abduction and forward flexion, and pain. After head and neck cancer surgeries, exercises should focus initially on range of motion of the shoulder and cervical muscles with stretching of the pectoralis muscles to prevent contractures.

Later, isometric exercises are used to strengthen the serratus anterior, rhomboids, and levator scapulae. Proper shoulder support and positioning help to decrease pain.[51]

CONCLUSION

Whether women with cancer were mild to moderate exercisers or competitive athletes premorbidly, many continue to exercise both during and after treatment. The exercise program, however, must be modified and individualized according to each woman. Even though the side effects of treatments, especially cancer-related fatigue, can impair exercise ability, women with cancer still experience significant benefits from exercise. Women with cancer can safely participate in exercise and recreational activities as long as guidelines and precautions are followed. More studies investigating exercise response in women with various types of cancer at different stages of disease and treatment would be informative. In addition, evaluation and comparison of exercise programs of variable exercise types, frequencies, intensities, and durations would help to determine the optimal exercise prescription for achieving maximal benefits without harmful consequences. The health care team should encourage all women with cancer to participate in an exercise program because of the many benefits, which include promoting confidence, independence, and sense of well-being, while decreasing side effects of treatments and improving quality of life.

REFERENCES

1. Parker SL, Tong T, Bolden S, et al. Cancer statistics, 1997. *CA Cancer J Clin.* 1997;47:5–27.

2. Ries LAG, Kosary CL, Hankey BF, et al. *SEER Cancer Statistics Review, 1973–1993: Tables and Graphs* (NIH Pub. 96–2789). Bethesda, MD: National Cancer Institute; 1995.

3. Elward K, Larson EB. Benefits of exercise for older adults. A review of existing evidence and current recommendations for general population. *Clin Geriatr Med.* 1992;8:35–50.

4. U.S. Department of Health and Human Services. *Physical Activity and Health: A Report of the Surgeon General.* Atlanta: U.S. Department of Health and Human Services Center for Disease Control and Prevention, National Center for Chronic Disease Prevention and Health Promotion; 1996:87–102.

5. Hershcopf RJ, Bradlow H. Obesity, diet, endogenous estrogens, and the risk of hormone sensitive cancer. *Am J Clin Nutr.* 1987;45:283–289.

6. Key TJ, Pike MC. The role of oestrogens and progestogens in the epidemiology and prevention of breast cancer. *Eur J Cancer Clin Oncol.* 1988;24:29–43.

7. Frisch RE, Wyshak G, Albright N, et al. Lower lifetime occurrence of breast cancer and cancers of the reproductive system among former college athletes. *Am J Clin Nutr.* 1987;45:323–335.

8. Nieman DC, Henson DA. Role of endurance exercise in immune senescence. *Med Sci Sports Exerc.* 1994;26:172–181.

9. Frisch R. Delayed menarche and amenorrhea in ballet dancers. *N Engl J Med.* 1980;303(1):17–19.

10. Frisch RE, Wyshak G, Albright NL, et al. Lower prevalence of breast cancer and cancers of the reproductive system among former college athletes compared to non-athletes. *Br J Cancer.* 1985;52:885–891.

11. Paffenbarger RS, Hyde RT, Wing AL, et al. Physical activity all-cause mortality, and longevity of college alumni. *N Engl J Med.* 1986;314(10):605–613.

12. Dorgan JF, Brown C, Barrett M, et al. Physical activity and risk of breast cancer in the Framingham Heart Study. *Am J Epidemiol.* 1994;139:662–669.

13. Thune I, Brenn T, Lund E, et al. Physical activity and the risk of breast cancer. *N Engl J Med.* 1997;18:1269–1275.

14. Willet WC, Browne ML, Bain C, et al. Relative weight and risk of breast cancer among premenopausal women. *Am J Epidemiol.* 1985;122:731–740.

15. Forney JP, Melewich L, Chen GT, et al. Aromatization of androstenedione to estrone by human adipose tissue in vitro. Correlation with adipose tissue mass, age and endometrial neoplasia. *J Clin Endocrinol Metab.* 1981;53:192–199.

16. Shephard RJ et al. Potential impact of physical activity and sport on the immune system—a brief review. *Br J Sports Med.* 1994;28(4):247–255.

17. Shepard RJ. Exercise in the prevention and treatment of cancer: An update. *Sports Med.* 1993;15:258–280.

18. Colditz GA, Cannuscio CC, Frazier Al. Physical activity and reduced risk of colon cancer: Implications for prevention. *Cancer Causes Control.* 1997;8:649–667.

19. MacFarlane G, Lowenfels A. Physical activity and colon cancer. *Eur J Cancer Prev.* 1994;3:393–398.

20. Smets EM, Garsen B, Schuster-Uitterhoeve ALJ, de Haes JCJM. Fatigue in cancer patients. *Br J Cancer.* 1993;68:220–224.

21. Knoff MT. Physical and psychological distress associated with adjuvant chemotherapy in women with breast cancer. *J Clin Oncol.* 1986;4(5):678–685.

22. Winningham ML, Nail LM, Barton Burke M, et al. Fatigue and the cancer experience: The state of the knowledge. *Oncol Nurse Forum.* 1994;21(1):23–36.

23. Fobair P, Hoppe RT, Bloom J, Cox R, Varghese A, Spiegel D. Psychosocial problems among survivors of Hodgkin's disease. *J Clin Oncol.* 1986;4:805–814.

24. Tierney AJ, Leonard RC, Taylor J, et al. Side effects expected and experienced by women receiving chemotherapy for breast cancer. *BMJ.* 1991;302:272.

25. Love RR, Leventhal H, Easterling DV, et al. Side effects and emotional distress during cancer chemotherapy. *Cancer.* 1989;63:604–612.

26. Nail LM. Coping with intracavitary radiation treatment for gynecologic cancer. *Cancer Pract.* 1993;1:218–224.

27. Ehlke G. Symptom distress in breast cancer patients receiving chemotherapy in the outpatient setting. *Oncol Nurs Forum.* 1988;15:343–346.

28. Haylock P, Hart L. Fatigue in patients receiving localized radiation. *Cancer Nurs.* 1979;2:461–467.

29. Quested K, Malec J, Harney R, et al. Rehabilitation program for cancer related fatigue: An empirical study. *Arch Phys Med Rehabil.* 1982;63:532.

30. Hettinger T. In: Thurwell MH, ed. *Physiology of Strength*. Springfield, IL: Charles C Thomas; 1961:1–84.

31. Droste C. Transient hypoalgesia under physical exercise: Relation to silent ischemia and implications for cardiac rehabilitation. *Ann Acad Med Singapore*. 1992;21:23.

32. Varrassi G, Bazzano C, Edwards WT. Effects of physical activity on maternal plasma β-endorphin levels and perception labor pain. *Am J Obstet Gynecol*. 1989;160(3):707–712.

33. Gurevich M. Exercise induced analgesia and the role of reactivity in pain sensitivity. *J Sports Sci*. 1994;12:549.

34. Dimeo F, Tilmann MH, Bertz H, et al. Effects of aerobic exercise on physical performance and incidence of treatment-related complications after high-dose chemotherapy. *Blood*. 1997;90(9):3390–3394.

35. Winningham ML, MacVicar MG. The effects of aerobic exercise on patient reports of nausea. *Oncol Nurs Forum*. 1988;15:447–450.

36. Mock V, Dow KH, Meares CJ, et al. Effects of exercise on fatigue, physical functioning, and emotional distress during radiation therapy for breast cancer. *Oncol Nurs Forum*. 1997;24(6):991–1000.

37. Dimeo FC, Stieglitz R, Novelli-Fischer U, et al. Effects of physical activity on fatigue and psychologic status of cancer patients during chemotherapy. *Cancer*. 1999;65(10):2273–2277.

38. MacVicar MG, Winningham JL, Nickel JL. Effects of aerobic interval training on cancer patients' functional capacity. *Nurs Res*. 1989;38:348–351.

39. Mock V. The benefits of exercise in women with breast cancer. In: Dow KH, ed. *Contemporary Issues in Breast Cancer*. Boston: Jones & Bartlett; 1996:99–106.

40. Young-McCaughan S, Sexton DL. A retrospective investigation of the relationship between aerobic exercise and quality of life in women with breast cancer. *Oncol Nurs Forum*. 1991;18:751–757.

41. Garden FH, Gillis TA. Principles of cancer rehabilitation. In: Braddom RL, ed. *Physical Medicine and Rehabilitation*. Philadelphia: WB Saunders; 1996:1199–1214.

42. Harpham WS. *Aftereffects of Cancer Treatments. After Cancer: A Guide to Your New Life*. New York: WW Norton and Company; 1994:95–164.

43. Piper B, Lindsey A, Dodd M. Fatigue mechanisms in cancer patients: Developing nursing theory. *Oncol Nurs Forum*. 1987;14(6):17–23.

44. Bruera E, MacDonald RN. Overwhelming fatigue in advanced cancer. *Am J Nurs*. 1988;88:99–100.

45. Meyers CA, Abbruzzese JL. Cognitive functioning in cancer patients. Effect of previous treatment. *Neurology*. 1992;42:434–436.

46. Schwartz AL, Winningham ML. Problems related to exercise reported by athletic breast cancer survivors. *Oncol Nurs Forum*. 1995;22(2):351.

47. Wiley LD, Reid DC, McKenzie DC. Evaluation of exercise tolerance before and after stage II breast cancer therapy in women [abstract]. *Med Sci Sports Exerc*. 1998;30(5):8159.

48. MacVicar MG, Winningham ML. Promoting the functional capacity of cancer patients. *Cancer Bull*. 1986;38:235–239.

49. Schwartz AL. Patterns of exercise and fatigue in physically active cancer survivors. *Oncol Nurs Forum*. 1998; 5(3):485–491.

50. American College of Sports Medicine. *Guidelines for Exercise Testing and Prescription*. 5th ed. Philadelphia: Lea & Febiger; 1995.

51. Hicks JE. Exercise for cancer patients. In: Basmajiian JV, Wolf SL, eds. *Therapeutic Exercise*. 5th ed. Baltimore: Williams & Wilkins; 1990:351–369.

52. Vallbona C. Bodily responses to immobilizations. In: Kottke FJ, Stillwell GK, Lehman JF, eds. *Krusen's Handbook of Physical Medicine and Rehabilitation*. 3rd ed. Philadelphia: WB Saunders; 1982:963–975.

53. Borg G. Perceived exertion as an indicator of somatic distress. *Scand J Rehabil Med*. 1970;2–3:92–98.

54. Winningham JL. Walking program for people with cancer. Getting started. *Cancer Nurs*. 1991;14:270–276.

55. Winningham ML, MacVicar MG, Burke CA. Exercise for cancer patients: Guidelines and precautions. *Physician Sportsmed*. 1986;14(10):125–134.

56. Unverferth DV, Balcerzak SP, Neidhart JA. Ventricular arrhythmias following intravenous cancer chemotherapy [abstract]. *Clin Res*. 1983;31(4):742A.

57. Meadows A, Hobbie W. The medical consequences of cure. *Cancer*. 1986;58:524–528.

58. Kissen MW. Risk of lymphedema following the treatment of breast cancer. *Br J Surg*. 1986;73:580.

59. Nelson PA. Recent advances in treatment of lymphedema of extremities. *Geriatrics*. 1966;21:162–173.

60. Wingate L. Efficacy of physical therapy for patients who have undergone mastectomies: A prospective study. *Phys Ther*. 1985;65(6):896–900.

61. Lotze MT, Duncan MA, Gerber LH, Woltering EA, Rosenberg SA. Early vs delayed shoulder motion following axillary dissection. *Ann Surg*. 1981;193(3):288–295.

62. Cooley ME, Erickson B. Rehabilitation. In: Fowble RL, Goodman E, Glick JH, Rosato EF, eds. *Breast Cancer Treatment: A Comprehensive Guide to Management*. St. Louis, MO: Mosby; 1991:571–583.

63. Duncan MA, Lotze M, Gerber LH, et al. Incidence, recovery and management of serratus anterior palsy after axillary node dissection. *Am J Phys Ther*. 1983;63:1243–1249.

64. Lynn JM. Rehabilitation and nursing care. In: Roses DF, ed. *Breast Cancer*. New York: Churchill Livingstone; 1999:625–633.

65. McKenzie DC. Abreast in a boat—a race against breast cancer. *CMAJ*. 1998;159(4):376–378.

66. Mandi A, Szepesi K, Morocz I. Surgical treatment of pathologic fractures from metastatic tumors of long bones. *Orthopedics*. 1991;14:59.

67. Nilsonne U. Surgery for bone metastases. *Acta Orthop Scand*. 1984;55:489–490.

68. Otis JC, Lane JM, Kroll MA. Energy cost during gait in osteosarcoma patients after resection and knee replacement and after above-the-knee amputation. *J Bone Joint Surg Am*. 1985;67:606–611.

69. McAnelly RD, Faulkner VW. Lower limb prostheses. In: Braddom RL, ed. *Physical Medicine and Rehabilitation*. Philadelphia: WB Saunders; 1996:289–320.

70. Mullen BD, McGinn KA. *Swimming and Other Diversions. The Ostomy Book: Living Comfortably with Colostomies, Ileostomies, and Urostomies*. Palo Alto, CA: Bull Publishing Company; 1992:241–249.

71. Dimeo F, Bertz H, Finke J, Fetscher S, Mertelsmann R, Keul J. An aerobic exercise program for patients with haematological malignancies after bone marrow transplantation. *Bone Marrow Transplant*. 1996;18:1157–1160.

CHAPTER 16

Pain and Headaches

Kerry Gill DeLuca and R. Norman Harden

INTRODUCTION

Epidemiological studies have noted that, in general, women report more pain than men.[1] For years, researchers have been exploring the relationship between gender and pain, but recently, the investigation into the gender difference in apparent perception of pain and expression of pain has intensified. Although most of the studies in both animal models and humans are not statistically compelling, a number of investigators have concluded that there appears to be an intrinsic difference between men and women when responding to painful stimuli.[2-7] Hypotheses to explain this theoretical difference include influence of gonadal hormones (possibly by effect on opioid receptors or by another mechanism),[6,8] gender difference in response to opioid analgesics,[6,7,9] and/or societal factors/gender roles affecting the expression of pain.[1] The exact mechanism explaining the apparent difference remains unknown.

Very little is available in the current literature specifically addressing pain in the woman athlete. In general, injury rates in women athletes are no higher than those in men athletes; injury patterns are more sport related than gender related.[10] Differences in pain response between male and female athletes may correlate with more general differences in pain response between men and women.

BASICS OF PAIN GENERATION AND TRANSMISSION

Anatomy and Physiology of Nociception

When discussing pain, one must distinguish between pain, which is a perception that can be influenced by various psychosocial factors, and nociception, which is the detection of damage or the threat of damage by nerve endings and the transmission of that information from the nociceptive transducer along peripheral nerves and spinal cord tracts to the brain.[11] Nociception may be modulated at many levels before cortical awareness of an unpleasant sensation.[12]

The free nerve endings that respond to damaging stimuli are called nociceptors, and their signals are carried by A-delta (thinly myelinated) and C fiber (unmyelinated) axons. (Using a separate classification, these small fibers are also described as type III and type IV fibers.)[13] Two different types of pain are distinguished: fast pain, characterized as a pricking sensation, carried by A-delta fibers, and slow pain, a burning sensation, carried by C fibers.[12] Table 16–1 displays characteristics of various sensory afferents. There are distinct types of nociceptors: mechanical nociceptors, which respond to strong, sharp mechanical stimuli; thermal nociceptors, which respond to temperatures greater than 45°C (human heat pain threshold); and polymodal nociceptors, which respond to many types of noxious stimuli.[13]

Skeletal muscle sensory receptors are chiefly mechanoreceptors and nociceptors, although some muscle receptors may be thermosensitive or chemosensitive.[12] Some muscle nociceptors have been theorized to be polymodal, because they are activated by both capsaicin and mechanical stimuli.[14]

Joint nociceptors are activated by hyperextension or hyperflexion. If sensitized by inflammation, they respond to smaller movements than those that usually activate these receptors.[12] Nociceptive information is transmitted to the gray matter of the spinal cord (laminae I, II, and V of the dorsal horn), where the information can be modulated (Figure 16–1). The nociceptive signal may be dampened by an inhibitory interneuron acting under the influence of a larger

Table 16–1 Sensory Nerve Classification

Fiber Group	Modality Transmitted	Diameter (µm)	Conduction Velocity (m/s)
A-alpha (myelinated)	Limb proprioception	13–20	80–120
A-beta (myelinated)	Touch, vibration Limb proprioception	6–12	35–75
A-delta (lightly myelinated)	Sharp, pricking pain	1–5	5–30
C (unmyelinated)	Slow, burning pain	0.2–1.5	0.5–2.0

nearby sensory fiber (A-beta) or from descending antinociceptive pathways. Spinal modulation of pain signals can also occur in the form of central sensitization, in which a noxious signal of sufficient intensity causes the coding of pain-signaling neurons for a given stimulus to be increased. In the dorsal horn, this windup phenomenon results from repeated stimulation of afferent fibers, resulting in an exaggerated response to a given stimulus.[15] From the level of entry into the spinal cord, pain is mediated by the spinothalamic tract, which conveys information to the thalamus and eventually to the cerebral cortex (Figure 16–2).[12,13] This pathway is responsible for the sensory-discriminative component of pain; however, a second aspect of pain response, the motivational-affective response, which includes attention and arousal, somatic and autonomic reflexes, and emotional changes, depends on activity in several ascending pathways, including spinothalamic, spinoreticular, and spinomesencephalic tracts.[12]

The descending control system regulating the transmission of nociceptive information is known as the endogenous analgesia system. This system is made up of several centers in the brain stem and descending pathways from these centers, including the periaqueductal gray, the locus ceruleus, and the medullary raphe nuclei. Stimulation of these centers inhibits nociceptive neurons at the brain stem and spinal cord levels. Endogenous analgesia can be subdivided into opioid analgesia, with endogenous opioid peptides (ß-endorphin, enkephalin, and dynorphin) as neurotransmitters, and nonopioid analgesia, with serotonin and catecholamines as neurotransmitters.[12]

The opiate-receptor-endorphin system has been shown to alter the perception of pain during high-intensity exercise with a benefit on performance.[16] Some forms of exercise are

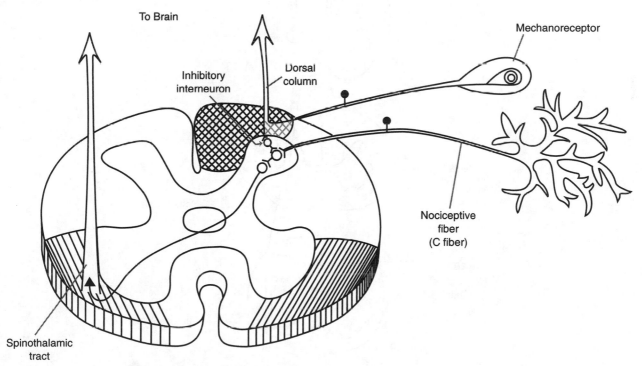

Figure 16–1 Sensory Input and Mechanism for Modulation of Nociceptive Signal at the Spinal Cord Level.

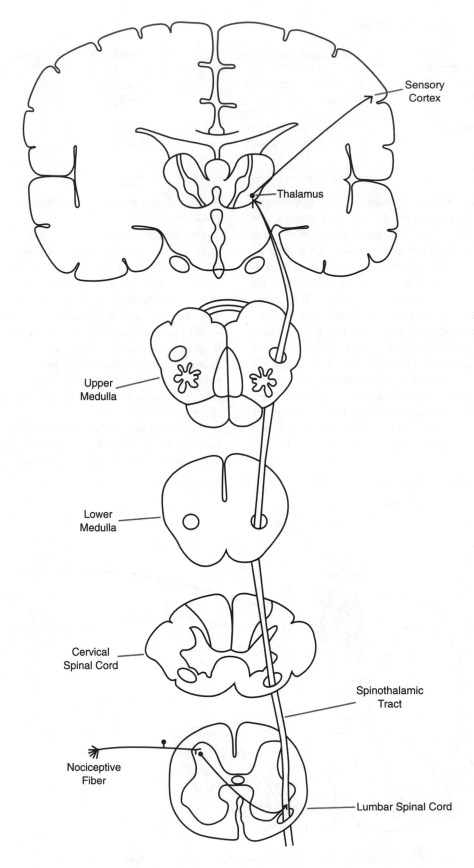

Figure 16–2 The Spinothalamic Tract Conveys Nociceptive Input to the Sensory Cortex.

also noted to produce a nonopiate form of analgesia (stress-induced analgesia).[12]

Pain Generators

In the presence of inflammation or tissue damage, neuropeptides that modulate pain are released onto the distal afferent fibers.[17] Neurotransmitters released from both damaged cells (bradykinin, histamine, prostaglandins, etc) and from free nerve endings (substance P, serotonin, prostaglandins), cause action potentials in the small unmyelinated C fibers and faster, lightly myelinated A-delta fibers. Prostaglandins, in particular, sensitize non-nociceptive thermal and mechanical transducers such that a hyperalgesic (allodynic) state occurs.[16] In animal models, prostaglandins E_2 and I_2, considered to be the most hyperalgesic prostaglandins, have been proven to lower the mechanical nociceptive threshold in an animal model,[18] whereas prostaglandin I_2 has been proven to be a mediator of inflammatory swelling and pain.[19] In both delayed-onset muscle soreness and endurance exercise (marathon running, triathlons), ultrastructural muscle damage is thought to be the cause of the inflammatory response.[16]

Inflammation causes decreased nociceptor threshold and increased neuronal activity (sensitization).[12] In animal studies of inflammation, A-delta and C fibers show a change in threshold after inflammation and decreased response to inflammatory agents after administration of anti-inflammatory medications.[14]

After inflammation, increased activity is noted in both primary afferent and dorsal horn neurons.[12] These neurons subsequently display increased responsiveness to both ongoing noxious and sometimes inocuous cutaneous stimuli, as well as increased background activity and expansion of the receptive field.[17]

Pain sensation from muscle nociceptors is usually duller (more difficult to localize) than pain sensed by nociceptors at the skin surface.[20] Muscle pain may also be referred to an area separate from the muscle sensing the nociceptive stimulus; this is known as referred pain.[20,21] Some researchers have categorized structures in order of sensitivity to nociception, from periosteum (most sensitive) followed by ligament, fibrous joint capsule, tendon, fascia, to muscle (least sensitive).[22] Others state that pain localization is more likely a function of tissue depth than tissue type[23] and that nociceptive stimuli sensed by superficial structures are easier to localize than those from deeper tissues.[23]

Muscle fibers with marked degenerative changes have been found more frequently in trapezius biopsy specimens of patients with work-related myalgia than in healthy subjects.[24] A study of healthy women with localized trapezius myalgia noted a change in fiber-type predominance, deficiency of oxidative enzymes, and lower capillary/fiber ratio compared with muscle samples from control patients.[25]

Women may be particularly affected by increased ligamentous laxity related to the presence of relaxin during the luteal phase of the menstrual cycle[26] and to the effects of relaxin and progesterone during pregnancy.[26,27] Changes in ligamentous structure and/or bony alignment related to this ligamentous laxity may be a source of pain.[26,27]

Irritation of the nerve root or peripheral nerve itself may occur as a result of mechanical compression (eg, as a result of a herniated nucleus pulposus or peripheral entrapment through soft tissues) or as a result of chemical irritation by mediators of inflammation. Sensations are described as tingling, burning, or sharp and may be associated with paresthesias.[28]

GENDER DIFFERENCES IN RESPONSE TO PAIN

Animal Models

Much of the scientific work done in the investigation of gender and pain has been done in rodent models. Results of these studies cannot be directly correlated to human models; in fact, results of animal studies in some areas of pain response are exactly opposite of results from human investigations.[29] In addition, there is a lack of consistent findings across laboratories, attributed, in part, to small population sizes and methodological variability among studies.[29] Although these limitations detract from the strength of the conclusions, the animal studies raise interesting points.

Studies have been done on the effects of gonadal hormones (estrogen, progesterone, etc) on the expression of pain behaviors in animals,[30,31] as well as what, if any, variations occur in that effect over the course of the menstrual cycle.[30–32] Testosterone has also been implicated as a modulator of gender-sensitive and gonadectomy-sensitive responses.[33]

Male and female rats are noted to react differently to nociceptive stimuli.[31] The intensity of the stimuli can be varied to selectively target opioid or nonopioid analgesia.[31,33] In the rat model, estrogen has been shown to be responsible for the impact of the estrous cycle on opioid but not on nonopioid analgesia.[30] There appears to be a two-way interaction between the gonadal hormones (eg., estrogen) and the opioids, with opioid peptides preventing the preovulatory surge of luteinizing hormone and ovulation, whereas estrogen decreases the postsynaptic sensitivity to endogenous opioids and attenuates μ-opioid and γ-aminobutyric acid (GABA)-B responses.[34] Investigators studying swim stress-induced analgesia (nonopioid analgesia) in the rat model found that female rats displayed a unique analgesia that differed significantly from that in the male rats. The findings point to a unique, female-specific, estrogen-dependent mechanism of stress-induced analgesia and indicate that gender must be considered a factor in pain research.[31]

In the rat model, neurons in the nociceptive-responsive regions of the spinal trigeminal nucleus and spinal gray matter have been shown to express estrogen receptor immunoreactivity.[35] In addition, aversive stimuli have been found to produce different patterns of expression of transcription factors in the hippocampus of male and female rats, suggesting that differences between genders include changes in those areas involved in cognition and emotion.[36]

Debate exists in the animal literature regarding pain response and the estrous cycle. Giamberardino et al[32] found enhancement of visceral pain sensitivity in the perimenstrual period, which differed from studies finding lower thresholds in proestrus/estrus. She explained that her findings agreed with prior studies looking at visceral pain but differed from data obtained from superficial somatic stimuli and postulated that the difference in afferent sensory source (deep vs superficial) might explain the difference in findings.

Some researchers have found gender differences in antinociception to be dependent on the type of opioid receptor tested and the dose of opioid used and postulate that the great methodological variability among animal studies may contribute to a lack of consensus in the literature.[37] Kappa opioid agonists have been found to produce greater antinociception in female rats.[37] Other researchers have found that male rats displayed significantly greater analgesia after administration of morphine (primarily a μ-receptor agonist).[38,39] In one study, the greater potency of morphine in males appeared to be due primarily to pharmacokinetic considerations, with morphine levels in the brains of males found to be 35% higher than those in females.[39]

Human Studies

Descriptive Studies

As noted earlier, epidemiological studies have documented that women report pain more frequently than men.[1] Some of the pain reports considered are from experiences unique to women (eg, menstruation, pregnancy, and labor). One questionnaire study noted that, at first glance, women did report more pain than men. However, when menstrual pain was eliminated, there was no difference in pain reporting between genders.[40] In that study, even when menstrual pain was eliminated, women reported childhood exposure to more pain models (individuals in their lives who expressed pain behaviors) and more female pain models than did men.

Hoping to understand the hormonal influence on pain response, investigators have looked at differences between pregnant and nonpregnant populations. Substance P is a mediator of inflammation released from nociceptive free nerve endings. Significantly lower serum levels of substance P–like immunoreactivity (SPLI) have been found in populations of pregnant women compared with nonpregnant women.[41] In that study, the presence of acute pain did not significantly alter the SPLI concentrations.

Experimental Studies

Experimental laboratory studies looking at gender and pain have focused on varied aspects of the puzzle, including sensitivity to noxious stimuli[2–4,42,43] and effects of hormones[6,8] or resting blood pressure[44] on pain response. In studies looking at response to noxious stimuli, both the type of stimulus applied and the measures used to quantify the response vary, making comparison among studies difficult. In addition, many of the studies are small, leading to questions of statistical power and generalizability of results.

In a comprehensive review of the literature specifically focused on gender differences in the responses to noxious stimuli, researchers concluded that the literature indicates that females exhibit greater sensitivity to noxious stimulation than males.[5] Because so many of the studies considered in that review were small, a follow-up meta-analysis of the same data was done; only 7 of the 34 previously reviewed articles were large enough to have adequate statistical power. The authors did, conclude, however, that females do appear to have greater sensitivity to experimentally induced pain.[45]

In a small study looking at the effect of variation in pain response across the menstrual cycle, investigators found that women were less sensitive to one type of noxious stimulus (ischemic pain) during the midfollicular phase compared with other phases of the menstrual cycle.[8] The authors also note that there was no change in ß-endorphin levels across the menstrual cycle and that both of their findings are consistent with previous studies. Other studies have found no association between menstrual cycle phase and pain response,[6,7] although many studies do not address the menstrual cycles of the participants at all.[3,4,42,44] Female hormones have also been thought to modulate the pain response (along with endogenous opioids) during pregnancy, because both animal and human studies have shown pregnant females to have higher pain thresholds than nonpregnant females.[46]

Investigation into the relationship between blood pressure and pain response also seems to indicate some gender difference. In a study looking at groups of normotensive men and women, resting blood pressure was inversely related to sensitivity to thermal and ischemic pain among men (higher blood pressure correlating with lower pain response). In that same study, women exhibited greater pain sensitivity on some, but not all, pain measures.[44]

In a small study using a thermal noxious stimulus, researchers showed a gender difference in perceived intensity, with women rating the stimulus as more intense than did the men. In this same study, positron emission tomography scanning was used to evaluate cortical activation after the stimulus and demonstrated a difference between genders in activation of contralateral forebrain structures, suggesting a gender difference in neural processing.[47]

Clinical Studies

A few studies done in the clinical setting focus on gender difference in pain reporting and produce conflicting results. A study looking at relatively larger numbers of both men and women of varying age groups (three populations studied, 30–100 men and women in each group) found no significant difference between genders in reports of pain.[48] A study done in an emergency department setting found that women reported more pain and were treated with more analgesics than men.[49]

Investigations into the gender differences in response to opioid analgesia have largely been done in the clinical setting.[6,7,9] Initial studies noted a difference in the analgesic effect of opioids that act at κ-receptors, but not in the effect of opioids that act at μ-receptors.[9] Further studies confirmed greater analgesic effect of opioids that act on κ-receptors (pentazocine,[7] butorphanol, and nalbuphine[6]) in women compared with the effect of these drugs in men. The physiological basis for the gender-related difference in analgesic response to κ-opioid agonists is not known. A review of the literature of gender response to opioid analgesia revealed that in most clinical studies of opioid use, done primarily with patient-controlled analgesia administration of μ-agonists, men consumed more opioids than women. Patient weight was found to not be statistically related. The review also examined the gender difference in response to κ-agonist opioids. The authors concluded that there is an intrinsic difference between genders in response to pain and opioid analgesics, but that certainly more research is needed.[50]

GENDER/PAIN ISSUES IN ATHLETES

Few studies specifically address the athlete's response to nociceptive stimuli. A small study looking at the difference

in response to cold stimuli between athletes and nonathletes found that both men and women athletes tolerated pain much better than nonathletes. No significant gender difference was noted among athletes in response to pain.[51] On the basis of the premise that laboratory studies of painful stimuli might not replicate the type of stressful environment encountered by the athlete in competition, one study tested athletes with noxious stimuli before and immediately after competition. In some cases, pain sensitivity decreased immediately after competition, whereas in other cases, responses to painful stimuli were actually heightened. There were no gender differences in these competition-related changes in pain sensitivity.[52]

HEADACHES IN WOMEN ATHLETES

Headaches represent a special pain problem that may affect women athletes or, in the case of migraine headaches, affect women more frequently than men.[53] The most common type of headache in men and women is episodic or chronic tension-type headache,[54,55] and some evidence exists that aerobic exercise has a protective effect against this type of head pain. When headache represents a referral of myofascial pain syndrome, there is a possibility that its incidence can be increased in athletes who have cervical and trapezial soreness from unaccustomed exercise.[56] The simple treatment for this is heat, ice, massage, and stretching. Nonsteroidal anti-inflammatory drugs (NSAIDs) can also be quite useful.

Although women are twice as likely to have migraine headaches, this disproportion only occurs in the menstrual years.[53] Premenstrual and postmenstrual females have the same incidence of migraines as men.[55] Little evidence exists regarding the impact of athleticism on the incidence of migraine, although runners were noted in one survey to have a higher incidence of migraine than the general population, 36% vs 17%.[57] Like chronic tension-type headache, there is anecdotal evidence that aerobic exercise may have a protective effect against the frequency of migraine,[57,58] although it apparently has no impact on the intensity or duration of migraine attacks. There are many new abortive agents available that are very effective in migraine, such as the $5HT_{1D}$ receptor agonists (ie, sumatriptan), and if the headache is frequent and intense enough, or lasts 1 to 2 days, it may be prudent to consider migraine prophylaxis.[59] β-blockers, calcium channel blockers, and tricyclics are the leading antimigraine prophylactic compounds.[55]

- Calcium channel blockers
- Tricyclic antidepressants

Clinical Guideline

The most likely type of headache to affect women athletes is the exertion-type headache.[60–63] These headaches have intense, sometimes migrainous, features and can follow minor exertion. They can range from very mild to severe headaches associated with infarction.[64] They are closely related to other types of headaches that are associated with the Valsalva maneuver: micturition, cough, sneeze, coital, and weightlifter's headaches are apparently of the same general class.[61,65] As a class, these headaches are sometimes called the indomethacin-responsive syndromes.[55,66] The name obviously implies one of the more dramatic treatments, and indomethacin treatment can have substantial impact on these exertion-type headaches. Unfortunately, chronic indomethacin treatment can have substantial side effects, such as gastrointestinal erosion, ulceration, and renal damage. If indomethacin therapy is entertained chronically or during an intense training period, it is important that patients be advised of the symptoms of gastritis and to observe their stool for changes suggesting melena (ie, dark, tarry stools). Renal function should be periodically checked. Indomethacin seems to be considerably more effective than other NSAIDs, and this may be based on its ability to decrease cerebrospinal fluid pressure and/or the fact that it crosses the blood–brain barrier better than any other nonsteroidal medication.[67] Naproxen sodium is a distant second choice in this condition. Calcium channel blockers have also been tried, and nimodipine would theoretically be the most effective (because it has the most dramatic effect on cerebral vasculature). However, it is currently a costly option. Nonpharmacological management may include gradual desensitization using a light Valsalva maneuver.

A rare cause of headache in the female athlete is commonly called footballers headache. This refers to soccer players who frequently head the ball, and apparently this minor trauma, particularly after a long history of repeated minor head injury, can precipitate substantial headaches. Again the headache can take on the characteristics of migraine or be more consistent with the episodic tension type.[53] Unfortunately, this type of headache can have some long-term association with a decline in cognitive abilities and in that context resembles dementia pugilistica. An analysis of technique and practice of neck strengthening exercises may be helpful. A move to a position where heading the ball is less likely may help; however, there is no position on the field where heading is never required (except perhaps goalie). Of course there is another risk associated with soccer or any sport, and that is the postconcussive headache.[55] Any blow to the head, particularly one associated with alteration or loss of consciousness, needs to be evaluated carefully. Multiple concussions in the same athlete are a very serious problem with potential long-term consequences.[68] Refer to Chapter 20 for guidelines on concussion management.

Headache Types

- Episodic/chronic tension headaches
- Migraine headaches
- Exertion/indomethacin-responsive headaches
- Footballers headache

Clinical Guideline

THERAPEUTIC CONSIDERATIONS

In the athletic population, pain treatment will most often be aimed at decreasing mild-to-moderate acute pain. Nonopioid analgesic medications are indicated as the first-line medications in the treatment of mild-to-moderate acute pain. This group of medications includes acetaminophen and the NSAIDs. Acetaminophen has analgesic and antipyretic, but no anti-inflammatory, properties. It is relatively safe and causes far fewer gastrointestinal side effects than NSAIDs but causes hepatotoxicity in patients with underlying liver disease and has nephrotoxic potential with long-term use.[69] If a condition with a component of inflammation is being treated, NSAIDs, with anti-inflammatory, in addition to analgesic and antipyretic properties, would be more appropriate. NSAIDs block the synthesis of prostaglandins and thereby decrease the sensitization of pain receptors.[16] In addition to their action in the periphery, NSAIDs may also have central analgesic[70] and antipyretic effects.[69] Side effects resulting from NSAID use, including gastrointestinal irritation, platelet dysfunction, and renal compromise, must be considered.[71] These side effects may be less of an issue with the use of selective cyclo-oxygenase inhibitors.[72]

Should adequate pain control not be achieved with nonopioid analgesia, low-potency opioid medications may be added for short-term use. Opioids, which act by binding to peripheral or central opioid receptors, are effective agents for treatment of severe pain.[73] Expected side effects include constipation, sedation, nausea, vomiting, and respiratory depression; mild-to-moderate side effects can be managed with complementary medication, whereas severe side effects can be reversed with naloxone.[73] Long-term use of opioids is controversial.[74]

Corticosteroids are potent anti-inflammatory agents and may be useful when pain is associated with inflammation. Their use must be balanced against the many system side effects that may result, particularly with longer term corticosteroid use.[75]

Anticonvulsants are more often used to treat neuropathic, often chronic, pain, and the mechanism of their action is

Commonly Used Pain in Medications

Type	Recommended Use	Common Side Effects
Acetaminophen	Pain	Hepatotoxicity
NSAIDs	Pain, inflammation	GI, renal, platelet function
Opioids	Pain	Nausea, constipation, cognitive
Corticosteroids	Inflammation, pain	GI, endocrine, cognitive
Antidepressants	Chronic pain	Anticholinergic, cognitive

Clinical Guideline

unknown. Possible hypotheses include membrane stabilization, effects on sodium or calcium channels, interaction with the GABA system, or inhibition of excitatory amino acids.[76] Antidepressants are also used to treat chronic pain. Their mechanism in this role is also not entirely understood, although it is hypothesized to be through modulation of serotonin and norepinephrine. Tricyclic antidepressants have been shown to be helpful in various conditions, whereas selective serotonin reuptake inhibitors have not been as widely studied and have more limited use in the treatment of pain.[77]

Nonpharmacological modalities should also be considered early in treating the pain patient. Cryotherapy (cold therapy) causes local vasoconstriction with reflexive vasodilation, decreased metabolic activity, and is useful in decreasing pain and muscle spasticity. Cryotherapy is often used for the first 48 hours after acute musculoskeletal injury and for symptomatic relief in painful soft tissue and articular inflammatory states.[78] Superficial heat, provided by hot packs or whirlpool (among others), causes increased blood flow and aids in pain control and muscle relaxation but may exacerbate acute inflammatory conditions.[78] Ultrasound, a deeper heating modality, is often used to treat the pain associated with tendinitis, degenerative arthritis, and subacute trauma.[79]

Biofeedback has been found to be effective in treating certain painful conditions, including tension and migraine headaches and low back pain.[80] A National Institutes of Health panel reviewed evidence regarding the use of biofeedback for chronic pain management and found that moderate evidence supported its use, especially in the area of headaches.[80]

A rehabilitation program designed to address musculoskeletal pain will contain elements of strength and flexibility training and aerobic exercise and will consist of the acute phase (in which pain and acute inflammation are treated), the recovery phase (in which manual techniques and mobilization may enhance proper tissue alignment for healing), and the maintenance phase.[79]

AREAS OF ONGOING RESEARCH

The gender biology of pain is a young field,[50] and further research is needed to answer questions ranging from the gender differences in opioid receptor pharmacology[37] to the mechanisms underlying the gender-related differences in pain response[5] to the role of psychosocial factors affecting gender-related response to pain.[81] Issues that are more relevant to athletes and that have yet to be fully explained include the effects of competition on the perception of pain and which pain modulatory mechanisms become activated during competition.[52] In addition, further research is needed to determine whether athletes are socialized in such a way that they tolerate greater pain, or whether personality traits lead certain people to athletics.[51]

Given that response to painful stimuli seems to be related to hormonal factors, an additional issue in female athletes would be the possible effect of menstrual irregularities, such as amenorrhea or luteal phase defects, on pain response.

The most important consideration is the clinical relevance of the research findings.[5,50] The research done in this area to date is fascinating and raises very interesting points, but how do the research findings translate into changes in the treatment of women athletes? Studies done with women athletes as subjects in a setting more closely resembling a training or competitive environment would seem to be more relevant to the care of the woman athlete.

CONCLUSION

The phenomenon of pain is a complex one, because the basic process of nociception, modulated at many levels and influenced by many factors, is further combined with psychosocial factors that influence the eventual experience of pain. Many aspects of the basic anatomy and physiology do not differ between genders, although recent research has been focused on and continues to raise questions about gender differences in the nociceptive process and experience of pain. At this point, it appears that significant gender differences exist between men and women in the experience of pain, but the exact mechanisms underlying these differences are not fully understood. Further information specifically about pain in the woman athlete remains to be discovered.

REFERENCES

1. Unruh AM. Gender variations in clinical pain experience. *Pain.* 1996;65:123–167.

2. Feine JS, Bushnell MC, Miron D, Duncan GH. Sex differences in the perception of noxious heat stimuli. *Pain.* 1991;44:255–262.

3. Fillingim RB, Maixner W, Kincaid S, Silva S. Sex differences in temporal summation but not sensory-discriminative processing of thermal pain. *Pain.* 1998;75(1):121–127.

4. Maixner W, Humphrey C. Gender differences in pain and cardiovascular responses to forearm ischemia. *Clin J Pain.* 1993;9(1):16–25.

5. Fillingim RB, Maixner W. Gender differences in the responses to noxious stimuli. *Pain Forum.* 1995;4(4):209–221.

6. Gear RW, Miaskowski C, Gordon NC, et al. Kappa-opioids produce significantly greater analgesia in women than in men. *Nat Med.* 1996;2(11):1248–1250.

7. Gear RW, Gordon NC, Heller PH, et al. Gender difference in analgesic response to the kappa-opioid pentazocine. *Neurosci Lett.* 1996;205(3):207–209.

8. Fillingim RB, Maixner W, Girdler SS, et al. Ischemic but not thermal pain sensitivity varies across the menstrual cycle. *Psychosom Med.* 1997;59:512–520.

9. Gordon NC, Gear RW, Heller PH, et al. Enhancement of morphine analgesia by the GABA B agonist baclofen. *Neuroscience.* 1995;69(2):345–349.

10. Pauls J. Soft tissue disorders: The female athlete. *Ortho Phys Ther Clin North Am.* 1996;5(1):137–166.

11. Mersky H, Bogduk N. *International Association for the Study of Pain (IASP) Classification of Chronic Pain.* 2nd ed. Seattle: IASP Press; 1994.

12. Berne RM, Levy MN, eds. *Physiology.* 4th ed. St. Louis, MO: Mosby; 1998:109–128.

13. Martin JH, Jessell TM. Modality coding in the somatic sensory system. In: Kandel ER, Schwartz JH, eds. *Neurosciences.* 3rd ed. New York: Elsevier; 1991:341–352.

14. Marchinetti P. Muscle pain: Animal and human experimental and clinical studies. *Muscle Nerve.* 1993;16:1033–1039.

15. Raja SN, Dougherty PM. Pain and the neurophysiology of somatosensory processing. In: Benzon HT, Raja SN, Borsook D, Molloy RE, Strichartz G, eds. *Essentials of Pain Medicine and Regional Anesthesia.* New York: Churchill Livingstone; 1999:2–6.

16. Miles M, Clarkson PM. Exercise-induced muscle pain, soreness, and cramps. *J Sports Med Phys Fitness.* 1994;34(3):203–216.

17. Sluka KA. Pain mechanisms involved in musculoskeletal disorders. *J Sports Phys Ther.* 1996;24(4):240–254.

18. Taiwo YO, Levine JD. Effects of cyclooxygenase products of arachidonic acid metabolism on cutaneous nociceptive threshold in the rat. *Brain Res.* 1990;537:372–374.

19. Murata T, Ushikubi F, Matsuoka T, et al. Altered pain perception and inflammatory response in mice lacking prostacyclin receptor. *Nature.* 1997;388(14):678–682.

20. Kellgren JH. Observations on referred pain arising from muscle. *Clin Sci.* 1938;3:175–190.

21. Travell JG, Simons DG. *Myofascial Pain and Dysfunction.* Baltimore: Williams & Wilkins; 1983:5.

22. Inman VT, Saunders JB. Referred pain from skeletal structures. *J Nerv Ment Dis.* 1944;99:660–667.

23. Kellgren JH. On the distribution of pain arising from deep somatic structures with charts of segmental pain areas. *Clin Sci.* 1939;4:35–46.

24. Sjogaard G, Sogaard K. Muscle injury in repetitive motion disorders. *Clin Orthop Rel Res.* 1998;351:21–31.

25. Kadi F, Waling K. Ahlgren C, et al. Pathologic mechanisms implicated in localized female trapezius myalgia. *Pain.* 1998;78(3):191–196.

26. Baker PK. Musculoskeletal origins of chronic pelvic pain. *Obstet Gynecol Clin North Am.* 1993;20(4):719–742.

27. Bullock-Saxton J. Musculoskeletal changes associated with the perinatal period. In: Sapsford R, Bullock-Saxton J, Markwell, eds. *Women's Health: A Textbook for Physiotherapists.* London: WB Saunders; 1998:134–161.

28. Martin L, Hagen N. Neuropathic pain in cancer patients: Mechanisms, syndromes, and clinical controversies. *J Pain Symptom Manage.* 1997;14(2):99–117.

29. Sternberg WF. Methodological and life span factors can modulate gender differences in the analgesic response to stress. *Pain Forum.* 1995;4(4):222–224.

30. Ryan SR, Maier SF. The estrous cycle and estrogen modulate stress-induced analgesia. *Behav Neurosci.* 1988;102:371–380.

31. Mogil JS, Sternberg WF, Kest B, Marelk P, Liebeskind JC. Sex differences in the antagonism of swim stress-induced analgesia: Effects of gonadectomy and estrogen replacement. *Pain.* 1993;53:17–25.

32. Giamberardino MA, Affaitati G, Valente R, Iezzi S, Vecchiet L. Changes in visceral pain reactivity as a function of estrous cycle in female rats with artificial ureteral calculosis. *Brain Res.* 1997;774(1–2):234–238.

33. Bodnar RJ, Romero MT, Kramer E. Organismic variables and pain inhibition: Roles of gender and aging. *Brain Res Bull.* 1988;21:947–953.

34. Kelly MJ, Loose MD, Ronnekleiv OK. Estrogen suppresses mu opioid and GABAB-mediated hyperpolarization of hypothalamic arcuate neurons. *J Neurosci.* 1992;12: 2745–2750.

35. Amandusson A, Hermanson O, Blomqvist A. Estrogen receptor-like immunoreactivity in the medullary and spinal dorsal horn of the female rat. *Neurosci Lett.* 1995;196:25–28.

36. Aloisi AM, Zimmerman M, Herdegen T. Sex-dependent effects of formalin and restraint on c-fos expression in the septum and hippocampus of the rat. *Neuroscience.* 1997;81(4):951–958.

37. Bartok RE, Craft RM. Sex differences in opioid antinociception. *J Pharmacol Exp Therap.* 1997;282(2):769–778.

38. Kepler KL, Standifer KM, Paul D, et al. Gender effects and central opioid analgesia. *Pain.* 1991;45:87–94.

39. Candido J, Lufty K, Billings B, et al. Effect of adrenal and sex hormones on opioid analgesia and opioid receptor regulation. *Pharmacol Biochem Behav.* 1992;42:685–692.

40. Koutantji M, Pearse SA, Oakley DA. The relationship between gender and family history of pain with current pain experience and awareness of pain in others. *Pain.* 1998;77(1):25–31.

41. Dalby PL, Ramanathan S, Rudy TE, et al. Plasma and saliva substance P levels: The effects of acute pain in pregnant and non-pregnant women. *Pain.* 1997;69:263–267.

42. Bush FM, Harkins SW, Harrington WG, Price DD. Analysis of gender effects on pain perception and symptom presentation in temporomandibular pain. *Pain.* 1993;53:73–80.

43. Robinson ME, Riley JL, Brown FF, Gremillion H. Sex differences in response to cutaneous anesthesia: A double blind randomized study. *Pain.* 1998;77(2):143–149.

44. Fillingim RB, Maixner W. The influence of resting blood pressure and gender on pain responses. *Psychosom Med.* 1996;58:326–332.

45. Riley JL, Robinson ME, Wise EA, Myers CD, Fillingim RB. Sex differences in the perception of noxious experimental stimuli: A meta-analysis. *Pain.* 1998;74:181–187.

46. Cogan R, Spinnato JA. Pain and discomfort thresholds in late pregnancy. *Pain.* 1986;27:63–68.

47. Paulson PE, Minoshima S, Morrow TJ, Casey KL. Gender differences in pain perception and patterns of cerebral activation during noxious heat stimulation in humans. *Pain.* 1998;76:223–229.

48. Lander J, Fowler-Kerry S, Hargreaves A. Gender effects in pain perception. *Percept Motor Skills.* 1989;68(3 pt 2):1088–1090.

49. Raftery KA, Smith-Coggins R, Chen AH. Gender-associated differences in emergency department pain management. *Ann Emerg Med.* 1995;26(4):414–421.

50. Miaskowski C, Levine J. Does opioid analgesia show a gender preference for females? *Pain Forum.* 1999;8(1):34–44.

51. Hall EG, Davies S. Gender difference in perceived intensity and affect of pain between athletes and nonathletes. *Percept Motor Skills.* 1991;73:779–786.

52. Sternberg WF, Bailin D, Grant M, Gracely RH. Competition alters the perception of noxious stimuli in male and female athletes. *Pain.* 1998;76:231–238.

53. Silberstein S, Merriam G. Sex hormones and headache 1999 (menstrual migraine). *Neurology.* 1999;53(Suppl 1):S3–S13.

54. Headache Classification Committee of the International Headache Society. Classification and diagnostic criteria for headache disorders, cranial neuralgias and facial pain. *Cephalgia.* 1988;8(Suppl 7):S10–S96.

55. Raskin NH. *Headache.* New York: Churchill Livingstone; 1988: 153–154, 215–228, 269–282.

56. Jaeger B. Head and neck pain. Myofascial pain and dysfunction. *Trigger Point Man.* 1999;1(2):237–484.

57. Swain R. Headache occurrence and classification among distance runners. *West Va Medl J.* 1999;95:76–79.

58. Lockett D-MC, Campbell JF. The effects of aerobic exercise on migraine. *Headache.* 1992;32:50–54.

59. Boyle, C. Management of menstrual migraine. *Neurology.* 1999; 53(Suppl 1):S14–S18.

60. Rooke ED. Benign exertional headache. *Med Clin North Am.* 1968; 52:801–808.

61. Williams SJ, Nukada H. Sport and exercise headache: Part 1. Prevalence among university students. *Br J Sports Med.* 1994;28:290–295.

62. Williams SJ, Nukada H. Sport and exercise headache: Part 2. Diagnosis and classification. *Br J Sports Med.* 1994;28:96–100.

63. Pascal J, Oterino A, Vasques-Barcaro A, Berciano J. Cough, exertional and sexual headaches: An analysis of 72 benign and symptomatic cases. *Neurology.* 1996;46:1520–1524.

64. Nassar L, Albano J, Padron D. Exertional headache in collegiate gymnast. *Clin Sports Med.* 1999;9(3):182–183.

65. Paulson GW. Weightlifter's headache. *Headache.* 1983;23:193–194.

66. Diamond S. Prolonged benign exertional headache: Its clinical characteristics and response to indomethacin. *Headache.* 1982; 22:96–98.

67. Sicuteri F, Michelacci S, Anselmi B. Termination of migraine headache by a new anti-inflammatory vasoconstrictor agent. *Clin Pharmacol Ther.* 1964;6:336–344.

68. Kelly JP, Rosenberg JH. Diagnosis and management of concussion in sports. *Neurology.* 1997;48:575–580.

69. Rummans TA. Nonopioid agents for treatment of acute and subacute pain. *Mayo Clin Proc.* 1994;69:481–490.

70. Taiwo YO, Levine JD. Prostaglandins inhibit endogenous pain control mechanisms by blocking transmission at spinal noradrenergic synapses. *J Neurosci.* 1988;8(4):1346–1349.

71. Drugs for pain. *Med Lett.* 1993;35(887):1–6.

72. Rofecoxib for osteoarthritis and pain. *Med Lett.* 1999;41(1056):59–62.

73. Fishman SM, Borsook D. Opioids in pain management. In: Benzon HT, Raja SN, Borsook D, Molloy RE, Strichartz G, eds. *Essentials of Pain Medicine and Regional Anesthesia.* New York: Churchill Livingstone; 1999:51–54.

74. Harden RN, Bruehl S. The use of opioids in treatment of chronic pain: An examination of the ongoing controversy. *J Back Musculoskel Rehab.* 1997;9:155–180.

75. Haynes RC, Murad F. Adrenocortical steroids. In: Gilman AG, Goodman LS, Rall TW, Murad F, eds. *The Pharmacologic Basis of Therapeutics.* 7th ed. New York: Macmillan; 1985:1463–1485.

76. Vu TH, Borsook D. Membrane stabilizers. In: Benzon HT, Raja SN, Borsook D, Molloy RE, Strichartz G, eds. *Essentials of Pain Medicine and Regional Anesthesia.* New York: Churchill Livingstone; 1999.66–69.

77. Borsook D, Fishman SM. Psychotropic drugs useful in pain treatment. In: Benzon HT, Raja SN, Borsook D, Molloy RE, Strichartz G, eds. *Essentials of Pain Medicine and Regional Anesthesia.* New York: Churchill Livingstone; 1999:63–65.

78. Weber DC, Brown AW. Physical agent modalities. In: Braddom RL, ed. *Physical Medicine and Rehabilitation.* Philadelphia: WB Saunders; 1996:449–463.

79. Prather H, Press JM, Young JL Physical medicine and rehabilitation approaches to pain management. In: Benzon HT, Raja SN, Borsook D, Molloy RE, Strichartz G, eds. *Essentials of Pain Medicine and Regional Anesthesia.* New York: Churchill Livingstone; 1999:115–118.

80. Haythornthwaite JA, Heinberg LJ. Psychological interventions for chronic pain. In: Benzon HT, Raja SN, Borsook D, Molloy RE, Strichartz G, eds. *Essentials of Pain Medicine and Regional Anesthesia.* New York: Churchill Livingstone; 1999:119–122.

81. Rollman GB. Gender differences in pain: Role of anxiety. *Pain Forum.* 1995;4(4):231–234.

CHAPTER 17

Breast Health in Active and Athletic Women

Sandra J. Hoffmann

INTRODUCTION

With the emergence of women as highly competitive and recreational athletes, specific health concerns of the female athlete have become more important. Little information about normal physiological changes of the breast that occur during puberty, pregnancy, lactation, or menopause is available to women, particularly those who want to become or remain physically active. Literature available to health care providers is minimal in typical sports medicine texts to counsel active and athletic women about appropriate breast injury prevention and treatment, breast pain, sports bras, and the relationship of physical activity to breast cancer. This chapter will review breast health, injury prevention, and treatment of breast problems commonly seen in active and athletic women.

BREAST ANATOMY AND DEVELOPMENT

Clinicians who care for female athletes need to be aware of common developmental breast anomalies. These include supernumerary nipples (polythelia) and, uncommonly, extra breasts (polymastia).[1,2] Polymastia, although a rare condition, may make fitting of sports bras difficult, and specially designed bras may be needed if surgical excision is not elected. Supernumerary nipples can be found anywhere along the milk lines from axilla to groin and can be irritated or chaffed during sporting activity. If problematic, surgical excision can be performed.[2]

Other developmental anomalies that are quite uncommon include the inverted nipple (increased risk of infection) and bifid nipple.[2] Athletes with unilateral absence of the breast (amastia) or Poland's syndrome (congenital unilateral absence of the pectoralis major muscle and overlying tissue) may require a specialized mastectomy bra for sporting activities.

Anatomically, the breast is located on the anterior chest wall over the pectoralis major muscle. Fifteen to 20 lobular glands are surrounded by adipose tissue with minimal connective tissue (Cooper's ligaments) (Figure 17–1). Variation between individuals is tremendous in size, contour, and density of the breast at maturity. Hormonal influences such as menses, pregnancy, lactation, oral or implanted contraceptives, and other hormonal supplements cause changes in the glandular components' shape and structure.[3,4] These changes often require a change in bra or cup size.

The nipples and areola are composed of smooth muscle fibers and sensory nerve endings that cause nipple erection in response to various thermal and sensory stimuli. Women should be encouraged to protect the nipple from irritation and chafing during cold weather or wind by wearing a nipple cup or placing an adhesive bandage over the nipple.

The breasts have an abundant blood supply from the internal mammary artery, thoracic aorta, and lateral pectoralis artery.[3] This abundant blood supply is an important consideration in treating athletic-related trauma such as lacerations and hematomas. Sensory nerve supply to the breast derives from the second to sixth intercostal nerves, except for a small area of skin over the upper portion of the breast, which is supplied by the supraclavicular nerve.[3] In backpackers or women who carry heavy purses, the first signs of "backpackers palsy" may be paresthesia over the breast. This should be treated with reduction in weight of the backpack or purse.

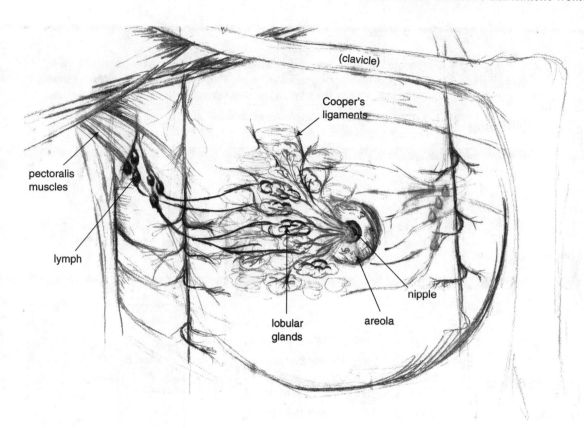

Figure 17–1 Anatomy of the Female Breast. The breast is composed of 15–20 lobules supported loosely by Cooper's ligaments (fascia), with abundant nerve and blood supply.

Development of breast buds (thelarche) and subsequent adult breasts occurs over a wide range of norms from age 8 to 13 and is followed in most women 1 to 3 years later with menarche. Female athletes follow the same expected bell curve for maturation and development of mature breast sizes as nonathletes: 15%, A cup; 30%, B cup; 25%, C cup; 25%, D cup; and 10%, DD cup.[5] Exercise cannot increase breast size because there is no muscle tissue in the breast itself, except in the nipple. Hypertrophy of the underlying pectoralis major muscle during athletic training may cause the breasts to appear larger. Because the breast is composed of mainly fatty tissue, exercise may actually decrease the breast size if it is vigorous enough to decrease overall body fat stores.

BREAST EXAMINATION

Most physicians who care for women advocate that self-breast examination education should be done as part of routine physical examinations and preventive services starting in adolescence (Figure 17–2).[1,2] For physicians who have longitudinal care of the adolescent athlete, introduction of self-breast examination (SBE) techniques at an appropriate physical and psychological developmental stage can help adolescents develop comfort with their bodies and sexuality.[1,2] In the collegiate population, use of the athletic preparticipation examination (PPE) as an opportunity to initiate health promotion activities such as SBE is encouraged. The PPE can also be an excellent opportunity to open discussion about sports bras as both protective gear and athletic clothing.

MASTALGIA

Many women have cyclic breast pain throughout their reproductive years. Cyclic mastalgia is thought by most to be exacerbated by estrogen, but progesterone excess can also exacerbate symptoms.

No evidence exists that participation in physical activity either promotes or prevents cyclic mastalgia. Treatment should consist primarily of a well-fitted, supportive sports bra and mild analgesics if needed. Hormonal manipulation should be tried if already on an oral contraceptive pill (OCP) or hormone replacement therapy (HRT). Other modalities such as treatment with danazol, selective estrogen receptor modulators (SERMs), or bromocriptine may be warranted. Dietary manipulation such as decreasing fat intake, daily intake of 400 IU of vitamin E, and abstinence from

Why

do the
Breast Self-Exam?

There are many good reasons for doing a breast self-exam each month. One reason is that it is easy to do and the more you do it, the better you will get at it. When you get to know how your breasts normally feel, you will quickly be able to feel any change, and early detection is the key to successful treatment.

Remember: A breast self-exam could save your breast--and save your life. Most breast lumps are found by women themselves, but in fact, most lumps in the breast are not cancer. Be safe, be sure.

When

to do
Breast Self-Exam

The best time to do breast self-exam is right after your period, when breasts are not tender or swollen. If you do not have regular periods or sometimes skip a month, do it on the same day every month.

How

to do
Breast Self-Exam

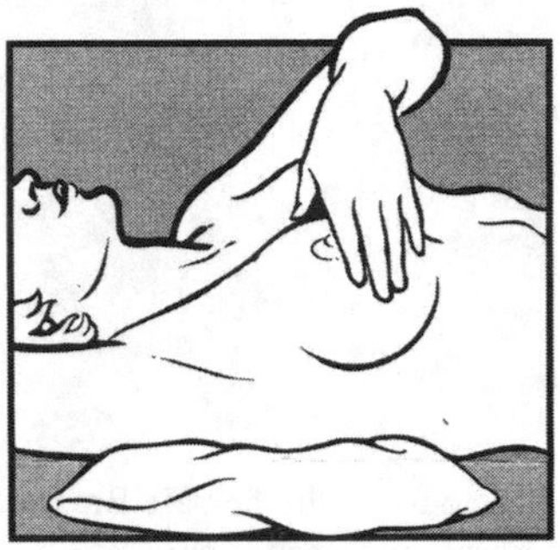

1. Lie down and put a pillow under your right shoulder. Place your right arm behind your head.

2. Use the finger pads of your three middle fingers on your left hand to feel for lumps or thickening in your right breast. Your finger pads are the top third of each finger.

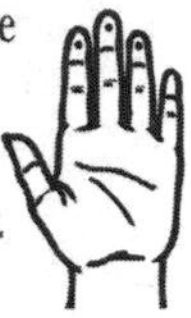

3. Press firmly enough to know how your breast feels. If you're not sure how hard to press, ask your health care provider. Or try to copy the way your health care provider uses the finger pads during a breast exam. Learn what your breast feels like most of the time. A firm ridge in the lower curve of each breast is normal.

4. Move around the breast in a set way. You can choose either the circle (**A**), the up and down (**B**), or the wedge (**C**). Do it the same way every time. It will help you to make sure that you've gone over the entire breast area, and to remember how your breast feels.

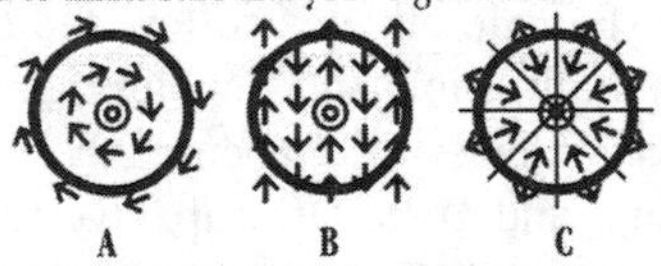

5. Now examine your left breast using right hand finger pads.

6. Repeat the examination of both breasts while standing, with one arm behind your head. The upright position makes it easier to check the upper and outer part of the breasts (toward your armpit). You may want to do the standing part of the BSE while you are in the shower. Some breast changes can be felt more easily when your skin is wet and soapy.

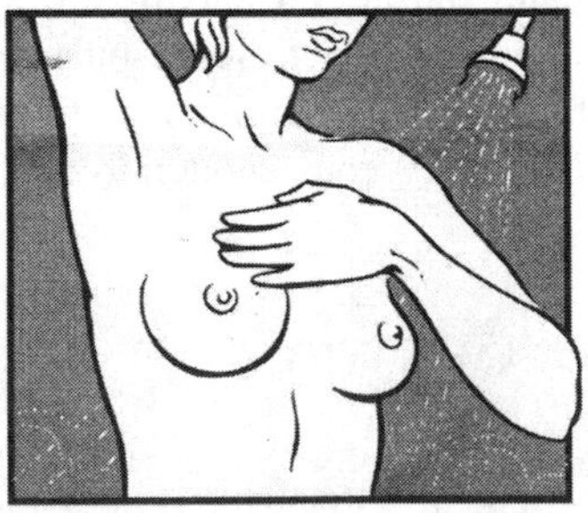

For added safety, you can also check your breasts for any dimpling of the skin, changes in the nipple, redness, or swelling while standing in front of a mirror right after your BSE each month.

If you find any changes, see your doctor right away.

Figure 17–2 Self-Breast Examination Technique. Starting at the upper-outer quadrant of the breast, the woman should be taught to feel in small, concentric circles encircling the breast in either a clockwise or counterclockwise fashion. Care should be taken to examine the areola and nipple carefully and to include the tissue close to the axilla.

caffeine may be overall healthy behaviors but has not specifically been shown to be effective in preventing or treating mastalgia.[4,6–8]

Treatment of Cyclic Mastalgia in Women

- Well-fitted sports bra
- Mild analgesics
- Hormonal manipulation
- OCPs
- HRT
- SERMs
- Danazol
- Bromocriptine
- Dietary manipulation

Clinical Guideline

Noncyclic mastalgia is commonly reported by women during physical activity.[9–15] A recent report suggests that reduction in breast motion and displacement decrease pain during exercise and that this can be accomplished with appropriate breast support.[14]

GALACTORRHEA

A number of causes of galactorrhea exist in nonpregnant women, none of which however are related directly to sports participation.[1,2] Milky discharge is usually physiological, but evaluation for organic factors is indicated in all cases. A thorough history and physical examination should be conducted, and any medications that could be contributing to the galactorrhea should be discontinued. Bloody or serous nipple discharge should be immediately evaluated and the patient referred to a breast specialist. Treatment of galactorrhea depends on the cause, and the reader is referred to further references for more specific therapies.[1–4]

BREAST HEALTH FOR ACTIVE PREGNANT AND LACTATING WOMEN

The literature on breast health issues in pregnant and lactating women who engage in physical activity and exercise is sparse. Physiological changes that occur in pregnancy include an increase in breast size caused by hormonal stimulation and milk production and an increased prominence of nipples, which are therefore more susceptible to injury.[16] It is imperative that exercising pregnant women have an appropriately fitting sports bra throughout their pregnancy. Because of the rapidly changing size of their breasts at various points in the pregnancy, it is recommended to refit their bra at 8- to 10-week intervals or at every trimester. Sports bras may be more comfortable throughout the pregnancy than conventional-type bras.

Studies done in lactating women who underwent submaximal exercise have found no change in breast milk composition.[17] Small increases in lactic acid and a decrease in immunoglobulin A have been found in breast milk up to 30 to 60 minutes after intense (85% max VO_2) aerobic exercise.[18,19] Whether any of these changes are clinically or physiologically significant to the developing infant is uncertain, and these data should not restrain lactating women from moderate aerobic exercise. It is suggested that women pump their breasts of milk before exercise, particularly for comfort. If they are concerned about any effects that exercise may have on the composition of breast milk, it is recommended they wait 1 to 2 hours after any maximal exercise before breastfeeding.

The American College of Obstetrics and Gynecology has published guidelines for exercise during pregnancy and the postpartum period.[20] Readers are referred to this guideline and Chapter 11 of this text for more details about exercise during pregnancy.

BREAST MASSES

Breast lumps or masses are a common occurrence and are frequently found by women during self-examinations or by their intimate partners during sexual activity. The causes of breast masses are numerous, with the incidence of each dependent primarily on age.

Common Causes of Breast Masses

- Breast cysts
- Breast abscess
- Hematomas
- Fat necrosis
- Gynecomastia
- Virginal hypertrophy
- Neurofibromatosis
- Benign tumors:
  Fibroadenoma
  Juvenile fibroadenoma
  Cystosarcoma phylloides
  Lipoma
- Malignant tumors:
  Adenocarcinoma
  Cystosarcoma phylloides
  Metastatic lesions

Clinical Guideline

Hematomas and fat necrosis resulting from trauma may be common sports-related breast masses. Breast abscesses resulting from poor moisture control and skin breakdown may also occur as a result of physical activity. Treatment of these conditions is described later in this chapter. The evaluation and treatment of nonsports-related breast masses are beyond the scope of this chapter, and the reader is referred to authoritative texts.[3] All women, including adolescents, should be taught SBE techniques.

PHYSICAL ACTIVITY AND BREAST CANCER PREVENTION

Epidemiological studies that have tried to determine a relationship between physical activity and breast cancer prevention have resulted in conflicting data, mostly caused by methodological concerns.[21–24] Many studies that have been undertaken did not define physical activity or exercise.[24] Many activity studies involving women have only looked at leisure time or occupational activities and failed to account for activity in the home or activity related to child care.[24] In addition, many studies did not adequately control for hormonal status of the women studied.[24]

In general, physical activity appears to decrease all cancer mortality in both men and women. Physical activity also appears to prevent the development of breast cancer in women.[21,25,26] Putative mechanisms include increase in natural killer cells and immunity, improvement in overall health behaviors, genetics, decrease in body fat, improved energy balance, decrease in insulin or insulin-like growth factors, and increased destruction of oxygen free radicals.[27] The effect of physical activity on ovarian and adipose tissue steroid synthesis and degradation and the use of exogenous steroids in the form of OCPs and HRT complicates many conclusions.

Putative Mechanisms by Which Physical Activity Decreases Cancer Risk in Active Women

- Increase in overall healthy behaviors
- Increase in natural killer cells
- Increase in immune system functioning
- Increase in destruction of oxygen free radicals
- Decrease in body fat stores
- Decrease in insulin and insulin-like growth factor-1
- Improved energy balance

Clinical Guideline

BREAST TRAUMA AND INJURY

Trauma and injury to breasts in female athletes reportedly are rare but do occur.[1,2,9,13,15,28–31] Breast injuries are suspected to be more common than actually reported by athletes. Underreporting is believed to be multifactorial and could be due to gender differences between female athletes

and male clinicians, general embarrassment, the athlete being uncomfortable talking about certain body parts, or the athlete thinking a breast injury is not important or serious. Underreporting may also be due to a perceived or real unwillingness or discomfort on the part of clinicians to discuss breast issues. Clinicians are encouraged during examinations for athletic and active women to set a tone that conveys caring for the woman's overall health and comfort in discussing sensitive health issues, including preventive measures for breast injuries.

Direct trauma to the breast can occur from objects such as balls, pucks, sticks, or other sporting equipment; other body parts; or directly falling onto the breast during sliding or diving for balls. Contusions are the result of superficial capillary rupture, and the accompanying swelling and ecchymosis are usually mild and resolve easily.[2] Treatment is ice and compression with padding in the sports bra as needed. Mild analgesics may be necessary. Infrequently, direct trauma can lead to hematomas, both superficial and deep. These may be quite painful because of swelling and the abundant nerve supply to the breast. Although most spontaneously resolve, needle aspiration under sterile conditions may be needed for control of pain or development of secondary infection.[2] A continuously worn bra, including at night, may help control pain until symptoms subside. Hematomas from severe trauma rarely lead to fat necrosis with residual scarring.[5] Trauma may also lead to Mondor's disease or superficial thrombophlebitis of breast veins.[1,2,5] Mondor's disease usually resolves with symptomatic treatment with mild heat and analgesics. If the condition persists or is associated with unilateral arm or facial swelling, further evaluation is warranted. In general, athletes can be reassured there is no evidence that breast trauma increases a woman's subsequent risk of breast cancer.[32]

Abrasions may occur from sliding, diving onto hard surfaces after balls, or from nipple rings or bra parts.[2] Athletes should be encouraged to remove nipple rings before all athletic activities. Abrasions should be washed thoroughly and treated symptomatically with mild analgesics. Cold therapy is usually not warranted and could be harmful. Compression may actually slow healing by increasing moisture and risk of secondary infections. Injured areas should be protected during subsequent athletic activity. Careful observation for signs of secondary infection and prompt treatment with antibiotics if infection develops are imperative.[2]

Breast lacerations may occur during sporting activities, particularly hockey and fencing. Lacerations should be thoroughly cleansed, then sutured with early (3 days) removal of sutures followed by Steri-Strips if needed. A compression dressing is imperative to prevent swelling and hematoma formation. Cold therapy and analgesics may be helpful. Continuous support with a bra should be provided until resolution of symptoms.[2] Nipple laceration sustained from nipple rings may require a surgical specialist to repair; therefore, all athletes should be encouraged to remove these before activity. As with all lacerations, tetanus toxoid should be updated.

The nipple is reported to be the most common site of sports injury.[2] Abundant smooth muscle fibers and sensory nerve endings in the nipple and areola cause nipple erection in response to various thermal and sensory stimuli. Prolonged contact of erect nipples with irritating material during exercise can lead to pain and bleeding.[9,13,15,33]

Treatment of Breast Contusions
- Cold therapy
- Mild analgesics
- Intermittent compression with sports bra

Treatment of Breast Hematomas
- Cold therapy
- Analgesics
- Continuous compression with sports bra
- Needle aspiration

Treatment of Breast Abrasions
- Thorough cleansing
- Mild analgesics
- Keep area *dry*
- Protection during subsequent activities
- Antibiotic therapy for secondary infections

Treatment of Breast Lacerations
- Thorough cleansing
- Analgesics
- Cold therapy
- Suture with early suture removal
- Compression and support with sports bra
- Tetanus toxoid
- Antibiotic therapy for secondary infections

Clinical Guideline

SPORTS BRAS

Bras are important protective equipment for female athletes participating in any sport and are as important to the recreational athlete as to competitive elite athletes. An appropriately designed sports bra should be aesthetic, comfortable, and functional for injury protection.

Sports Bras in Injury Protection and Prevention

Although not frequently reported by athletes, breast injuries do occur. Protection from impact injuries can be ac-

complished with padding, although cotton and other materials commonly used for this purpose often retain moisture and can lead to irritation, chafing, and infection.[2,34] If padding is used, it should be lined on both sides with a "wickaway" material.

Protection is particularly important in contact sports such as martial arts and boxing, fencing in which there is use of a sharp instrument, and sports in which objects are hurled at high speeds such as ice hockey, softball, lacrosse, and cricket. Use of polyurethane plastic nipple cups, breast cups, or full chest shields is recommended.[2] Nipple and breast cups can be placed between two sports bras, a sports bra and a lactation bra, or placed in specially designed bras for that purpose (Figure 17–3). Full polyurethane chest shields can also be worn over a sports bra. If used, the shields should be custom fitted for each athlete. Full chest shields are expensive protective gear and can cost upwards of several hundred dollars, whereas nipple and breast cups are relatively inexpensive. Which form of protection an athlete chooses is an individual decision based on protective needs, comfort, and aesthetics.

Sports Bra Design and Fit

The ideal sports bra should be made of a material that is nonabrasive; hypoallergenic; has secure straps; and is without seams, ridges, or hooks, particularly over the breast itself (Figure 17–4).[1,2,5,10,11,34–40] Whether the material is all synthetic or a synthetic-cotton blend depends on personal preference and exercise intensity. Weather conditions may also influence choice, because cotton will retain moisture and heat better. In choosing any particular type of material, moisture control away from the skin and protection from wind and cold are imperative to prevention of skin and nipple irritation, chafing, and subsequent infection.

A properly fitted sports bra is essential for both comfort and injury protection. The bra should fit firmly enough around the chest and breasts to control motion but not too tight to cut off breathing. When properly fitted, the entire upper body should move as one unit. The bra should have enough horizontal stretch to allow it to be placed over the shoulders but have minimal vertical stretch to keep the shoulder straps from slipping and breast motion to a minimum. A "Y" or modified Y design of the shoulder and back provides the most security (Figure 17–5).[2]

Sports bras come in two basic designs, compression and encompassing. The compression type fits best for women with A and B cup size or bust sizes less than 38 inches (Figure 17–6).[2] These bras are sold in almost any sporting goods store and are usually sized as S, M, L, and XL rather than by bust and cup size. Not all compression style bras that are marketed as "sports bras" are actually designed for use in sporting activities. Care should be taken to test bras for

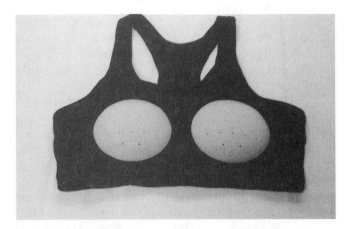

Figure 17–3 Protective Breast Cups and Sports Bra.

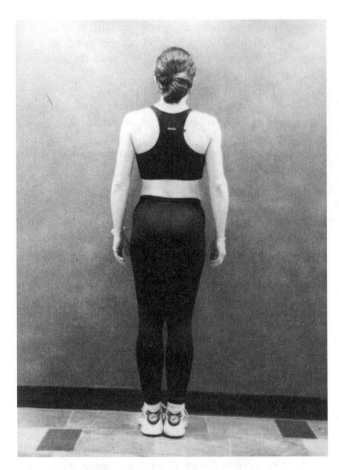

Figure 17–5 Sports Bra with "Y"-Shaped Back.

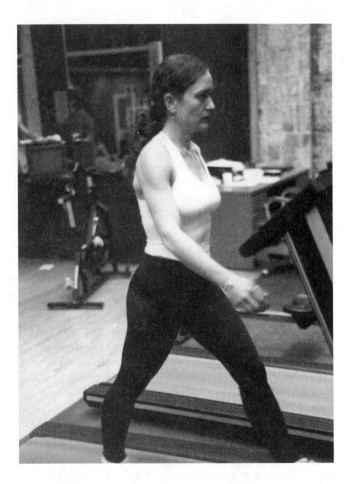

Figure 17–4 Ideal Sports Bra with Secure Straps, Hypoallergenic Material, with "Wick-away" Material Next to the Skin. Note there are no seams, hooks, or ridges over the breast.

support before purchasing. Conversely, encompassing bras in which each breast is separately supported are designed primarily for women with larger busts and cup sizes (Figure 17–7). These bras, which were once difficult to find, are becoming more readily available in stores, specialty catalogs, and Internet sites that specialize in sports and women. Encompassing bras are sold according to chest and cup sizes similar to nonsports bras. Proper measurements for encompassing bra sizing should be taken without clothing over the chest and largest part of the breasts (bust size), and around the chest just below the most inferior portion of the breasts (chest size). Cup size is determined by the difference of the chest and bust size. A 0- to 2-inch difference corresponds to an "A" cup, with each incremental 2-inch difference corresponding to the next larger cup size. Thus a 4- to 6-inch difference between bust and chest measurements would correspond to a "C" cup.

Regardless of the type and material composition of a sports bra, it is imperative that the athlete try it on before making a purchase. With the bra on the upper body, the athlete should jump with hands placed on top of the breast to check for breast motion.[5] A series of shoulder shrugs and

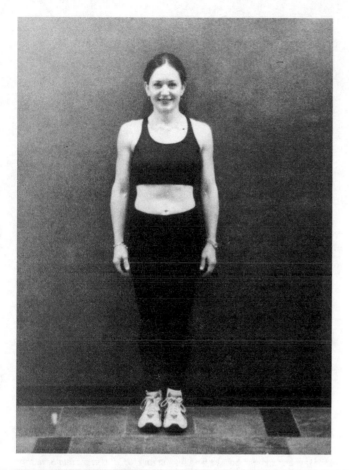

Figure 17–6 Typical Compression-Style Sports Bra.

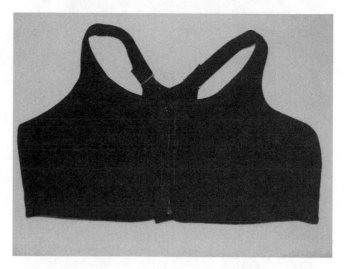

Figure 17–7 Typical Encompassing-Style Sports Bra.

quick overhead motion similar to the "crawl" swimming stroke can help determine whether the shoulder straps are secure. It is suggested the athlete try on several styles and sizes to determine the most comfortable for each individual. With any 10 pound or more change in weight, it is recommended that the athlete be remeasured to ensure continued proper fit and protection.[2]

CONCLUSION AND FUTURE RESEARCH

More attention is needed in several areas regarding breast health in active and athletic women. Foremost, explaining the relationship between physical activity and breast cancer has tremendous public health implications and is an area deserving of more research.[23,24,27]

Little research has been conducted in sports bra design, particularly for women with larger bust or cup sizes. Research on applying newer principles of biomechanics, motion detection, and material development that provide firm breast support while maintaining comfort is needed.[5,12,14]

Research on breast symptoms and breast injuries in women, especially while participating in athletics, is scarce.[5,14,28,34,41] At our institution studies are currently under way to attempt to explain breast injury incidence and prevalence in various recreational and competitive sports. In addition, we are attempting to explain the factors that determine reporting of breast injuries to health care professionals.

REFERENCES

1. Greydanus DE, Parks DS, Farrell EG. Breast disorders in children and adolescents. *Pediatr Clin North Am.* 1989;36(3):601–638.

2. Greydanus DE, Patel DR, Baxter TL. The breast and sports: Issues for the clinician. *Adolesc Med: State Art Rev.* 1998;9(3):1–18.

3. Bland KI, Vezeridas MP, Copeland III EM. Breast. In: Schwartz SI, et al, eds. *Principles of Surgery.* New York: McGraw-Hill;1999:533–593.

4. McCool WF, Stone-Condry M, Bradford H. Breast health care: A review. *J Nurse-Midwifery.* 1998;43(6):406–430.

5. Hindle WH. The breast and exercise. In: Hale RW, ed. *Caring for the Exercising Woman.* New York: Elsevier Science;1991:83–92.

6. Fitzpatrick L. Selective estrogen receptor modulators and phytoestrogens: New therapies for the postmenopausal women. *Mayo Clin Proc.* 1999;74:601–607.

7. Holliday HW, Blamey RW. Drugs for breast pain. *Br Med J (Clin Res Ed.).* 1981;282:1159.

8. O'Brien S, Abukhalil IEH. Randomized controlled trial of the management of premenstrual syndrome and premenstrual mastalgia using luteal phase-only danazol. *Am J Obstet Gynecol.* 1999;180(1):18–23.

9. Levit F. Joggers nipples. *N Engl J Med.* 1977; 297:1127.

10. Lorentzen D, Lawson L. Selected sports bras: A biomechanical analysis of breast motion while jogging. *Phys Sportsmed.* 1987;15(5):128.

11. Lorentzen D, Lawson L. Best health-support bets for active breasts: Researchers rate 8 sports bras. *Self Health Watch.* 1987;5:1.

12. Mason BR, Page KA, Fallon K. An analysis of movement and discomfort of the female breast during exercise and the effects of breast support in three cases. *J Sci Med Sport.* 1999;2(2):134–144.

13. Otis CL. Women and sports: Breast and nipple injuries. *Sports Med Dig.* 1988;10:7.

14. Page KA, Steele JR. Breast motion and sports brassiere design. Implications for future research. *Sports Med.* 1999;27(4):205–211.

15. Powell B. Bicyclists nipples. *JAMA.* 1983;249:2457.

16. Bedinghaus JM. Care of the breast and support of breast-feeding. *Primary Care.* 1997;24(1):147–160.

17. Dewey KG, Lovelady CA, Nommsen-Rivers LA, et al. A randomized study of the effects of aerobic exercise by lactating women on breast-milk volume and composition. *N Engl J Med.* 1994;330(7):449–453.

18. Prentice A. Should lactating women exercise? *Nutr Rev.* 1994;52:358–360.

19. Wallace JP, Inbar G, Ernsthausen K. Infant acceptance of postexercise breast milk. *Pediatrics.* 1992;89:1245–1247.

20. American College of Obstetrics & Gynecology. Exercise during pregnancy and the postpartum period. *ACOG Technical Bull.* 1994;189:1–5.

21. Friedenreich CM, Rohan TE. A review of physical activity and breast cancer. *Epidemiology.* 1995;6:311–317.

22. Frisch RE, Wyshank G, Albright NL, et al. Lower prevalence of breast cancer and cancers of the reproductive system among former college athletes compared to nonathletes. *Br J Cancer.* 1985;52:885–891.

23. Hoffman-Goetz L, Husted J. Exercise and breast cancer: Review and critical analysis of the literature. *Can J Appl Physiol.* 1994;19(3):237–252.

24. Kiningham R. Physical activity and the primary prevention of cancer. *Primary Care.* 1998;25(2):515–536.

25. Sesso H, Paffenbarger RS, Lee I. Physical activity and breast cancer risk in the college alumni health study (United States). *Cancer Causes Control.* 1998;9:433–439.

26. Thune I, Brenn T, Lund E, et al. Physical activity and the risk of breast cancer. *N Engl J Med.* 1997;336:1269–1275.

27. Hoffman-Goetz L, Apter D, Demark-Wahnefried W, et al. Possible mechanisms mediating an association between physical activity and breast cancer. *Cancer.* 1998;83(S):621–628.

28. Alleyne JMK, O'Conner CE. Breast care and athletics: Identifying the incidence of breast-related complaints in women exercisers. *Clin J Sports Med.* 1999;9(2):111.

29. Gillette J. When and where women are injured in sports. *Phys Sportsmed.* 1975;3(5):61–70.

30. Haycock CE, Gillette JV. Susceptibility of women athletes to injury. Myths vs. reality. *JAMA.*1976;236:163.

31. Whiteside P. Men's and women's injuries in comparable sports. *Phys Sportsmed.* 1980;8(3):130.

32. Monkman GR, Orwoll G, Ivins JC. Trauma and oncogenesis. *Mayo Clin Proc.* 1974;49:157–163.

33. Haycock CE. Supportive bras for jogging. *Med Aspect Hum Sexuality.* 1980;14:3–6.

34. Gehlsen G, Stoner LJ. The female breast in sports and exercise. *Med Sport Sci.* 1987;24:13–22.

35. Adrian MJ. Proper clothing and equipment. In: Haycock CE, ed. *Sports Medicine for the Athletic Female.* Oradell, NJ: Medical Economics Book Division;1980:61.

36. Gehlsen G, Albohm M. Evaluation of sports bras. *Phys Sportsmed.* 1980;8:88–97.

37. Lee J. Sport support. *Women's Sports Fitness.* 1995;17:72–73.

38. Sports bras. *Women's Sports Fitness.* 1995;17(1):72.

39. Stamford B. Sports bras and briefs. Choosing good athletic support. *Phys Sportsmed.* 1996;24(12):99–100.

40. Walzer E. Sports support. *Women's Sports Fitness.* 1980;12:66–68.

41. Barton MB, Elmore JG, Fletcher SW. Breast symptoms among women enrolled in a health maintenance organization: Frequency, evaluation, and outcome. *Ann Intern Med.* 1999;130:651–657.

Bone Metabolism—Bone Loss and Injury in the Female Athlete

Lorraine A. Fitzpatrick

BONE REMODELING

Macro Architecture of the Skeleton

The skeleton is made up of multiple tissues, which include bone, cartilage, fat, connective tissue, hematopoietic bone marrow, nerves, and vessels. The skeleton provides three major functions: to provide mechanical support, to protect vital organs, and to serve as a metabolic reservoir of calcium and phosphate. Bone is classified as cortical or cancellous (trabecular) but is made up of the same cellular elements and matrix proteins. Distinct structural and functional differences exist between the two classifications. Cortical bone is dense and compact and makes up 60% of the skeleton. Cortical bone provides structural stability, which is largely present in the shafts of long bones. Twenty percent of the skeleton is made up of cancellous bone, which is more metabolically active and contains a higher surface area.

Cellular and Matrix Components

Osteoblasts are cells that form unmineralized bone (osteoid) through the production of collagenous and noncollagenous proteins. Osteoblasts are derived from primitive mesenchymal cells. Osteoblasts contain a specific isoform of alkaline phosphatase that can be localized in the plasma membrane of the osteoblast. This ectoenzyme is used as a histological marker, but its function remains ill defined.

The author wishes to thank Ms. Ruth Kiefer for her excellent editorial assistance and Mr. Sean Harrison for formulation of the figures.

A clear association between enzymatic activity and bone formation has been demonstrated, and measurement of the serum level of the isoenzyme of alkaline phosphatase specific to bone can aid in the diagnosis of various metabolic bone diseases. Elevated enzyme activity is used as a marker of bone formation and occurs during growth, during fracture healing, or in diseases with high bone turnover. The osteoblast regulates bone formation, which includes the synthesis and internal processing of type I collagen; the secretion and extracellular processing of collagen; the formation of microfibrils, fibrils, and fibers from collagen; matrix maturation; and the nucleation of hydroxyapatite crystals to form a calcified matrix.[1] Regulation of these processes by the osteoblast is an area of intense investigation, and many hormones and growth factors alter the function of the osteoblasts.

Osteocytes are osteoblasts that have been incorporated into matrix. The contact among the osteocytes is maintained by cellular processes that convert mineralized tissue. Osteocytes are responsible for the exchange of nutrients that occurs within the calcified bone matrix.

Osteoclasts are multinucleated cells that are responsible for bone resorption. Osteoclasts are derived from the monocyte-macrophage lineage and formed by the fusion of progenitor cells. Osteoclasts are highly polarized and are histologically distinct, because they contain an average of 10 to 15 nuclei. Osteoclasts must attach to the bone surface for resorption to occur. The integrins are cell surface proteins on the osteoclast that interact with the RGD sequence (ARG-GLY-ASP) on several noncollagenous bone matrix proteins. Osteoclasts attach by means of the integrins to the bone matrix proteins, and bone resorption occurs.[2]

Type I collagen provides the structural framework for calcification in bone. Breakdown products of type I collagen include pyridinoline and deoxypyridinoline. These urinary metabolites are used as biochemical markers in the assessment of bone resorption ("cross-links"). Another marker, N-telopeptide (NTx), is both a serum and urine marker that is also used as a measurement of bone resorption.

The ground substance of bone consists of proteoglycans and glycoproteins that have a high ion-binding capacity and are important to calcification. Noncollagenous matrix proteins make up 10% to 15% of the matrix such as osteopontin, bone sialoprotein, osteocalcin, osteonectin, biglycan, and decorin. These proteins serve important functions in bone modeling and remodeling. One noncollagenous protein, osteocalcin, is used as a serum marker of bone formation.[3]

Regulation of Bone Formation and Resorption

Bone is a dynamic tissue that undergoes constant remodeling. Remodeling serves two important functions. The remodeling process renews the skeleton and provides regulation of calcium homeostasis. Bone remodeling units (BRUs) are groups of cells that occur at discrete locations and in different phases of bone growth. The changes in bone matrix and mineral content that take place during normal development and aging are functions of BRUs. In the classic view of remodeling, the cycle contains three phases: activation, resorption, and formation (Figure 18–1). The cycle is initi-

ated with the recruitment of osteoclast precursors to become osteoclasts. Resorption begins by the osteoclasts; the area is then invaded by preosteoblasts that differentiate into osteoblasts. These cells form a new matrix that becomes mineralized. In the normal skeleton, a complete remodeling cycle takes 100 days in cortical bone and 200 days in trabecular bone. The term "coupling" is supplied to the linked activation of osteoclast-mediated bone resorption and bone formation by osteoblasts. Changes in bone mass result from an imbalance between the amount of bone resorbed and the amount of bone formed. Bone remodeling is regulated by polypeptide, steroid, and thyroid hormones and by numerous locally produced cytokines and growth factors.[4]

Phases of Bone Remodeling

- Activation: Osteoclasts recruited to bone surface
- Resorption: Osteoclasts dissolve/resorb bone mineral
- Formation: Osteoblasts are recruited and lay down matrix

Clinical Guideline

Regulation of Bone Remodeling by Parathyroid Hormone, 1,25(OH)$_2$ Vitamin D, and Calcitonin

Parathyroid hormone, 1,25(OH)$_2$ vitamin D, and calcitonin influence bone remodeling. Parathyroid hormone stimu-

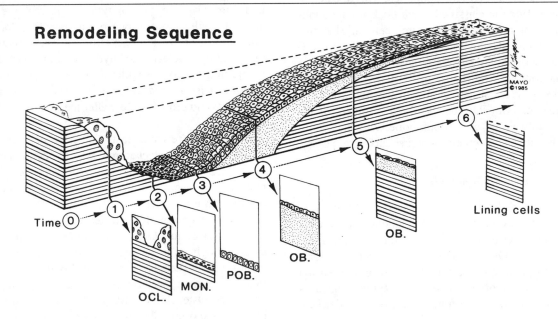

Remodeling Sequence

Time (0) — 1 — 2 — 3 — 4 — 5 — 6

OCL.   MON.   POB.   OB.   OB.   Lining cells

Figure 18–1 Longitudinal and Cross-Sectional Representation of the Bone Remodeling Unit in Cancellous Bone. Five phases are distinguishable: 1, osteoclast-mediated bone resorption; 2, resorption by mononuclear cells; 3, migration of preosteoblasts and differentiation into osteoblasts; 4, osteoid deposition; and 5, mineralization. MON., mononuclear cells; OB., osteoblasts; OCL., osteoclasts; POB., preosteoblasts.

lates differentiation of progenitor cells to form mature osteoclasts. It enhances bone resorption by the osteoclast and stimulates matrix production by the osteoblast. Thus, when serum calcium levels fall, the increase in parathyroid hormone that occurs directly affects bone by increasing bone resorption and enhancing bone formation. In patients with an excess of parathyroid hormone, there is a large increase in bone remodeling. $1,25(OH)_2$ Vitamin D is also a potent stimulator of bone resorption. $1,25(OH)_2$ Vitamin D stimulates osteoclast progenitors to differentiate and overall increases the number and activity of osteoclasts. Calcitonin was initially described due to its ability to cause contraction of the osteoclast cell membrane, and this activity correlates with inhibition of bone resorption.

ESTROGEN AND BONE

Cellular Effects of Estrogen

Estrogen receptors are present on the cells responsible for bone formation (osteoblasts) and bone resorption (osteoclasts). Estrogen has direct effects on the osteoblast, increases cell proliferation, and enhances expression of genes that encode for growth factors, cytokines, enzymes, and matrix proteins that alter bone remodeling. In cell culture systems, for example, estrogen stimulates the synthesis of transforming growth factor-β, insulin-like growth factor-1 (IGF-1), and the IGF binding proteins. Estrogen inhibits the production of cytokines associated with bone resorption that are released by osteoblasts such as interleukin (IL)-1, IL-6, and IL-11. Production of some of the important proteins in bone remodeling, such as bone morphogenic protein-6 and osteoprotegerin, is regulated by estrogen. Estrogen deficiency is associated with an increase in the maturation of osteoblasts and osteoclasts, resulting in an increase in bone remodeling. The role of the estrogen receptors (ERα and ERβ) in the human skeleton is under active investigation. In a male patient with an inactive mutated ERα, osteopenia and lack of closure of the epiphysis were two clinically relevant findings (see In Vivo Effects of Estrogen on Bone).[5]

The major action of estrogen on the skeleton is inhibition of bone resorption and occurs through indirect actions of estrogen on osteoclasts through its action on osteoblasts. Some evidence in avian, rabbit, and human species suggests direct action by regulation of specific genes. Estrogen also induces apoptosis (programmed cell death), reducing the lifespan of the osteoclast. It has been proposed that the synergy of several cytokines such as IL-6, IL-1, IL-2, tumor necrosis factor-α (TNF-α), and others enhance osteoclast recruitment, differentiation, and activity. The blockage of production of these cytokines by osteoblasts prevents the bone resorption noted in the estrogen-deficient state.

One of the most potent inhibitors of osteoclastogenesis is osteoprotegerin (OPG). The natural ligand for OPG (OPG-L) is related to the cytokine TNF and identical to TRANCE/RANKL, a factor that enhances T-cell growth and function of dendritic cells. OPG-L may be the putative "coupling factor" that enhances cross-talk from bone marrow cells to osteoblasts or osteoclast progenitors. OPG is strongly regulated by estrogen and may provide evidence for the protection afforded to the skeleton by estrogen.[6–8]

Estrogens are essential for skeletal maturation and consolidation. Bone cells contain estrogen receptors that respond to endogenous or exogenous estrogen. Estrogens decrease bone resorption through actions on the osteoclast. Recently, estrogens have been shown to decrease the synthesis of cytokines such as IL-1 and IL-6, which normally stimulate bone resorption. Inhibition of cytokine synthesis may be an important mechanism by which estrogen decreases bone resorption.

Effects of Estrogen on Bone

- Increases osteoblast proliferation
- Enhances gene expression of growth factors and cytokines
- Increases synthesis of matrix proteins
- Slows maturation of osteoblasts and osteoclasts
- Inhibits bone resorption*
- Induces apoptosis of osteoclasts
- Inhibits cytokine production that enhances osteoclast recruitment, differentiation, and activity
- Inhibits release of bone-resorbing cytokines released by osteoblasts
- Induces apoptosis of osteoclasts
- Inhibits cytokine production that enhances bone resorption
- Enhances skeletal maturation and consolidation
- Responsible for accretion and maintenance of bone mineral
- Determines normal skeletal proportions

*Major effect of estrogen

Clinical Guideline

In Vivo Effects of Estrogen on Bone

Our understanding of the role of estrogen in human skeletal maturation has increased markedly with the recognition of two genetic disorders. One patient, a 27-year-old man, presented with tall stature, progressive genu valgum, and continued linear growth. Skeletal maturation was greatly delayed at 15 years, and osteoporosis was confirmed by dual-energy x-ray absorptiometry (DEXA). Levels of follicle-stimulating hormone, luteinizing hormone, estradiol, and estrone suggested estrogen resistance, which was confirmed to be due to a missense mutation in the estrogen receptor.[5] This patient demonstrated that estrogen is essential for skeletal maturation and mineralization.

A second set of patients with aromatase deficiency has been described.[9,10] These patients are unable to convert androgens to estrogens. The male patient had estrogen insensitivity with normal sexual maturity, tall stature (204 cm), delayed skeletal maturation, eunuchoid proportions, and osteopenia. Plasma levels of testosterone, androstenedione, and 5α-dihydrotestosterone were markedly elevated. Administration of exogenous estrogen resulted in rapid accretion of bone mineral density (BMD) and cessation of linear growth. These patients demonstrate that estrogens are essential for the accretion and maintenance of BMD and mass and for normal skeletal maturation and proportions.

DETERMINANTS OF PEAK BONE MASS

During puberty, BMD more than doubles at sites such as the lumbar spine.[11] This sequence is delayed by 2 years in males, resulting in a prolonged growth period in males. The result is a larger increase in bone size and cortical thickness in males compared with females. The gain in statural height and bone mass accretion is asynchronous such that the peak of statural growth velocity precedes peak bone mass. In healthy, Caucasian women with adequate nutrition, peak BMD is completed before the end of the second decade.[11–13]

Determinants of Peak Bone Mass

- Genetics (up to 80%)
- Diet
- Physical activity
- Hormonal status

Clinical Guideline

Determinants of peak bone mass are multifold. Genetics plays a large role, but the specific genetic determinants have yet to be defined. Although epidemiological and twin studies suggest that heritable factors account for up to 80% of the variability in BMD,[14,15] other factors responsible for peak bone mass include diet, physical activity, and hormonal status.

Peak bone mass is a significant predictor of risk for the development of osteoporosis. In a study of young (18–35 years of age) Caucasian women, BMD of the hip and lumbar spine was positively correlated with weight, height, body mass index, and level of physical activity. BMD of the hip correlated with dietary intake of calcium. Hip BMD was negatively correlated with amenorrhea of >3 months duration, caffeine intake, and age. For peak BMD, weight, age,

level of physical activity, and family history were independent predictors.[16]

Numerous studies have identified relationships among the level of protein intake, calcium-phosphate metabolism, and BMD on the risk of osteoporotic fracture.[17,18] Undernutrition during growth can severely impair bone development. In animal studies, protein deficiency produces reduced bone mass and strength. Similar correlations can be found with calcium intake and BMD. In prepubertal identical twins, calcium supplementation of 700 mg/day over and above a dietary intake of 950 mg/day significantly enhanced the rate of BMD gain (Figure 18–2).[19] The long-term effects of calcium supplement on the attainment of peak bone mass during the second decade of life remain unknown.

The effect of exercise during the accreditation of peak bone mass has not been well studied. In a large group of elite prepubertal girls (3 years of high-level sport training), BMD in gymnasts was statistically greater than the control group or in age- or anthropometric-matched swimmers.[20] In a study of the subjects who were long-term (>20 years) athletes, aged 42 to 50 years, amount of impact correlated with BMD.[21]

NUTRITION AND BONE

Recommendation of good nutrition for adolescent girls is intuitive; however, how to influence behavior of this age group that is greatly influenced by peer pressure remains problematic. Puberty is a period of enormous skeletal growth, and approximately 40% of peak bone mass in girls is obtained at this time.[12] In American women, for example, 90% of total body bone mineral content was attained by age 17 years, and 99% was attained by 26 years of age.[22]

Bone health can be compromised by excessive thinness from the lack of appropriate nutrition. In addition, excessive exercise or eating disorders leading to disruption of the hypothalamic-pituitary-ovarian axis and less weight-bearing load on the skeleton can also compromise skeletal growth. (See Chapter 19, The Female Athlete Triad.)

Calcium Intake

The importance of adequate calcium intake during growth and adolescence cannot be underestimated (see section "Determinants of Peak Bone Mass"). Adequate calcium intake has been a key determinant of peak bone mass in adolescent women. Cross-sectional studies have implicated a role for calcium in establishment of peak BMD. Prospective observational studies have confirmed the relationship in prepubertal girls. In postmenopausal women, the relationship is less definitive because of the low bone turnover (~1% in those more than 5 years postmenopausal). Recommendations of maximal calcium intake have varied in the past few years (see Clinical Guideline). Intervention trials have

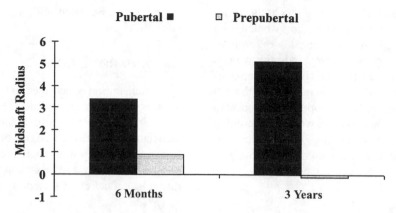

Figure 18–2 Calcium Supplementation in Prepubertal Girls. This 3-year, double-blind, placebo-controlled trial evaluated the effect of calcium supplementation (1000 mg/day of calcium citrate malate) on bone mineral density in 70 pairs of identical twins with a mean age of 10 ± 2 years. In each pair, one twin served as a control. Bone mineral density was measured at the radius, hip, and spine. The mean daily calcium intake of twins on placebo was 908 mg and in twins on calcium supplement was 1612 mg. The data are expressed as mean differences within twin pairs. The twins receiving calcium supplements had significantly greater increases in bone mineral density at both radial sites and in the lumbar spine after 3 years. After 3 years, the differences in increases of two of three femoral sites also approached significance. In prepubertal children whose average dietary intake of calcium approximated the recommended dietary allowance, calcium supplementation enhanced the rate of increase in bone mineral density. *Source*: Reprinted with permission from C. Johnston et al., Calcium Supplementation and Increase in Bone Mineral Density in Children, *The New England Journal of Medicine*, Vol. 327, pp. 82–87. Copyright (c) 1992 Massachusetts Medical Society. All rights reserved.

generally confirmed that calcium attenuates bone loss in a calcium-depleted women.

Several additional studies stress the importance of diet in the preadolescent. In a 10-year longitudinal study, bone mass as assessed by quantitative ultrasound of the calcaneus in 18- to 19-year-olds correlated with preadolescent intake of calcium and magnesium. Using dietary history of milk intake from early childhood to 12 years of age, a positive correlation was found between milk ingestion and BMD at the spine, total body, and radius.[23]

Vitamin D

Adequate vitamin D is essential for the maintenance of bone health. Vitamin D plays an important role in calcium homeostasis and facilitates absorption of dietary calcium. Reduced synthesis of vitamin D as a result of liver or kidney disease, low sunlight exposure, or diminished intestinal absorption can contribute to vitamin D deficiency. Several studies have highlighted the association of hip fracture and vitamin D status. In one report, supplemental vitamin D (700

Optimal Calcium Intake

Group	Estimated Optimal Daily Calcium Intake
Infants (birth–6 mo)	400 mg/day
(6–12 mo)	600 mg/day
Young children (1–5 yr)	800 mg/day
Older children (6–10 yr)	800–1200 mg/day
Adolescents and young adults (11–24 yr)	1200–1500 mg/day
Women (25–50 years)	1000 mg/day
Pregnant or lactating women	1200 mg/day
Postmenopausal women on estrogen replacement therapy	1000 mg/day
Postmenopausal women receiving no estrogen replacement therapy	1500 mg/day
Men (25–65 years)	1000 mg/day
Men and women over 65 years	1500 mg/day

Clinical Guideline

IU) in healthy elderly women slowed bone loss at the femoral neck.[24] In a cohort of community-dwelling women with osteoporosis admitted for hip replacement, lower levels of 25-hydroxyvitamin D were present compared with women without osteoporosis admitted for elective joint replacement when adjusted for age and estrogen intake. Parathyroid hormone levels were higher in the osteoporotic group with fractures compared with the osteoporotic women undergoing elective joint replacement. These data suggest that occult vitamin D deficiency may be common in community-dwelling postmenopausal women and increase fracture risk.[25]

Vitamins and Trace Metals

Vitamins C and K and the minerals manganese, copper, and zinc are co-factors for enzymes involved in the modification of various constituents of bone matrix. It is unknown whether acquired adult deficiencies of any of these minerals in humans play a role in the pathogenesis of osteoporosis. There is no known role for vitamin C in osteoporotic bone fragility, although vitamin C is necessary for collagen cross-linking. Vitamin K is a co-factor necessary for gammacarboxylation of several bone matrix proteins, including osteocalcin. In patients with osteoporosis, osteocalcin may be undercarboxylated in patients with osteoporosis. Whether vitamin K deficiency per se causes bone fragility is unknown; however, deficiency of vitamin K is rare and easily treatable.

Other Nutrients

Phosphorus, sodium, and protein may influence bone metabolism by their effects on calcium homeostasis. Specific effects of calcium on the development of peak bone mass are described in the preceding section. Low calcium/phosphorus ratios are associated with bone loss in animals, but the response in humans is less clear-cut.[26] Chronic overuse of sodium chloride may contribute to the bone loss through loss of urinary calcium. High protein intake also promotes hypercalciuria,[27] but further work is necessary to fully understand these complex relationships and minimal dose to cause skeletal damage.

ORAL CONTRACEPTIVES AND OSTEOPOROSIS

Although many studies support the use of hormone replacement therapy (HRT) in the prevention of bone loss in the postmenopausal woman, few studies evaluate the use of oral contraceptives in the premenopausal woman. In a population-based case study of hip fracture among Swedish women, use of oral contraceptives was associated with a 25% reduction in hip fracture in the postmenopausal years. Higher doses of estrogen (≥ 50 μg of ethynylestradiol per

tablet) were associated with a 44% lower risk of hip fractures.[28]

HRT AND BONE LOSS

Administration of estrogen to the postmenopausal women reduces skeletal turnover and the rate of bone loss (Figure 18–3).[29] Epidemiological data suggest that estrogen use is associated with a decreased risk of fracture. These retrospective studies suggest that risk reduction averaged on the order of 50%. In the few and less-than-perfect prospective studies that exist, reduction of vertebral fracture risk may be as high as 75%.

Estrogens primarily reduce the rate of bone loss; hence, administration early in menopause will preserve more bone mass. Data suggest that estrogen administration reduces the rate of bone loss in menopausal women independent of age.[30] Although older textbooks suggest that the effective dose of oral estrogen is 0.625 mg (conjugated equine estrogen or its equivalent), more recent data suggest that as little as 0.3 mg of oral estrogen may maintain bone mass.[31,32] Different types of estrogen (estradiol, esterified estrogen, conjugated equine estrogen, and transdermal preparations) have all been effective in preserving bone. The effects of estrogen continue for as long as treatment continues, but bone loss occurs rapidly when treatment is discontinued.

At present, little evidence exists that the addition of progestin to HRT would have a negative impact on the effect of estrogen on the skeleton (Figure 18–3).[29] The 19-nortestosterone derivative, norethindrone acetate, is a synthetic progestin used in combination with estrogen. The 19-norprogestin derivatives may have an additive effect for the preservation of bone mass. Measurements of bone mass by DEXA to monitor patients are useful aids to enhance compliance with HRT and assess efficacy of treatment.

BONE LOSS DURING LACTATION

Despite the fact that a large transfer of calcium from mother to child occurs during nursing, few studies evaluate the effects of lactation on the maternal skeleton. Surprisingly, however, nulliparity is a risk factor for the development of osteoporosis. One prospective study evaluated 26 lactating and 8 nonlactating women longitudinally for 7 months postpartum. Average calcium intake from diet and supplements in lactating women was 1300 to 1500 mg/day compared with 775 to 975 mg/day in nonlactating women. Parathyroid hormone, calcium, and estradiol levels were lower in the lactating women compared with postpartum, nonlactating women. Lactating women had a 4% decline in spine BMD between 0.5 and 3 months postpartum, which returned to initial values postweaning. These results (in a small number of subjects) suggest that in well-nourished

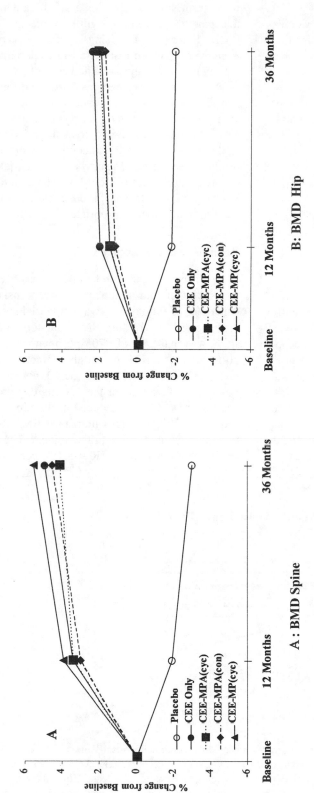

Figure 18–3 Postmenopausal Estrogen-Progestin Intervention Trial. This 3-year, multicenter, randomized, double-blinded placebo-controlled clinical trial assessed the effects of hormone therapy on bone mineral density of the spine and hip of postmenopausal women. A total of 875 healthy women aged 45–64 were recruited at seven clinical centers. Patients were treated with placebo, conjugated equine estrogens (CEE), 0.625 mg/day alone; CEE, 0.625 mg/day, plus medroxyprogesterone acetate (MPA), 10 mg/day for 12 days/month; CEE, 0.625 mg/day, plus MPA, 2.5 mg daily or CEE, 0.625 mg/day plus micronized progesterone (MP), 200 mg/day for 12 days/month. Participants assigned to the placebo group lost an average of 1.8% of spine BMD and 1.7% of hip BMD at 36 months. Those assigned to active regimens of estrogens or estrogen and progestogen gained BMD at both sites ranging from 3.5% to 5.0% increases in spinal BMD and a total mean increase of 1.7% BMD in the hip over a 36-month period. A, unadjusted mean percent change in bone mineral density in the spine by treatment assignment and visit: adherent PEPI participants only. B, unadjusted mean percent change in bone mineral density in the hip by treatment assigned and visit: adherent PEPI participants only.

women, bone loss that occurs during lactation recovers post-weaning.[33]

In an age-stratified random sample of Caucasian women in Rochester, Minnesota, the total duration of breastfeeding and duration of breastfeeding per child were not associated with bone loss. Breastfeeding for more than 8 months was associated with bone mineral loss at selected sites. No consistent effects were observed after adjusting for gravidity or parity, age at menarche or first delivery, use of oral contraceptives, or estrogen replacement therapy (ERT).[34] On the basis of this study, young women with low BMD are advised not to breastfeed for longer than 8 months.

SELECTIVE ESTROGEN RECEPTOR MODULATORS AND BONE METABOLISM

Tamoxifen and BMD

The effect of tamoxifen citrate, a synthetic-anti-estrogen, on BMD has been evaluated in several trials. In one published study of postmenopausal women, tamoxifen slightly increased BMD (0.61%) in the lumbar spine over 2 years compared with the loss (−1.0%) that occurred in the placebo-treated group. Radial BMD decreased to the same extent in both groups.[35] Results of the Breast Cancer Prevention Trial have been analyzed with respect to BMD and fracture risk. In this trial, 13,388 women with ages ranging from 35 to 70 were followed for 4 years. In postmenopausal women, tamoxifen caused a small increase in spine BMD. At the hip, there was an increase in BMD in year 1 that was not

present in year 2. The results in premenopausal women were surprising. There was a significant fall in BMD in the spine; there were no significant changes in trochanteric BMD (Figure 18–4). Using a growth curve analysis, premenopausal women lost bone while taking tamoxifen more rapidly than the placebo-treated controls.[36]

These studies have demonstrated the differences in estrogen-replete versus estrogen-deplete states. Generalizations about the selective estrogen receptor modulator (SERM) class of compounds should be avoided. Additional randomized studies designed for osteoporotic women are needed to resolve these issues. Meanwhile, women taking tamoxifen for breast cancer prevention should be monitored with serial BMDs, other risk factors for bone loss eliminated, and treatment initiated when appropriate.

Raloxifene and Fracture Risk

Raloxifene, a cousin to tamoxifen, has been approved for the prevention and treatment of osteoporosis. The Multiple Outcomes of Raloxifene Evaluation trial specifically evaluated the risk of fracture in postmenopausal women. The study was made up of 7705 postmenopausal women aged 30 to 80 years. Risk of vertebral fracture was reduced at both doses of raloxifene: for the 60 mg/day group, relative risk (RR) = 0.7, and for the 120 mg/day group, RR = 0.5. Fracture risk was not reduced at the hip or at other sites. Raloxifene (60 mg/day) increased BMD by 2.1% in the femoral neck and 2.6% in the spine.[37] The risk of venous thromboembolism was RR = 3.1%, comparable with that

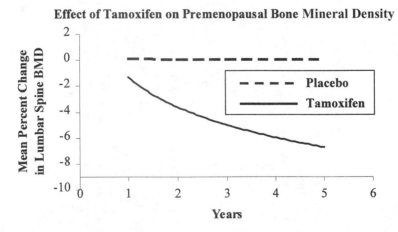

Effect of Tamoxifen on Premenopausal Bone Mineral Density

Figure 18–4 Effect of Tamoxifen on Bone Mineral Density at the Lumbar Spine in Premenopausal Women. The effect of tamoxifen was evaluated in premenopausal and postmenopausal women as part of the Breast Cancer Prevention Trial. Women were selected for increased breast cancer risk and randomly assigned to placebo or tamoxifen with an average follow-up of 4 years. Hip and lumbar spine BMD were measured in a subgroup of 135 premenopausal and postmenopausal women. In postmenopausal women, tamoxifen versus placebo therapy was associated with a small but significant gain in lumbar spine BMD in years 1 and 2. However, in premenopausal women (shown in figure), tamoxifen was associated with significant losses at the lumbar spine in years 1, 2, and 5. There was a similar trend in hip BMD.

of estrogen. Raloxifene did not cause vaginal bleeding or mastalgia and was associated with a lower incidence of breast cancer.

The SERMs such as tamoxifen and raloxifene offer alternatives to traditional HRT. Long-term risk/benefit ratios are not established, and thus choices must be made on an individual basis. New SERMs may be developed for prevention of breast cancer and treatment of osteoporosis. Each SERM may have differential effects on premenopausal versus postmenopausal women in the prevention of breast cancer and preservation of bone mass.

PHYTOESTROGENS AND BONE MINERAL DENSITY

Estrogen-like compounds are found in many foodstuffs. Soy products contain isoflavones (genistein and daidzein) and coumestrans (coumestral). Data on the effects of soy on bone are limited. In ovariectomized rats fed soy protein, BMD of the spine and femoral bone density were greater than controls.[38] In another study, rats injected with coumestrol had significantly less ovariectomy-induced bone loss.[39]

In one placebo-controlled trial, hypercholesterolemic postmenopausal women were given isoflavone-enriched soy protein (40 g/day) or casein in a double-blind, randomized trial. No significant differences were noted in the casein-treated group or the group ingesting only 56 mg/day of isoflavones. In the group of postmenopausal women ingesting 90 mg of isoflavone, significant increases in BMD of the spine ($P<0.05$) were noted.[40] In premenopausal women, there is a good deal of confusion regarding the potential benefit or risk of phytoestrogens on bone. In premenopausal women, vegetarians have lower BMD than omnivores. Other interesting data regarding the effects of the SERMs suggest differential effects on bone in premenopausal and postmenopausal subjects (see Tamoxifen and BMD). No evidence for fracture reduction in a clinical setting exists for the phytoestrogens. Epidemiological data are flawed by confounding variables including genetics. Randomized, controlled clinical trials are needed to assess the safety and efficacy of these potentially important compounds.[41]

BUILDING BONE WITH EXERCISE

Numerous cross-sectional studies support the concept that high levels of physical activity are associated with increased bone density in the eumenorrheic female. Literature supports increased BMD in female bodybuilders,[42] soccer players,[43] basketball players,[44] volleyball players,[44] runners,[45] college-aged,[46,47] and former gymnasts.[48]

Randomized longitudinal studies have confirmed these findings in premenopausal and postmenopausal women.

However, recommendations for specific guidelines regarding the optimal time and type of training to enhance bone formation are problematic. Studies have demonstrated positive, negative, and neutral effects on the skeleton in response to resistance training. Other forms of exercise such as walking or running provide a large number of loading cycles. Krall and Dawson-Hughes[49] examined the effect of walking on the lumbar spine and whole body BMD in healthy postmenopausal women who were participating in a vitamin D supplementation trial. Women who walked >7.5 miles/week had higher whole body and trunk BMD compared with women who walked <1 mile/week.

Until the 1990s, few prospective intervention trials of the effect of exercise on bone mass were completed. In general, with weight-bearing exercise, gains in BMD of the lumbar spine approximate 1.5% (Figure 18–5).[50] Little improvement is usually noted at the hip.[51,52] An excellent editorial by R. Marcus[52] reviews the differences in load-bearing that occur at the hip compared with the spine.

Maximizing peak bone mass is an important strategy for the prevention of osteoporosis. When walking, the load imposed on the skeleton is one body weight. This increases to three to four body weights during jogging. Gymnastics training provides even higher impact loading strains on the skeleton (Figure 18–6). The impact of load on the skeleton is confirmed in several well-designed studies of college-age athletes. Taaffe et al.[45] monitored longitudinal changes in BMD in collegiate women gymnasts and compared these results with those found in controls and swimmers. The percentage change in BMD of the lumbar spine was significantly greater in gymnasts than in swimmers or controls. For a cohort followed for 12 months, gymnasts gained 2.3% at the lumbar spine compared with swimmers (−0.3%) or controls (−0.4%). Changes at the femoral neck were also greater in gymnasts than in swimmers or controls. These findings were independent of hormonal status and emphasized the role of impact loading on bone formation.

In comparison of matched controls to runners, runners had increased BMD. However, gymnasts had higher lumbar spine BMD compared with runners, suggesting that impact is an important regulator of skeletal BMD. This is in contrast to swimmers, who were not weight bearing, and had lower BMD compared with controls despite upper body exercise with hand weights. These studies emphasized the type of impact necessary to increase BMD.[50,52]

On the basis of studies like these, Bassy and coworkers[53] developed an impact exercise program for healthy women. The exercise program consisted of 50 vertical jumps per day providing an estimated three to four body weights per jump. Premenopausal women experienced an increase in femoral and trochanteric BMD of 2% to 3% after 5 months of exercise. Postmenopausal women, on or off HRT, had no change in BMD measurements. Although this study sug-

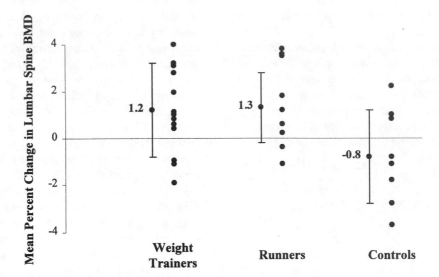

Figure 18–5 Controlled Exercise Intervention Trial in Young Athletes. This study is a controlled exercise intervention trial in a group of healthy college women who were randomly assigned to a control group or to a program of progressive training in jogging or weight lifting. Fifty-two women, mean age 19.9 years, in good health and with regular menstrual cycles, participated in the exercise sessions. For weight training, subjects performed a circuit of 14 exercises 3 times a week under supervision. Running schedules were designed for each subject on the basis of her 1.5 mile walk/run time. Mileage increases were restricted to 10% per week. The control subjects did not change their baseline physical activity patterns. Significant group-trial interactions were observed for lumbar spine BMD. Responses in the exercise groups did not differ from each other but were significantly greater than those of the control subjects.

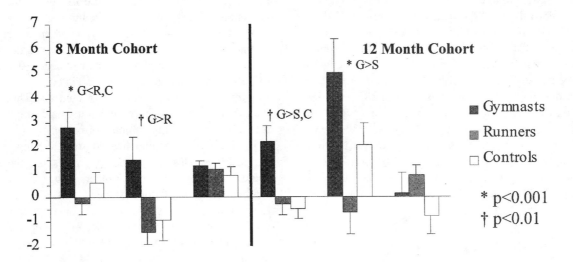

Figure 18–6 Gymnastics training and high-impact loading strains on the skeleton. To examine the role of gymnastics, longitudinal changes in regional and whole body BMD in collegiate women gymnasts and competitive athletes such as runners and swimmers were studied. Twenty-six gymnasts, 36 runners, and 14 nonathletic women were followed over an 8-month period. In a second cohort, 8 gymnasts, 11 swimmers, and 11 nonathletic women were followed over a 12-month period. The results indicate that BMD at lumbar spine and femoral neck increased dramatically as a result of mechanical loading characteristic of gymnastics training in college-aged women. This suggests that high-impact loading underlies the high BMD values characteristic of women gymnasts. Gymnasts from both cohorts experienced gains in femoral neck BMD compared with runners and swimmers. Changes for runners or controls and swimmers or controls were not different form one another and not significantly different compared with 0.

gests that there may be a decreased responsiveness with aging, the duration of the study may not have been sufficient to see changes in BMD. One study provided evidence that older women may gain bone by resistance exercise. Kerr et al.[54] conducted a 1-year study of bicycle exercise in postmenopausal women. One leg served as the control, whereas the other was exposed to increase in resistance. The hip on the side with progressive increase in resistance had a 2% increase in BMD compared with the control side. The difference in these studies may be due to the different types of impact: muscle-generated forces in the bicycle training compared with impact absorption during jumping. One additional difference was the progressive loading in the protocol of Kerr that stresses the importance of training in untrained subjects.[52]

The role of resistance training in bone metabolism remains less well defined. Resistance training improves muscle hypertrophy, muscle strength, and functional mobility.[55] With stronger muscles, better balance and coordination occur, resulting in fewer falls, and fewer falls result in fewer fractures. Does resistance training increase BMD? This question is more difficult to assess. In one prospective study of healthy, older women aged 65 to 79 years, neither high- nor low-resistance training altered hip or spine BMD over a 1-year period (Figure 18–7).[56] Resistance training in pre-menopausal women results in different findings, perhaps because of the presence of estrogen (Figure 18–8).[51]

Estrogens and Exercise

Mechanical loading of the skeleton and interactions with estrogen have been topics of interest for many years. Concepts developed by Frost[57] suggested a "mechanostat" in bone to assess skeletal load. Normal levels of estrogen are associated with the estrogenic response of the skeleton to load. In the amenorrheic athlete, the inadequate levels of estrogen prevent the response to load, and high load levels are necessary to prevent osteoporosis or osteopenia. Recent studies of athletes with low levels of estrogen and high loading activity indicate that even in response to high loads, the bone loss occurs.

The role of estrogen in weight-bearing exercise cannot be underestimated. Rencken et al.[58] studied amenorrheic and eumenorrheic athletes aged 17 to 39 years. In this case-control study, BMD was significantly lower at all sites except the fibula. Duration of amenorrhea and body weight predicted BMD at the femoral neck, trochanter intertrochanteric region, and the tibia (Figure 18–9). BMD was altered in these amenorrheic athletes even in skeletal sites receiving high impact load. Similar findings have been confirmed in

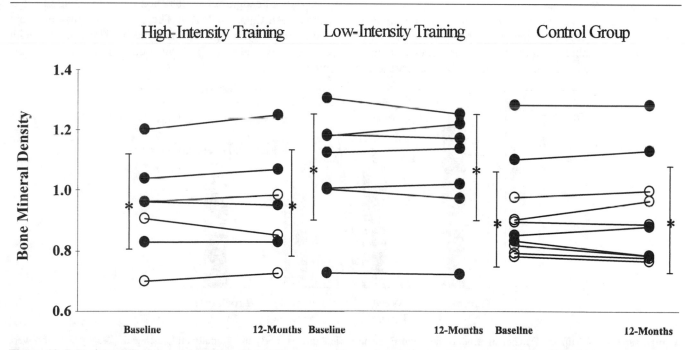

Figure 18–7 Resistance Training and BMD in Older Women. In a 12-month resistance training program in healthy older women, subjects were assigned to high-intensity, low-intensity, or control group. Most lower strength and BMD of the lumbar spine and total hip were measured at baseline and 12 months. Group differences in BMD change were not significant. In this study, high-intensity and low-intensity resistance training regimens increased muscle strength but not lumbar spine or total hip BMD in healthy older women (aged 65–79 years). Open circles represent women not on hormone replacement therapy. Filled circles represent individuals taking hormone replacement therapy.

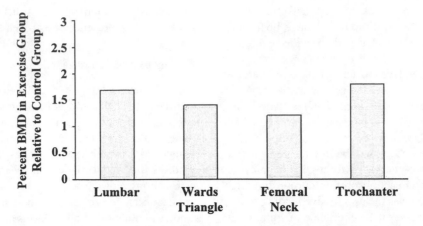

Figure 18–8 BMD and Resistance Training in Premenopausal Women. This study was designed to assess the effects of resistance exercise on total bone mineral density in premenopausal women aged 28–39. Subjects were randomly assigned to an exercise or control group. BMD increased significantly above baseline at the lumbar spine for the exercise group at 18 months compared with controls. Trochanter BMD also increased significantly over this time. Overall, these results support the use of strength training for increasing muscular strength with smaller differences in regional bone mineral density in the premenopausal population.

amenorrheic long-distance runners compared with their eumenorrheic counterparts.[59] The free estradiol index (derived as the ratio of estradiol to sex hormone–binding globulin) was significantly lower in the amenorrheic runners, even though estradiol levels were not different compared with eumenorrheic long-distance runners.

Most studies have not demonstrated a positive impact of exercise in increasing cancellous bone volume. Many confounding variables, including oligomenorrhea or amenorrhea, can influence bone metabolism. One observational

prospective study suggested that women who were ovulating had increased cancellous BMD as measured by quantitative computed tomography. By analyzing ovulation patterns, effects on spinal cancellous BMD were associated with luteal length; women with the shortest luteal phase experienced a significant 3.6% bone loss. In addition, exercise also influenced BMD. The greater the distance ran, the more likely bone loss was to occur. Thus, luteal length and activity were independent predictors of BMD in this model.[60]

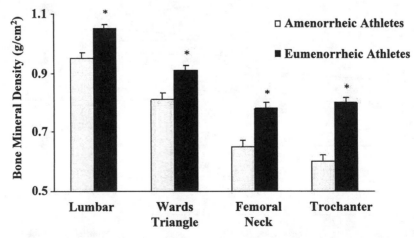

Figure 18–9 Bone Mineral Density in Amenorrheic and Eumenorrheic Athletes. Forty-nine female athletes, aged 17–39 years who were competitive or recreational runners, had their bone mineral density measured. All participated in some form of weight-bearing activity such as aerobics, basketball, weight training, or dance. A minimum of 45 minutes of activity 4 days a week was required. There were 23 amenorrheic women and 16 eumenorrheic women. There were no significant differences between the groups in age, height, weight, calcium intake, or training regimen. Amenorrheic athletes had a later age of menarche and significantly more months of amenorrhea. This study indicates that weight-bearing exercise does not offset the negative effect of decreased estrogen production on the skeleton of amenorrheic athletes.

HRT and Exercise

The lack of estrogen during menopause has profound effects on bone loss. Increased resorption of bone occurs, and osteoclast numbers and activity increase during estrogen deficiency. Intestinal absorption of calcium and renal absorption of calcium are also decreased by the lack of estrogen. The administration of ERT influences all the endocrine and paracrine effects on bone and increases the bone loss associated with menopause. Estrogens stimulate the differentiation and activity of osteoblasts and inhibit osteoclast-mediated bone resorption. The rate of bone loss is approximately 3% in the first 5 years after menopause and falls to approximately 1% per year thereafter.

Several prospective clinical trials have evaluated the effect of exercise on bone in the postmenopausal woman taking HRT. These studies provide conflicting data regarding exercise in the estrogen-replete woman. Some studies demonstrate no effect of exercise compared with estrogen alone; other studies demonstrate increased bone density in the HRT plus exercise group compared with HRT alone. Many reasons exist for these discordant results. The type and quality of the exercise have profound influence on the outcome. Second, women who take HRT, including those who volunteer for clinical protocols, are in general better health and have fewer adverse risk factors for bone loss. Many of the exercise studies are not of long enough duration to affect a change in BMD, and lack of precision of BMD measurements may make small increments difficult to detect. One additional problem may reside in bone turnover in the early postmenopausal woman: the effect of estrogen is greatest in the first few years after menopause because of high bone turnover. The large increment gained in bone mass by the administration of estrogen may attenuate any effect of exercise in the perimenopausal and early postmenopausal years.

OSTEOPOROSIS

Osteoporosis is defined as the loss of normally mineralized bone. Osteoporosis is characterized by low bone mass and microarchitectural deterioration of bone (Figure 18–10). The result is bone fragility with an increaseed risk of fracture. The advent of noninvasive radiological techniques that measure bone density has led to the widespread recognition and diagnosis of this disorder. Bones are structurally weak, and there is an associated loss of trabecular bone, enlargement of the medullary space, cortical porosity, and a reduction in cortical thickness. The reduction in bone mass and changes in bone architecture are associated with an increased risk of fracture, which results in pain and deformity. Low bone mass and nontraumatic or atraumatic fractures are features of osteoporosis. The excessive bone loss that characterizes the pathogenesis of osteoporosis results from abnormalities in the bone remodeling cycle.

Epidemiology of Osteoporosis

It is currently estimated that between 13% and 18% of postmenopausal Caucasian women in the United States have osteoporosis, and an additional 30% to 50% have low bone density at the hip. Osteoporosis affects an enormous number of people, and its prevalence will increase as the population ages. On the basis of data from the National Health and Nutrition Examination Survey III, it is estimated that more than 10 million people in the United States have osteoporosis of the hip, whereas 19 million have low bone mass as measured at the hip. One of every two Caucasian woman will experience an osteoporotic fracture sometime during her lifetime. There is also a significant risk for nonwhite women, although the risk is lower.

The most serious outcome of osteoporosis is hip fracture. Other common sites of fractures include the vertebrae (spine) and distal forearm (wrist). Hip fracture can result in up to 20% excess mortality within 1 year. Up to 25% of hip fracture patients may require long-term institutional care, and only one-third regain the level of independence that they experienced before the fracture. Vertebral fractures cause significant complications, including height loss, kyphosis, and back pain. Activity may be limited because of height changes, and cosmetic effects may prevent clothing from fitting well and erode self-esteem. Multiple thoracic fractures can result in restrictive lung disease and abdominal pain and distress.

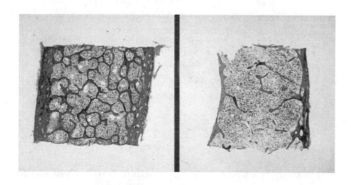

Figure 18–10 Histology of Normal and Osteoporotic Bone. Histological section of bone from a normal 47 year old woman (left) and an osteoporotic 52-year-old woman (right). On the normal biopsy, you can see two thick cortical surfaces with serpiginous trabecular bone within the marrow space. In the osteoporotic individual, the cortical surfaces are narrowed. The volume of bone overall is reduced in both the cortical and trabecular compartments. Connectivity between the trabecular bone and cortical surfaces is poor, and isolated bone islands are present.

The economic burden of osteoporotic fractures is tremendous. Direct medical expenditures for 1995 exceeded $13.8 billion for the cost of fracture care. By the year 2040, one estimate suggests that the number of hip fractures and their costs will triple.

Definition of Osteoporosis by Bone Mineral Density

Measurement of Bone Mineral Density

Evaluation of a patient for osteoporosis at this time remains somewhat controversial. The National Osteoporosis Foundation (NOF) has provided guidelines as to who should have a BMD determination. At the time of menopause, all women should be evaluated for fracture risk. Risk factors for osteoporosis can be modifiable in some cases. Bone mineral testing is recommended in patients under the age of 65 with one or more risk factors or patients who have had a fracture. All postmenopausal women over the age of 65 should be tested for osteoporosis.

BMD can establish or confirm a diagnosis of osteoporosis, predict future fracture risk, and monitor changes in BMD during therapy. The lower the BMD, the greater the risk for fracture.

Measurements of BMD at any skeletal site have been valuable to predict fracture risk. BMD of the hip is the best predictor of hip fractures. The measurement of BMD at the hip also predicts fractures at other sites. BMD is expressed as a relationship to two normative values: the expected BMD for patient's age and sex, termed the T-score or "young normal" and BMD of adults of the same age and sex termed the Z-score. The difference between a patient's score and the normal value is expressed as a standard deviation (SD) above or below the mean. The T-score declines in parallel with a steady drop in bone mass that occurs with aging. Most guidelines use the T-score for clinical decision making.

The DEXA method of bone density measurement is currently the "gold standard" and can be measured at the hip or spine. DEXA scans can be completed in a few minutes with a radiation exposure that is approximately one-tenth of a standard chest x-ray film. At present, several peripheral measurements of the calcaneus or finger are available. Quantitative ultrasound (QUS) measurement of bone density may be performed in the heel, tibia, patella, or other peripheral sites. QUS is a radiation-free technique that evaluates bone density and structure. Broadband ultrasound attenuation measures scatter and absorption of sound waves and reflects density, microarchitecture, and elasticity of bone. Other measurements obtained with ultrasound include spread of sound and velocity of bone, which reflect bone density. Ultrasound measurements are generally not as precise as DEXA but may predict fracture risk well. These tests are useful for screening, but it is currently recommended that patients with a low BMD determined by ultrasound should have a confirmatory BMD by DEXA scan.

BMD Should Be Performed on:

1. All postmenopausal women less than the age of 65 who have one or more additional risk factors for osteoporotic fracture
2. All women age 65 and older
3. Postmenopausal women who present with fracture
4. Women who are considering therapy for osteoporosis in whom BMD testing would facilitate the decision
5. Women who have been on hormone replacement therapy for prolonged periods

Clinical Guideline

The diagnosis of osteoporosis is currently based on guidelines developed by the World Health Organization (WHO) or the NOF. Both sets of guidelines used peak bone mass as normative data. Osteoporosis is defined as –2.5 (WHO) or –2.0 (NOF) standard deviations below the mean.

On the basis of WHO criteria, Melton[61] estimated that 16.8 million (54%) postmenopausal Caucasian women have osteopenia, and 9.4 million (30%) have osteoporosis.

Definition of Osteoporosis by T-Score

WHO*		NOF†
<–1.0	Normal	<–1.0
–1.0 to –2.5	Osteopenia	–1.0 to –2.0
>–2.5	Osteoporosis	>–2.0
–2.5 SD with one or more fragility fractures	Severe osteoporosis	—

Definition is based on T-score, the standard deviation below the young adult mean.
*World Health Organization.
†National Osteoporosis Foundation.

Clinical Guideline

These different definitions of osteoporosis have led to some controversy as to when to intervene with treatment. Caution should be observed if measuring BMD in a younger person. Someone who is 17 years old, for example, may not have reached peak bone mass yet and thus be below the mean compared with the older, age-based control.

Juvenile Osteoporosis

Idiopathic juvenile osteoporosis occurs in prepubertal patients and is progressive in nature. Bone formation proceeds normally, but ostcoclast activity is increased. Osteoporosis becomes evident in the thoracic and lumbar spine and manifests as anterior wedging and concave deformities of vertebral bodies. The disorder is self-limited, and slipped capital femoral epiphyses may be present. Symptoms begin with an insidious onset of pain in the lower back, hips, and feet. There may be knee and ankle pain and fractures of the lower extremities. Both sexes are affected equally, and supportive care is recommended in anticipation of a spontaneous recovery with the onset of puberty.

Regional Osteoporosis

Regional osteoporosis has been found as an incidental finding on radiographs. This may occur in patients with reflex sympathetic dystrophy syndrome or in patients whose limbs have been immobilized for more than 4 weeks. The genesis is unclear, but injured axons show increased sensitivity to norepinephrine or other substances that may be associated with the underlying process.

Postmenopausal Osteoporosis

Peak adult bone mass is obtained at age 20 to 30, after which point age-related bone loss occurs (see section on "Determinants of Peak Bone Mass"). With normal aging, the impairment of coupling between bone resorption and formation becomes progressive, so that with each cycle the deficit between resorption and formation becomes exaggerated.

Effects of Estrogen Deficiency During Menopause on Bone Health

↑ Osteoclast-mediated bone resorption
↑ Ostcoclast recruitment
↑ Osteoclast activity
↓ Intestinal absorption of calcium
↓ Renal reabsorption of calcium
↓ Matrix synthesis by osteoblasts

Clinical Guideline

Bone loss is an asymptomatic process, and the key to prevention of osteoporosis is early identification of subjects at greatest risk. The development of peak bone mass is primarily under genetic control, and the variance in bone mass does not change with age. This may explain why fracture prevalence incidences are greatest in those with a low bone mass at any age.[62]

Osteoporosis in the absence of fractures is otherwise asymptomatic. Osteoporosis does not result in delayed fracture union, and if nonunion or delayed union occurs, conditions other than osteoporosis should be considered. Osteoporotic vertebral fractures may occur in the absence of acute symptoms. Vertebral fractures are associated with a loss of stat-

ure and progressive kyphosis. Anatomical changes become more pronounced as more vertebral bodies fracture. The abdomen and, in severe cases, the lower hips protrude. The distorted body image may result in an altered self-image, vague gastrointestinal problems, respiratory problems, and depression. If acute symptoms occur with vertebral fracture, immobilization, appropriate analgesia, vertebroplasty, and kyphoplasty are the mainstays of treatment.

SECONDARY OSTEOPOROSIS

Secondary osteoporosis is defined as bone loss resulting from specific well-defined clinical disorders. Many times reversible causes of bone loss are not considered in a patient with low BMD. A recent study suggested that up to one third of patients with osteoporosis had a secondary cause. For this reason, it is important to rule out these causes of bone loss before finalizing decisions regarding treatment. Secondary osteoporosis may be due to endocrine disorders, medications, immobilization, disorders of the gastrointestinal or biliary tract, or renal disease.

Secondary Causes of Osteoporosis

- Acromegaly
- Adrenal atrophy in Addison's disease
- Amyloidosis
- Ankylosing spondylitis
- Chronic obstructive pulmonary disease
- Congenital porphyria
- Cushing's syndrome
- Endometriosis
- Epidermolysis bullosa
- Gastrectomy
- Gonadal insufficiency (primary or secondary)
- Hemachromatosis
- Hemophilia
- Hyperparathyroidism
- Hyperthyroidism
- Hypophosphatasia
- Idiopathic scoliosis
- Insulin-dependent diabetes mellitus
- Lymphoma and leukemia
- Malabsorption syndromes
- Mastocytosis
- Multiple myeloma
- Multiple sclerosis
- Nutritional disorders
- Osteogenesis imperfecta
- Parenteral nutrition
- Pernicious anemia
- Rheumatoid arthritis
- Sarcoidosis
- Severe liver disease
- Thalassemia

- Toxicosis
- Tumor secretion of parathyroid hormone–related peptide

Clinical Guideline

In this section, osteoporosis associated with drug therapy and endocrine disorders will be described.

Drugs Associated with Bone Loss

- Aluminum
- Anticonvulsants
- Cigarette smoking
- Cytotoxic drugs
- Excessive alcohol
- Excessive thyroxine
- Glucocorticoids and adrenocorticotropin
- Gonadotropin-releasing hormone agonists
- Heparin
- Lithium
- Tamoxifen (in the premenopausal patient)
- Vitamins A and E

Clinical Guideline

Secondary Osteoporosis Associated with Drug Therapy

Glucocorticoids

Decalcification of the skeleton was recognized as a clinical feature of Cushing's disease as early as 1932. Glucocorticoid excess results in diffuse bone loss and may affect trabecular bone more than cortical bone. The osteopenia is due to suppression of osteoblast function, inhibition of intestinal calcium absorption leading to secondary hyperparathyroidism, and increased osteoclast-mediated bone resorption. Bone loss is also promoted by direct stimulation of renal excretion of calcium by glucocorticoids. Hypogonadism may occur with the suppressive effects of glucocorticoids on the hypothalamic-pituitary axis.

Bone density is reduced in 40% to 60% of patients with an endogenous glucocorticoid excess, and pathological fractures have been observed in 16% to 67% of them. Short-term studies have indicated that glucocorticoid-induced bone loss appears greater in the first 6 to 12 months of therapy. The minimum dose of glucocorticoids associated with rapid bone loss is not established, but some studies indicate that as little as 5 or 7.5 mg of prednisone per day produces considerable bone loss. Glucocorticoid-induced osteoporosis is more severe in patients younger than 15 years, older than 50 years, and in postmenopausal women.

Serum and urine biochemical indices in patients with glucocorticoid-induced osteopenia are generally normal. Serum immunoreactive parathyroid hormone levels may be normal or mildly elevated. Serum alkaline phosphatase (bone fraction) activity and osteocalcin levels decline steadily after the initiation of glucocorticoid therapy. Urinary calcium excretion may be increased during the first several months to years of steroid therapy because of the direct calciuric effect of glucocorticoids on the kidney.[62]

Anticonvulsant Medications

Bone disease associated with anticonvulsant therapy has been considered a form of osteomalacia. High turnover of osteoporosis is often present, and in its florid form, bone changes such as osteopenia and fractures are associated with hypocalcemia, hypophosphatemia, and muscle weakness. Rickets has been observed in children taking anticonvulsant medication. Usually, however, minimal biochemical abnormalities are present, which include increased circulating levels of parathyroid hormone and skeletal changes such as deficits in cortical bone mass. Several studies have recently been reported that indicate the anticonvulsant-induced bone disease may reflect a rapid remodeling state. Alterations and hepatic metabolism of vitamin D, such that inactive polar metabolites are produced, have been demonstrated in epileptic subjects. A decrease in the available stores of 25-hydroxyvitamin D, leading to decreased intestinal calcium absorption, could explain a compensatory secondary hyperparathyroidism that occurs.

Miscellaneous Medications Associated with Osteoporosis

Other medications have been associated with the development of osteoporosis. Methotrexate has been implicated as a cause of bone loss, but in most studies, other drugs have been administered or the gonadal status of the patients has been altered, making definitive conclusions difficult. The zealous administration of exogenous thyroid hormone has been associated with osteopenia. Clinical relevance of osteoporosis associated with excessive thyroid hormone has been examined in terms of development of fractures, but the data remain controversial. Heparin has been implicated in the suppression of bone formation.

Endocrine Disorders Associated with Secondary Osteoporosis

Hyperthyroidism

Both thyroid insufficiency and excess lead to alterations in bone mass. Thyroid hormone increases the creation of new BRUs with an enhancement of remodeling activity. Thyrotoxicosis is associated with increased bone resorption. Even mildly excessive doses of thyroid hormone may prevent bone loss, but this raises the clinical specter of iatrogenic hyperthyroidism. Published evidence indicates that minimally excessive long-term thyroid hormone replacement can bring about a decrease in cortical bone mass.

Primary Hyperparathyroidism

Parathyroid hormone is responsible for stimulating calcium homeostasis through its action on target cells in the bone and kidney. Primary hyperparathyroidism is a common disorder and usually asymptomatic. Parathyroid hormone itself has devastating effects on the skeleton, although severe bone involvement osteitis fibrosa cystica is now uncommon. The hallmark of skeletal involvement in primary hyperparathyroidism is an increase in bone turnover rate. Parathyroid hormone has a preference for cortical bone over trabecular bone, and cortices are thin or excessively porous, whereas cancellous bone volume is relatively well maintained in primary hyperparathyroidism. Fracture rates are higher in patients with primary hyperparathyroidism compared with community-dwelling controls.[64] If the patient has surgery for asymptomatic primary hyperparathyroidism, remarkable gains in BMD occur postoperatively.[65]

Acromegaly

Elevated concentration of growth hormone causes acceleration of bone turnover. In patients with acromegaly, the frequency of osteoporosis or fractures does not appear to be increased. However, in some studies, bone mass has proved to be increased, and elevated $1,25(OH)_2D_3$ levels have been noted. When osteoporosis occurs in acromegaly, the bone in this setting shows unusual architecture and composition. There is usually a very low trabecular bone volume, whereas the mean trabecular plate thickness is strikingly increased.

Cushing's Syndrome

Hypercortisolism is a well-recognized risk factor for the development of osteoporosis. This occurs in exogenous (see section on Glucocorticoids) or iatrogenic hypercortisolism and where trabecular bone tends to be lost in preference to cortical bone. If Cushing's syndrome is cured surgically, some of the bone loss is reversible.

Insulin-Dependent Diabetes Mellitus

Low BMD is associated with insulin-dependent diabetes mellitus. No increase in the incidence of fracture versus the incidence in a nondiabetic population has been noted, but the incidence of stress fractures in foot bones is greater in diabetic patients than in nondiabetic patients. Bone formation rates are low in patients with diabetes mellitus, and the reduction in bone turnover rate may cause the bone to be more fragile, resulting in the risk of fracture in a subset of patients.

Miscellaneous Causes of Secondary Osteoporosis

Immobilization

Immobilization causes a rapid and diffuse bone loss. The nature and mechanics of normal bone stress have been intensely studied. When healthy adults are placed on bedrest, hypercalciuria develops and persists for months. Whole body mineral loss of about 0.5% per month can occur, and remineralization begins once ambulation is resumed. Data from space flights have revealed the critical importance of gravitational stress. Despite frequent strenuous exercise, astronauts in weightless orbit have impressive hypercalciuria and a negative calcium balance. In bedridden patients, lumbar spine mineral content decreases by 0.9% per week, which is equivalent to a 45% loss per year. Bone mineral content can be restored within 4 months once subjects start to walk again. The primary loss of mineral from bone stems from a suppressed parathyroid-vitamin D axis.

In a recent study in which normal subjects underwent 12 weeks of bedrest, bone mineral density declined at the spine by −2.9% and at the hip by −3.8%. Bedrest resulted in a significant increase in urinary calcium and phosphorus and in serum calcium. Bone histomorphometric studies revealed a suppression of osteoblast surfaces and increased bone resorption. Eroded surfaces increased. Surprisingly, serum biochemical markers of bone formation did not change, but biochemical markers of bone resorption have a significant increase during bed rest that declined toward normal during reambulation.[66]

Vitamin A and Vitamin E

Hypervitaminosis A results in weakness, emotional lability, musculoskeletal pain, headache, pseudotumor cerebri, and osteopenia. Serum alkaline phosphatase activity may be elevated, and elevation of both hepatic and bone isoenzymes may be present.

Marrow-Related Disorders

Cancellous and endocortical bone surfaces are in close opposition to the bone marrow, and disorders of bone marrow can produce profound changes in bone. Plasma cell dyscrasia such as multiple myeloma and macroglobulinemia are associated with bone disorders caused by an increase in bone-resorbing cytokines such as IL-1, TNF, and lymphotoxin. Other disorders such as leukemia, lymphomas, and systemic mastocytosis can result in osteoporosis. Chronic anemia such as sickle cell anemia and β-thalassemia associated with bone loss and bone diseases are common features of Gaucher's disease and Niemann-Pick disease.

Metabolic Bone Disease Associated with Gastrointestinal and Biliary Tract Disorders

Impaired absorption or catabolism or both of vitamin D and its metabolites and malabsorption of calcium can occur in subjects with gastrointestinal tract disorders. Secondary hyperparathyroidism occurs and is characterized by an increased surface area and volume of unmineralized tissue. The most common finding in patients with gastrointestinal tract disorders and bone disease is low turnover osteoporosis. Protein and other micronutrient deficiencies may contribute to this. Secondary hyperparathyroidism is a consistent feature in these vitamin D–deficient patients with accelerated loss of cortical bone.

TRAUMA

Strategies for reducing fracture risks include increasing peak bone mass and reducing the bone loss that occurs associated with estrogen deficiency in the postmenopausal years. Multiple factors have an impact on fracture risk, including diet, genotype, physical activity, reproductive status, and low bone mass. For every 1 standard deviation decline in BMD, fracture risk increases twofold.[62]

Fracture Repair

When trauma occurs, the skeleton attempts to restore functional and anatomical integrity. As with any injured tissue, adult bone tissue reverts to basic undifferentiated mesenchymal tissue, which is followed by wound closure and scar formation. What is unusual about the skeleton is that the scar tissue of bone is bone and the repair of the skeletal tissue is basically the formation of normal bone development and growth.

The initial repair tissue formed is called callus, which is ultimately modeled into normal bone. Like growing bone, callus is dynamic and undergoes rapid structural changes. Callus is made up of fibrous tissue, woven bone, and cartilage. Mechanical stress and oxygen tension are important determinants in cell differentiation. Intermittent stress favors cartilage formation. In suitably immobilized fractures, membranous bone forms, whereas in free fractures, endochondral bone forms as a predominant feature.

Phases of Fracture Healing

- Inflammatory: Damaged tissue creates inflammatory cellular response. Connective tissue organizes and vascular network forms. Osteoblasts deposit immature, woven bone.
- Reparative: Orderly formation of callus. Woven bone is replaced with cartilage and ossified elements.
- Modeling: Fracture site strengthens by replacement and shaping of bone along lines of stress. Restoration of medullary cavity.

Clinical Guideline

Fracture healing can be divided into three phases: inflammatory, reparative, and modeling. The inflammatory phase begins immediately after trauma, where in the first 5 days after injury, the necrotic and damaged tissue generates an inflammatory cellular response. Connective tissue invades and eventually replaces (organizes) the hematoma. A rich vascular network develops around the fracture zone. Blood flow around the fracture increases, and dilated capillary spaces become engorged with blood and with stasis and passive congestion develops. Osteoblasts differentiate from the undifferentiated mesenchymal tissue and immature woven bone is deposited. The first signs of mineralization are visible radiographically after 14 days.

The reparative phase of fracture healing is characterized by the more orderly secretion of callus, the removal and replacement of immature woven bone through the process of cartilage differentiation, and endochondral ossification. Clinical union is achieved when the callus is sufficiently developed to allow weight bearing or similar stress usually at around 4 weeks after injury. The fracture continues to strengthen during the modeling phase.

The modeling phase involves the realignment and mechanical shaping of bone and callus along the lines of stress. The final stage of fracture healing results in restoration of the medullary cavity in bone marrow. Clinical healing precedes the anatomical reconstitution, and extensive remodeling will continue for years.

The sequence of events that takes place during fracture healing is important in the subsequent management of patients with fractures. Although the hematoma is not essential for fracture healing, it plays a metabolic role in inducing the formation of granulation tissue. The greater the hematoma formation, the more cellular and robust is the callus that is formed. Therefore, the hematoma should not be disturbed. Large necrotic bone fragments must be removed by osteoclast activity and may impede callus formation. Sequestered bone fragments may need to be surgically removed. Skeletal muscle is richly vascular and contributes extensively to the development of the callus; therefore injured soft tissue should not be disturbed. Poor fracture healing typically occurs in the superficial bones that have little or no adjacent musculature such as the tibia.

Complications of Fracture Healing

Nonunions

The time it takes for most fractures to heal is surprisingly uniform. When fractures take longer than usual but show signs of progressive healing, this is considered a delayed union. A nonunion occurs when the fracture remains unhealed and shows no signs of further healing. Numerous factors may contribute to delayed union or nonunion, which include the location of the fracture, soft tissue damage, tissue interposition, bone loss, and wound contamination or infection. The incidence of delayed union is unknown, and the incidence of nonunion is estimated to occur in 5% of all long-bone fractures. Nonunion rarely occurs in bones of the axial skeleton, the skull, ribs, vertebrae, scapulas, or pelvis.

Fibrous Union

The distal pretibial and carpal navicular bones have relatively poor blood supply and little associated subcutaneous tissue and muscle. These areas may have difficulty establishing the normal vascular network at the fracture zone. Poor blood supply to a fracture site promotes primitive scar tissue rather than callous formation. The bridge between the two fractured bone fragments is consequently filled with an avascular fibrous connective tissue rather than the usual bone and cartilage elements of the callus. In some cases, electrical stimulation of the fracture has dramatically improved the response of these fibrous nonunions to treatment.

Stress Fractures

Stress fractures are a common overuse injury in female athletes. Stress fractures can occur as a result of increased stress on bone or normal stress on weakened bones (Figures 18–11 to 18–13). Insufficiency fractures occur when normal physiological stress is applied to bone with abnormal elastic or mineral properties. Fatigue fractures are defined when abnormal stress is applied to normal bone. Stress (fatigue) fractures can result from repetitive cycle loading of bone. Insidious pain, which worsens with exercise, is frequently the presentation of a stress fracture. Occasionally, periosteal thickening, swelling, or redness may be present at the site of fracture. Clinical diagnosis is frequently adequate; imaging modalities can confirm the diagnosis (Figure 18–8). Plain radiographs are of little use for diagnosis. On MRI, periosteal and marrow edema and the fracture line can be visualized. The major treatment is rest, and most stress fractures heal in 6 to 8 weeks. Fractures of the navicular or anterior tibia cortex are particularly prone to nonunion and may take longer to heal. The resumption of physical activity should be judged by symptoms. Often other physical activity can be assumed during the rest period such as swimming, weight training, or cycling to maintain fitness.

Stress Fractures

Bone scan is frequently positive at the time of clinical presentation (or within 24 hours) of fracture. Plain radiograph visualization may not occur for 2 to 10 days after injury.

Clinical Guideline

Tibial Stress Fractures

In military recruits, upper third postmedially is the most common site of stress fracture.
In young athletes, the junction of the mid and lower thirds is the site of most common involvement.
Ballet dancers are more likely to injure the midshaft.
Resolution may take several weeks to months of reduced activity.

Clinical Guideline

Insufficiency Fractures Can Occur in Patients with the Following Abnormal Bone:

- Osteoporosis
- Rheumatoid arthritis
- Osteomalacia/rickets
- Paget's disease
- Hyperparathyroidism
- Renal osteodystrophy
- Radiation therapy
- Steroid use

Clinical Guideline

Stress fractures present a unique set of problems in the high-performance athlete. Several studies have attempted to identify risk factors associated with stress factors, but little success has been achieved to date. In a case-control study of 49 female soldiers with confirmed stress fractures, physical activity, prior calcium intake, and bone density were compared as predictors of stress fractures. Only a weak relationship with prior activity was observed, and no association with calcium intake or bone density was noted.[67]

The importance of "pacing" during training to prevent injury was demonstrated in a group of female Australian Army recruits. In the 1991 to 1992 time period, pelvic stress fracture incidence was 11.2% compared with an incidence of 0.1% in male recruits (1992–1993). Preventive strategies included reduction of march speed, softer surfaces for running, and promotion of individual step length instead of

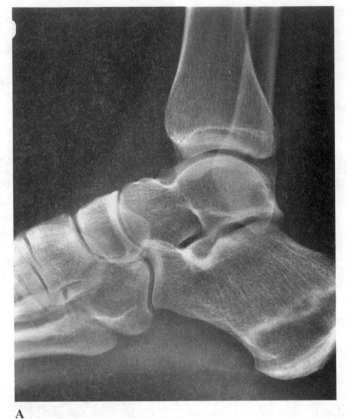

A

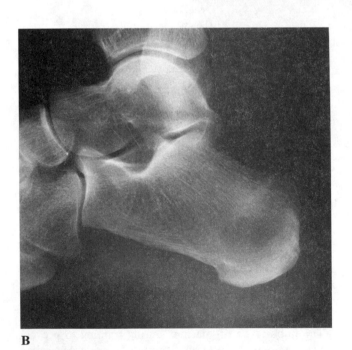

B

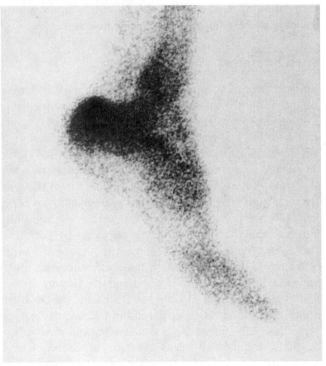

C

Figure 18–11 A, left calcaneal stress fracture. This 29-year-old woman had left heel pain develop after several long walks and jumping rope. The initial radiograph was normal. After 5 to 6 weeks of persistent pain, a left calcaneal stress fracture was noted. B, radiography of right ankle of a 51-year-old woman who had pain develop 5 hours after her aerobics class. C, bone scan of calcaneal stress fracture. The bone scan shows increased uptake in all three phases, consistent with stress fracture of the calcaneous.

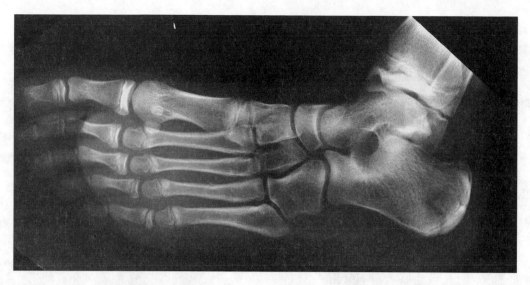

Figure 18–12 Metatarsal Fracture in a 12-Year-Old Competitive Figure Skater. The patient had a recent change in her training regimen. There is a nondisplaced fracture of the right fourth metatarsal consistent with a stress fracture.

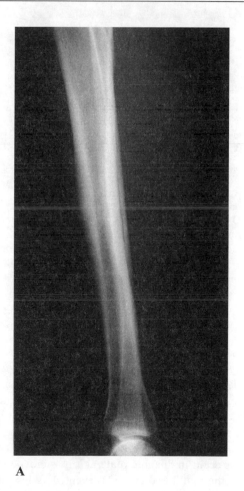

A

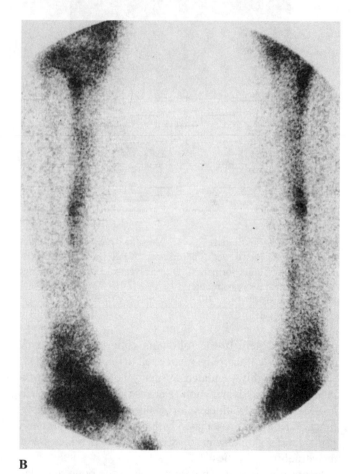

B

continues

Figure 18–13 A, tibial stress fracture in a 34-year-old woman with tibial pain bilaterally for 18 months. She had been jogging 5 miles per day for 18 months. Cortical thickening with central lucent transverse defect midshaft of the tibiae. B, bone scan showing bilateral uptake in the tibia, consistent with stress fractures.

continued

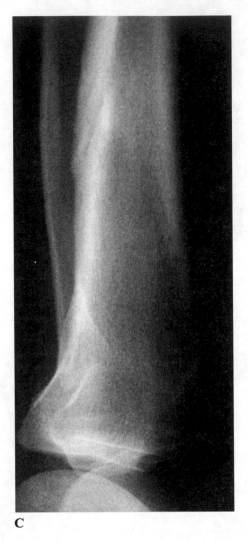

C

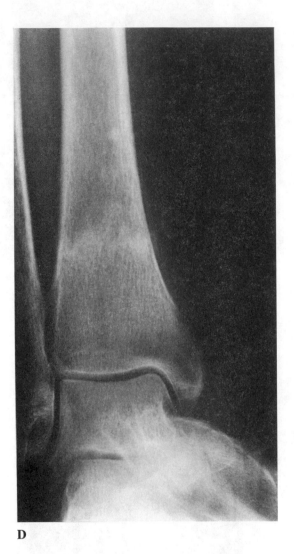

D

Figure 18–13 (continued) C, a 15-year-old woman cross-country runner who had leg pain for 6 weeks. She was restricted from running and jumping. This 6-week radiograph reveals healing stress fracture involving posterior medial aspect of the right tibia with minimal periosteal new bone formation. D, a 57-year-old runner with right foot pain. Linear band sclerosis in the right distal tibial metaphysis is consistent with a stress fracture.

marching in step. In the following cohort of 161 female recruits, pelvic fracture incidence fell to 0.6% ($P < 0.001$).[68]

BMD is highly regulated by many hormones and cytokines. Menstrual dysfunction can cause significant reduction in BMD in female athletes. Increasing severity of menstrual function is linearly associated with declining BMD and may explain the high incidence of stress fractures in athletes with menstrual irregularities.[69]

Stress fractures may not be related to the bone remodeling cycle in athletes. Recently, in a 12-month prospective study of 46 female and 49 male track and field athletes, no differences in bone turnover were detected by biochemical markers in the 20 athletes who sustained a stress fracture compared with their matched comparison group.[70] Thus, one is unable to predict "at risk" individuals by measurements of serum osteocalcin, pyridinium cross-links (Pyr and D-Pyr) or NTx of type I collagen.

Elite rowers may experience rib fractures, especially associated with long-distance training and heavy load per stroke. Fractures occur in the anterolateral to posterolateral aspects of ribs 5 through 9 and can be prevented by less use of the serratus anterior and external oblique through a truncated arm pullthrough and decreased by leg back position at the end of the stroke.[71] Stress fractures of the ribs have also been

Fatigue Fracture: Defined as Abnormal Muscular Stress Applied to Bone with Normal Elastic Resistance

Location	Cause of fracture
Coracoid process of the scapula	Trap shooting
Ribs	Golf, coughing
Distal shaft of the humerus	Throwing ball
Femoral neck	Ballet, running
Femoral shaft	Ballet, marching, long-distance running, gymnastics
Obturator ring of the pelvis	Running, gymnastics
Patella	Hurdling
Tibial shaft	Ballet, jogging
Calcaneus	Jumping, parachuting
Metatarsal (commonly second metatarsal)	Marching, stomping on the ground, ballet

Clinical Guideline

described in golfers and swimmers. Stress fractures of the metatarsals or tibia can be seen in skaters and most commonly occurs in the take-off leg. Conservative management with rest usually provides an adequate outcome.

Another 12-month prospective study identified risk factors for stress fractures in female track and field athletes aged 17 to 26 years. Significant risk factors included a lower BMD, history of menstrual disturbance, a discrepancy in leg length, less lean mass in the lower limb, and a lower fat diet.[72]

Diagnosis of stress fractures should be considered in the active elderly patient. In a retrospective study of 30 stress fractures in elderly patients enjoying noncompetitive sporting events such as marching or running, diagnosis was delayed or incorrect, because the stress fracture was mistaken for another condition.[73]

REFERENCES

1. Fitzpatrick LA. Metabolic and nontumorous bone disorders. In: Damjanov I, Linder L, eds. *Anderson's Pathology.* St. Louis, MO: Mosby; 1996:2574.

2. Roodman GD. Cell biology of the osteoclast. *Exp Hematol.* 1999;27:1229–1241.

3. Robey PG, Fedarko NS, Hefferan TE, et al. Structure and molecular regulation of bone matrix proteins. *J Bone Mineral Res.* 1993;8:S483–S487.

4. Raisz LG. Physiology and pathophysiology of bone remodeling. *Clin Chem.* 1999;45:1353–1358.

5. Smith EP, Boyd J, Frank GR, et al. Estrogen resistance caused by a mutation in the estrogen-receptor gene in a man. *N Engl J Med.* 1994;331:1056–1061.

6. Spelsberg TC, Subramaniam M, Riggs BL, Khosla S. The actions and interactions of sex steroids and growth factors/cytokines on the skeleton. *Mol Endocrinol.* 1999;13:819–828.

7. Oursler MJ. Estrogen regulation of gene expression in osteoblasts and osteoclasts. *Crit Rev Eukaryotic Gene Expression.* 1998;8:125–140.

8. Jilka RL. Cytokines, bone remodeling, and estrogen deficiency: A 1998 Update. *Bone.* 1998;23:75–81.

9. Conte FA, Greenbach MM, Ito Y, Fisher CR, Simpson ER, et al. A syndrome of female pseudohermaphroditism, hypergonadotropic hypogonadism, and multicystic ovaries associated with missense mutations in the gene encoding aromatase (P450arom). *J Clin Endocrinol Metab.* 1994;78:1287–1292.

10. Morishima A, Grumbach MM, Simpson ER, Fisher C, Qin K. Aromatase deficiency in male and female siblings caused by a novel mutation in the physiological role of estrogen. *J Clin Endocrinol Metab.* 1995;80:3689–3698.

11. Theintz G, Buchs B, Rizzoli R, Slosman D, Clavier H, Sizonen K. Longitudinal monitoring of bone mass accumulation in healthy adolescents: Evidence for a marked reduction after 16 years of age at the levels of lumbar spine and femoral neck in female subjects. *J Clin Endocrinol Metab.* 1992;75:1060–1065.

12. Matkovic V, Jelic T, Wardlaw GM, Ilich JZ, Goel PK, Wright JK. Timing of peak bone mass in Caucasian females and its implication for the prevention of osteoporosis: Inference from a cross-sectional model. *J Clin Invest.* 1994;93:799–808.

13. Rizzoli R, Bonjour J-P. Determinants of peak bone mass and mechanisms of bone loss. *Osteoporos Int.* 1999;2:S17–S23.

14. Pocock NA, Eisman JA, Hopper JL, Yeates MG, Sambrook PN, Eberl S. Genetic determinants of bone mass in adults: A twin study. *J Clin Invest.* 1987;80:706–710.

15. Evans RA, Marel GM, Lancaster EK, Kos S, Evans M, Wong SY. Bone mass is low in relatives of osteoporotic patients. *Ann Intern Med.* 1988;109:870–873.

16. Rubin L, Hawker GA, Peltekova VD, Fielding LJ, Ridout R, Cole DEC. Determinants of peak bone mass: Clinical and genetic analyses in a young female Canadian cohort. *J Bone Mineral Res.* 1999;14:633–643.

17. Orwoll ES. The effects of dietary protein insufficiency and excess on skeletal health. *Bone.* 1992;13:343–350.

18. Bonjour JP, Schurch MA, Rizzoli R. Nutritional aspects of hip fractures. *Bone.* 1996;18:S139–S144.

19. Johnston CC Jr, Miller JZ, Slemenda CW. Calcium supplementation and increases in bone mineral density in children. *N Engl J Med.* 1992;327:82–87.

20. Courteix D, LesPessailles E, Loiseau Perers S, Obert P, Germain P, Benhamou CL. Effect of physical training on bone mineral density in prepubertal girls: A comparative study between impact-loading and non-impact-loading sports. *Osteoporos Int.* 1998;8:152–158.

21. Dook JE, James C, Henderson NK, Price RI. Exercise and bone mineral density in mature female athletes. *Med Sci Sports Exerc.* 1997;29:291–296.

22. Teegarden D, Lyle RM, Proulx WR, Martin BR. Peak bone mass in young women. *J Bone Mineral Res.* 1995;10:711–715.

23. Teegarden D, Lyle RM, Proulx WR, Johnston CC, Weaver CM. Previous milk consumption is associated with greater bone density in young women. *Am J Clin Nutr.* 1999;69:1014–1017.

24. Dawson-Hughes B, Harris SS, Krall EA, Dallal GE, Falconer G, Green CL. Rates of bone loss in postmenopausal women randomly assigned to one of two dosages of vitamin D. *Am J Clin Nutr.* 1995;61:1140–1145.

25. LeBoff MS, Kohlmeier L, Hurwitz S, Franklin J, Wright J, Glowacki J. Occult vitamin D deficiency in postmenopausal US women with acute hip fracture. *JAMA.* 1999;281:1505–1511.

26. Calvo MS, Park YK. Changing phosphorus content of the U.S. diet: Potential for adverse effects on bone. *J Nutr.* 1996;126:1168S–1180S.

27. Heaney RP, Recker RR. Effects of nitrogen, phosphorus, and caffeine on calcium balance in women. *J Lab Clin Med.* 1982;99:46–55.

28. Michaelsson K, Baron JA, Farahmand BY, Persson I, Ljunghall S. Oral-contraceptive use and risk of hip fracture: A case-control study. *Lancet.* 1999;353:1481–1484.

29. Anonymous. Effects of hormone therapy on bone mineral density: Results from the Postmenopausal Estrogen/Progestin Interventions (PEPI) Trial. The Writing Group for the PEPI. *JAMA.* 1996;276:1389–1396.

30. Lindsay R, Tohme JF. Estrogen treatment of patients with established postmenopausal osteoporosis. *Obstet Gynecol.* 1990;76:290–295.

31. Recker RR, Davies KM, Dowd RM, Heaney RP. The effect of low-dose continuous estrogen and progesterone therapy with calcium and vitamin D on bone in elderly women: A randomized, controlled trial. *Ann Intern Med.* 1999;130:897–904.

32. Genant HK, Lucas J, Weiss S, et al. Low-dose esterified estrogen therapy: Effects on bone, plasma estradiol concentrations, endometrium, and lipid levels. *Arch Intern Med.* 1997;157:2609–2615.

33. Krebs NF, Reidinger CJ, Robertson AD, Brenner M. Bone mineral density changes during lactation: Maternal, dietary, and biochemical correlates. *Am J Clin Nutr.* 1997;65:1738–1746.

34. Melton LJ, Bryant SC, Wahner HW, et al. Influence of breast feeding and other reproductive factors on bone mass later in life. *Osteoporos Int.* 1993;3:76–83.

35. Love RR, Mazess RB, Barden HS, et al. Effects of tamoxifen on bone mineral density in postmenopausal women with breast cancer. *N Engl J Med.* 1992;326:852–856.

36. Burshell AL, Anderson SJ, Leib ES, Johnston CC, Costantino JP. The effect of tamoxifen on pre and postmenopausal bone. *J Bone Mineral Res.* 1999;14:S158.

37. Ettinger B, Black DM, Mitlak BH, et al. Reduction of vertebral fracture risk in postmenopausal women with osteoporosis treated with raloxifene: Results from a 3-year randomized trial. *JAMA.* 1999;282:637–645.

38. Arjmandi BH, Alekel L, Hollis BW, et al. Dietary soybean protein prevents bone loss in an ovariectomized rat model of osteoporosis. *J Nutr.* 1996;126:161–167.

39. Draper CR, Edel MJ, Dick IM, Randall AG, Martin GB, Prince RL. Phytoestrogens reduce bone loss and bone resorption in oophorectomized rats. *J Nutr.* 1997;127:1795–1799.

40. Potter SM, Baum JA, Teng H, Stillman RJ, Shay NF, Erdman JW Jr. Soy protein and isoflavones: their effects on blood lipids and bone density in postmenopausal women. *Am J Clin Nutr.* 1998;68:1375S–1379S.

41. Vincent A, Fitzpatrick LA. Soy isoflavones: Are they useful in menopause? *Mayo Clinic Proc.* 2000; 75:1174–1184.

42. Heinrich CH, Going SB, Pamenter RW, Perry CD, Boyden TW, Lohman TG. Bone mineral content of cyclically menstruating female resistance and endurance trained athletes. *Med Sci Sports Exerc.* 1990;22:558–563.

43. Alfredson H, Nordstrom P, Lorentzon R. Total and regional bone mass in female soccer players. *Calcif Tissue Int.* 1996;59:438–442.

44. Risser WL, Lee EJ, LeBlanc A, Poindexter HB, Risser JM, Schneider V. Bone density in eumenorrheic female college athletes. *Med Sci Sports Exerc.* 1990;22:570–574.

45. Taaffe DR, Robinson TL, Snow CM, Marcus R. High-impact exercise promotes bone gain in well-trained female athletes. *J Bone Mineral Res.* 1997;12:255–260.

46. Kirchner EM, Lewis RD, O'Connor PJ. Bone mineral density and dietary intake of female college gymnasts. *Med Sci Sports Exerc.* 1995;27:543–549.

47. Robinson TL, Snow-Harter C, Taaffe DR, Gillis D, Shaw J, Marcus R. Gymnasts exhibit higher bone mass than runners despite similar prevalence of amenorrhea and oligomenorrhea. *J Bone Mineral Res.* 1995;10:26–35.

48. Kirchner EM, Lewis RD, O'Connor PJ. Effect of past gymnastics participation on adult bone mass. *J Appl Physiol.* 1996;80:226–232.

49. Krall EA, Dawson-Hughes B. Walking is related to bone density and rates of bone loss. *Am J Med.* 1994;96:20–26.

50. Snow-Harter C, Bouxsein ML, Lewis BT, Carter DR, Marcus R. Effects of resistance and endurance exercise on bone mineral status of young women: A randomized exercise intervention trial. *J Bone Mineral Res.* 1992;7:761–769.

51. Lohman T, Going S, Pamenter R, et al. Effects of resistance training on regional and total bone mineral density in premenopausal women: A randomized prospective study. *J Bone Mineral Res.* 1995;10:1015–1024.

52. Marcus R. Exercise: Moving in the right direction. *J Bone Mineral Res.* 1998;13:1793–1796.

53. Bassey EJ, Rothwell MC, Little JJ, Pye DW. Pre- and postmenopausal women have different bone mineral density responses to the same high impact exercise. *J Bone Mineral Res.* 1998;13:1805–1813.

54. Kerr D, Morton A, Dick I, Prince R. Exercise effects on bone mass in postmenopausal women are site-specific and load-dependent. *J Bone Mineral Res.* 1996;11:218–225.

55. Fiatarone MA, Marks EC, Ryan ND, Meredith CN, Lipsitz LA, Evans WJ. High-intensity strength training in nonagenarians: Effects on skeletal muscle. *JAMA.* 1990;263:3029–3034.

56. Pruitt LA, Taaffe DR, Marcus R. Effects of a one-year high-intensity versus low-intensity resistance training program on bone mineral density in older women. *J Bone Mineral Res.* 1995;10:1788–1795.

57. Frost HM. The role of changes in mechanical usage set points in the pathogenesis of osteoporosis. *J Bone Mineral Res.* 1992;7:253–261.

58. Rencken ML, Chesnut CH, Drinkwater BL. Bone density at multiple skeletal sites in amenorrheic athletes. *JAMA.* 1996;276:238–240.

59. Pettersson U, Stalnacke BM, Ahlenius GM, Henriksson-Lasrsen K, Lorentzon R. Low bone mass density at multiple skeletal sites, including the appendicular skeleton in amenorrheic runners. *Calcif Tissue Int.* 1999;64:117–125.

60. Petit MA, Prior JC, Barr SI. Running and ovulation positively change cancellous bone in premenopausal women. *Med Sci Sports Exerc.* 1999;31:780–787.

61. Melton LJ. How many women have osteoporosis now? *J Bone Mineral Res.* 1995;10:175–177.

62. Heaney RP. Pathophysiology of osteoporosis. *Am J Med Sci.* 1996;312:251–256.

63. Fitzpatrick LA. Glucocorticoid-induced osteoporosis. In: Marcus R, ed. *Osteoporosis.* Boston: Blackwell Scientific Publications; 1994:202.

64. Khosla S, Melton LJ, Wermers RA, Crowson CS, O'Fallon WM, Riggs BL. Primary hyperparathyroidism and the risk of fracture: A population-based study. *J Bone Mineral Res.* 1999;14:1700–1707.

65. Silverberg SJ, Shane E, Jacobs TP, Siris E, Bilezikian JP. A 10-year prospective study of primary hyperparathyroidism with or without parathyroid surgery. *N Engl J Med.* 1999;341:1249–1255.

66. Zerwekh JE, Ruml LA, Gottschalk F, Pak CY. The effects of twelve weeks of bed rest on bone histology, biochemical markers of bone turnover, and calcium homeostasis in eleven normal subjects. *J Bone Mineral Res.* 1998;13:1594–1601.

67. Cline AD, Jansen GR, Melby CL. Stress fractures in female army recruits: Implications of bone density, calcium intake, and exercise. *J Am Coll Nutr.* 1998;17:128–135.

68. Pope RP. Prevention of pelvic stress fractures in female army recruits. *Milit Med.* 1999;164:370–373.

69. Tomten SE, Falch JA, Birkeland KI, Hemmersbach P, Hostmark AT. Bone mineral density and menstrual irregularities: A comparative study on cortical and trabecular bone structures in runners with alleged normal eating behavior. *Int J Sports Med.* 1998;19:92–97.

70. Bennell KL, Malcolm SA, Brukner PD, et al. A 12-month prospective study of the relationship between stress fractures and bone turnover in athletes. *Calcif Tissue Int.* 1998;63:80–85.

71. Karlson KA. Rib stress fractures in elite rowers: A case series and proposed mechanism. *Am J Sports Med.* 1998;26:516–519.

72. Bennell KL, Malcolm SA, Thomas SA, et al. Risk factors for stress fractures in track and field athletes. A twelve-month prospective study. *Am J Sports Med.* 1996;24:810–818.

73. Carpintero P, Berral FJ, Baena P, Garcia-Frasquet A, Lancho JL. Delayed diagnosis of fatigue fractures in the elderly. *Am J Sports Med.* 1997;25:659–662.

CHAPTER 19

The Female Athlete Triad

Sheila A. Dugan

INTRODUCTION

Over the last several decades, women's participation in organized athletics has grown tremendously. Although the health benefits of regular exercise are innumerable, vigorous exercise can put some women at risk for serious health consequences, whether at the recreational, high school, collegiate, Olympic, or professional level. Excessive weight loss can lead to menstrual dysfunction with detrimental effects on bone density. The term "female athlete triad," developed at the 1984 American College of Sports Medicine (ACSM) course, describes the interrelatedness of disordered eating, amenorrhea, and premature osteoporosis in female athletes. Research into amenorrhea, disordered eating, and osteoporosis in female athletes has been ongoing. Associated injuries and illnesses such as stress fractures and infertility continue to be the subject of investigation.

In the early 1990s, the ACSM established the Task Force on Women's Issues in Sports Medicine. This panel of experts developed an action plan to improve the understanding and awareness of the prevention, recognition, and treatment of eating disorders, amenorrhea, and osteoporosis. In 1997, the ACSM position stand on the triad was published.[1] Today, the Strategic Health Initiative for Women, Sport and Physical Activity, a committee of the ACSM, continues the focus on the female athlete triad with ongoing research, education, and training. Their goal is that all individuals supporting women's participation in sports, including coaches, teachers,

I am grateful for the efforts of the Spaulding Rehabilitation Hospital librarians, Ms. Terry O'Brien, and Ms. Terry Cucuzza. Without their assistance, I would not have been able to complete this project.

administrators, parents, and health care practitioners, be well versed on the prevention, recognition, and treatment of the triad. There continue to be many unanswered questions regarding causation, frequency, and management of the triad. Thankfully, top rate research continues on all fronts. Because numerous researchers and participants in this initiative have personal experience with the female athlete triad, emotion fuels the research and debate.

DISORDERED EATING

The first component of the female athlete triad is disordered eating. This includes a spectrum of abnormal or unhealthy eating habits seen in athletes from poor or under-nutrition (or "malnutrition") to occasional bingeing or purging to clinically diagnosable anorexia nervosa or bulimia nervosa. An individual does not need to meet the Diagnostic and Statistical Manual of Mental Disorders (DSM) IV criteria[2] for eating disorders to have severe medical morbidities. In her review, Smith[3] lists behavioral signs suggestive of disordered eating, including preoccupation with weight, expression of concerns about weight or criticisms of one's body, frequent trips to the restroom around mealtime, and compulsive exercise. In Rosen et al's[4] review of female college athletes, 32% of the 182 athletes studied performed at least one unhealthy weight-control behavior for at least 1 month, including self-induced vomiting; laxative, diuretic, or diet pill use; biweekly bingeing; or excessive weight loss.

Disordered eating can stem from an athlete's attempt to con-trol her body weight. An athlete naturally focuses on her body weight. Weight is a pertinent factor to consider in athletic performance and one that is under the control of the individual. For example, a runner's weight has a direct impact on the work she will be doing during her race. Performance can be reduced or enhanced on the basis of weight and body fat percentage. Drinkwater[5] reviewed the range of women's body fat percentages when athletes in different sports were measured. The lowest percentages of body fat were seen in pentathletes (11.0%) and runners (12.8%–18.3%), whereas the highest were seen in swimmers (14.6%–24.7%) and skiers (17.3%–22.7%). Likely, this sports-specific variation in body composition reflects the body's adaptations for performance enhancement. She also analyzed the various methods of measurement of body fat and cautioned the reader about the limitations of using equations for predicted anthropometric measurements and applying "norms" from the population at large to the specific population of female athletes being studied. Models and actresses currently exemplifying the "aesthetic ideals" have 10% to 15% body fat compared with 22% to 26% for normal weight healthy women.[6]

From a broader health perspective, individuals frequently consider the role of exercise in weight control. Many individuals exercise alone or in combination with dietary restrictions to reduce their body fat. Some evidence exists that exercise may suppress the appetite.[7] In most sports, athletes often concern themselves with the role of weight in exercise or, more aptly, performance. In some instances, this concern can be extreme, resulting in excessive weight loss that can depress performance and, in the worst case, impair the athlete's health. The possible role of the training itself suppressing the appetite and adding to a disordered eating behavior may be significant and warrants further research.

Alterations in eating behaviors can occur on a continuum from a simple imbalance in energy input (nutrition) versus output (activity) to frank eating disorders such as anorexia nervosa (AN) and bulimia nervosa (BN). The DSM IV definitions of AN and BN are shown in the Clinical Guidelines. Athletes may consume fewer nutrients than the recommended daily allowance and limit protein intake.[8] Carbohydrate restriction is another version of dieting promoted in the older Scarsdale or newly popular Atkins diet. Iron and calcium intake may be limited in vegetarian athletes and can be detrimental to the growing athlete. Kopp-Woodroffe et al[9] review the issue of the bioavailability of iron in female athletes.

Definitions of Anorexia and Bulimia Nervosa[2]

- Anorexia Nervosa is defined as:
  Weight 15% below expected
  Morbid fear of fatness
  "Feeling" fat when thin
  Amenorrhea
- Bulimia Nervosa is defined as:
  Binge eating twice per week for at least 3 months

Loss of control over eating
Purging behavior
Overconcern with body shape.

Clinical Guideline

Diagnostic Criteria for Anorexia Nervosa[2]

A. Refusal to maintain body weight at or above a minimally normal weight for age and height (eg, weight loss leading to maintenance of body weight less than 85% of that expected; or failure to make expected weight gain during period of growth, leading to body weight less than 85% of that expected).

B. Intense fear of gaining weight or becoming fat, even though underweight.

C. Disturbance in the way in which one's body weight or shape is experienced, undue influence of body weight or shape on self-evaluation, or denial of the seriousness of the current low body weight.

D. In postmenarcheal females, amenorrhea, ie, the absence of at least three consecutive menstrual cycles. (A woman is considered to have amenorrhea if her periods occur only following hormone, eg, estrogen, administration.)

Clinical Guideline

Source: Reprinted with permission from the *Diagnostic and Statistical Manual of Mental Disorders, Fourth Edition.* Copyright 1994 American Psychiatric Association.

Diagnostic Criteria for Bulimia Nervosa[2]

A. Recurrent episodes of binge eating. An episode of binge eating is characterized by both of the following:
   (1) eating, in a discrete period of time (eg, within any 2-hour period), an amount of food that is definitely larger than most people would eat during a similar period of time and under similar circumstances.
   (2) a sense of lack of control over eating during the episode (e.g., a feeling that one cannot stop eating or control what or how much one is eating).

B. Recurrent inappropriate compensatory behavior in order to prevent weight gain, such as self-induced vomiting; misuse of laxatives, diuretics, enemas, or other medication; fasting; or excessive exercise.

C. The binge eating and inappropriate compensatory behaviors both occur, on average, at least twice a week for 3 months.

D. Self-evaluation is unduly influenced by body shape and weight.

E. The disturbance does not occur exclusively during episodes of Anorexia Nervosa.

Clinical Guideline

Source: Reprinted with permission from the Diagnostic and Statistical Manual of Mental Disorders, Fourth Edition. Copyright 1994 American Psychiatric Association.

Morbidity and Mortality Associated with Eating Disorders

- Medical
  Renal and electrolyte (ie, increased blood urea nitrogen, hyper/hypokalemia)
  Cardiac (ie, arrhythmia, orthostatic hypotension, cardiomyopathy)
  Endocrine (ie, hypothalamic-pituitary axis, LH & FSH abnormalities)
  Metabolic (ie, osteoporosis, osteopenia, vitamin deficiencies)
  Gastrointestinal (ie, pain, impaired motility, superior mesenteric artery syndrome)
  Dermatological (ie, lanugo-like hair, dry skin, calluses, drug eruptions)
  Pulmonary (ie, pneumomediastinum, subcutaneous emphysema)
  Hematological (ie, anemia, leukopenia, thrombocytopenia)
  Dental (ie, decalcification, enamel erosion)
- Psychological
  Anxiety
  Lethargy
  Depression and suicide
  Substance abuse

Clinical Guideline

The plethora of medical and psychological conditions associated with AN and BN, leading to mortality and morbidity, are summarized in the Clinical Guideline. It is paramount that these conditions be recognized, worked up, and treated because of the severe and life-threatening associated medical problems. In his article on eating disorders in athletes, Katz[10] concludes that 40% of all patients treated for an eating disorder recover, 30% show moderate improvement, and 30% have a chronically debilitating course (including the 5% to 10% who die of the illness). Consequently, long-term treatment of disordered eating is necessary.

Some studies of women who participate in endurance sports, such as long distance running, demonstrated a discrepancy in energy balance that was attributed to metabolic efficiency in these athletes.[11] However, other researchers concluded that this discrepancy may be related to under-reporting on food diaries by the athletes rather than a true energy imbalance.[12] Long-term balance between energy intake and expenditure is necessary to maintain a stable body weight. This balance may also be crucial in preventing exercise-induced changes in luteinizing hormone (LH). Loucks and others[13] studied the effects of energy availability on LH. When the diet of women was restricted, the LH pulse frequency decreased and the overnight LH pulse amplitude increased. This mirrored previous findings in amenorrheic athletes in regard to LH.[14] Loucks et al concluded that these athletes consumed diets similar to sedentary women despite much higher levels of energy expenditure; this leads to an energy debt.

Frequency of Eating Disorders

Almost 5% of women in industrialized societies can be expected to have an eating disorder sometime in their life.[10] Studies of female athletes identified disordered eating in 16% to 64% of these athletes.[4,15,16] Clinicians, parents, coaches, and members of the sports medicine team must have a high degree of suspicion for disordered eating in female athletes.

Clinical Guideline

Female athletes may be more prone to eating disorders developing than nonathletes. Although the prevalence of eating disorders in the population is 5%,[10] there is a wide range of prevalence in studies of female athletes, from 16% to 64%.[4,15,16] This range reflects differences in how the disordered eating was defined, which sports the athletes participated in, and how the data were collected. It may be that the same personality traits that help an athlete excel in sports—goal-directed behavior, commitment, and perfectionism—predispose them to disordered eating. Bolen[17] reminds us that disordered eating often goes undetected, likely leading to prevalence figures that underestimate the problem.

Norwegian elite female athletes studied by Sundgot-Borgen[18] had a higher prevalence of eating disorders when participating in sports emphasizing leanness or specific weight. Athletes with eating disorders began sports-specific training and dieting earlier than control athletes. Trigger factors for the onset of eating disorders included prolonged periods of dieting, weight fluctuations, increased training volume, and traumatic events. Men participating in sports with weight classification may also be at increased risk for disordered eating.

High-Risk Sports According to the ACSM Position Stand on the Female Athlete Triad[1]

- Sports with subjective scoring
- Endurance sports
- Sports requiring contour-revealing apparel
- Sports requiring prepubertal body habitus
- Sports with weight classifications

Clinical Guideline

At times, pressure from coaches, parents, or peers can bring about extreme weight loss.[19] In their 1994 article, Nattiv et al[20] reported on the declining height and weight trends of the US Women's Olympic gymnastic team over the last three decades. Outside of the athletic arena, the young female athlete continues to be at risk for disordered eating, especially when one considers the concurrent societal pressures coming to bear in the adolescent years. The pubertal female in the United States is faced with an increased body fat percentage compared with her male peers in a culture that emphasizes thinness in women.

Other risk factors for the development of disordered eating include a family history of obesity or eating disorder. Athletes should be screened regarding their eating habits, including content and frequency of meals, in addition to questions regarding abnormal behaviors such as self-induced vomiting and bingeing. Concurrent psychological stressors should be explored; female athletes with a limited or unhealthy support system can be at higher risk of disordered eating, such as occurs when living away from home at college.

Although eating disorders and subsequent amenorrhea and osteoporosis have been shown to occur in conjunction with one another, significant scientific and clinical research continues to establish the links that interrelate these disorders. Athletes will continue to monitor their weight and body composition to maximize their performance and can benefit from an enhanced understanding of disordered eating and how it compromises health. Athletic department personnel, family, and sports medicine practitioners should monitor female athletes for any signs of disordered eating. Education on healthy eating habits should be readily available.

AMENORRHEA

The second component of the female athlete triad is amenorrhea. As noted earlier with disordered eating, there is a spectrum of menstrual abnormalities seen in female athletes that can lead to health risks. Various definitions of menstrual irregularities are used in the myriad of studies and reviews that have been done on this topic; this increases the complexity of comparing the results. Although amenorrhea is a key component of the triad, some of the other issues to consider in the gynecological history of the female athlete are oligomenorrhea, delayed menarche, and inadequate luteal phase. Fertility is obviously adversely affected during the period of amenorrhea and possibly beyond.

Classification of Amenorrhea[21]

- Amenorrhea: the absence of menstruation for 6 months or longer
- Primary amenorrhea: the failure of menses to start initially
- Secondary amenorrhea: the absence of menstruation in a woman who previously menstruated
- Oligomenorrhea: irregular periods, usually occurring every 2 to 5 months; the interval between periods must be longer than 40 days but shorter than 6 months
- Hypomenorrhea: a reduction in the number of days or amount of menstrual flow
- Eumenorrhea: normal menses
- Delayed onset of menstruation: primary amenorrhea after the age of 16

Clinical Guideline

As a means of standardizing future research, the International Olympic Committee has agreed to the definition of amenorrhea as one menstrual period or less per year.[22] The prevalence of secondary amenorrhea is 2% to 5% in the general population. Because of inconsistencies in defining secondary amenorrhea, the prevalence in studies of female athletes has varied from 3.4% to 66%.[23–25]

At puberty, there is a change in sensitivity of the hypothalamic-pituitary-ovarian (H-P-O) axis, as depicted in Figure 19–1. The hypothalamic neurons that release gonadotropin-releasing hormone (GnRH) become less sensitive to the suppressive effect of the gonadal steroids; pulsatile LH secretion increases in response to the increased intermittent GnRH discharges. This causes the gonads to increase production of sex steroids, leading to changes in secondary sex characteristics. The shift in hypothalamic sensitivity is related to adrenal maturation, by means of dehydroepiandrosterone (DHEA), DHEA sulfate, and androstenedione. Regular ovulatory cycles directed by the hypothalamic release of GnRH develop over several years.

Many factors modulate the amplitude and frequency of GnRH release, including catecholamines, γ-aminobutyric acid, dopamine, prolactin, cortisol, thyroid hormones, endorphins, and estrogen, among others.[26] In her book on women and sports, Wells[27] summarized the many studies done regarding hormonal levels in eumenorrheic versus amenorrheic athletes with a comprehensive table. These studies demonstrated differences between eumenorrheic and amenorrheic athletes in sex steroids, LH and FSH, cortisol, and prolactin among other hormones. In many instances, conflicting results were found. Explanations for the range of results included improper handling of serum samples, failure to account for diurnal variation, and disparity of the populations studied.

The Clinical Guideline lists the age of menarche in adolescent girls participating in different sports and with training initiated at different stages. De Souza et al[26] concluded that not only is exercise associated with a later age of menarche, but the level and timing of training vis-à-vis menarche are directly correlated. Higher intensity of training initiated at an

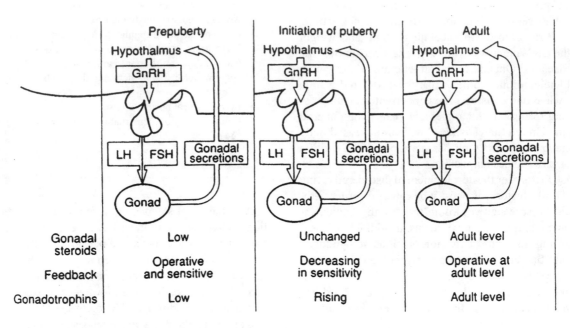

Figure 19–1 Change in Sensitivity of the Hypothalamic-Pituitary-Ovary Axis at Puberty.

earlier age was correlated with later onset of menarche. The later age of menarche of female athletes found in previous studies may have illustrated some predisposition of females with delayed menarche to sports participation. Malina[28] suggested that the physical characteristics associated with late-maturating girls may be advantageous for athletic performance. She also suggested a socialization process may occur in the early-maturing girl that shifts her interests away from sports.

Age of Menarche in Populations of Athletes

Population	Age of Menarche (yr)
Sedentary controls	12.7
High school athletes	13.1
College athletes	13.0
Olympic athletes	13.7
Ballet dancers	15.4
Athletes trained before menarche	15.0
Athletes trained after menarche	12.6

Clinical Guideline

Exercised-associated or athletic amenorrhea is a diagnosis of exclusion. Other causes of amenorrhea must be ruled out first.

Clinical Guideline

Causes of Amenorrhea[22]

- Pregnancy
- Abnormalities of the reproductive tract
- Ovarian failure
- Pituitary tumors or abnormalities
- Hypothalamic amenorrhea
- Chronic anovulation
- Polycystic ovarian disease

Clinical Guideline

Athletic amenorrhea has been linked to several mechanisms of reproductive disorder but is most likely a subset of hypothalamic dysfunction. Frisch and McArthur[29] proposed that a critical minimum weight was necessary for the onset and maintenance of normal menstrual cycles. Therefore, excessive or sudden weight loss could lead to amenorrhea. They hypothesized that a minimal amount of stored, easily mobilized energy is necessary for ovulation and menstrual cycles. It is most likely that it is a loss of energy availability rather than absolute weight that accounts for menstrual abnormalities. Loucks et al[14] determined that high volumes of training may diminish GnRH pulsatility. This differs from AN-related amenorrhea in which excessive weight loss causes the H-P-O axis to revert to its prepubertal state.

In their 1984 review of athletic amenorrhea, Loucks and Horvath[30] focused on secondary amenorrhea. They concluded that the mechanism by which exercise affects the menstrual cycle had not been delineated and cautioned the reader about methodological errors in the studies reviewed. They affirmed the link between athletic amenorrhea and the H-P-O axis on the basis of studies of amenorrheic female athletes demonstrating low basal estrogen levels, low or normal gonadotropin levels, and decreased gonadotropin responsiveness to GnRH administration.

Bullen et al[31] showed that the intensity and rapidity of training are crucial in perturbing menstrual function. Menstrual disorders were induced in untrained women with strenuous exercise. This induction is particularly relevant in younger women with a more susceptible H-P-O axis.

Although many of the details of the menstrual cycle have been worked out, the direct effect of exercise on hypothalamic function has not been defined. In their 1991 review, De Souza and Metzger[32] compare the weight loss–and exercise-associated menstrual dysfunction in anorexic patients and athletes. They concluded that the mechanisms of reproductive dysfunction in amenorrheic athletes differed from anorexic patients. Stress has been shown to play a role in the amenorrhea associated with anorexia nervosa from hypercortisolism and abnormalities of cortisol and thyroid hormone metabolism. Although the mechanism has not been defined, athletes also have mild hypercortisolism. This may be related to psychological stress, exercised-induced stress, or weight loss. Regardless of the mechanism, changes in the pulsatile release of GnRH in female athletes led to menstrual irregularity, shortened luteal phase, anovulation, and amenorrhea, all of which negatively affect fertility.

A more recent review of exercise-related menstrual irregularities (ERMI) by De Cree[33] rejected older hypotheses of hyperprolactinemia or critical weight as the cause for ERMI. He cited more recent hypotheses linking energy deficiency or catecholestrogen to hypothalamic amenorrhea as more tenable. He thoroughly summarized the feasibility of the catecholestrogenic hypothesis, linking ERMI to changes in estrogen levels by way of mediators such as insulin-like growth factors and intracerebral catecholamines. The energy deficiency data including changes in thyroid hormones and leptin are reviewed. He suggested that future studies should use radioisotope tracers to further delineate the metabolic processes associated with ERMI.

Exercise-induced amenorrhea is second only to pregnancy as the most common reason for secondary amenorrhea in young women.[22]

Clinical Guideline

Clearly, amenorrhea is a significant condition that should be identified and worked up. If one works with female athletes, she will interact with women with this condition. Once

pregnancy is ruled out, exercised-induced amenorrhea is the next most common cause of amenorrhea in young women.[22] Short- and probable long-term effects of amenorrhea on fertility must be seriously considered, as well as issues of bone health like osteoporosis and stress fracture. As in postmenopausal women, exposure to a hypoestrogenic state causes maximal bone loss early in its course. Early identification and prevention of amenorrhea are crucial.

OSTEOPOROSIS

The third component of the triad is osteoporosis. Osteoporosis in young female athletes refers to either inadequate bone formation or premature loss of bone mass. There may be inadequate bone formation because young amenorrheic female athletes in their late teens and 20s are not building peak bone mass. Some of the major determinants of peak bone mass such as body mass index and estrogen exposure are directly influenced by disordered eating and amenorrhea.

The World Health Organization (WHO) Classification of Osteoporosis[34] (based on bone mineral density [BMD] measurement *t* score [expressed as a percentage value of young healthy adults])

- Normal bone density: BMD within 1 standard deviation (SD) or less of the youthful norm
- Osteopenia: BMD between 1 and 2.5 SDs below the youthful norm
- Osteoporosis: BMD greater than 2.5 SDs below the youthful norm
- Severe osteoporosis: BMD more than 2.5 SDs below the youthful norm in the presence of one or more fragility fractures

Clinical Guideline

Clinical Guideline

Normative data for bone density of adolescent girls are not yet available, limiting the ability to adequately define pathological bone loss in this age group.

Clinical Guideline

Premature osteoporosis leads to an increased risk for stress fractures and other more devastating fractures of the hip or spine. In the setting of secondary amenorrhea, a young athlete can have a decline in bone density similar to that of a postmenopausal woman.[35] Figure 19–2 depicts the changes in the skeletal structure of postmenopausal osteoporotic women.

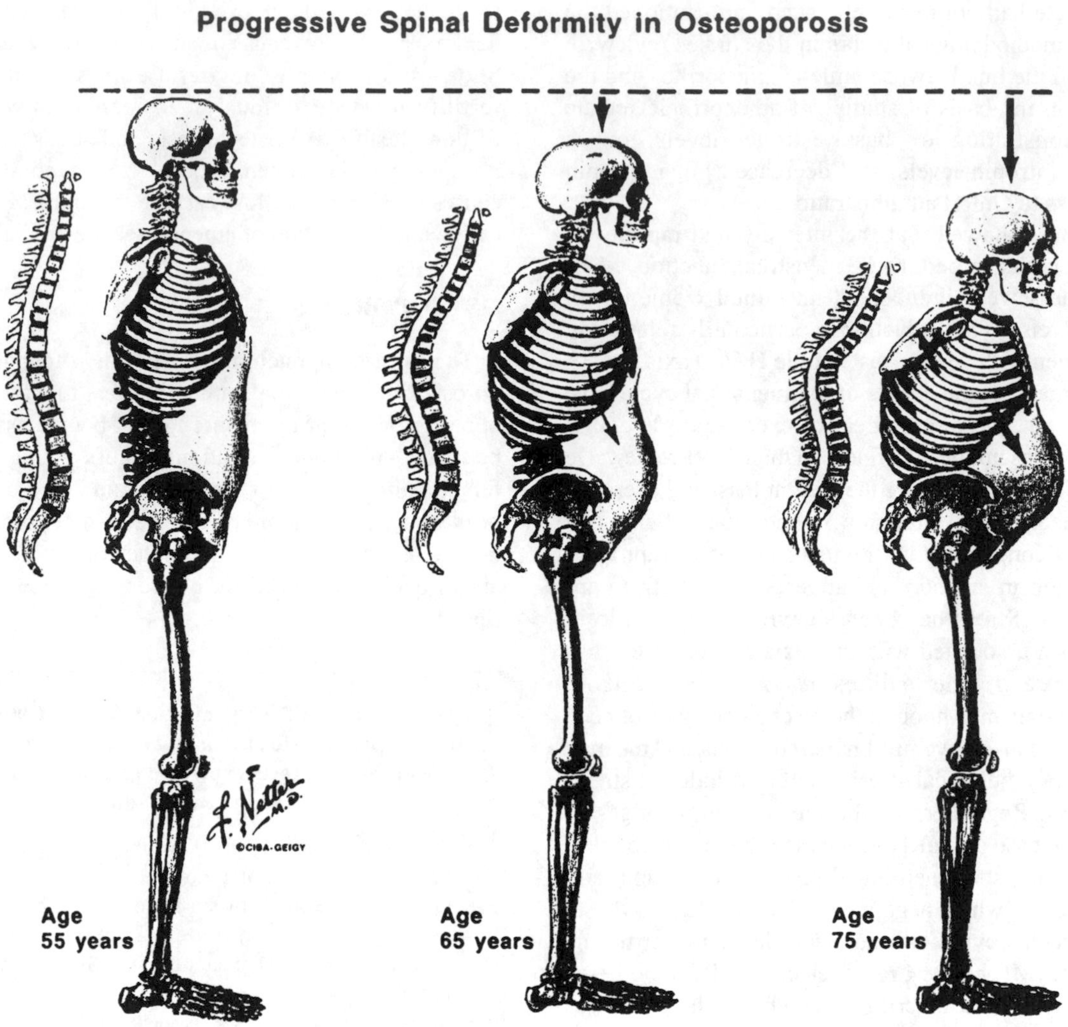

Progressive Spinal Deformity in Osteoporosis

Figure 19–2 Changes in Spinal Structure and Posture in Postmenopausal Women Resulting from Compression Fractures. Note the loss of height, abdominal distention, and progressive thoracic kyphosis.

Drinkwater[35] found that the BMDs in 25-year-old amenorrheic runners were similar to 50-year-old women. Initial studies reported that the premature decline of BMD could recover with the return of menses or with estrogen replacement with oral contraceptive pills (OCPs), but more recent investigations revealed that this bone loss may be irreversible.[36] In women of all ages, circulating estrogens support bone maintenance by means of effects on calcium metabolism.

Prior et al[37] showed that spinal bone density correlated with ovulatory disturbances and postulated that progesterone deficiency may also play a role in premature osteoporosis. However, this effect was not specific to exercising women. Inadequate progesterone production can cause luteal sup-

pression, another menstrual disorder seen in female athletes. Shangold et al[38] argued that this is an early phase along the spectrum of exercised-induced menstrual dysfunction.

Drinkwater et al[39] expressed concern over the residual negative effect on bone density of hypoestrogenic states like amenorrhea and oligomenorrhea. This loss of bone density was most impressive at the lumbar vertebral body. A more recent study by Keen and Drinkwater[36] arrived at the more worrisome conclusion that this bone loss may be irreversible. That showed that even after 6 to 10 years of resumption of normal menses or use of OCPs, amenorrheic and oligomenorrheic athletes did not demonstrate significantly improved vertebral BMD compared with eumenorrheic athletes over the same period. The data were not as clear for the femoral neck BMD. These findings moderated the enthusiasm for an earlier study that showed a small increase in lumbar BMD after the resumption of menses for 14 months in former amenorrheic athletes.[40] Jonnavithula et al[41] studied 30 women over 2 years comparing dancers with a control group of sedentary individuals. They showed that although the exercising amenorrheic subjects demonstrated increased bone density before the return of normal menses, bone mass remained below control values.

A delay in menarche and prolonged intervals of amenorrhea were shown to predispose ballet dancers to scoliosis and stress fracture.[42] A study by Myburgh et al[43] concluded that low BMD in amenorrheic athletes was not limited to the axial skeleton. Of note, body mass failed to predict bone density; menstrual history significantly predicted BMD at axial and appendicular sites. They concluded that female athletes with amenorrhea may be at long-term risk of both vertebral and appendicular fractures.

Multiple studies have been done in regarding the increased risk of female athletes for stress fracture.[44-46] Lloyd et al[47] looked at premenopausal women runners and collegiate athletes and concluded that those with absent or irregular menses were at increased risk of musculoskeletal injuries while engaged in active training. OCP use provided a protective effect because the likelihood of injury was negatively correlated with OCP use. Myburgh et al[48] showed that fewer athletes with fractures were using OCPs than athletes without fractures. In addition, athletes without stress fractures had a higher intake of calcium than those with stress fractures. Carbon et al[49] compared nine elite runners with stress fractures to matched controls without stress fractures and found significant differences in the number of menses per year (less in fracture group) and the age of onset of menses (delayed in fracture group). All athletes had femoral neck BMD values within the 95% confidence limit for nonathletic women. They concluded that stress fracture risk in elite runners was independent of BMD.

Exercise positively modulates the health of bone by providing a mechanical stimulus for osteogenesis.[50,51] Dalsky[52] showed that athletes have a higher BMD than sedentary controls. Weight-bearing exercise helps build and maintain peak bone mass and is recommended for the prevention and treatment of postmenopausal osteoporosis. A recent study by Petit et al[53] demonstrated that spinous cancellous bone is positively affected in eumenorrheic women by running and luteal phase length. These factors acted independently.

Site-specific increases in BMD have been shown in gymnastics, rowing, and figure skating, even in amenorrheic athletes.[54-56] This is due to mechanical loading that stimulates local osteogenesis. For instance, amenorrheic rowers had higher lumbar BMD than amenorrheic runners or dancers. It may be that this type of site-specific loading compensates for the underlying loss of BMD related to the amenorrhea. However, Pettersson et al[57] concluded in their study of amenorrheic runners that weight-bearing activity alone did not compensate completely for the decline in bone density even in weight-bearing bones.

Exercise is a mainstay in peak bone density development and maintenance. In the setting of the amenorrheic athlete, exercise can be detrimental, causing loss of bone structure and injury. Osteoporosis may be tempered locally with site-specific maintenance or increase in bone density on the basis of the type of sport. This phenomenon could possibly be exploited in closely monitored exercise regimens. Calcium plays an important role in osteoporosis prevention and treatment, as well as stress fracture prevention. More extensive research is needed in the prepubertal and pubertal female athlete regarding bone loss, including establishing normative data for bone density. This population is particularly at risk for exercised-induced menstrual abnormalities and the skeletal sequelae reviewed earlier as a result of an immature H-P-O axis.

MANAGEMENT

History and Physical Findings that Suggest Risk of Female Athlete Triad

- History:
  Disordered eating behaviors
  Menstrual irregularity
  Previous fractures
  Weight fluctuations
  Symptoms of depression
- Physical findings:
  Lanugo (fine downy hair)
  Salivary gland enlargement
  Cardiac arrhythmias
  Facial hair
  Pain with palpation or vibration over bone

Clinical Guideline

Coaches, administrators, and members of the sports medicine team must be informed of the presenting signs and symptoms of eating disorders, amenorrhea, and osteoporosis to maximize identification of women at risk for or affected by the triad. The United States Olympic Committee and ACSM consensus statement, prepared in June 1999 by a panel of coaches and scientists, recommends that coaches refer any female athlete exhibiting any signs of the triad to a health care professional. Furthermore, they recommend that coaches have a referral network of medical, counseling, and nutrition experts. Athletes at risk for the female athlete triad are also identified during screening or preparticipation

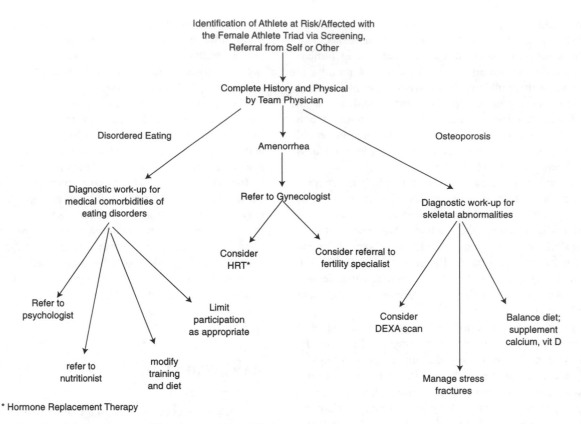

Figure 19–3 Overview of Management of the Female Athlete Triad.

history and physical examinations. Once affected or at-risk individuals are identified, appropriate work-up and referral are recommended. Refer to Figure 19–3 for an overview.

Eating Disorders

As noted in the previous section on eating disorders, individuals supporting female athletes must be vigilant in identifying affected women. Only then can treatment be initiated. Training techniques requiring frequent weighing or punitive measures for weight gain should be avoided because they have been shown to predispose women to disordered eating.[20] Involvement of a registered dietitian with a background in sports is critical.

Beyond individual psychotherapy, family and group therapy are frequently used. Family issues can be causative and must be addressed, especially in the adolescent athlete who resides at home. A behavior modification program can be helpful for changing aberrant eating habits. Any suicidal ideation should be appropriately addressed, with consideration for psychiatric hospitalization. Psychiatric referral for medication management may be necessary.

The extent of medical work-up and intervention is based on the comorbidities listed in the Clinical Guideline. Appropriate electrolyte repletion and monitoring of any electrocardiogram abnormalities are mandatory. Once medically cleared to play, participation may be dependent on weight gain. A verbal or written contract may facilitate weight gain by the athlete.[58]

Principles of Treatment of Eating Disorders[10]

- An earlier intervention increases the likelihood of response.
- Treatment must be individually tailored and based on phase, severity, and setting.
- Multimodal treatment is better than unimodal.
- The treatment team must be flexible in its approach.

Clinical Guideline

Hospitalization Criteria in an Athlete with an Eating Disorder[59]

- Weight loss below 30% of normal
- Cardiac, blood pressure, electrolyte, or fluid status compromise
- Failed outpatient treatment

Clinical Guideline

Amenorrhea

Menstrual dysfunction in the female athlete requires a medical evaluation. As noted earlier, this should not be considered a benign condition. A referral to a gynecologist familiar with athletes is most effective. An athlete may not understand the associated health risks and may even avoid a medical work-up. She may prefer the convenience of not menstruating. If she is sexually active, she may incorrectly assume amenorrhea provides protection against pregnancy. This may not be the case; she may resume an ovulatory cycle and become pregnant even before menstruating.

It is beyond the scope of this text to review a complete work-up for amenorrhea. The evaluation includes a detailed menstrual history. In the sexually active female, pregnancy should be ruled out. In the female using OCPs, withdrawal of the OCP should result in the return of menses; if this does not occur within 6 months, an amenorrhea work-up is required. Hirsutism, acne, and other signs of androgen excess may be present in polycystic ovarian syndrome. Vaginal dryness or hot flashes may be present with premature ovarian failure. An individual or family history of anosmia may suggest an isolated GnRH deficiency. The physical examination should include Tanner staging, body fat estimate, thyroid, breast, and pelvic examination. Laboratory testing should include pregnancy, thyroid function, and hormonal testing. Depending on the individual athlete, other diagnostic testing including progestin challenge, endometrial biopsy, magnetic resonance imaging of the pituitary, and/or pelvic sonography, among others, may be pertinent.

In the management of amenorrhea, a gynecologist or reproductive endocrinologist consultation is strongly recommended. Treatment of amenorrhea is based on the results of the laboratory and diagnostic testing noted earlier. In regard to athletic amenorrhea (with other causes ruled out), Marshall[22] recommends that the athlete decrease exercise intensity and gain a small amount of weight. This may not be an option in elite athletes. A balanced diet providing adequate calories is non-negotiable. Calcium intake should be at least 1500 mg daily along with 400 to 800 IU of vitamin D. If menses does not spontaneously return, hormone replacement should be considered. If the patient is sexually active but does not desire conception, OCPs will provide estrogen exposure and contraception. If she desires conception, other causes of infertility should be ruled out before proceeding to ovulation induction under the care of her gynecologist or fertility specialist. Options for ovulation induction include clomiphene citrate, Pergonal, or intravenous pump infusion of GnRH. Pump infusion is less likely to cause multiple births.[60]

Controversy continues regarding the use of estrogen replacement in place of the return of naturally occurring menses. Drinkwater[35] suggests that optimal treatment for the female athlete triad results in the spontaneous return of menses after activity modification and weight gain. If menses does not return within 2 to 3 months, hormone replacement therapy (HRT) should be considered. In the case of eating disorders, the return of menses can be a strong motivating force in successful treatment; this stimulus for weight gain may be eliminated if OCPs are prescribed and the menstrual cycle is restored pharmacologically. If HRT is necessary, estrogen and progesterone given in physiological doses do not suppress the H-P-O axis cyclical nature like OCPs will and may be more appropriate. Shangold[61] recommends giving both estrogen and progesterone because unopposed estrogen can cause endometrial hyperplasia. She states that HRT should be initiated within 6 months of the onset of the amenorrhea.

Ongoing research should focus on the difference in bone density if amenorrheic athletes are treated with physiological doses of estrogen and progesterone versus OCPs versus resumption of normal menses; identifying a difference would have implications for the management of athletic amenorrhea. Furthermore, clinical trials on when to initiate HRT would also help guide clinical decisions. Current recommendations for female adolescents who have had only a few cycles before loss of menses include delaying estrogen replacement until age 16. As Vereeke West[62] notes, the management of female adolescents with exercise-induced amenorrhea is more speculative. She recommends modifying dietary and training habits with follow-up every 3 to 6 months. Estrogen replacement therapy is recommended in the setting of stress fracture. Per the recommendations listed earlier, young athletes need aggressive medical management to return menses initially without pharmacological intervention and must be followed closely. If this approach fails, consideration for estrogen replacement may be warranted.

Osteoporosis

As noted earlier, a detailed history including diet and menstrual history is pertinent for osteoporosis risk factor assessment. Other risk factors for postmenopausal osteoporosis such as caffeine intake or smoking have not been fully explored in young female athletes. A history of stress fractures or other fractures is pertinent to the decision to initiate a more comprehensive work-up and treatment.

At present, the most accurate noninvasive method of bone mass evaluation is dual energy x-ray absorptiometry. The amount of x-ray exposure for the subject is less than 5 mrem/scan.[63]

Clinical Guideline

Even in the setting of clinically diagnosed osteoporosis (refer to WHO classification earlier), specific guidelines for activity or training intensity are not possible. As discussed previously, weight-bearing exercise stimulates osteogenesis and should be continued. Site-specific increases in bone density have been demonstrated in multiple sports and may be crucial to maintenance of bone density at these sites. A decrease in training intensity and volume is recommended in conjunction with an increase in calorie and calcium intake to resolve an energy debt. In the setting of osteoporosis, calcium intake should equal 1500 mg/day, and vitamin D intake should equal 400 to 800 IU/day. As detailed previously, estrogen replacement therapy with physiological doses or OCPs should be considered in amenorrheic athletes who are unsuccessful with attempts at nonpharmacological interventions to return normal menses.[61,63]

Management of Osteoporosis

- Appropriate weight-bearing exercise
- Decrease intensity of exercise
- Supplement calcium and vitamin D
- Resumption of menses or consider estrogen replacement
- Manage stress fractures as appropriate

Clinical Guideline

PREVENTION

As with most medical problems, particularly with severe associated morbidity and mortality, prevention is the best approach. Strategies on preventing the triad are repeatedly identified by the ACSM as key to minimizing its impact. Ideally, these strategies are aimed at preventing all three components of the triad. In the setting of an identified eating disorder or exercise-related menstrual disorder, prevention of the associated components of the triad is the most appropriate goal. Providing an open, self-empowered, and caring environment for athletes enhances their willingness to discuss personal matters, especially as pertains to disordered eating, such as dissatisfaction with body shape or family dysfunction. Identifying and treating disordered eating can prevent the associated menstrual and bone metabolism disorders. Similarly, identifying exercise-induced amenorrhea and providing treatment before the development of osteoporosis are important.

Educational material is available from the ACSM and National Collegiate Athletic Association and should be prominently displayed in locker rooms and training areas. Principles of proper hydration and nutrition should be presented in required team meetings and reinforced during practice, competition, and team meals. Calcium supplementation in conjunction with normal estrogen levels and exercise may maximize peak bone mass in early adult years.[35] Annual gynecological examinations are indicated after puberty not only to prevent triad-related health consequences but for cancer prevention.

This information about the female athlete triad needs to reach the athlete. This is most likely to occur if teachers, coaches, athletic administrators, parents, team physicians, and trainers are well informed. Further studies to define the origin and pathophysiology of the triad and the most effective prevention and treatment strategies are needed. This chapter provides a platform for the reader to begin or further his or her own educational, clinical, and research efforts relative to the female athlete triad. As one carries the message of the health benefits of exercise, one should also spread the word about this serious but preventable health problem.

REFERENCES

1. American College of Sports Medicine Position Stand. The female athlete triad. *Med Sci Sports Exerc.* 1997;29:i–ix.

2. American Psychiatric Association. *Diagnostic and Statistical Manual of Medical Disorders: IV.* Washington, DC: The Association; 1994:539–550.

3. Smith AD. The female athlete triad: Causes, diagnosis and treatment. *Phys Sport Med.* 1996;24:67–86.

4. Rosen LW, McKeag DB, Hough DO, et al. Pathogenic weight-control behavior in female athletes. *Phys Sport Med.* 1986;14:79–86.

5. Drinkwater BL. Women and exercise: Physiological aspects. *Exerc Sport Sci Rev.* 1984;12:21–51.

6. Wilfley DE, Grilo CM, Brownell KD. Exercise and regulation of body weight. In: Shangold MM, Mirkin G, eds. *Women and Exercise: Physiology and Sports Medicine.* 2nd ed. Philadelphia: FA Davis; 1994:427–454.

7. Oscai LB. The role of exercise in weight control. *Exerc Sport Sci Rev.* 1973;1:103–123.

8. Warren MP, Shangold MM. *Sports Gynecology: Problems and Care of the Athletic Female.* Cambridge, MA: Blackwell Scientific Publications; 1997.

9. Kopp-Woodroffe SA, Manore MM, Dueck CA, Skinner JS, Matt KS. Energy and nutrient status of amenorrheic athletes participating in a diet and exercise training intervention program. *Int J Sport Nut.* 1999;9:70–88.

10. Katz JL. Eating disorders. In: Shangold MM, Mirkin G, eds. *Women and Exercise: Physiology and Sports Medicine.* 2nd ed. Philadelphia: FA Davis; 1995:292–312.

11. Brownell KD, Steen SN, Wilmore JH. Weight regulation practices in athletes: Analysis of metabolic and health effects. *Med Sci Sports Exerc.* 1987;19:546–556.

12. Edwards JE, Lindeman AK, Mikesley AE, Stager JM. Energy balance in highly trained female endurance runners. *Med Sci Sports Exerc.* 1993;25:1398–1404.

13. Loucks AB, Heath EM. Dietary restriction reduces the luteinizing hormone (LH) pulse frequency during waking hours and increases LH pulse amplitude during sleep in young menstruating women. *J Clin Endocrinol Metab.* 1994;78:910–915.

14. Loucks AB, Mortola JF, Girton C, Yen SS. Alterations in the hypothalamic-pituitary-ovarian and the hypothalamic-pituitary-adrenal axes in the athletic women. *J Clin Endocrinol Metab.* 1989;68:402–411.

15. Dummer GM, Rosen LW, Heurner WW. Pathogenic weight-control behavior of young competitive swimmers. *Phys Sport Med.* 1987;15:75.

16. Sundgot-Borgen J. Prevalence of eating disorders in elite female athletes. *Int J Sport Nutr.* 1993;3:29.

17. Bolen JD. Differentiating healthy from unhealthy behaviors in active and athletic women. In: Agostini R, ed. *Medical and Orthopedic Issues of Active and Athletic Women.* Philadelphia: Hanley and Belfus Inc; 1994:102–107.

18. Sundgot-Borgen J. Risk factors for the development of eating disorders in female elite athletes. *Med Sci Sport Exerc.* 1994;26:414–419.

19. Yeager KK, Agostini R, Drinkwater B. The female athlete triad: Disordered eating, amenorrhea, osteoporosis. *Med Sci Sports Exerc.* 1993;25:775–777.

20. Nattiv A, Agostini R, Drinkwater B, Yeager KK. The female athlete triad: The inter-relatedness of disordered eating, amenorrhea, and osteoporosis. *Clin Sport Med.* 1994;13:405–418.

21. Wentz AC. Amenorrhea: Evaluation and treatment. In: Jones HW, Wentz AC, Burnett LS, eds. *Novak's Textbook of Gynecology.* 11th ed. Baltimore: Williams & Wilkins; 1988:351.

22. Marshall LA. Clinical evaluation of amenorrhea in active and athletic women. *Clin Sports Med.* 1994;13:371–387.

23. Shangold M, Rebar RW, Wentz AC, Schiff I. Evaluation and management of menstrual dysfunction in athletes. *JAMA.* 1990;263:1665.

24. Feicht CB, Johnson TS, Martin BJ, Sparkes KE, Wagner WW. Secondary amenorrhea in athletes. *Lancet.* 1978;2:1145.

25. Otis CL. Exercise-associated amenorrhea. *Clin Sports Med.* 1992;11:351.

26. De Souza MJ, Arce JC, Metzger DA. Endocrine basis of exercised-induced amenorrhea. In: Costa DM, Guthrie SR, eds. *Women and Sport: Interdisciplinary Perspectives.* Champaign, IL: Human Kinetics; 1995:185–210.

27. Wells CL. *Women, Sport & Performance: A Physiological Perspective.* 2nd ed. Champaign, IL: Human Kinetics; 1991:111–113.

28. Malina RM. Menarche in athletes: A synthesis and hypothesis. *Ann Human Biol.* 1983;10:1–24.

29. Frisch RE, McArthur JW. Menstrual cycles: Fatness as a determinant of minimum weight for height necessary for their maintenance or onset. *Science.* 1974;185:949–951.

30. Loucks AB, Horvath SM. Athletic amenorrhea: A review. *Med Sci Sports Exerc.* 1985;17:56–72.

31. Bullen BA, Skrinar GS, Beutins IZ, vonMering G, Turnbull BA, McArthur JW. Induction of menstrual disorders by strenuous exercise in untrained women. *N Engl J Med.* 1985;312:1349–1353.

32. De Souza MJ, Metzger DA. Reproductive dysfunction in amenorrheic athletes and anorexic patients: A review. *Med Sci Sports Exerc.* 1991;23:995–1007.

33. De Cree C. Sex steroid metabolism and menstrual irregularities in the exercising female: A review. *Sports Med.* 1998;25:369–406.

34. Kanis JA, Melton LJ, Christiansen C, Johnston CC, Khattaev N. The diagnosis of osteoporosis. *J Bone Miner Res.* 1994;9:1137–1141.

35. Drinkwater BL. The female athlete triad. Presented at the 13th annual conference on exercise sciences and sports medicine: Women, exercise and sport; March 26–27, 1999; San Juan, Puerto Rico.

36. Keen AD, Drinkwater BL. Irreversible bone loss in former amenorrheic athletes. *Osteoporos Int.* 1997;7:311–315.

37. Prior JC, Vigna YM, Schechter MT, Burgess AE. Spinal bone loss and ovulatory disturbances. *N Engl J Med.* 1990;323:1221–1227.

38. Shangold M, Freeman R, Thysen B, Gatz M. The relationship between long-distance running, plasma progesterone, and luteal phase length. *Fertil Steril.* 1979;31:130–133.

39. Drinkwater BL, Bruemner B, Chestnut CH. Menstrual history as a determinant of current bone density in young athletes. *JAMA.* 1990;263:545–548.

40. Drinkwater BL, Nilson K, Chestnut CH, Bremner WJ, Shainholtz S, Southwertz MB. Bone mineral density after resumption of menses in amenorrheic athletes. *JAMA.* 1986;256:380–382.

41. Jonnavithula S, Warren MP, Fox RP, Lazaro MI. Bone density is compromised in amenorrheic women despite return of menses: A 2-year study. *Obstet Gynecol.* 1993;81:669–674.

42. Warren MP, Brooks-Gunn J, Hamilton LH, Warren F, Hamilton WG. Scoliosis and fractures in young ballet dancers: Relation to delayed menarche and secondary amenorrhea. *N Engl J Med.* 1986;314:1348–1353.

43. Myburgh DH, Bachrach LK, Lewis B, Kent K, Marcust R. Low bone mineral density at axial and appendicular sites in amenorrheic athletes. *Med Sci Sports Exerc.* 1993;25:1197–1202.

44. Barrow G, Saha S. Menstrual irregularity and stress fracture in collegiate female distance runners. *Am J Sports Med.* 1988;16:209–216.

45. Marcus R, Cann C, Hadvig P, et al. Menstrual function and bone mass in elite women distance runners: Endocrine and metabolic factors. *Ann Intern Med.* 1985;102:158–163.

46. Bennell KL, Brukner PD. Epidemiology and site specificity of stress fractures. *Clin Sports Med.* 1997;16:179–196.

47. Lloyd T, Triantafyllou SJ, Baker ER, et al. Women athletes with menstrual irregularity have increased musculoskeletal injuries. *Med Sci Sports Exerc.* 1986;18:374–379.

48. Myburgh KH, Hutchins J, Fataar AB, Hough SF, Noaker TD. Low bone density is an etiologic factor for stress fracture in athletes. *Ann Intern Med.* 1990;113:754–759.

49. Carbon R, Sambrook PN, Deakin V, et al. Bone density of elite female athletes with stress fractures. *Med J Aust.* 1990;153:373–376.

50. Drinkwater BL. Weight-bearing exercise and bone mass. *Phys Med Rehab Clin North Am.* 1995;6:567–578.

51. Snow-Harter CM. Bone health and prevention of osteoporosis in active and athletic women. *Clin Sports Med.* 1994;13:389–404.

52. Dalsky GP. Effect of exercise on bone: Permissive influence of estrogen and calcium. *Med Sci Sports Exerc.* 1990;22:281–285.

53. Petit MA, Prior JC, Barr SI. Running and ovulation positively change cancellous bone in premenopausal women. *Med Sci Sports Exerc.* 1999;31:780–787.

54. Robinson TL, Snow-Harter C, Taaffe DR, Gillis D, Shaw J, Marcus R. Gymnasts exhibit higher bone mass than runners despite similar prevalence of amenorrhea and oligomenorrhea. *J Bone Mineral Res.* 1995;10:26–35.

55. Wolman RL, Clark P, McNally E, Harres M, Reeve J. Menstrual state and exercise as determinants of spinal trabecular bone density in female athletes. *BMJ.* 1990;301:516.

56. Slemenda CW, Johnston CC. High intensity activities in young women: Site specific bone mass effects among female figure skaters. *Bone Miner.* 1993;20:125.

57. Pettersson U, Stalnacke BM, Ahlenius GM, Henriksson-Larsen K, Lorentzon R. Low bone mass density at multiple skeletal sites, including the appendicular skeleton in amenorrheic runners. *Calcif Tissue Int.* 1999;64:117–125.

58. Nattiv A, Yeager K, Drinkwater B, Agostini R. The female athlete triad. In: Agostini R, ed. *Medical and Orthopedic Issues of Active and Athletic Women.* Philadelphia: Hanley and Belfus; 1994:169–174.

59. Johnson MD. Disordered eating. In: Agostini R, ed. *Medical and Orthopedic Issues of Active and Athletic Women.* Philadelphia: Hanley and Belfus; 1994:141–151.

60. Claman P, Seibel MM. Ovulation induction: GnRH. In: Seibel MM, ed. *Infertility.* Norwalk, CT: Appleton & Lange; 1990:333–350.

61. Shangold M. Menstruation. In: Shangold M, Mirkin G, eds. *Women and Exercise: Physiology and Sports Medicine.* 2nd ed. Philadelphia: FA Davis; 1988:129–145.

62. Vereeke West R. The female athlete: The triad of disordered eating, amenorrhoea and osteoporosis. *Sports Med.* 1998;26:63–71.

63. Snow-Harter C. Athletic amenorrhea and bone health. In: Agostini R, ed. *Medical and Orthopedic Issues of Active and Athletic Women.* Philadelphia: Hanley and Belfus; 1994:164–168.

PART IV

Health and Wellness

CHAPTER 20

Medical Screening and Clearance

Nadya Swedan and Suzanne Meth

INTRODUCTION

The requirement of a preparticipation physical evaluation (PPE) before participation in scholastic or organized athletics has created generally accepted guidelines for this screening process. Sensitivity, specificity, efficiency, and cost-effectiveness have been studied with the development of unisex standards for health care providers. Most recommendations, however, do not accommodate for either sex or activity. Comprehensive women's sports medicine screening and clearance guidelines must accommodate for not only organized team sports, but also other fitness activities, including dance, yoga, aerobics, adventure, and recreational activities. Often, the specific needs of athletic girls and women are overlooked by organized screening processes. Clinical experience and recent trends have aided in development of the guidelines specific to active women presented in this chapter.

THE PREPARTICIPATION PHYSICAL EVALUATION

It is quite common that the PPE is the only medical contact an uninjured young athlete will have; studies suggest that 80% receive no other medical evaluation.[1-3] Expectations of the PPE are to screen presumably healthy active girls and women for major medical and musculoskeletal problems in an efficient, consistent manner. Health risks and musculoskeletal impairments and weaknesses can be assessed, rehabilitation or precautions prescribed, and future injuries and illnesses prevented. Unique to women at all ages, gynecological and nutritional history is invaluable; screening for eating disorders, amenorrhea, and osteoporosis must be included. The high frequency of these disorders in female athletes and associated health risks make identification vital to present and future health, along with performance, of the athlete. While general applications are for competitive and scholastic athletes, girls and women of all ages and fitness levels should also undergo preparticipation medical screening and clearance. A recent survey revealed that only 40% of health and fitness facilities use any form of cardiovascular health screening.[4] Ideally, universal guidelines for gender-specific pre-athletic health screening will become the standard rather than the exception.

Goals of a Comprehensive Preparticipation Screening

Goals include the following:
—assess general health
—identify risks to participation in her activity
—assess past injuries and residual deficits, pain, or weaknesses
—identify health-threatening behaviors (eating, sleeping, substance abuse, performance enhancers)
—screen for signs or symptoms of disordered eating
—establish inventory of overall fitness
—identify muscle imbalances or weakness that may need to be strengthened
—identify impairments in environmental management including balance, vision, hearing
—assess posture and alignment
—ensure appropriate gynecological and breast health care
—provide referral to appropriate health care professionals, including specialists, therapists, athletic trainers, and psychologists if needed

—prevent injuries by prescribing specific training goals

—provide a confidential arena for athlete to address health concerns

—establish and reinforce physician-patient relationship and trust

—collect emergency medical information

—establish a sports/health care network to improve performance

—meet legal and insurance requirements of governing athletic bodies

Clinical Guideline

Types of Evaluation

Cost, availability of appropriately trained personnel, school, state or athletic governing bodies, and athlete preference contribute to the format in which the preparticipation evaluation takes place. Formal screening arranged by the school or sports organization is usually set up as a station examination in one location, during or around a practice session. Personal physician exams occur when the school or organization does not have these resources available and are the common method of preparticipation screening in adults.

The station examination is both cost-effective and time-efficient, allowing screening of large numbers of athletes. Multiple health care providers are involved, often including ancillary staff, nurses, athletic trainers or therapists, and physicians. The station examination is conducive to more sports-specific physicals, because the providers are usually knowledgeable in sports medicine. The inclusion of athletic trainers can assist in comprehensiveness of the musculoskeletal examination. Stations are usually numbered and correspond to the history form for easy reference during examination. Usually, the first station is for intake of history forms, height and weight, and Snellen's test. Further stations are usually for medical examination, including screening head, eyes, ears, nose, and throat; chest auscultation; and abdominal examination; the musculoskeletal station exam can also include a brief skin assessement. If available, athletes should briefly be encouraged to also meet privately with a nutritionist and psychologist. Communication between all levels is encouraged, and coaches and team trainers should be present to facilitate compliance with specific referrals, modifications, or precautions. Limits to the station examination are that of privacy and time because of the nature of the group setting.

Personal physicians who complete the preparticipation examinations are usually pediatricians, family physicians, or internists. Privacy and continuity of medical care are important benefits of this type of examination. Further physician referral, if needed, is usually appropriately followed. Although screening for serious medical risks is quite thorough, evaluation of musculoskeletal and sports-specific issues can be weak due to less specific knowledge and training in sports behavior and risks.[5]

Guidelines of PPE

The PPE as a screening, prevention, and performance-enhancing tool has been developed as a unisex examination. Standardization of prevention and clearance exams were first established in 1992 as a monograph produced by the American Academy of Family Physicians, American Academy of Pediatrics, American Medical Society for Sports Medicine, American Orthopedic Society for Sports Medicine, and American Osteopathic Academy of Sports Medicine, with a second edition in 1997[2]. In 1996, the American Heart Association consensus panel developed specific cardiovascular screening protocols.[6,7] Obtaining both of these publications is recommended for more detailed guidelines on meeting legal requirements of preparticipation screening. As these widely accepted guidelines do not address gender differences, this chapter provides more specific recommendations for evaluating female athletes.

Ideally, preparticipation physicals should be performed yearly with records maintained on each athlete; standard recommendations currently are for every 2 years with interim history. State scholastic regulations, athletic program, and health club screening requirements vary widely. The athlete should be encouraged to communicate with coaches, trainers, and the team physician regarding injuries, illnesses, or new medications. It is our responsibility as sports health care providers to enforce medical clearance before beginning a new sport or exercise program, particularly in women who have not exercised in the past.

To allow time for treatment, management, and evaluation of any identified limitations to sports participation, the PPE should be performed 6 to 8 weeks before the start of season training. Coaches or trainers who will be working with the athletes should be available to allow communication and establish preseason goals, particularly for athletes with musculoskeletal or health limitations. In some states, health care professionals other than physicians can clear athletes for participation. However, it is still recommended that each athlete has contact with a physician or appropriately skilled nurse practitioner or physician's assistant. Each provider should be familiar with the demands and expectations of the PPE, as well as guidelines for clearance.

As each exam should be individualized, certain populations require additional attention. For example, disabled athletes should be screened for bowel and bladder, tone, and skin integrity. Proper equipment and ambulatory devices are essential; consultation with the athlete's physiatrist or primary care physician is recommended.

In screening dancers and skaters, particular attention should be paid to posture, lower extremity alignment, ankles and feet, and body composition. More specific guidelines for preparticipation dance evaluations are available in the literature.[8] Again, one cannot overemphasize the importance of a thorough history of eating patterns and nutrition at all ages, because eating disorders and body image concerns often begin in grade school.

The History

A comprehensive history allows for a more efficient and effective screening process; approximately 70% of potential medical and musculoskeletal injury risks can be identified by history alone.[9–11] A recent study at Stanford University[1] demonstrated the use of an internet Web site to collect medical, musculoskeletal, menstrual, nutrition, sleep, and social history information. This information was summarized into a two-page form for easy physician reference (Exhibit 20–1). Sensitivity and specificity for an accurate history were thereafter calculated as 97% and 99.7%, respectively.[1(p 1733)] Participating physicians agreed this history format improved screening and medical care, focused the examination, and allowed for more efficient examination time.

A thorough gynecological history in adolescent and postadolescent women is essential because it can reflect overall health status, hormonal status, pregnancy, and other health risks. Preventive behaviors and the importance of examinations including pelvic, Pap smears, and breast examinations should be reinforced and discussed. The prevalence of athletic amenorrhea and oligomenorrhea should not prevent a physician from overlooking other medical causes. These can include pregnancy, prolactin-secreting pituitary tumors, thyroid disorders, and virilizing syndromes.[12(p 60)] Other considerations include anabolic steroid use or other performance-enhancing medications. Primary amenorrhea after the age of 16 and absence of menses for 6 months or longer should be referred to a specialist.[13]

Behavioral signs of eating disorders include excessive training time, preoccupation with restriction of food, hyperactivity, depression, elimination of foods or food groups, unusual meal patterns, wearing layers of loose clothing, obsession with thinness, drug abuse, and denial of low bodyweight.[14(pp 295–296)] Physical complaints in the history can include muscle cramping, easy bruising (from hypokalemia), cold intolerance, hair loss, fainting, and gastrointestinal complaints, including constipation, bloating, and heartburn.[15] Comments made on weight intake should be noted for appropriateness. On physical examination, body weight 15% less than that expected for height is suggestive of anorexia.[14(p 295)]

Exhibit 20–2 is an extensive history form that can be modified for age. In girls less than the age of 18, health and immunization histories should be completed or reviewed and signed by the parent/legal guardian. Social history and lifestyle questions are to be answered separately from the section signed by parents to protect confidentiality in young women. In adults, the section for parental consent can be removed and all questions combined; thus, this form can serve as a thorough evaluation for women athletes at all ages and levels.

The Examination

The medical clearance examination should include general assessment, age-appropriate medical examination, and sports-appropriate musculoskeletal examination. For each station or examination component, the relevant history should be reviewed verbally with the athlete. Positive history and red flags should be addressed during the examination. General assessment includes physique, overall appearance, height, and weight. Weight should be taken in privacy, and its importance as an identifying value downplayed. Inappropriate comments from the athlete should be noted (such as a very thin athlete feeling she weighs too much); these athletes and those expressing weight concerns should be referred to the nutritionist and/or psychologist. Refer to Exhibit 20–3 for an outline of an examination intake form.

Ketone breath, frail appearance, and poor skin and nail health are indicative of malnutrition and anorexia. Lanugo (fine body and facial hair) may also be present.[15(p 604)] Bulimic behavior is associated with characteristic physical signs,[12(p 64)] including subconjunctival hematomas, tooth enamel erosion, and gingival and oral mucosal damage resulting from repeated vomiting. Russell's sign, lacerations on the knuckles secondary to vomiting, has also been described as a marker of bulimia.[16] Parotid gland enlargement, resulting in a "chubby-cheeked" appearance is also common; the cause of this physical sign is suspected to be parotid stimulation by repeated vomiting.[16(p 107)]

Certain settings, populations, and sports require more detailed attention to certain exam aspects, appropriate to activity.[17] For example, contact and field sports participants require focused vision, pupil, and neurology exams[17(pS341)]; an inner ear examination should be performed in swimmers; musculoskeletal exams can also be focused such as a thorough foot and ankle exam in dancers and runners.

An appropriate cardiovascular screening examination includes blood pressure, cardiac auscultation both seated and supine, and palpation of femoral artery pulses. Blood pressure guidelines should be age appropriate, less than 135/85 for ages 10 and older, and 125/75 if under the age of 10.[18(p 9)] If elevated, blood pressure should be repeated at the end of the examination. All diastolic murmurs, systolic murmurs greater than grade III, and murmurs that worsen with the Valsalva maneuver require cardiology referral.[18(p 9)] A midsystolic

Exhibit 20–1 Summary Report of History Questionnaire Responses Requiring Physician Attention[1(p 1730)]

Stanford University PPE Medical History Summary

Name	Varsity Athlete	Medical History Date	00/00/00
Sport(s)	Soccer	Form ID	0000
Class	Freshman	Scholarship	Yes

Gender	Female	**ALLERGIES**
Date of Birth	00/00/00	Environmental: pollen
Age	20	
Height (inches)	63	
Weight (lbs)	117	

CURRENT MEDICATIONS	Dose	Frequency
Motrin	200mg	2x a day
Claritin	10mg	daily

MEDICAL HISTORY FOR PAST 12 MONTHS

Head & Neck:	Nil
Eyes:	Wears glasses/contacts Wears them during training or competition
	Eye exam in past 12 months
Lungs:	Nil
Heart:	heart murmur Investigations:
	Exercise induced: cough Echocardiogram—heart murmur
Abdomen:	Nil
Genitourinary:	Nil
Menstrual:	No pelvic exam/pap smear in the past 12 months: Age at menarche: 12
	Most recent menstrual period: <1 month ago
	Number of periods: >12
	Longest time between periods: 1–3 month(s)
	Average duration of period: 1–5 days
Neurology:	migraine headaches
Skin:	Nil
Other:	heat exhaustion/heat stroke
	chickenpox
	two normal eyes, ears, kidneys

SURGICAL HISTORY FOR PAST 12 MONTHS

Site	Date	Reason
mouth	9/97	wisdom teeth extraction

Form ID: 0000

continues

Exhibit 20–1 continued

Stanford University PPE Medical History Summary

ORTHOPAEDIC HISTORY FOR PAST 12 MONTHS

		Current				Current
Neck:	Nil		Thigh:	quadriceps strain/injury		
Back:	Nil		Knee:	tendonitis		Yes
Shoulder:	AC separation		Lower leg:	shin splints		Yes
Elbow:	Nil		Ankle:	sprain		
Arm:	Nil			instability		Yes
Hand:	Nil		Foot:	Nil		
Pelvis:	Nil		Other injuries:	Nil		
Treated in past year:	shin splints ankle sprain	Yes	Brace/Orthotics:	Uses brace/splint/sleeve Uses orthotics Nil		

FAMILY HISTORY

SUDDEN DEATH IN FAMILY <50 YRS OF AGE: Yes—heart attack

Heart attack:	Mother/Father		Diabetes:	Nil
Heart abnormality:	Nil		Kidney disease:	Nil
Marfan syndrome:	Nil		Arthritis:	Nil
Hypertension:	Grandparent		Cancer:	Grandparent
High cholesterol:	Grandparent		Epilepsy:	Nil
Bleeding disorder:	Mother/Father		Psychiatric disorder:	Nil
Sickle cell anemia:	Nil			

HEALTH HABITS

Nutrition:	avoids meat
Safety:	Nil
Smoking:	Has not smoked in past year
Alcohol:	Beer: 1 per week
	Wine: 1 per week
	Liquor: 1–3 per month
Physician consult requests:	weight control
	stress

Form ID: 0000

Exhibit 20–2 History Intake Form To Be Reviewed with Athlete

Name_____ Age _____ DOB _____

Sports you play _____

Address _____ Phone _____

School or place of employment _____

Emergency contact: Name _____ Phone _____ Work phone _____

Your physician's name _____ Address_____ Phone _____

Please list answers to the following questions as best you can.

How many days a week do you train? _____

How many hours a day do you train (include playing time, practice, weight training)?_____

What goals do you have for this season? _____

When is your next competitive event?_____

Where do you have pain, if any? _____

Do you feel you have any muscle weakness? If so, where?_____

List medical problems _____

Do you have any allergies (include foods, insects, medicines, etc.) _____

What medications do you take? _____

What pain relievers do you take ? _____

What herbs or supplements do you take? _____

Have you had any surgeries? _____

When was your last doctor's visit? _____ For what? _____

Do you, your parents, or siblings have a heart condition? _____

What age did you first get your period? _____

How many periods have you had in the past year? _____

Regarding your periods, you usually get them every ____ weeks; they usually last _____ days.

When did your last period end? _____

When did you last have a pelvic examination/Pap smear? _____

When did you last do a self-breast examination? _____

Please circle appropriate response.   *Examiner's comments*

Do you feel you tire during exercise more easily than others? . . . . Yes   No

Have you ever been short of breath? . . . . Yes   No

Have you ever passed out during or after exercise? . . . . Yes   No

Have you ever been told you have a heart murmur? . . . . Yes   No

Do you ever feel chest pain? . . . . Yes   No

continues

Exhibit 20–2 continued

Please circle appropriate response. *Examiner's comments*

Do you ever get heart racing or feel your heart skip beats? .... Yes No

Has anyone in your family died from a heart condition before age 50? .... Yes No

Have you ever had wheezing? .... Yes No

Do you cough a lot during exercise or otherwise? .... Yes No

Do you get a lot of colds or sinus problems? .... Yes No

Have you ever had an illness lasting longer than 1 week? .... Yes No

Were you ever hospitalized overnight? If yes, for what/<u>when</u> _____ ..... Yes No

Have you ever had a sudden rash or hives? .... Yes No

Have you ever hit your head hard enough to pass out? .... Yes No

Have you ever felt light-headed or dizzy? .... Yes No

Do you have headaches? .... Yes No

Have you ever had a seizure? .... Yes No

Have you ever lost your memory? .... Yes No

Have you ever felt numb or tingly anywhere? If yes, <u>where</u> _____ .... Yes No

Do you experience muscle cramps? .... Yes No

Does anyone in your family have a muscular or nerve disease? .... Yes No

Do you ever have frequent diarrhea or constipation? .... Yes No

Have you ever had bloody stools? .... Yes No

Do you bruise easily? .... Yes No

Do you eat three meals a day? .... Yes No

Do you drink at least 8 glasses of water, juice, or sports drink a day? .... Yes No

Do you take vitamins or supplements? .... Yes No

Do you have any eating concerns? .... Yes No

Do you want to weigh more or less than you do now? .... Yes No

Have you ever been on a weight-loss diet? .... Yes No

Have you ever been diagnosed with an eating disorder? .... Yes No

Do you have any cuts, bruises, rashes, or open sores now? .... Yes No

Have you ever had swelling of a joint or limb? .... Yes No

Have you had any fractures, joint dislocations, or sprains? .... Yes No

Do you have any vision problems? .... Yes No

Do you wear glasses or contacts? .... Yes No

Have you ever had frostbite? .... Yes No

Have you ever passed out from heat or dehydration? .... Yes No

Do you need any special equipment (brace, orthotics, retainer, hearing aid)? .... Yes No

Have you ever been restricted from play for health reasons? .... Yes No

Have you ever been denied medical clearance to participate in a sport? .... Yes No

Immunizations (please list most recent date)

Tetanus _____ Measles _____ Mumps _____ Hep B _____ Varicella (chickenpox) _____ Rubella _____

Athlete's signature _____ Print name_____ Date _____

Parent/legal guardian signature _____ Print name_____ Date _____

continues

Exhibit 20–2 continued

The following questions should be completed privately by the athlete before the medical examination (the answers will remain confidential):

Do you smoke? _____ If yes, how many packs a day?_____	Yes	No
Do you drink alcohol? _____ If yes, how often? _____	Yes	No
Have you ever used any street drugs?	Yes	No
Do you wear a seatbelt?	Yes	No
Do you wear a helmet?	Yes	No
Do you sleep well?	Yes	No
Do you feel stressed out?	Yes	No
Do you ever vomit after eating?	Yes	No
Do you ever use laxatives?	Yes	No
Do you ever take diuretics?	Yes	No
Have you ever taken anything to help you lose weight?	Yes	No
Have you ever taken anything to help you gain muscle or strength?	Yes	No
Have you ever taken anything to keep you awake or alert?	Yes	No
Would you like to speak confidentially about your weight?	Yes	No
Would you like to speak confidentially about sexual concerns?	Yes	No
Do you have a foul-smelling vaginal discharge?	Yes	No
Do you have any pelvic pain?	Yes	No
Would you like to speak confidentially about stress?	Yes	No

click with or without a late systolic murmur is common in mitral valve prolapse. In athletes with long, lean builds, Marfan's syndrome should also be considered. Femoral artery pulse quality should be assessed to rule out coarctation of the aorta.[7(p 855)] Lung auscultation, abdominal palpation for organomegaly, assessment of radial and femoral pulses, and assessment of skin integrity is advised.

Functional assessment of the neuromusculoskeletal system requires review of past injuries. The examiner should consider that musculoskeletal histories may lack some detail, because often an athlete will forget events such as a mild head injury or ankle sprain. In those athletes who do have a history of injury, the examination should be more specific. The musculoskeletal examination should include posture, alignment, gait, strength, and range of motion and ideally should be sports specific with attention to areas at highest risk of injury (refer to Appendix A for guidelines). Standard screening examinations have been established and described in various publications. These include the 13-step musculoskeletal examination,[18(pp 9–17)] the 2-minute orthopaedic

examination,[13(pp 42–47)] and the 90-second orthopaedic screening examination.[10(pS69),19(p421)] Neurological evaluation of muscle stretch reflexes, cranial nerves, and coordination should be more thorough in athletes with a history and increased risk of head injury.

Further Evaluation

Diagnostic testing is recommended only if the history and physical examination detect potential health risks. In a young, healthy athletic population, it is agreed that there are no cost-effective benefits to routine laboratory screening, including blood work, urinalysis, or cardiopulmonary testing, such as electrocardiogram, echocardiogram, or stress testing.[2(p7)] Cardiac referral should be recommended in an athlete with reported exercise intolerance, syncope or near syncope, chest pain, arrhythmia, and family history of cardiac or unknown cause of death before age 50.[20(p 638)] In women older than 50, stress testing should be considered.[21(p S349)] (Refer to Chapter 14 for further details regarding cardiac issues.)

Exhibit 20–3 Examination Intake Form

Athlete's name_____ Age_____ Date _____

Height_____ Weight_____ Athletic Activity_____

B/P_____ P_____ R_____

Vision R 20/_____ L 20/_____ with glasses/contacts/protective eyewear

Pupils _____ R/L PERRLA _____ Abnormalities _____

Ears   R/L TM_____   Abnormalities_____   Nose/throat   Wnl_____ Abnormalities_____

Heart   sit_____   stand_____   Vasalva_____

Femoral pulses   2+   1+   Trace 0   Distal Cap._____ refill_____ Wnl_____   Other_____

Lungs   CTA_____   Abnormalities _____

ABD   Wnl_____   Abnormalities _____

Skin   Wnl_____   Abnormalities _____

Gait   Wnl_____   Deficits _____

Balance   Wnl_____   Deficits _____

Posture   Wnl_____   Deficits _____

Spine   Wnl_____   Deficits _____

Upper extremity strength   Wnl_____   Deficits _____

Lower extremity strength   Wnl_____   Deficits _____

Range of motion   Wnl_____   Deficits _____

Reflexes   Biceps_____   Knees_____ Other _____

Flexibility   Wnl_____   Hypermobility_____ Deficits_____

Clearance (check one) ____ unrestricted for athletic activity identified above

_____ limited clearance with recommendations below

_____ not cleared for referrals

Recommendations: _____

_____

Clearance to be deferred to: _____

Athlete referred to: _____Pending: _____

Examiner's signature: _____Date _____

Examiner's printed name: _____ Office phone _____

Urine drug screening occurs routinely in elite and professional athletes by the governing athletic bodies (see Chapters 23 and 24). Team physicians and athletic health care providers should be aware of the policies on banned medications and substances. Human immunodeficiency virus and hepatitis screening is rarely required, and only in a few contact sport settings; however, athletes with a history of exposure should be encouraged to undergo voluntary testing.

Clearance

According to the 1997 manual, *Preparticipation Physical Evaluation*, 2nd ed., 0.3% to 1.3% of athletes are denied clearance during the PPE, and 3.2% to 13.5% are referred for further evaluation.[2(p1)] Exhibit 20–4 provides the established guidelines for medical conditions and sports participation. In a comprehensive study of PPEs done at the Mayo Clinic,[19] vision, musculoskeletal, cardiac, and weight-diet factors were the greatest reasons for referral before clearance, in decreasing order.[19(p 424)] As this study did not differentiate between genders, it can be speculated that female athletes would have a higher prevalence of clearance issues related to weight-diet.

To respect confidentiality, the athlete and parent/legal guardian should be informed of limited or restricted clearance status in a private setting with a health care provider to answer questions. Before the health care provider may release this information to the athletic organization, school, coaches, or trainers, authorization from the athlete or parent/guardian is required.[2(p 30)] Specific legal guidelines vary from state to state, but an athlete may have the right to participate in a sport *against medical advice*. In these instances, proper forms must be completed by the athlete and the parent or legal guardian if necessary to absolve the physician of any legal responsibilities.[2(p 43)]

TYPE OF ATHLETIC ACTIVITY

Type of sport is important in determining clearance. Although an athlete may be precluded from certain activities, she can usually be redirected to another. Level of contact in sports is an important consideration, as well as strenuousness. Specifically, an athlete who has had three episodes of loss of consciousness should be directed to less contact sports (refer to Exhibit 20–4). In 1999, *JAMA* published studies evaluating mild traumatic brain injury (MTBI) rates in high school sports. Risks were higher in male athletes with an overall rate of 1.8 male:1 female MTBI per 100 player seasons. Highest reported rates in girls occurred in soccer (1.4) and girls' basketball, in which girls' injury rates were higher than boys (1.04 vs .75).[22] In addition, there was a reported higher level of learning disability and decreased performance on neuropsychological testing in students who had one or more concussions.[23]

Level of contact, as well as risk for falls, is an important consideration in pregnant athletes. Physicians should discourage pregnant women from participating in sports with any level of contact (Exhibit 20–5); they should avoid prolonged strenuous exercise and maintain hydration and body temperature at optimum levels. Scuba diving and exercising at altitudes greater than 8000 ft is prohibited (refer to Chapter 11 for further guidelines on exercise in pregnancy).

Some girls and women are better adapted at certain sports; repetitive activities a body is not designed for can lead to chronic overuse injuries. For example, a heavy-set, large-boned girl is likely to find it easier to excel at crew or volleyball rather than gymnastics or marathon running. Analyzing running styles, extensive training, and appropriate strengthening and stretching can make marathon running easier to achieve; however, the greater force of impact with each stride in a larger woman versus a smaller woman may increase risk of long-term injuries. Genetics play a major role in this determinant; girls should be encouraged at a young age to participate in various activities to promote balance of muscle strength, adaptation, and flexibility. In addition, they will likely eventually discover an athletic activity that they both enjoy and excel at.

TEAM PHYSICIAN DUTIES

Responsibilities of the team physicians include managing medical and musculoskeletal problems and providing athletic event coverage for early assessment of acute injuries. There are many advantages of having a team physician, most notably continuity and consistency of health care. Athletes develop trust in their providers, an important aspect of medical treatment in girls and women. Also, education and training to prevent medical and musculoskeletal risk factors lessen the frequency of chronic and complicated medical and musculoskeletal issues. Communication between physician, coach, trainer, and athlete is essential and is facilitated with consistently available professionals. Ultimately, readiness for and return to play is the decision of the athlete's team and/or personal physician. Protocols should be established to clarify assessment and treatment of injuries.

During the season, musculoskeletal injuries are the greatest limitation to practice or competition, affecting approximately one-third of athletes at some time.[19(p 419)] With respect to acute illness, fever and diarrhea are contraindications because of impaired hydration and thermoregulation.[2(p 31)] Other contraindications include respiratory diseases that limit adequate ventilation and endurance, wounds that cannot be covered, and contagious viral or skin infections (refer to Chapter 13 for further considerations). Eye injuries must also be evaluated and protective eyewear worn if necessary. In severe cases of eating disorders, participation should not be allowed until treatment ensues. Stress fractures, particularly those associated with the female athlete triad, should be treated as carefully as traumatic fractures with modified activity and complete evaluation of activity tolerance.

Musculoskeletal injuries must be evaluated and treated with specific goals. Before return to play, strength and range of motion should be at least 85% to 90% of normal, and the athlete should be without pain or instability. Neurological conditions including burners, stingers, and concussions must be evaluated thoroughly and future play recommended with respect to prior head injuries or concussions (see Clinical Guideline). Prudent medical care includes a low threshold for referral to a specialist in the event of repeated injuries or persistent symptoms.

Team or covering physicians can be liable for allowing play during threatening or inclement weather, on dangerous surfaces, or with faulty equipment.[10(pS68)] There has been

Exhibit 20–4 Medical Conditions and Sports Participation

This exhibit is designed to be understood by medical and nonmedical personnel. In the "Explanation" section below, "needs evaluation" means that a physician with appropriate knowledge and experience should assess the safety of a given sport for an athlete with the listed medical condition. Unless otherwise noted, this is because of the variability of the severity of the disease or of the risk of injury among the specific sports, or both.

Condition	May Participate
Atlantoaxial instability* (instability of the joint between cervical vertebrae 1 and 2)	**Qualified Yes**
Explanation: Athlete needs evaluation to assess risk of spinal cord injury during sports participation.	
Bleeding disorder*	**Qualified Yes**
Explanation: Athlete needs evaluation.	
Cardiovascular diseases	
Carditis (inflammation of the heart)	**No**
Explanation: Carditis may result in sudden death with exertion.	
Hypertension (high blood pressure)	**Qualified Yes**
Explanation: Those with significant essential (unexplained) hypertension should avoid weight and power lifting, body building, and strength training. Those with secondary hypertension (hypertension caused by a previously identified disease), or severe essential hypertension, need evaluation.	
Congenital heart disease (structural heart defects present at birth)	**Qualified Yes**
Explanation: Those with mild forms may participate fully; those with moderate or severe forms, or who have undergone surgery, need evaluation.‡	
Dysrhythmia (irregular heart rhythm)	**Qualified Yes**
Explanation: Athlete needs evaluation because some types require therapy or make certain sports dangerous, or both.	
Mitral valve prolapse (abnormal heart valve)	**Qualified Yes**
Explanation: Those with symptoms (chest pain, symptoms of possible dysrhythmia) or evidence of mitral regurgitation (leaking) on physical examination need evaluation. All others may participate fully.	
Heart murmur	**Qualified Yes**
Explanation: If the murmur is innocent (does not indicate heart disease), full participation is permitted. Otherwise, the athlete needs evaluation (see " Congenital heart disease" and "Mitral valve prolapse" above.	
Cerebral palsy*	**Qualified Yes**
Explanation: Athlete needs evaluation.	
Diabetes mellitus*§	**Yes**
Explanation: All sports can be played with proper attention to diet, hydration, and insulin therapy. Particular attention is needed for activities that last 30 minutes or more.	
Diarrhea¶	**Qualified No**
Explanation: Unless disease is mild, no participation is permitted, because diarrhea may increase the risk of dehydration and heat illness. See "Fever" below.	
Eating disorders	
Anorexia nervosa, Bulimia nervosa	**Qualified Yes**
Explanation: These patients need both medical and psychiatric assessment before participation.	
Eyes	
Functionally one-eyed athlete, loss of an eye, detached retina, previous eye surgery, or serious eye injury	**Qualified Yes**
Explanation: A functionally one-eyed athlete has a best corrected visual acuity of <20/40 in the worse eye. These athletes would suffer significant disability if the better eye was seriously injured as would those with loss of an eye. Some athletes who have previously undergone eye surgery or had a serious eye injury may have an increased risk of injury because of weakened eye tissue. Availability of eye guards approved by the American Society for Testing Materials (ASTM) and other protective equipment may allow participation in most sports, but this must be judged on an individual basis.	
Fever¶	**No**
Explanation: Fever can increase cardiopulmonary effort, reduce maximum exercise capacity, make heat illness more likely, and increase orthostatic hypotension during exercise. Fever may rarely accompany myocarditis or other infections that may make exercise dangerous.	

continues

Exhibit 20–4 continued

Condition	May Participate
Heat illness, history of	**Qualified Yes**
Explanation: Because of the increased likelihood of recurrence, the athlete needs individual assessment to determine the presence of predisposing conditions and to arrange a prevention strategy.	
HIV Infection¶	**Yes**
Explanation: Because of the apparent minimal risk to others, all sports may be played that the state of health allows. In all athletes, skin lesions should be properly covered, and athletic personnel should use universal precautions when handling blood or body fluids with visible blood.	
Kidney: absence of one	**Qualified Yes**
Explanation: Athlete needs individual assessment for contact/collision and limited contact sports.	
Liver, enlarged	**Qualified Yes**
Explanation: If the liver is acutely enlarged, participation should be avoided because of risk of rupture. If the liver is chronically enlarged, individual assessment is needed before contact/collision or limited contact sports are played.	
Malignancy*	**Qualified Yes**
Explanation: Athlete needs individual assessment.	
Musculoskeletal disorders	**Qualified Yes**
Explanation: Athlete needs individual assessment.	
Neurologic	
History of serious head or spine trauma, severe or repeated concussions, or craniotomy	**Qualified Yes**
Explanation: Athlete needs individual assessment for contact/collision or limited contact sports, and also for noncontact sports if there are deficits in judgment or cognition. Recent research supports a conservative approach to management of concussion.	
Convulsion disorder, well controlled	**Qualified Yes**
Explanation: Risk of convulsion during participation is minimal.	
Convulsive disorder, poorly controlled	**Qualified Yes**
Explanation: Athlete needs individual assessment for contact/collision or limited contact sports. Avoid the following noncontact sports: archery, riflery, swimming, weight or power lifting, strength training, or sports involving heights. In these sports, occurrence of a convulsion may be a risk to self or others.	
Obesity	**Qualified Yes**
Explanation: Because of the risk of heat illness, obese persons need careful acclimatization and hydration.	
Organ transplant recipient*	**Qualified Yes**
Explanation: Athlete needs individual assessment.	
Ovary: absence of one	**Yes**
Explanation: Risk of severe injury to the remaining ovary is minimal.	
Respiratory	
Pulmonary compromise including cystic fibrosis*	**Qualified Yes**
Explanation: Athlete needs individual assessment, but generally all sports may be played if oxygenation remains satisfactory during a graded exercise test. Patients with cystic fibrosis need acclimation and good hydration to reduce the risk of heat illness.	
Asthma	**Yes**
Explanation: With proper medication and education, only athletes with the most severe asthma will have to modify their participation.	
Acute upper respiratory infection	**Qualified Yes**
Explanation: Upper respiratory obstruction may affect pulmonary function. Athlete needs individual assessment for all but mild disease. See "Fever" above.	
Sickle cell disease	**Qualified Yes**
Explanation: Athlete needs individual assessment. In general, if status of the illness permits, all but high-exertion, contact/collision sports may be played. Overheating, dehydration, and chilling must be avoided.	
Sickle cell trait	**Yes**
Explanation: It is unlikely that individuals with sickle cell trait (AS) have an increased risk of sudden death or other medical problems during athletic participation except under the most extreme conditions of heat, humidity, and possibly increased altitude. These individuals, like all athletes, should be carefully conditioned, acclimatized, and hydrated to reduce any possible risk.	

continues

Exhibit 20–4 continued

Condition	May Participate
Skin: boils, herpes simplex, impetigo, scabies, molluscum contagiosum Explanation: While the patient is contagious, participation in gymnastics with mats, martial arts, wrestling, or other contact/collision or limited contact sports is not allowed. Herpes simplex virus probably is not transmitted via mats.	Qualified Yes
Spleen, enlarged¶ Explanation: Patients with acutely enlarged spleens should avoid all sports because of risk of rupture. Those with chronically enlarged spleens need individual assessment before playing contact/collision or limited contact sports.	Qualified Yes
Testicle: absent or undescended Explanation: Certain sports may require a protective cup.	Yes

* *Not discussed in text of the monograph.*
† *See table 4.*
‡ *Mild, moderate, and severe congenital heart disease are defined in 26th Bethesda Conference: Recommendations for determining eligibility for competition in athletics with cardiovascular abnormalities. January 6-7, 1994. Med Sci Sports Exerc 1994;26(10 suppl):S246–253.*
§ *Well controlled.*
¶ *AAP recommendation as indicated; see text for qualifications by other commentators.*

no documented evidence of gender differences in overall tolerance of extreme exercise climates, although men actually have greater incidences of exertional heat stroke.[24](p 336) With the exception of a greater frequency of heat edema and Raynaud's phenomenon, self-limiting clinical entities,[24] women are equally able to tolerate temperature differences. Cold tolerance is aided by larger muscle mass, due to increased shivering and heat production. The average greater amount of muscle mass in men is thought to be compensated for by increased subcutaneous fat in women.[25](p359)

Sports Concussion Guidelines

Grade of Concussion

Grade 1	Grade 2	Grade 3
Transient confusion	Transient confusion	Any loss of consciousness
No loss of consciousness	No loss of consciousness	Evaluation in ER
Concussion symptoms <15 min	Concussion symptoms >15 min	May need CT or MRI

Management of First Concussion

Remove from game	Remove from game	If LOC lasts seconds, no play until symptom free × 1 wk
Examine immediately and at 5-min intervals	Examine on site and frequently	If LOC lasts minutes, no play until symptom free × 2 wk
May return to game if symptoms resolve in 15 min	No play until symptom free × 1 wk	If abnormal, CT/MRI—end of season
	MD examination after 1 wk symptom free	
	If symptoms > 1 wk, CT or MRI	

Management of Second Concussion

2nd Gr 1—remove from play	2nd Grade 2—no play until symptom free (rest and exertion) × 2 wk	2nd Gr 3—no play until symptom free 1 mo or longer based on MD decision
Return when symptom free × 1 wk	If any CT/MR abnormality—end of season	

Clinical Guideline

Exhibit 20–5 Classification of Sports by Contact

Contact/Collision	Limited Contact	Noncontact
Basketball	Baseball	Archery
Boxing*	Bicycling	Badminton
Diving	Cheerleading	Body building
Field hockey	Canoeing/kayaking (white water)	Canoeing/kayaking (flat water)
Football	Fencing	Crew/rowing
Flag	Field	Curling
Tackle	High jump	Dancing
Ice hockey	Pole vault	Field
Lacross	Floor hockey	Discus
Martial arts	Gymnastics	Javelin
Rodeo	Handball	Shot put
Rugby	Horseback riding	Golf
Ski jumping	Racquetball	Orienteering
Soccer	Skating	Power lifting
Team handball	Ice	Race walking
Water polo	In-line	Riflery
Wrestling	Roller	Rope jumping
	Skiing	Running
	Cross-country	Sailing
	Downhill	Scuba diving
	Water	Strength training
	Softball	Swimming
	Squash	Table tennis
	Ultimate Frisbee	Tennis
	Volleyball	Track
	Windsurfing/surfing	Weight lifting

* Participation not recommended by the AAP. The AAFP, AMSSM, AOASM, and AOSSM have no stand against boxing.

Winter Temperature/Wind Chill Guidelines Precautions[10](p 568)

T<50° F/10° C increasesd risk for hypothermia

T<31° F/–1° C increased risk for frostbite

T<–4° F/–20° C skiing events canceled

Clinical Guideline

BODY IMAGE AND HEALTH MAINTENANCE

The pressures of both society and athletic performance, particularly in aesthetic sports, result in a frequent occurrence of eating disorders and related health risks in female athletes. Denial and unrealistic images of body appearance often prevent the athlete from recognizing the problem herself. In a study of "lean and fit" regularly exercising women, 77% wanted to lose weight; 57% were dieting.[26](p 47)

Coaches, trainers, family members, friends, and fellow teammates can assist in identifying inconsistencies or deficits resulting from poor health and nutrition. Sports health staff have the responsibility not only of clearing the athlete for participation but also for educating them on prevention and identification of risk-taking and injury promoting behavior. A study in the Florida schools in 1998 revealed that 86% of eating disorders begin before the age of 21.[27](p 51) This study evaluated the positive efficacy of training school professionals to identify students at risk of eating disorders.

Summer Heat/Humidity Precautions[24](pp 334,337)

T > 86°F/humidity > 90%, heat precautions should be taken

T > 95° F, evaporation is cooling mechanism, less effective in high humidity

Clinical Guideline

The importance of screening and monitoring girls and women for eating disorders cannot be underestimated; the earlier in life this problem is addressed, the more likely it can be effectively treated.[12(p 63)] Unfortunately, many girls and women hide their anorexic or bulimic behaviors quite well. (Refer to Exhibit 20–6 for guidelines on additional screening questions helpful in identifying girls and women at risk.) Bulimic behavior can be present in athletes of normal weight; physical signs of vomiting and frequent trips to the bathroom, particularly after eating, are revealing. The Eating Disorder Inventory Questionnaire[28–30] has also been implemented as a screening tool for abnormal eating behaviors in certain settings. Specific to bulimia, an eating disorder screening examination is also available.[31] In girls and women who do not fall into specific categories, the classification of Eating Disorder Not Otherwise Specified should also be considered.[32] Early education, identification, and intervention with nutritional education and counseling are effective in preventing chronic destructive behaviors. Referral to a multidisciplinary eating disorder clinic is essential to addressing the many associated physical and psychological complications.

Nutrition habits, weight desires, and menstrual history should be periodically evaluated. Although an estimated 30% of dancers and marathon runners report amenorrhea or oligomenorrhea,[12(p 60)] classic cases of anorexia nervosa are always associated with secondary amenorrhea.[12(p64),14(p296)] Careful interview may reveal the denial that is seen with eating disorders. Referral to a nutritionist or sports psychologist may also unveil unhealthy patterns. Reminding athletes that muscles and bones need fuel for optimum performance and enforcing the importance of meals, snacks, and fluids is encouraged.

Girls and young women should also be educated in the consequences of amenorrhea and oligomenorrhea and be made aware of the possibility of pregnancy, despite lack of menses. A preprinted list of adolescent clinics, counselors, and nutritionists or peer support groups should be available at all times and on completion of the PPE. In addition, names and phone numbers of physicians, health clinics, specialty clinics, and planned parenthood or family planning centers should be available and used appropriately for follow-up care.

CONCLUSION

Sports health care providers must take their responsibilities seriously. Whether in a private association, or school athletic setting, sports-specific appropriate medical screening and follow-up will decrease incidence of illness and injury. The ability to establish trust and communication, as well as consistency and follow-up, is an invaluable tool. Education and awareness of issues unique to female athletes are essential. It is anticipated that standards of screening in all athletic settings, such as the 1998 joint position statement by the American College of Sports Medicine and American Heart Association: Recommendations for Cardiovascular Screening, Staffing, and Emergency Policies at Health/Fitness Facilities,[4] should be implemented and used. As Dr. Cantwell describes: "Physicians always need to function in an atmosphere of uncertainty. We need to meet certain practice guidelines in the region where we work."[16(p S342)] Currently, there are not enough solid data to establish specific black-and-white guidelines. We can practice within our best limits of time, cost, knowledge, experience, and conscience. As research continues, and girls and women increase their participation in athletic activities, evaluation, treatment, and prevention will become more effective and focused, ultimately decreasing the amount of chronic health-impairing behaviors. Applying the knowledge gained in studying the elite athletic population to a broader fitness population will benefit women at all levels.

Exhibit 20–6 Useful Questions in Eliciting a History of an Eating Disorder

- What is the most you've ever weighed? When was that?
- What is the least you've ever weighed? When was that?
- What do you think you should weigh?
- Many women try different ways to control their weight. What have you tried?
- Have you ever had a binge, or "pig out?" What makes up a binge? How much, how often? What ends the binge? Any triggers that you can identify that lead to a binge?
- Have you ever made yourself vomit? How many times per day? Any relation to meals? How long has this occurred?
- Have you ever used laxatives, diuretics, diet pills, caffeine? (Ask each separately.) How much, how often, and what time frame?
- What do you do for exercise? How much, how often? How stressed do you feel if you miss a workout?
- Can you tell me what you ate in the past 24 hours? How many bites of _____?

REFERENCES

1. Peltz JE, Haskell W, Matheson GO. A comprehensive and cost-effective preparticipation exam implemented on the world wide web. *Med Sci Sports Exerc.* 1999;31:1727–1740.

2. American Academy of Family Physicians, American Academy of Pediatrics, American Medical Society for Sports Medicine, American Orthopaedic Society for Sports Medicine, American Osteopathic Academy of Sports Medicine. *Preparticipation Physical Evaluation.* 2nd ed. Minneapolis: The Physician and Sportsmedicine; 1997.

3. Tanner SM. Preparticipation examination targeted for the female athlete. *Clin Sports Med.* 1994;13:337–353.

4. American College of Sports Medicine. Joint position statement by the American College of Sports Medicine and American Heart Association: Recommendations for Cardiovascular Screening, Staffing, and Emergency Policies at Health/Fitness Facilities. *Med Sci Sports Exerc.* 1998;30:1009–1018.

5. Glover DW, Maron BJ, Matheson GO. The preparticipation physical examination: Steps toward consensus and uniformity. *Physician Sportsmed.* 1999;27:29–34.

6. American Heart Association. Cardiovascular preparticipation screening of competitive athletes (scientific statement). *Med Sci Sports Exerc.* 1996;28:1445–1452.

7. American Heart Association. Cardiovascular preparticipation screening of competitive athletes (scientific statement). *Circulation.* 1996;94:850–856.

8. Schon LC, Biddinger KR, Greenwood P. Dance screen programs and development of dance clinics. *Clin Sports Med.* 1994;13:865–882.

9. Myers A, Sickles T. Preparticipation sports examination. *Adolesc Med.* 1998;25:225–236.

10. Smith J, Wilder RP. Musculoskeletal rehabilitation and sports medicine. 4. Miscellaneous sports medicine topics. *Arch Phys Med Rehabil.* 1999;80:S68–89.

11. Carek PJ, Futrell M, Hueston WJ. The preparticipation physical examination history: Who has the correct answers? *Clin J Sport Med.* 1999;9:124–128.

12. Bergfeld JA, Martin MC, Shangold MM, Warren MP. Women in athletics: Five management problems. *Patient Care.* 1987;21:60–64.

13. Johnson MD. Preseason sports examination for women. In: Agostini R, Titus S, eds. *Medical and Orthopedic Issues of Active and Athletic Women.* Philadelphia: Hanley & Belfus; 1994:35–49.

14. Katz JL. Eating disorders. In: Shangold MM, Mirkin G. *Women and Exercise: Physiology and Sports Medicine.* 2nd ed. Philadelphia: FA Davis; 1994:292–312.

15. Gidwani GP, Rome ES. Eating disorders. *Clin Obstet Gynecol.* 1997;40:601–615.

16. Daluiski A, Rahbar B, Meals RA. Russell's sign: subtle hand changes in patients with bulimia nervosa. *Clin Orthop Rel Res.* 1997;343:107–109.

17. Cantwell JD. Preparticipation physical evaluation: Getting to the heart of the matter. *Med Sci Sports Exerc.* 1998;30:S341–S344.

18. Tanner SM. Preparticipation evaluation. In: Teitz C. *The Female Athlete.* Rosemont, IL: American Academy of Orthopedic Surgeons; 1997:1–23.

19. Smith J, Laskowski ER. The preparticipation physical examination: Mayo Clinic experience with 2,739 examinations. *Mayo Clin Proc.* 1998;73:419–429.

20. Snider RK, ed. Preparticipation athletic evaluation. In: *Essentials of Musculoskeletal Care.* Rosemont, IL: American Academy of Orthopaedic Surgeons Editorial Board; 1997:635–638.

21. MacAuley D. Does preseason screening for cardiac disease really work? The British perspective. *Med Sci Sports Exerc.* 1998;30:S345–S350.

22. Powell JW, Barber-Foss KD. Traumatic brain injury in high school athletes. *JAMA.* 1999;282:958–963.

23. Collins MW, Grindel SH, Lovell MR, et al. Relationship between concussion and neuropsychological performance in college football players. *JAMA.* 1999;282:964–970.

24. Foyster P. Heat and cold. In: Agostini R, Titus S, eds. *Medical and Orthopedic Issues of Active and Athletic Women.* Philadelphia: Hanley & Belfus; 1994:333–346.

25. Beerman G. Scuba diving and the marine environment. In: Agostini R, Titus S, eds. *Medical and Orthopedic Issues of Active and Athletic Women.* Philadelphia: Hanley & Belfus; 1994: 355–362.

26. Wilfley DE, Grilo CM. Brownell KD. Exercise and regulation of body weight. In: Shangold MM, Mirkin G. *Women and Exercise: Physiology and Sports Medicine.* 2nd ed. Philadelphia: FA Davis; 1994:27–54.

27. Chally PS. An eating disorders prevention program. *JCAPN.* 1998;11:51–60.

28. Lauder TD, Williams MV, Campbell CS, Davis GD, Sherman RA. Abnormal eating behaviors in military women. *Med Sci Sports Exerc.* 1999;31:1265–1271.

29. Olson MS, Williford HN, Richards LA, et al. Self-reports on the eating disorder inventory by female aerobic instructors. *Percept Motor Skills.* 1996;82:1051–1058.

30. O'Connor PJ, Lewis RD, Kirchner EM, Cook DB. Eating disorder symptoms in former female college gymnasts: Relations with body composition. *Am J Clin Nutr.* 1996;64:840–843.

31. Wade T, Tiggemann M, Martin N, Heath A. A comparison of the eating disorder examination and a general psychiatric schedule. *Aust N Z J Psychiatry.* 1997;31:852–857.

32. Schwitzer AM, Bergholz K, Dore T, Salimi L. Eating disorders among college women: Prevention, education, and treatment responses. *JACH.* 1998;46:199–207.

CHAPTER 21

Sports Nutrition

Marlisa Brown

Nutrition provides the fuel the body converts into the energy needed to sustain life. In sports medicine, medical nutrition therapy is used to help speed recovery and to increase performance by targeting intake to a specific health problem or goal. This chapter will outline the basics of nutrition to allow further understanding of sports nutrition in the female athlete.

ENERGY-PROVIDING NUTRIENTS

Carbohydrates

Carbohydrates supply 4 calories per gram. Carbohydrates are found in grains, fruits, and vegetables. Controversy exists as to the amount of carbohydrate a person may need, high carb, low carb, no carb. The truth is carbohydrates supply energy for the body's muscles, and under normal circumstances are the number one fuel source for the brain.[1] Also body tissues and red blood cells use almost all of their energy from glucose, the breakdown product of carbs.

Carbohydrate supplies energy for muscles and it is the No. 1 fuel source for the brain.

Clinical Guideline

Special thanks to Jodi Wright, RD, Catherine Brittan, MS, RD, CDN, and Jacqueline Guiterrez, MS, RD, CDN, for their support in the development of this chapter.

Stored carbohydrate is kept in the muscles and liver in the form of glycogen and is converted to glucose as needed. The stored glycogen makes up approximately 325 g in the muscles and 90 to 110 g in the liver.[2] Glycogen stored in muscle can be converted directly to energy for the muscle. Glycogen in the liver can be converted to glucose for the body when needed. The glycogen stored by the body supplies approximately 1500 to 2000 calories of energy (glycogen has 4 calories per gram). This amount of stored energy is approximately enough to power a 20-mile run. During a marathon, athletes speak of "hitting the wall"; this is when their glycogen stores have been exhausted.

Different types of simple or monosaccharide carbohydrates include glucose, fructose, and galactose. Disaccharides include sucrose, maltose, and lactose.

Sucrose = Glucose + Fructose
Maltose = Glucose + Glucose
Lactose = Glucose + Galactose

Simple carbohydrates (monosaccharides) do not need to be broken down, and they may cause a quicker increase in blood glucose levels than disaccharides. Usually, the more processed a food is, or the more broken down a food, the more simple sugars it contains. The more whole the food is the more complex. For example, apple juice is more simple than applesauce and applesauce is more simple than a whole apple; whole wheat bread is more complex than white bread. The easiest way to explain this is that if it is harder to chew the food, it is usually more complex.

Determining Carbohydrate Needs

Most athletes consume far too little carbohydrate.

Clinical Guideline

The carbohydrate content of one's diet should be 50% to 60% of the total calories daily.[3] If one was consuming a 2000 calorie diet and 50% of calories were coming from carbohydrates, that would be 1000 calories divided by 4 calories per gram, and that is 250 g of carbohydrate per day. The recommendations for carbohydrate intake for athletic women range from 50% to 70% of the diet. The one fact that seems to be consistent is that most athletes consume far too little carbohydrate than needed.[4–6]

Fiber

Fiber is the indigestible part of a plant. The American Dietetic Association (ADA) and the National Cancer Institute recommend a daily intake of 25 to 35 g, or 10 to 13 g/1000 calories.[7,8] Fiber has many functions within our body, some of which include stool bulk, softness, and transit time. Fiber when combined with high-carbohydrate foods may slow the rate at which carbohydrates are absorbed into the bloodstream.[3] Foods providing good sources of fiber include whole grains, especially bran, beans, whole fruits, and vegetables.

Protein

Protein is the building block for body tissues and body fluid status.

Clinical Guideline

Protein foods contain 4 calories per gram, and are needed to repair and build body tissues. Good sources of low-fat protein include lean meats, fish, poultry without skin, low-fat dairy, and beans. Nuts and seeds also contain protein, but they are higher in fat. Protein is essential in the production of enzymes, hormones, and other substances the body uses. Protein helps regulate water balance and helps make muscles contract. Amino acids are the building blocks of proteins. All proteins we eat are a combination of amino acids that our bodies break down and rebuild again into proteins. Twenty amino acids make up protein, nine of these are essential and must be supplied by consumption.

Determining Protein Needs

While athletes may have higher protein needs than the general population, protein needs are often not as high as expected.

Clinical Guideline

The Recommended Dietary Allowances (RDA) state that protein needs are 0.8 g/kg of body weight. Therefore, if a woman weighs 140 lb/2.2 kg = 63.64 kg × 0.8 g of protein, she requires 50.9 g of protein. If 5 ounces of protein in the form of meat, fish, poultry, beans, or cheese are consumed, the woman will get 35 g of protein. Add two servings of dairy for 16 g of protein and 4 servings of grains for 12 g protein. The total protein here is 63 g, with minimal servings of protein, dairy, and starch. This exceeds the 50.9 g recommended for her body weight.

The American Dietetic Association (ADA) states protein needs are 1 g/kg of body weight. Therefore, for the same 63.64-kg person the requirement would be 63.64 g of protein, which is the same amount calculated from the dietary intake previously.

Both these protein recommendations may be underestimated for athletes.[9–12] Some studies cite needs as high as 1.2 to 1.7 g/kg.[9,11] Endurance athletes may have to take in additional protein to help repair damaged muscle fibers. The total amount of protein is approximately 1.2 to 1.6 g/kg/day.[9] Body builders may benefit from up to 1.6 to 1.7 g/kg.[9] At 1.6 g/kg the same 140-pound woman would need 101.83 g of protein (63.64 kg × 1.6 g of protein = 101.83 g protein). By consuming 8 ounces of protein (56 g), three servings of dairy (24 g of protein), and seven servings of starch (21 g of protein), the total protein intake is 101 g. As can be seen even on the higher protein estimates of a medium-weight woman, it is not difficult at all to meet protein needs. Excess protein consumed beyond what the body needs will be stored as body fat.

Lipids or Fats

Fats contain 9 calories per gram. Foods that supply fats include butter, olive oil, other oils, cream, sour cream, cheese, red meat, and many other foods. Many foods contain hidden fats. The American Heart Association recommends that diets should have 30% or fewer of their calories coming from fat.[13] This means that on a 2000-calorie diet, less than 600 calories or 66.7 g of fat per day should be consumed. High-fat diets, especially those high in saturated fats, have been shown to increase the risk of many diseases, including high cholesterol, high triglycerides, diabetes, hypertension, and obesity.[13] Saturated fats are found in meats with a high fat content such as red meats and poultry skin; and high-fat dairy products like butter, cream, and whole milk. To reduce saturated fat intake low-fat dairy can be used, poultry skins can be removed, lean meats can be chosen, and vegetable oils can be substituted for high saturated fat choices like butter. One teaspoon of oil contains 45 to 50 calories and 5 grams of fat.

All fats are combinations of saturated, polyunsaturated, and monounsaturated fats. Some fats are higher in one type and hence their name. For example, olive and canola oils are higher in monounsaturated fatty acids; therefore they are called monounsaturated oils. Monounsaturated fats when substituted for saturated fats in a low-fat diet have been shown to lower total cholesterol without lowering high-density lipoprotein (HDL) cholesterol (known as the good cholesterol).[14]

Fat has many benefits that should not be overlooked. Fat provides energy; helps transport fat-soluble vitamins like A, D, K, and E; depress gastric secretions; and slow the emptying time of the stomach. They also help promote satiety.[3] Diets too low in fat can lead to an essential fatty acid deficiency and nutrient deficiencies.[15] Women athletes in a quest to keep thin may consume diets too low in fat. Long-term effects of these diets may not be totally understood as of yet. For these reasons the World Health Organization has set the lower limit for fat consumption at 15% of calories.[16] Excess calories of fat or any other kind are stored as body fat, and some body fat is needed for good health. Adipose or fat tissue helps hold the body organs and nerves in position, protects against traumatic injury, and shock. In addition it can insulate the body for better temperature regulation, and stored fat can be an excellent source of energy for athletes.[3]

Alcohol

Alcohol is not recommended for athletes.

Clinical Guideline

Alcohol provides 7 calories per gram consumed. Alcohol is not recommended for athletes because of its limited nutritional value and dehydrating effects. Many athletes believe that it reduces tension; therefore, they feel as if they are performing better.[17] However, McNaughton and Preece[18] found that alcohol did not act as an ergogenic acid, but rather adversely affected performance of runners. Alcohol also affects the body's ability to adapt to exercise in cold environments. Even moderate levels of blood alcohol can impair the thermoregulation of the body during exercise in cold temperatures.[19] In general, women have smaller body sizes and may not be able to tolerate alcohol as well as men.

ESTIMATING MACRONUTRIENT NEEDS

If a person has been maintaining his or her body weight without losing or gaining any weight, an analysis of his or her intake would determine total calorie needs. Adding or subtracting 500 calories per day should provide a 1-pound weight gain or loss per week. This type of adjustment is not recommended for those with eating disorders, because their obsession with calories and weight is part of their problem. The best way to calculate calories consumed is to feed a person in a closed environment and perform a computerized nutrient analysis on the basis of intake. Because it is rarely possible to feed a person in a controlled environment, a food record is another method for determining calories. A 3-day intake is preferred over a 1-day intake, because it better indicates a typical pattern. In a 3-day record there should be typical days in a row including 1 weekend day and 2 work days; again a computerized nutrient analysis would be used to determine calories consumed.

Depending on the activity, age, metabolism, and so forth, the amount of calories for two women of seemingly the same needs may be radically different. For the purpose of this text I will discuss two other popular methods for calculating calories.

Food records provide maximum clinical insight into nutrition needs and habits.

The Harris Benedict Method (1919)[20]

This method uses an equation to determine resting energy expenditure (REE) multiplied by an activity factor to give the total energy expenditure (TEE). It is often used in hospitals and nursing homes to determine the caloric needs of patients. Roza and Shizgal[21] revised the method in 1984.

The revised Harris Benedict equation for females is:

REE (kcal) = 447.6 + 9.2 (W) + 3.1 (H) − 4.3 (A) X activity factor

(Where W = weight in kg, H = height in cm, and A = age in years)

Activity factors:
1. Restricted: 1.0
2. Sedentary: 1.2
3. Aerobic (3X/week): 1.3
4. Aerobic (5X/week): 1.5
5. Aerobic (7X/week): 1.6
6. True athlete: 1.7

For instance let us look at a 25-year-old woman who weighs 140 pounds, is 5'7" tall, and is aerobically active 5 times per week:

Convert weight in pounds to weight in kilograms by dividing pounds by 2.2

140 lb/2.2 = 63.64 kg

Convert height in inches to height in cm by multiplying inches by 2.54

5'7" = 67 inches × 2.54 = 170 cm

REE = 447.6 + 9.2 (63.64) + 3.1 (170) − 4.3 (25)

REE = 1452.6 calories (kcal)

TEE = 1452.6 × 1.5

TEE = 2178.9 kcal

Therefore, this woman requires approximately 2200 calories to maintain her current weight.

The Total Energy Expenditure (TEE) Rule of Thumb Method[22]

This method assumes that a certain number of calories are expended per kilogram of body weight. The body weight in kilograms is multiplied by a number of calories on the basis of the activity and weight status of the individual.

	Sedentary	Moderate	Active
Overweight	20–25 kcal/kg	30 kcal/kg	35 kcal/kg
Normal weight	30 kcal/kg	35 kcal/kg	40 kcal/kg
Underweight	30 kcal/kg	40 kcal/kg	45–50 kcal/kg

Let us take the same 25-year-old woman as in the Harris Benedict example. She weighs 140 pounds and is moderately active (aerobic 5 times per week).

Convert weight in pounds to weight in kilograms by dividing pounds by 2.2

140 lb/2.2 = 63.64 kg

TEE = 63.64 × 35 kcal/kg

TEE = 2227.4

As can be seen, the calculations are about the same. She would require approximately 2200 calories a day to maintain her weight.

FLUIDS AND ELECTROLYTES

Water

Cold beverages are absorbed faster.

Clinical Guideline

Water is essential in any sports activity or physical exertion. Water is located everywhere within our bodies, and it is essential in many body functions, these including transporting nutrients and waste products to and from the cells through the bloodstream. Water is essential for adequate blood volume. Water helps cool the body and is essential

in virtually every body system. To quicken absorption time, cold drinks pass faster into the intestinal track.[23–24]

For every pound of body weight lost after an event, it is important to drink 16 ounces of fluid. It is important not to rely on thirst alone.

Clinical Guideline

How Much Fluid Is Needed

A 150-pound athlete could lose as much as 1½ quarts of fluid in an hour. To try to maintain fluid balance the following fluid recommendations are made.[25]

1. 2 cups of fluid 2 to 2½ hours before event.
2. 2 additional cups of fluid 15 minutes before a workout.
3. ½ to 1 cup of fluid every 14 to 20 minutes during an event.
4. After the event, drink 2 cups of fluid for every pound lost.
5. Continue to consume fluids throughout the day.

Dehydration

Dehydration, even in its mildest sense, would have an effect on the body. Some of the symptoms of dehydration include dark or strong-smelling urine, headache, muscle aches, and dry skin. Another symptom of dehydration is body weight loss. Dehydration of as little as 2% loss of body weight may result in impaired physiological and performance responses.[26] This means that in a woman who weighs 140 pounds, dehydration with consequences occurs with a 2- to 3-pound weight loss. For each pound of weight lost, two 8-ounce cups of fluid have been lost. Therefore, athletes should regularly weigh themselves before and after exercise to make sure they have replenished the fluids lost during exercise. The athlete should not depend on thirst to know when to consume fluids. By the time they feel thirsty, they may already be dehydrated. The reason for this is that a loss of 1½ to 2 liters of fluid is needed before the thirst mechanism kicks in. However, a loss of this magnitude will already have an impact on the body's ability to regulate temperature. The loss of water by the body leads to greater heat storage, causing a reduced sweat rate and skin blood flow. This causes the body's core temperature to rise. The athlete may also have a reduced ability to tolerate heat strain.[27] Exhaustion may coincide with high body temperature.[28]

In most cases, water is the preferred beverage of choice.

Clinical Guideline

Besides affecting the body's ability to regulate temperature, dehydration can also affect performance. If the athlete is dehydrated before exercise (hypohydration), aerobic endurance performance is reduced. Hypohydration results in a reduced blood volume, particularly if diuretics or sauna exposure induces it. Dehydration that occurs as a result of exercise increases body temperature, heart rate, and perceived exertion. Therefore, it reduces the aerobic performance of the athlete. These effects also seem to be related to a reduced blood volume.[29] Reduced blood volume concentrates the blood and may lead to increased cholesterol, triglycerides, blood glucose, and blood pressure. The reduction of blood volume reduces the muscle blood flow as well. Therefore, the athlete may fatigue more quickly because of increased carbohydrate oxidation and lactate production.[28] This means that the body is depending more on carbohydrate for fuel rather than fat because the blood cannot supply enough oxygen to the muscle. The use of fat as a fuel in exercise requires a large volume of oxygen. As carbohydrate is used, the body produces the acid lactate. This causes the burning feeling in muscle that makes the exercise stop.

Heat Stroke

Heat stroke is a medical emergency that occurs when the body's core temperature rises too high. It is the failure of the body to regulate heat brought on by excessively high body temperature. This can occur as a result of dehydration. When the thermoregulation of the body fails, sweating usually ceases, the skin becomes dry and hot, body temperature rises to approximately 106°F or higher, and the circulatory system is strained. If left untreated, the individual will die because of the collapse of the circulatory system and damage to the central nervous system. Symptoms may be subtle. Steps to reduce body temperature include alcohol rubs, application of ice packs, and/or whole body immersion in cold water.

When Water Alone Is Not the Best Choice: Hyponatremia

When sodium and glucose are available in fluids, it greatly enhances absorption.[23,30] The amount of carbohydrate needed is about 30 to 70 g/h, which is approximately a ½ to 1 cup of an 8% carbohydrate solution every 15 to 20 minutes.[31] The carbohydrate concentration needs to be at 6% to 8% to enter the bloodstream at a similar rate as water. The carbohydrate content may lead to improved performance. Less than 5% carbohydrate may not be adequate for in-creased performance and greater than 10% carbohydrate may lead to diarrhea, nausea, and cramps.[32] To determine the percentage of carbohydrate in a sports drink, divide the carbohydrate grams by the serving size amount (in milliliters) and then multiply by 100. For example, if the drink has 14 g of carbohydrate in an 8-ounce serving (240 mL), it is 5.8% carbohydrate.

$$[14 \text{ g}/240 \text{ mL}] \times 100 = 5.8\%$$

Carbohydrate taken during performance of events longer than 1 hour may offer an energy advantage compared with water alone.[33] In certain conditions excessive fluid intake in the form of plain water may be a problem. It may result in hyponatremia or "water intoxication," considered to exist when serum sodium levels drop below 136 mEq/L^{-1}. It occurs when large amounts of sodium are lost through prolonged sweating coupled with the dilution of existing extracellular sodium through fluid ingestion of water alone.[34] Sweat losses that may cause extreme sodium losses are often seen in hot and humid weather conditions.

Factors that Augment Hyponatremia

- Prolonged high-intensity exercise in hot weather.
- Poor fitness level associated with sweat production containing high sodium concentrations.
- Beginning physical activity in a sodium-depleted state because of a salt-free or low-sodium diet or use of a diuretics.
- Frequent and prolonged ingestion of sodium-free fluid during periods of excessive fluid loss.

Clinical Guideline

Hyponatremia is characterized by symptoms such as headache, confusion, malaise, nausea, cramping, and in severe cases seizures, coma, pulmonary edema, and possibly death. To prevent hyponatremia, include sodium and glucose in the rehydration drink, if exercise lasts longer than 1 hour or during extremely hot or humid days. This drink would facilitate the intestinal water uptake by means of the glucose sodium transport mechanism.

Electrolytes

Electrolytes are minerals that dissolve in the body as electrically charged particles called ions. The minerals that are considered to be electrolytes are sodium, potassium, and chloride. During exercise, these minerals are lost in sweat. If the loss is extreme, it may lead to impairment of nerve conduction to muscle fibers (including those of the heart). However, it is generally not necessary to supplement electrolytes unless exercise is intense and of long duration. For a fluid loss of less than 6 pounds of body weight, electrolytes are readily replenished by adding a slight amount of salt to food. A small amount of salt may be beneficial in that it may enhance the absorption of water by the body. Most sports drinks contain a small amount of salt.[1]

MICRONUTRIENTS AND SUPPLEMENTS

NOTE: Most women have calorie intakes that are not high enough to provide some of the needed nutrients.

Clinical Guideline

The energy intake of most female athletes may be insufficient to support estimated requirements of nutrients.[4,35] As a result, intakes of iron, calcium, vitamin B_{12}, zinc, magnesium, folate, vitamin B_6, and vitamin E may be lower than the recommended dietary allowances.[4,36–40] There may also be an increased need of nutrients such as B_{12} and iron. The metabolism of vitamin B_{12} may be altered in ultraendurance runners.[41] Iron loss in sweat may contribute to the iron deficiency seen in some endurance runners.[42] Therefore, it is important for the female athlete to be counseled on eating a balanced diet that supplies the recommended dietary allowances. Recently, the national research counsel released reports on Dietary Reference Intakes (DRI), which are intended to update and expand the RDAs. The DRIs are different from the RDAs in that they focus more on benefits of healthy eating rather than preventing deficiency. The DRIs include four categories of reference intakes. These are the RDA, Adequate Intakes (AI), Established Average Requirement, and Tolerable Upper Intake Levels.

The RDAs are the intakes that meet the nutrient needs of almost all healthy individuals in a specific age and gender group. It is used to guide individuals to achieve adequate nutrient intake to decrease the risk of chronic disease. The AIs are estimated average requirements that are set when an RDA cannot be determined. The Estimated Average Requirement is the intake that meets the established nutritional need of half the individuals in a specific group. The Tolerable Upper Intake Level is the maximum intake by an individual that is unlikely to pose risks of adverse health effects in almost all healthy individuals.[43–44] Table 21–1 gives the RDAs or AIs of the needs for females from the ages 4 to 70. The chart also includes in the requirements for pregnant and lactating females.

The best method to ensure adequate intake of nutrients is to eat a balanced diet. One reason for this is that vitamins synthesized in a laboratory are no better than vitamins found naturally in food. The one exception to this is folate. The supplemental form of folate found in fortified foods and in supplements is a form that is better absorbed by the body.[45]

When a diet is deficient, vitamin supplements may improve performance; however, it is unlikely that vitamin supplements will improve performance when the diet is adequate.[37] Generally, athletes or anyone who supplements vitamins should do so with caution, because there are no regulations on how supplements are prepared. Also, vitamins may be taken in levels that are toxic. This generally does not occur when taken in food form. Rather, toxicity can occur when it is supplemented in their diet. This is one reason why the new DRIs include the tolerable upper intake level.[44] Caution should be taken when supplements containing fat-soluble vitamins are being taken. These fat-soluble vitamins (A, D, E, and K) are stored in the liver and may build up to toxic levels if taken in amounts much greater than the RDAs or AIs. Other supplements may cause problems as well.

Iron

At times supplements may be beneficial to an athlete, particularly if the woman is deficient. Iron deficiency has been shown to lower V_{O_2}max (maximum oxygen uptake) and endurance in rats.[46] A similar finding in male athletes was discovered by Celsing et al.[47] When the anemic male athletes had their hemoglobin return to normal through blood transfusions, there was an increase in V_{O_2}max and endurance. These studies imply that if a person is deficient in iron, the ability to use oxygen and perform exercise for long bouts is diminished. By correcting the deficiency, the athlete will have improvement in oxygen uptake and endurance. All women are at risk of iron deficiency because of their menstrual cycle; add in the intensive exercise an athlete performs and the risk increases. Iron deficiency may be prevented if all athletes with low serum ferritin levels are given controlled iron supplements, as long as the iron deficiency is not due to a disease state.[48]

Calcium

Other beneficial supplements are those that improve the athlete's bone strength. This is particularly important in female athletes that are amenorrheic. These athletes should be encouraged to consume adequate amounts of calcium (usually deficient in female athletes), vitamin D, vitamin K, and phosphorus. Calcium is essential for bone strength. Vitamin D is needed for the body to use calcium. Vitamin K has been found to help calcium-binding capacity in low-estrogen female athletes.[49] Phosphorous is much like calcium in that it is essential for bone strength. These nutrients are best taken in food form. The most abundant sources of calcium are dairy products. It is also found in green leafy vegetables, tofu, canned fish with bones, and fortified beverages like orange juice. Vitamin D is found in milk, egg yolk, salmon, tuna, and sardines. It is also produced in the skin when the

Table 21–1 Daily Reference Intakes: Recommended Dietary Intakes and Adequate Intakes* for Females

Females by Age	Fat-Soluble Vitamins					Water-Soluble Vitamins								Minerals					
	Vit. A	Vit. D*	Vit. E	Vit. K	Vit. C^	Thiamin	Riboflavin	Niacin	Vit. B6	Folate	Vit. B12	Panthothenic acid*	Biotin*	Calcium	Phosphorus	Magnesium	Iron	Zinc	Iodine
Unit	RE	µg	mg	µg	mg	mg	mg	mg	mg	µg	µg	mg	µg	mg	mg	mg	mg	mg	µg
4–8	500	5	7	30	45	0.6	0.6	8	0.6	200	1.2	3	12	800	500	130	10	10	90
9–13	800	5	11	45	50	0.9	0.9	12	1.0	300	1.8	4	20	1300	1250	240	15	12	150
14–18	800	5	15	55	60	1.0	1.0	14	1.2	400†	2.4	5	25	1300	1250	360	15	12	150
19–30	800	5	15	60	75	1.1	1.1	14	1.3	400†	2.4	5	30	1000	700	310	15	12	150
31–50	800	5	15	65	75	1.1	1.1	14	1.3	400†	2.4	5	30	1000	700	320	15	12	150
51–70	800	10	15	65	75	1.1	1.1	14	1.5	400†	2.4‡	5	30	1200	700	320	10	12	150
>70	800	15	15	65	75	1.1	1.1	14	1.5	400	2.4‡	5	30	1200	700	320			
Pregnant <19	800	5	15	65	80	1.4	1.4	18	1.9	600§	2.6	6	30	1300	1250	400	30	15	175
19–30	800	5	15	65	85	1.4	1.4	18	1.9	600§	2.6	6	30	1000	700	350	30	15	175
31–50	800	5	15	65	85	1.4	1.4	18	1.9	600§	2.6	6	30	1000	700	360	30	15	175
Lactating <19	1300	5	19	65	115	1.5	1.6	17	2.0	500	2.8	7	35	1300	1250	360	15	19	200
19–30	1300	5	19	65	120	1.5	1.6	17	2.0	500	2.8	7	35	1000	700	310	15	19	200
31–50	1300	5	19	65	120	1.5	1.6	17	2.0	500	2.8	7	35	1000	700	320	15	19	200

*Note: This table presents the Recommended Dietary Allowances (RDAs) and the Adequate Intakes (AIs) followed by an asterisk. The RDAs and the AIs may both be used as goals for individual intake.

^Smokers should increase intake of Vitamin C by 35 mg/day.

†It is recommended that all women capable of becoming pregnant consume 400 µg of synthetic folic acid from fortified foods and/or supplements in addition to intake from food folate from a varied diet.

§It is assumed that women will continue taking 400 µg of folic acid until their pregnancy is confirmed and they enter prenatal care.

‡Since 10% to 30% of older people may malabsorb food-bound B12 it is advisable for those older than 50 years to meet their RDA mainly by taking foods fortified with B12 or a B12 containing supplement.

skin is exposed to sunlight. Vitamin K is found in oils, wheat bran, and green leafy vegetables. Phosphorus is found in milk, meat, poultry, and fish.

Carbohydrate Loading

Supplementation by athletes also occurs in other ways; for instance, some athletes use foods to help improve athletic performance. One such practice is carbohydrate loading used by endurance athletes to enhance glycogen stores to maintain high-intensity exercise. (Without glycogen, the athlete must either stop the exercise or reduce the pace drastically.) Carbohydrate loading is not necessary for exercise that lasts less than 1 hour, because carbohydrate intake and glycogen stores are generally considered adequate for this amount of exercise.[50] The plan for increasing muscle glycogen stores is done in two steps, depletion and loading. It is started approximately 1 week before competition.[1]

Plan for Carbohydrate Loading

1. Depletion
   a. Day 1: Exhaustive exercise performed to deplete muscle glycogen in specific muscles that are being used in competition (i.e., runners must deplete stores by running).
   b. Days 2, 3, and 4: Low-carbohydrate food intake (high percentages of protein and lipid in the diet).
2. Carbohydrate loading
   a. Days 5, 6, and 7: High-carbohydrate food intake/ normal percentage of protein in the daily diet, while slowly decreasing exercise intensity and duration.
   b. Competition day: Follow high-carbohydrate pre-competition meal.

Clinical Guideline

Some characteristics should be considered before attempting this procedure. For instance, this is inappropriate for athletes with diabetes, renal disorders, or heart disease, because all of these diseases cannot handle major modification in macronutrients. Another consideration is that water is bound to glycogen (2.7 g/1 g muscle glycogen).[1] This means that the athlete may feel "heavy" and uncomfortable. The water may act as a benefit later in the exercise, because the body releases it during glycogen breakdown. For temperature regulation the body can then use this freed water. Carbohydrate loading may only be effective in exercise bouts that are intense and prolonged. The last thing to consider about carbohydrate loading is that it may only benefit athletes who regularly train in endurance sports. It is this author's clinical opinion that it is better to just maintain a regular diet high in complex carbohydrates to achieve maximal performance.

Other "Performance" Supplements

Athletes often use other supplements to improve performance such as branched-chain amino acids (BCAA), medium-chain triglyceride (MCT) oil, creatine, carnitine, and caffeine. However, it seems that there is no special food that will allow athletes to perform better.[51] Davis et al.[52] recently found that there was no benefit to the addition of BCAA on high-intensity endurance running. In 1998, Jeukendrup et al.[53] found that ingesting MCT oil may provoke gastrointestinal problems that would then lead to decreased exercise performances. In 1999, Rauch et al.[54] compared the use of a mixed sports bar (7 g fat, 14 g protein, and 19 g carbohydrates) with just a carbohydrate supplement with the same calorie content to see whether it would improve ultraendurance cycling performance. They found that the ingestion of the sports bar enhanced fat metabolism but impaired the subsequent high- intensity time trial performance of the cyclists. In general, there are thousands of supplements on the market. Some of them help, some hurt, and some do nothing.

PRECOMPETITION MEALS

It is better not to eat high-fat foods before a workout.

Clinical Guideline

Eating the proper pre-event meal can provide needed nutrients to get one through the event with the energy needed. Because fat slows gastric emptying and may keep food in the stomach longer, it is best not to have a lot of fatty foods before an event. Timing is also important for larger meals. Larger meals should be eaten 3 to 4 hours before an event to allow for absorption. Smaller meals, 1 to 2 hours before an event are better tolerated. They allow for better digestion, provide for additional muscle glycogen, increased blood sugar, and better gastric emptying.[2] Before long-term aerobic events, an additional 50 to 100 g of carbohydrate up to 1 hour before the event may be helpful.[55] Consuming a meal that has a moderate glycemic index and is also high in fiber 45 minutes before a long exercise bout may increase exercise capacity.[56] Studies are controversial, however. In one study, the ingestion of 40 g of carbohydrate, 30 minutes before cycling did not improve workout intensity.

Glycemic index is an index that measures the amount of glucose that appears in the blood after the consumption of a food compared with that of sugar. Many things such as fiber content, digestion rate, and fat content can affect the glycemic index of a food.[58] Therefore, a food with a high glycemic index such as potatoes may cause a more rapid increase in blood glucose compared with a food with a low glycemic index. In comparison, a food with a low glycemic index such as milk will cause a slow rise in blood glucose. Foods are divided into those that have a high glycemic index (glucose, bread, potatoes, breakfast cereal, sports drinks), a moderate glycemic index (sucrose, soft drinks, oats, tropical fruits such as bananas and mangos), or a low glycemic index (fructose, milk, yogurt, lentils, pasta, and fruits such as apples and oranges).

Large pre-event meals should be taken 3 to 4 hours before an event; small meals 1 to 2 hours before an event are better.

Clinical Guideline

Athletes must heed caution with experimental foods. Many times, to gain the edge, athletes have experimented right before a big event with horrible results. Advise athletes to experiment only during practices.

Be careful with trying new foods before an event. Stick with foods that you know agree with you.

Clinical Guideline

Possible Preworkout Meals

1. Pasta (red sauce) with chicken and vegetables
2. Roast beef with baked potato and veggies
3. Macaroni and low-fat cheese
4. Cereal with skim milk
5. Bagel with low-fat cheese

These are just some suggestions and by all means not a complete list. Note that all choices above are low in fat, high in carbohydrates, and moderate in protein.

Clinical Guideline

INTAKE DURING EXERCISE

Endurance athletes may need to consume additional calories during an event to maintain energy levels. Foods that are consumed during an event must be easy to hold, temperature stable, easy to eat, and provide adequate amounts of calories for limited intake.

Foods that May Be Eaten during an Event

- Food and energy bars
- Food gels
- Some shakes and sports drinks

Clinical Guideline

POSTCOMPETITION MEALS

After an event, it is important to replace calories, fluids, electrolytes, and carbohydrates lost during the competition. Timing is everything, because replacing carbohydrates immediately after exercise provides better absorption. Consuming carbohydrate-rich food immediately after exercising helps speed replenishment.[59]

It is important to try to replace carbohydrates and fluids lost during an event as soon as possible.

Clinical Guideline

The amount of needed carbohydrate consumed will vary according to the intensity and length of time of the workout and the size of the athlete. In general, the amount of carbohydrate-rich foods should be between 50 and 100 g, within a 2-hour period after the event or workout session; this leads to the greatest glycogen synthesis (the storage of carbohydrate in the liver for future needs). Repeat as needed in 2-hour intervals.[60]

Foods Containing Approximately 50 g of Carbohydrate:

- 1 large bagel
- 12 oz of juice
- 2 large bananas
- 2 English muffins
- 2 large baked potatoes
- 1 cup of baked beans
- 2 fruit yogurts

Clinical Guideline

FAD DIETS

Fad diets have been around for many years. These diets may be poor for many reasons but mainly because they promote failure. Fad diets do not work. They are not designed for permanent weight loss. Types of recent fads diets will be discussed.

Warning Signs of Fad Diets

- Promise of a quick weight loss. This is usually caused by water loss that occurs with the loss of glycogen, lean muscle mass, or sodium.
- Rituals or prohibitions of entire food groups such as eat only fruit for breakfast or cut out all starchy carbohydrates. This results in nutritional deficiency.
- They are often billed as cure-alls.
- They do not support long-term lifestyle changes. Many people go back to their old habits and regain the weight.

Clinical Guideline

Low-Carbohydrate Diets

Low-carbohydrate diets cause the liver to perform gluconeogenesis (the production of glucose from carbon). The carbon comes mainly from the breakdown of lean protein containing body mass. Because protein tissue holds water, when the body releases protein, it also releases water, causing a rapid weight loss. In this process the body also uses fatty acids. When fatty acids are used in this manner, ketone bodies are formed.[57] Therefore, another name for this type of diet is ketogenic. Ketones are acid bodies that can cause bad breath, high blood acid, and kidney problems. Other possible problems include poor absorption of calcium and phosphorus and a slowed metabolism because of the loss of lean muscle mass.

A few examples of the ketogenic diet are the Atkin's New Revolution, the Zone, and the Scarsdale diet. In 1984, before the Zone diet, Porcello[61] found that ketogenic diets were inappropriate for athletes because of problems that can occur with the resulting dehydration and hyponatremia. The Zone diet is the latest to join the ranks. It promises a change in the body's insulin/glucagon ratio through the alteration of macronutrients in a 40% protein/30% carbs/30% fats division. This diet is likely to affect the ratio of pancreatic hormone release. In a review of literature on this theory, it was found that little human evidence exists to support the theory and that the Zone diet may be more ergolytic than ergogenic to athletes.[62]

Low-Fat Diets

The very low-fat diets are very high-carbohydrate diets. They allow only 5% to 10% of the calories to come from fat. This type of diet is really not too dangerous although individuals on these diets may not get enough of the essential fatty acids needed from their diet. (See the section on "Lipids or Fats.") This type of diet is difficult to follow, because it is mainly grains, fruits, and vegetables with very little meat, poultry, fish, dairy, or fat. An example of this diet is the Pritikin diet.

Novelty Diets

This category includes diets like the grapefruit diet or the cabbage soup diet. The theory behind many of these diets is that after eating one food for so long, dieters will become bored and in theory reduce calorie intake. The major risk with this type of diet is nutritional deficiency. Novelty diets also have high drop out rates.

Generally speaking, fad diets are not good because they are hypocaloric (low in calories). These cannot meet the training needs of the athlete. They will promote loss of lean muscle mass and carbohydrate stores.[61] The best method for weight loss is to follow sound nutrition and participate in regular physical activity.

OBESITY

Greater that 120% of ideal body weight is considered clinically obese. It is important, however, when determining appropriate body size to not just look at a chart but to consider many factors.

Factors To Consider in Assessing Obesity

- Obesity in a family
- Bone structure
- Muscle tone
- How the weight is distributed
- Body goals for the specific activity

Clinical Guideline

Obesity can help lead to many health problems, including hypertension, cardiovascular disease, diabetes, and some types of cancer. It is difficult to sometimes address why some people are obese and others are not; it is not always as clear as how much someone is eating. Some individuals have metabolisms that are much slower than others. Some recent research has found that in some individuals obesity may be related to a malfunctioning gene. This gene causes the release of a hormone leptin to the hypothalamus that tells the brain how much fat tissue the body has. The brain then releases other hormones to regulate metabolism. If leptin is not released or the brain is insensitive to it, the body thinks that there is not enough fat storage. Therefore, the brain slows down metabolism, and fat is stored more easily.[63]

Certainly there are athletic women who consumed far less than nonathletic women the same age and weight who gained weight at an unusually fast pace compared with others. It is excess calories that will produce weight gain, but the excess does not necessarily mean overeating. Excess calories more than you burn will increase your body weight 1 pound for every 3500 calories no matter what the source.

Treatment should include thorough medical work-up including thyroid studies. Nutrition expertise with a registered dietitian is essential.

Managing Weight Loss

- Evaluate calorie intake.
- Evaluate amount of protein, fat, carbohydrate, and fluids consumed.
- Rework meal plan based on assessment.
- Find a way of documenting and evaluating intake.
- Set a realistic weight goal. Some individuals may never be "thin" or a weight that is considered "normal" for their height.
- Provide a supportive environment. If the individual feels out of control, she may need psychological assistance.
- Never criticize or make the woman feel uncomfortable about her weight or any setbacks.

Clinical Guideline

EATING DISORDERS

There are different types of eating disorders. Anorexia nervosa is characterized by a refusal to maintain body weight at or greater than a minimally normal weight for age and height. Individuals with anorexia nervosa often have an intense fear of fatness and a distorted body image. Bulimia nervosa is characterized by binge eating and purging. These individuals may also have a distorted body image. Anorexia and bulimia are driven by an intense fear of gaining weight. Weight loss in these individuals is accomplished by reducing calorie intake and extensive or compulsive exercise.

Generally, the problem with eating disorders in the athletic population is that they are not consuming the adequate amount of calories. This has several effects on the body. Not only does metabolism slow down in response to starvation, nutritional deficiencies may develop. Most serious is consequences of insufficient calorie intake is the Female Athlete Triad: the female athlete may stop menstruating because of the decrease in fat tissue in the body. In response the body does not produce enough estrogen. When this occurs, there is early bone loss. This may lead to an increased risk of stress fractures.[64] (Refer to Chapters 18 and 19). These problems may seem slight; however, the individual with an eating disorder is at great risk for serious medical problems, some of which are fatal. Mortality rates have been reported between 1% and 18%.[65] The major cause of death in individuals with eating disorders is attributed to water and electrolyte abnormalities.[66]

All individuals working with physically active women should be educated about eating disorders and should develop strategies for preventing, identifying, and treating the problem.[67] It is important to keep in mind that eating disorders are complex diseases and that treating them requires a team of health professionals. The team should include a physician, a psychologist, and a registered dietitian. These diseases should not be dealt with by individuals who have little experience in the complexities of the disease. By no means should just one individual deal with them.

TEEN YEARS

Teens often have low intake of some nutrients as a result of high intake of fast foods and changes in lifestyle and eating behavior. Many teens have been shown to have low intakes of iron, calcium, riboflavin, and vitamin A.[68] Some adolescents skip meals, eat at fast food restaurants, and may use drugs, all of which contribute to decreased nutrient intake and absorption. The most important nutritional aspect when working with teenage girls is to emphasize the importance of getting enough calcium. These years are optimal for peak bone development. They should be encouraged to get at least three to four servings of dairy products a day to help achieve this goal. Iron is also of concern. Counseling these girls on how to obtain the optimal amount of iron in their diet is also importantant. This can be achieved by explaining which foods contain the most available iron such as meat, poultry, and fish.

PREGNANCY

Women planning a pregnancy may want to consult with their OB/GYN before conception to start taking prenatal vitamins. Many women do not know they have conceived until a month or more into their pregnancy, and certain nutrient needs are essential at this time. Supplementation of 400 µg of folic acid per day before and during early pregnancy has been show to radically reduce the incidence of neural tube defects.[45,69]

During pregnancy calorie needs are increased to meet the metabolic demands of the pregnancy and fetal growth. The 1989 RDA recommends an additional intake of 300 calories per day.[70] The intake of these extra calories should be added only in the second and third trimesters, unless the body reserves are depleted at the onset of pregnancy. With the pregnant athlete, it is important to advise about the adequate intake of energy, because excessive exercise and inappropriate intake could lead to suboptimal maternal weight gain and poor fetal growth.[71] The pregnant athlete should be advised to eat enough to satisfy physiological appetite and support appropriate weight gain.

Additional energy needs may be met by consuming four dairy servings a day. The daily consumption of whole grain breads and cereals, leafy green and yellow vegetables, and fresh and dried fruits should be encouraged to provide the additional minerals, vitamins, and fiber needed at this time. Water is very important during pregnancy to prevent constipation. Women should be counseled on getting at least six to eight 8-ounce glasses of water a day.

MENOPAUSE

Menopause is a time in a woman's life when the reproductive hormones decrease. This leads to the loss of bone. Exercise helps women slow bone loss associated with this time in life. At this time, the recommendation is for postmenopausal women to get adequate calcium and vitamin D. These women should also engage in weight-bearing exercise.

Another issue with older women is the absorption of vitamin B_{12}. Many people have problems absorbing vitamin B_{12} later in life. The recommendation is for individuals older than 50 years of age to meet the RDA for vitamin B_{12} by eating foods fortified or by taking a supplement of vitamin B_{12}.

HEALTHY SNACKING

Healthy snacking is important in any athlete's meal plan. Often hectic schedules provide little time for balanced meals, and snacking can help provide good dietary intake. Also, snacking can help prevent cravings that sometimes lead us to overeat.

Small frequent meals provide fuel throughout the day and do not overwork the digestive system, enabling the body to maintain normal blood glucose levels without peaks. A balanced snack high in complex carbohydrates, moderate in protein, and low in fat with a good source of dietary fiber is optimal for a balanced diet. Some recommendations for good snacks include:

Healthy Snacks

- Cereal with skim milk
- Pumpernickel bagel with low-fat cheese and tomato
- Whole grain bread with turkey, grilled chicken, or roast beef
- Whole grain pita with mixed veggies, tuna, and light mayonnaise

Clinical Guideline

SPECIAL NEEDS AND WHERE TO GET HELP

If a woman athlete is experiencing any problems with her weight, gastrointestinal function, blood pressure, cholesterol, triglycerides, anemia, calcium intake, performance, energy level, skin, or menstruation cycle, a thorough history and physical examination including blood work is recommended. After the evaluation, the patient should be referred to a registered dietitian with copies of any relevant medical information. Refer to Appendix 21–A for dietetic resources and support with nutritional concerns.

REFERENCES

1. McArdle WD, Katch FI, Katch VL. *Exercise Physiology: Energy, Nutrition, and Human Performance.* 4th ed. Baltimore: Williams & Wilkins; 1996:5–33, 472.

2. Felig P, Wahrin J. Fuel homeostasis in exercise. *N Engl J Med.* 1975;293:1078–1084.

3. Mahan KL, Escott-Stump S. *Krause's Food, Nutrition, and Diet Therapy.* 9th ed. Philadelphia: WB Saunders; 1996:54, 403–423, 502, 692.

4. Hawley JA, Dennis SC, Lindsay FH, Noakes TD. Nutritional practices of athletes: are they sub-optimal? *J Sports Sci.* 1995;13:S75–S81.

5. van Erp-Baart AM, Saris WH, Binkhorst RA, Vos JA, Elvers JW. Nationwide survey on nutritional habits in elite athletes, Part I: energy, carbohydrate, protein, and fat intake. *Int J Sports Med.* 1989;10(Suppl 1):S3–S10.

6. Neiman DC, Butler JV, Pollett LM, Dietrich SJ, Lutz RD. Nutrient intake of marathon runners. *J Am Diet Assoc.* 1989;89:1273–1278.

7. Slavin JL. Implementation of dietary modifications. *Am J Med.* 1999;106:46S–49S.

8. Warber J, Haddad E, Hodgkin G, Lee J. Dietary fiber content of a six-day weighed military ration. *Milit Med.* 1995;160:438–442.

9. Lemon PW. Effects of exercise on dietary protein requirements. *Int J Sport Nutr.* 1998;8:426–447.

10. Phillips SM, Atkinson SA, Tarnopolsky MA, MacDougall JD. Gender differences in leucine kinetics and nitrogen balance in endurance athletes. *J Appl Physiol.* 1993;75:2134–2141.

11. Tarnopolsky MA, Atkinson SA, MacDougall JD, Chesley A, Phillips S, Schwarcz HP. Evaluation of protein requirements for trained strength athletes. *J Appl Physiol.* 1992;73:1986–1995.

12. Meredith CN, Zackin MJ, Frontera WR, Evans WJ. Dietary protein requirements and body protein metabolism in endurance-trained men. *J Appl Physiol.* 1989;66:2850–2856.

13. American Heart Association. Dietary guidelines for healthy American adults: a statement for physicians and health professionals by the Nutrition Committee. *Circulation.* 1988;7:721A–724A.

14. Ginsberg HN, Barr SL, Gilbert A, et al. Reduction of plasma cholesterol levels in normal men on an American Heart Association Step I diet

or a Step II diet with added monounsaturated fat. *N Engl J Med.* 1990;322:574–579.

15. Schaefer EJ, Lichtenstein AH, Lamon-Fava S, et al. Body weight and low-density lipoprotein cholesterol changes after consumption of a low-fat ad-libitum diet. *JAMA.* 1995;274:1450–1455.

16. Food and Agriculture Organization. *Fats and Oils in Human Nutrition: Report of a Joint Expert Consultation* (WHO/FAO). 1994. FAO Paper 57.

17. Houmard JA, Langenfeld ME, Wiley RL, Siefert J. Effects of the acute ingestion of small amounts of alcohol upon 5-mile run times. *J Sports Med Phys Fitness.* 1987;27:253–257.

18. McNaughton L, Preece D. Alcohol and its effects on sprint and middle distance running. *Br J Sports Med.* 1986;20:56–59.

19. Graham T. Alcohol ingestion and man's ability to adapt to exercise in a cold environment. *Can J Appl Sport Sci.* 1981;6:27–31.

20. Harris JA, Benedict FG. *A Biometric Study of Basal Metabolism in Man.* Publication No. 279. Washington DC: Carnegie Institute of Washington; 1919.

21. Roza AM, Shizgal HM. The Harris Benedict equation reevaluated. *Am J Clin Nutr.* 1984;40:168–182.

22. Escott-Stump S. *Nutrition and Diagnosis-Related Care.* 4th ed. Baltimore: Williams & Wilkins; 1998:715.

23. Murray R. The effects of consuming carbohydrate-electrolyte beverages on gastric emptying and fluid absorption during and following exercise. *Sports Med.* 1987;4:322–351.

24. Costill DL, Saltin B. Factors limiting gastric emptying during rest and exercise. *J Appl Physiol.* 1974;37:679–683.

25. American Dietetic Association. *Winning Sports Nutrition: The Athlete's Guide to Healthy Eating.* Oct 1997. Brochure prepared for Healthtouch.

26. Kleiner SM. Water: an essential but overlooked nutrient. *J Am Diet Assoc.* 1999;99:200–206.

27. Sawka MN. Physiological consequences of hypohydration: exercise performance and thermoregulation. *Med Sci Sports Exerc.* 1992;24:657–670.

28. Gonzalez-Alonso J, Calbet JA, Nielsen B. Metabolic and thermodynamic responses to dehydration-induced reduction in muscle blood flow in exercising humans. *J Physiol.* 1999;520 Pt 2:577–589.

29. Barr SI. Effects of dehydration on exercise performance. *Can J Appl Physiol.* 1999;24:164–172.

30. Murray R, Bartoli W, Stofan J, Horn M, Eddy D. A comparison of the gastric emptying characteristics of selected sports drinks. *Int J Sport Nutr.* 1999;9:263–274.

31. Harkeins C, et al, eds. *Sports Nutrition: A Guide for the Professional Working with Active People.* 2nd ed. Chicago: The American Dietetic Association; 1993.

32. Davis JM, Burgess WA, Slentz CA, Bartoli WP, Pate RR. Effects of ingesting 6% and 12% glucose/electrolyte beverages during prolonged cycling exercise in the heat. *Eur J Appl Physiol.* 1988;57:563–569.

33. Sherman WM. Metabolism of sugars and physical performance. *Am J Clin Nutr.* 1995;62:228S–241S.

34. Applegate EA. Nutritional considerations for ultra endurance performance. *Int J Sport Nutr.* 1991;1:118–126.

35. Frentsos JA, Baer JT. Increased energy and nutrient intake during training and competition improves elite triathletes' endurance performance. *Int J Sport Nutr.* 1997;7:61–71.

36. Weight LM, Jacobs P, Noakes TD. Dietary iron deficiency and sports anemia. *Br J Nutr.* 1992;68:253–260.

37. Haymes EM. Vitamin and mineral supplementation to athletes. *Int J Sport Nutr.* 1991;1:146–169.

38. Keith RE, O'Keefe KA, Alt LA, Young KL. Dietary status of trained female cyclists. *J Am Diet Assoc.* 1989;89:1620–1623.

39. Deuster PA, Kyle SB, Moser PB, Vigersky RA, Singh A, Schoomaker EB. Nutritional survey of highly trained female runners. *Am J Clin Nutr.* 1986;44:954–962.

40. Moffatt RJ. Dietary status of elite female high school gymnasts: inadequacy of vitamin and mineral intake. *J Am Diet Assoc.* 1984;84:1361–1363.

41. Singh A, Evans P, Gallagher KL, Deuster PA. Dietary intakes and biochemical profiles of nutritional status of ultra marathoners. *Med Sci Sports Exerc.* 1993;25:328–334.

42. Brotherhood JR. Nutrition and sports performance. *Sports Med.* 1984;1:350–389.

43. National Academy of Sciences. Dietary reference intakes. *Nutr Rev.* 1997;55:319–326.

44. National Academy of Sciences. Uses of the dietary reference intakes. *Nutr Rev.* 1997;55:327–331.

45. Centers for Disease Control. Recommendations for the use of folic acid to reduce the number of cases of spinal bifida and other neural tube defects. *MMWR Morbid Mortal Wkly Rep.* 1992;41:2–7.

46. Davies KJ, Donovan CM, Refino CJ, Brooks GA, Packer L, Dallman PR. Distinguishing effects of anemia and muscle iron deficiency on exercise bioenergetics in the rat. *Am J Physiol.* 1984;246:E535–E543.

47. Celsing F, Blomstrand E, Werner B, Pihlstedt P, Ekblom B. Effects of iron deficiency on endurance and muscle enzyme activity in man. *Med Sci Sports Exerc.* 1986;18:156–161.

48. Nielsen P, Nachtigall D. Iron supplementation in athletes: current recommendations. *Sports Med.* 1998;26:207–216.

49. Craciun AM, Wolf J, Knapen MHJ, Brouns F, Vermeer C. Improved bone metabolism in female elite athletes after vitamin K supplementation. *Int J Sports Med.* 1998;19:479–484.

50. Sherman WM, Costill DL, Fink WJ, Miller JM. Effect of exercise-diet manipulation on muscle glycogen and its subsequent utilization during performance. *Int J Sports Med.* 1981;2:114–118.

51. Economos CD, Bortz SS, Nelson ME. Nutritional practices of elite athletes: practical recommendations. *Sports Med.* 1993;16:381–399.

52. Davis JM, Welsh RS, De Volve KL, Alderson NA. Effects of branched-chain amino acids and carbohydrates on fatigue during intermittent, high-intensity running. *Int J Sports Med.* 1999;20:309–314.

53. Jeukendrup AE, Thielen JJ, Wagenmakers AJ, Brouns F, Saris WH. Effect of medium-chain triglycerol and carbohydrate ingestion during exercise on substrate utilization and subsequent cycling performance. *Am J Clin Nutr.* 1998;67:397–404.

54. Rauch HG, Hawley JA, Woodey M, Noakes TD, Dennis SC. Effects of ingesting a sports bar versus glucose polymer on substrate utilization and ultra-endurance performance. *Int J Sports Med.* 1999;20:452–457.

55. Sherman WM, Peden MC, Wright DA. Carbohydrate feedings 1 h before exercise improves cycling performance. *Am J Clin Nutr.* 1991;54:866–870.

56. Kirwan JP, O'Gorman D, Evans WJ. A moderate glycemic meal before endurance can enhance performance. *J Appl Physiol.* 1998;84:53–59.

57. Palmer GS, Clancy MC, Hawley JA, Rodger IM, Burke LM, Noakes TD. Carbohydrate ingestion immediately before exercise does not improve 20 km time trial performance in well trained cyclists. *Int J Sports Med.* 1998;19:415–418.

58. Wardlaw GM, Insel PM. *Perspectives in Nutrition*. 3rd ed. St. Louis, MO: Mosby; 1996:104, 238, 319.

59. Burke LM, Collier GR, Hargreave SM. Muscle glycogen storage after prolonged exercise: effect of the glycemic index of carbohydrate feedings. *J Appl Physiol*. 1993;75:1019–1023.

60. Sherman WM. Metabolism of sugars and physical performance. *Am J Clin Nutr*. 1995;62:228S–241S.

61. Porcello LA. A practical guide to fad diets. 1984;3:723–729.

62. Cheuvront SN. The Zone diet and athletic performance. *Sports Med*. 1999;27:213–228.

63. Considine RV, Sinha MK, Heiman ML, et al. Serum immunoreactive-leptin concentrations in normal-weight and obese humans. *N Engl J Med*. 1996;334:292–295.

64. Warren MP, Stiehl AL. Exercise and female adolescents: effects on the reproductive and skeletal systems. *J Am Med Womens Assoc*. 1999;54:115–120, 138.

65. Thompson RA, Trattner-Sherman R. *Helping Athletes with Eating Disorders*. Champaign, IL: Human Kinetics; 1993.

66. Brownell KD, Rodin J, Wilmore JH. Prevalence of eating disorders in athletes. In: Brownell KD, Rodin J, Wilmore JH, eds. *Eating, Body Weight and Performance in Athletes: Disorders of Modern Society*. Philadelphia: Lea & Febiger; 1992:128–143.

67. West RV. The female athlete. The triad of disordered eating, amenorrhea and osteoporosis. *Sports Med*. 1998;26:63–71.

68. Centers for Disease Control and Prevention. Daily dietary fat and total-food-energy intakes, NHANES III, Phase 1, 1988–91. *JAMA*. 1994;271:1309.

69. MRC Vitamin Research Group. Prevention of neural tube defects: results of the Medical Research Council Vitamin Study. *Lancet*. 1991;338:131–137.

70. Food and Nutrition Board, National Research Council, NAS. *Recommended Dietary Allowances*. 10th ed. Washington, DC: National Academy Press;1989.

71. Jarski RW, Trippett DL. The risks and benefits of exercise during pregnancy. *J Fam Pract*. 1990;30:185–189.

Dietetic Resources

Total Wellness, Inc.
Marlisa Brown, MS, RD, CDE, CDN
160 Howells Rd.
Bay Shore, NY 11706
(516) 666–4297
Fax (516) 666–5284

The American Dietetic Association
216 West Jackson Boulevard
Chicago, IL 60606–6995
Consumer Nutrition Hot Line
(800) 366–1655
Online: http://www.eatright.org

American A]llergy Association
P.O. Box 7273
Menlo Park, CA 94026–7273

American Cancer Society
1599 Clifton Road NE
Atlanta, GA 30329
(800) 227–2345

American Diabetic Association
1660 Duke Street
Alexandria, VA 22314
(800) 232–3472

American Heart Association
7272 Greenville Avenue
Dallas, TX 75231
(800) AHA-USA1 ([800] 242–8721)

Anorexia Nervosa and Associated Disorders Inc.
P.O. Box 7
Highland Park, IL 60035
(847) 831–3438

Food Allergy Network
10400 Eaton Place
Suite 107
Fairfax, VA 22030
(703) 691–3179

National Cancer Institute
National Institutes of Health
31 Center Drive
Building 31, Room 10A07
Bethesda, MD 20892
(800) 4-CANCER ([800] 422–6237)

National Diabetes Information Clearinghouse
1 Information Way
Bethesda, MD 20892–3560
(301) 654–3327

National Digestive Diseases Information Clearinghouse
2 Information Way
Bethesda, MD 20892–3570
(301) 654–3810

National Kidney and Urologic Diseases Information Clearinghouse
3 Information Way
Bethesda, MD 20892–3580
(301) 654–4415

Psychology and the Injured Female Athlete

Doreen Greenberg

"In the middle of every difficulty lies opportunity."
—Albert Einstein

INTRODUCTION

In some ways, the female athlete is better prepared for dealing with an injury than her nonathlete counterpart. After all, she has spent a great deal of time tolerating discomfort in rigorous training, pushing herself to meet her goals, and overcoming failures. But because there has been such large investment of time, sweat, energy, glory, and tears in her sport, dealing with an injury sometimes proves to be a formidable task.

Rehabilitation means both mental and physical recovery from injury. The athlete's reaction to her injury is based more on her perception of what this injury means than on the actual physical injury itself. Possible outcomes may include a quick return to action, a long absence from competition, or an end of a career. It is the athlete's personal interpretation of what is happening to her that has the greatest influence on her psychological response.

The female athlete is unique in certain psychosocial respects. She has had to learn to overcome gender barriers and obstacles to accomplish her athletic goals. Most women in sports today will tell you that they have had to prove their worthiness in the sports world. They have had to create opportunities where none existed. Oftentimes they have had to fight for training time and space. Sometimes, they have had to defend their fit and strong image. It has been a challenge to earn respect as an athlete. It has taken a lot to be in control.

The injury may foster uncomfortable feelings for the female athlete of feeling out of control. In light of the long battle for deference and acceptance, an injury may send her emotionally tumbling. These feelings could be incomparable to anything she has felt before. The injury could be a real threat to her independence and self-esteem. For the sports medicine team, there is a need for understanding, not only the athlete's personal history, but also the general struggle of women in sports.

The sport psychology consultant (SPC) can play an indispensable role in the rehabilitation process. The philosophy expressed here emphasizes a speedy, safe return to sport of an emotionally and physically healthy athlete. This chapter contains information from some of the leading professionals in the field, summation of the existing research literature, anecdotal insights, and treatment recommendations in the following areas:

- psychological predisposition to injury
- psychological reaction to injury
- assessment and intervention
- sport psychology strategies for effective rehabilitation
- the sports psychologist in the sports medicine clinic

PSYCHOLOGICAL PREDISPOSITION TO INJURY AND INJURY RISK

One focus of recent research in the sport injury field has been the discovery of factors that expose an athlete to potential injury. Investigators have tried to determine not only what might lead to injury but also how we can make athletes less vulnerable and more resilient. What they have found are significant psychosocial antecedents to injury vulnerability. These factors have been positively associated with an increased risk of injury.[1,2] Although we cannot predict with any certainty which athletes will have this problem, we can look at the significant variables that might predispose an athlete to injury: stress and the stress response, personality factors, coping resources, and cultural factors.

The Stress-Injury Relationship

The main hypothesis of the stress-injury model is that athletes, who have a history of many stressors and few coping resources and are faced with a significant competitive situation, will be more prone to injury.[2,3] Therefore, when placed in a severe training session or a critical competitive event, the overstressed athlete may react with higher physiological activation and a disruption in normal athletic performance. This response may predispose the athlete to a sports injury.

The anxiety-producing factors earmarked as injury risk variables range from major to minor stresses in life. When we talk of major life events, we are concentrating on the year before the competitive season. Major events include such changes as death of someone close, relationship dissolution, moving, previous injury, sponsorship/funding difficulties, loss in athletic standing, and problems with coaches. Daily hassles, frustrations, irritations, and changes can also contribute to the athlete's overall stress-response level.

Major Life-Stress Events for Athletes

- Death of someone close
- Relationship dissolution
- Moving
- Previous injury
- Sponsorship/funding difficulties
- Loss in athletic standing
- Problems with coaches

Clinical Guideline

The stress-injury response is similar to the life stress-illness response that has been well researched in the medical and health community.[3,4] The stress leads to cognitive and physical adaptations, increased stress on the body, and then an increased risk for illness or injury. There is increased muscle tension, heightened distraction, a narrowing of the visual field, a decrease in self-confidence, and a disruption in concentration.

Personality Factors

There are certain personality characteristics that seem to exacerbate the stress response. These may put the athlete at risk for injury.[2–4] Athletes with a strong, internal locus of control are less likely to be injured. There has been some evidence that athletes with a higher level of competitive trait anxiety may be more vulnerable to injury.[4,5]

A positive state of mind seems to be significantly related to decreasing injury vulnerability. Perhaps, remaining optimistic may buffer the effects of the stress response. This would enable the athlete to stay relaxed and focused. Conversely, negative mood states, such as anger, aggression, and high pessimism have been associated with an increase in injury.

Personality Traits Associated with Injury Risk

- Poor locus of control
- High competitive anxiety
- Negative mood state
- High pessimism
- Anger
- Aggression

Clinical Guideline

Coping Resources

There is strong evidence of the impact that an athlete's coping resources, such as problem solving and social support, have on injury vulnerability.[2,4] How does the athlete usually handle disturbing situations? It is important to discover the athlete's problem-solving abilities and her capacity to think clearly under stressful situations.[1] The athlete's social support may be a critical factor in buffering the effects of life stressors.[1,3,6] Who does she typically turn to in the face of adversity? Can she depend on them for support?

The athlete needs to have a repertoire of stress management skills to cope with all the anxieties of sports competition. Other behaviors, such as proper sleeping, eating, and relaxation patterns, are directly related to psychological coping skills.

Cultural Factors

Many athletes are unwilling to quit because of pain, fatigue, illness, or injury, despite the discomfort. The belief is that their only choice is accepting the physical risk.[7] There has been a tradition in the male sports world of embracing sacrifice and pain as part of the price to pay for being a competitive athlete. Increasingly, more and more female athletes are accepting this doctrine that striving for success means sacrificing one's body.[7]

THE ATHLETE'S PSYCHOLOGICAL REACTIONS TO INJURY

Reactions to sports injury are as diverse as the women who participate in sports. This variety is due to the wide range of individual perceptions and expectations. For some, the injury may be a catastrophe, for others an inconvenience. What does this injury mean to this individual's life? This injury can mean a loss of identity, loneliness, separation, and a loss of confidence.[3,6]

Brewer[8] identified a cognitive appraisal model relevant to the athlete's psychological response. This model of psychological reaction to injury has replaced the traditional grief response model. It accounts more for individual differences. It includes looking at personal factors, such as disposition, and at situational factors, such as social environment. It also focuses on the athlete's personal interpretation of the injury rather than the injury itself. The athlete's cognitive appraisal determines her emotional response. Her emotional response determines her behavioral response to rehabilitation.

Effective rehabilitation is contingent on a precise evaluation of the athlete's situation. Prompt recognition of emotional distress may facilitate the athlete's safe return to sports participation.[4,9–10] The first step in any change process is awareness. Awareness will help the athlete gain an understanding of what is happening to her, both physiologically and emotionally.

Assessment

Rather than asking the injured athlete to fill in the blanks of an indifferent questionnaire, it is recommended here that someone on the sports medicine team do a quick emotional assessment face to face. The purpose of this in-person appraisal is to get a complete picture. The psychological evaluation needs to include her verbal and nonverbal responses to some important questions. Take note of her verbal tone, her body posture, the muscles of her face, and the look in her eyes as she is answering your questions. These communication forms are all tools to help assess the mood of the athlete.

It is often difficult to self-evaluate one's emotions during a crisis. Therefore, asking the injured party to pinpoint an emotional label by selecting it from a list becomes an arduous task. The "quick assessment tool" is used as an initial interview with the injured athlete. The following questions can help the sports medicine team gain some insight to the importance of sport participation in her life, how much she knows about the injury and recovery process, and the injury's effect on her mood and temperament.

Quick Assessment Tool—10 Questions To Ask the Injured Athlete:

- What are your reasons for participating in sports?
- Do you consider yourself a competitive or recreational athlete?

- How important is sports participation in your life?
- What were your specific athletic goals for this season/year?
- Have you been injured before? How did you handle it?
- What effect do you think your injury will have on the team?
- How much distress do you feel about your injury?
- What have your moods been like since the injury?
- How are you handling the pain?
- What are your expectations for recovery?

Clinical Guideline

Cognitive Appraisal

Once the initial quick assessment is concluded, a more in-depth dialogue should take place. The comprehensive assessment has two purposes. The first goal of assessment is to ascertain the athlete's level of distress. Naturally, any injury will add stress to the athlete's life. It is the amount of grief, worry, and anguish that is significant and whether it interferes with the athlete's daily functioning.

The second goal is to enlist the athlete's available coping resources.[4]

Through the interview process, you will get a sense of the athlete's general attitude, whether it is positive and optimistic or gloomy and apprehensive. It is important to learn about her previous stress management experiences, as well.

As with the previous quick questions, attention should be paid to nonverbal clues, as well as to the answers. Please keep in mind that these questions are intrusive and may cause discomfort. It is always better to "back-off" than pursue the answers to clearly disturbing questions. Remember that you are in the process of establishing and maintaining a trusting relationship.

The focus should be on the individuality of the injured athlete. It all comes down to perception. It is essential to explore how the athlete is interpreting this injury. Female athletes may derive a large component of their self-worth from their perceived athletic competence.[11] What does the athlete think this injury means to her? The perceived impairment of sport performance is the most important factor in psychological evaluation. It is this perception of the significance of injury that is the foundation of her emotional and behavioral responses.[3,12] Communication is so important at this point; athletes sometimes underestimate the disruption and short-term effects of the injury compared with the estimate of medical professionals.[13]

The athlete's perception of the significance of injury is the foundation of her emotional and behavioral responses.

Clinical Guideline

The information gathered in the interview will help in strategy planning. Does the athlete need immediate help with psychological skills for pain management? Will compliance with rehabilitation be an issue? Is it evident that the athlete appears to be "in the dark" about her treatment and rehabilitation? Is there a danger of severe mood disturbance. Are anxiety and depression a real concern?

Any woman who becomes an athlete has her own distinctive personality traits. Yet, there are also some characteristics that are universal to successful female athletes. Research has shown us that female athletes tend to be more assertive, in control, independent, and self-reliant than their nonathletic counterparts.[1] Is being out of control a threat to her mental status?

How does she perceive that this impairment/loss will affect her lifestyle? Is being a successful athlete the primary component of her identity and self-worth? Special attention needs to be paid to athletes with repetitive injuries over a prolonged period of time. These injuries particularly affect self-esteem and coping behavior. Research shows us that chronically injured athletes accept less social support and use more escape/avoidance behavior. Although female patients, in general, tend to self-disclose and seek social support more readily, chronically injured female athletes tend to avoid coping with the injury more than males.[14,15]

Cognitive appraisal of injury investigates the athlete's ego involvement in sport. Take a look at her fears about returning, missing training, or letting down the team. Are there any secondary gains to being injured? Has this injury become a face-saving measure or a safe way to end an unhappy experience? Explore, together, the following questions:

Cognitive Appraisal Questions

- How do you perceive this injury?
- Is it a disaster?
- Do you feel courageous?
- Is this injury an annoyance?
- Is it a relief from training and competition?
- Is it better than the embarrassment of poor performance?
- Is this a loss that you may not recover from?

Clinical Guideline

The sports medicine team needs to look at changes in the athlete's life since the injury. What roles are family, friends, teammates, and coaches still playing in her life? How confident is she about returning to the playing field? Personal history is a valuable tool. Ask about a previous catastrophe or major disappointment in her life. How did she handle it?

Grief Reaction

It is difficult to predict an athlete's emotional reaction to injury. Injured athletes are likely to exhibit significant mood changes that fluctuate throughout rehabilitation. Moods can range from feeling stressed to feeling devastated. There seems to be more mood disturbance with competitive athletes than recreational athletes.[6,16] One of the most helpful questions to ask an athlete is, "Describe your mood since the injury." Compare this information to the athlete's description of her emotional state before the injury.

Trauma reaction is normal. It is not unusual for athletes who have an injury to be concerned about complete recovery. Does the grief reaction seem normal to you on the basis of this athlete's emotional investment in her sport?[8,17] Does the athlete have a good sense of what actually happened during the injury? Does she have any memory lapses? Keep in mind that traditionally women have had greater psychological trauma with an injury that causes some physical unsightliness.[4] How much identity loss is associated with this injury?[6]

Signs of Poor Adjustment

Getting the blues is a normal reaction. A continued, depressed and anxious mood is not. Research demonstrates that physically injured athletes experience a period of emotional distress that in some cases may be severe enough to warrant clinical intervention. For some athletes being injured was found to result in a depressed mood state, greater anxiety, and lower self-esteem immediately after the injury and months later.[18] Research findings show that severe and chronic injuries can cause heightened emotional responses.[15] Athletes can have increased levels of depression, and anger and can develop a prolonged mood disturbance.[1,19,20]

There are warning signs of abnormal reaction and potentially serious psychological distress. Evidence of several of these manifestations may indicate referral to a psychological counselor. Note that the following reactions may be similar to one's reaction to pain.

Warning Signs of Psychological Distress

- Sleep disruption
- Poor eating
- Difficulty concentrating
- Easy to anger
- Feelings of agitation/nervousness
- Excessive guilt
- Feelings of hopelessness
- Withdrawal from teammates, family, and friends
- Poor adherence to rehabilitation

Clinical Guideline

Negative Addiction

Injury can be the side effect of a negative addiction to exercise and sport. These athletes are more at risk for mood disturbance such as elevated anxiety or depression. The addicted athlete will often continue training and competing when it is clearly contraindicated for physical and psychological health reasons.[6,9]

Withdrawal symptoms will typically occur within 24 hours of not training for her sport. These include symptoms of depression and anxiety, sleep disturbance, and irritability. There may be strong emotions associated with the incapacity to tolerate cessation of sport activity. "The fundamental characteristic of the addicted athlete is the need to perform a given activity regularly in order to maintain emotional equilibrium."[4(p 203)]

Anecdotal Testimony

Female athletes are more compliant and seem to have a better locus of control than their male counterparts, according to Nicholas DiNubile, MD, an orthopaedic surgeon specializing in sports medicine for elite and professional athletes. He finds this evident in the pain tolerance levels of his female athlete patients after reconstructive knee surgery. His female patients seem to have a better "work ethic" regarding physical therapy and recovery.

He senses a distinct difference in responses between competitive, elite level male and female athletes. In his experience, female athletes have been more willing to acknowledge and express their grief reaction. He believes that these feelings, after trauma, are a useful part of the course of recovery. According to Dr. DiNubile, once they have expressed their anguish, female athletes are ready to move beyond the grief and take on an important role in the rehabilitation process.

Dr. DiNubile learned a valuable lesson about taking female athletes seriously from an elite-level track and field star that he was treating. One of the top high school hurdlers in the country, she suffered an anterior cruciate ligament tear during her senior year in high school. Although he recommended reconstructive surgery, she chose conservative management and rehabilitation, because it was not her landing leg. The doctor believed that it was a risky decision; she wanted a quick return to her important senior year of competition. This athlete made the right decision for her, earning a full scholarship to a top university. After reaching her goal, she had the reconstructive surgery. Dr. DiNubile believes that it took a lot of courage, not only to pursue her goal but also to stand up to the medical team.

Carole Oglesby, PhD, is a certified consultant in sport psychology and world-renowned expert on women's sports issues. Along with all the advances in women's sports, Dr.

Oglesby sees a serious problem that has evolved with the advent of gender equity. Historically, male athletes have had a tradition of taking risks and ignoring pain and injury to achieve their competitive goals. It is all part of the "mythic hero" concept. Some highly motivated athletes train themselves to endure anything. This concept influences athletes' perceptions about injury. Dr. Oglesby now sees female athletes exhibiting these behaviors. Complete denial of pain and injury is not appropriate for anyone's sport! It is essential to educate athletes about which types pain to ignore and to which types of pain one should respond.

Another problem area that Dr. Oglesby sees is the misconception that some coaches have about their female athletes. There seems to be a common viewpoint among some coaches, according to Dr. Oglesby, about how much one should push an athlete to the edge. Some believe that one must "drive" an athlete as much as possible. They believe that there will always be a "natural safety mechanism" that will stop the athlete and protect her from harm. The athlete will know (mystically) when it is too much and will voluntarily cease the activity herself. Dr. Oglesby is often amazed by how compliant these athletes are to their coach's demands. This was evident in the elite-level female rowers who rowed until ribs cracked and then went on with their training with the injury. Their "protective devices" got suspended when honoring the coach's demands.

PSYCHOLOGICAL TREATMENTS FOR INJURED ATHLETES

Pepitas and Danish[6] describe three distinct phases of the injury process: crisis, rehabilitation, and recovery target date. Immediately after the onset of injury, it is important to help the athlete deal with emotional distress, including fear and denial. This is also a time of establishing rapport and trust with the athlete and evaluating her emotional status. After this initial crisis period, the athlete needs help with motivation and frustrations and "coping with the ups and downs of rehabilitation."[6(p 268)] The final phase deals with the doubts and apprehensions about returning to competition and fear of reinjury.

Psychological interventions can influence the speed of recovery after injury. Research findings demonstrate that athletes who use psychological skills recover faster than athletes who do not.[3,16] Success at coping with the injury, fostering compliance, and preparing the athlete for reentry to the sports domain involves the education of the athlete and offering her psychological skills training.

Once the assessment has taken place, the next step is fully educating the athlete about injury and recovery. After this, the next stage is teaching the athlete mental skills to cope with loss, pain, mood disturbance, and adherence to rehabilitation, with the ultimate goal to ensure a safe and rapid recovery.

Treatment Issues

How should the injured female athlete be treated? Much has been written about the differential medical treatment for women in the United States. Research seems to point to a link between the inequity of a woman's health care treatment and her subordinate status in our culture.[21] There remain many gender stereotypic attitudes in medical decision making.[21] Some medical personnel have attributed complaints to emotional rather than physical causes. This attitude can also have consequences for the female athlete in the sports medicine clinic.

Communication remains a big concern. Both physicians and patients bring biases and stereotypical thinking to the medical encounter. Traditionally, male physicians have reported liking male patients more than they like female patients, and patients expect to be able to talk more openly to female physicians.[22]

Female athletes' concerns need to be taken just as seriously as their male counterparts. How much of her self-worth and self-esteem is defined by her sports participation? It is critical to know how much her sense of self depends on her athletic status.[1] By inquiring about this significance and the consequence of ceasing participation, the physician and staff will gain a better understanding of the individual female athlete. This means breaking through the gender biases and gaining knowledge about how much her self-worth is wrapped up in her sport.

In this way, the rehabilitation team and the athlete will all be working toward the same goals. The athlete will come to fully trust the process. The staff can also give some personal responsibility to her for her own recovery. This is an ongoing process. Dr. DiNubile states that the physician needs to continually check in with the mental state of the athlete, because she has lost the connection to and feedback from the team. She needs the sports medicine team to fill this role. Dr. DiNubile states that the treating physician is not just a bystander; he or she plays an important role in setting the emotional tone of rehabilitation.

Education

It is imperative for the injured athlete to fully understand both the nature of the injury and the rehabilitation process. This is one important way for the sports medicine team to get the athlete committed to the recovery process. A great deal of anxiety stems from uncertainty and feeling out of control. Fully educating the athlete about recovery will help to eliminate uncertainties and misconceptions.

The Clinical Management list that follows is a general blueprint for injury education.

Topics of Injury Education

- Basic anatomy of the injured area
- Physical changes caused by injury
- Active and passive rehabilitation methods
- Mechanisms by which rehabilitation methods work
- Description of diagnostic and surgical procedures (if necessary)
- Potential problems with pain and how to cope with these
- Differentiation of benign pain from dangerous pain
- Guidelines for independent use of modalities (ie, heat, cold)
- Plan for progressing active rehabilitation (eg, resistance training)
- Anticipated timetable for rehabilitation
- Possibility of treatment plateaus
- Purposes of medication with emphasis on consistent use as prescribed
- Potential side effects of medication with encouragement to report these to the physician
- Rationale for limits on daily physical activities during healing
- Guidelines for the use of braces, orthotic devices, and crutches
- Injury as a source of stress and a challenge to maintaining a positive attitude
- Rehabilitation as an active collaborative learning process
- Deciding when to hold back and when to go all-out
- Long-term maintenance and care of healing the injury

Clinical Guideline

Social Support

The athlete's support system can have a tremendous influence on the athlete's recovery process. The support of the team, the coach, family, and friends can facilitate psychological adaptation.[6] Are they being negative and cultivating doubts in the athlete? Is she able to discuss her feelings with them? Promote social interactions with team members to continue throughout rehabilitation. Encourage the coach to keep the athlete an active member of the team.

Psychological Skills Development

Athletes are used to pushing their bodies to the maximum and taking risks. Make use of this ability when designing the rehabilitation game plan. The sports medicine staff have an opportunity to help the athlete make a psychological commitment to healing. Through training and practice of psychological skills for sport, the athlete can learn to better cope with the injury. Psychological interventions have been used successfully by athletes to foster faster healing.[3,4,16,23–25]

Most skills training in sports psychology is based on cognitive-behavioral techniques. These strategies include goal-setting, relaxation training, concentration instruction, positive self-talk, cognitive restructuring, negative thought stoppage, and imagery rehearsal. Some procedures are discussed below.

Psychological Skills for Injury Rehabilitation

- Goal-setting
- Relaxation training
- Concentration instruction
- Positive self-talk
- Cognitive restructuring
- Negative thought stoppage
- Imagery rehearsal

Clinical Guideline

Goal Setting

Short- and long-term goals can simplify the planning process and help the athlete stay motivated during rehabilitation.[6] For the injured athlete, setting realistic, positive, and attainable goals can be the first step in regaining control over her situation. It is a way of establishing realistic expectations. It is a way to help the athlete become more future oriented. It can also be a way to monitor progress. For the athlete and therapy team it can be a "road map to recovery."[26(p 30)]

Setting daily goals for healing and recovery was found to be most effective for injured athletes.[24] By setting a positive goal, the athlete is indicating an expectation of success. Two important questions that can get the athlete started on her goal-setting task are:

- "What do you want to achieve?"
- "What is stopping you?"

Cognitive Reframing

What the athlete says to herself during recovery from injury is an important determinant of her behavioral responses. Athletes can be taught to control negative thinking. Positive self-talk can be practiced. A suggestion is to let the athlete write down her thoughts and select out the negative statements. She could then be given the assignment of substituting positive statements or reframing the negative ones.

Another method of getting rid of negative self-talk is "thought stoppage." After helping the athlete become aware

of the negative thoughts, she is given a trigger to interrupt her undesirable thinking. The trigger can be a word, a phrase, or a physical action, such as pinching her fingers.

Affirmation statements have been successful in helping to eliminate negative thinking. These are contrived statements echoing a positive thought and phrased as if it were already true.

Modeling technique is another useful strategy for restructuring cognitions about injury and recovery. The athlete can view videotape testimony of athletes with similar injury experiences who have had successful rehabilitation.

Cognitive Reframing

- Controlling negative thinking
- Substituting positive statements
- Thought stoppage
- Affirmation statements
- Modeling technique

Clinical Guideline

Mental Rehearsal

Athletes can learn to control their visual images, as well. Imagery rehearsals can help the athlete anticipate the challenges of the recovery process. Typically, the SPC and the injured athlete would work together to manufacture a challenging rehabilitation scenario. Perhaps it would be a difficult physical therapy session that might result in emotional distress for the athlete. By incorporating all the senses into this detailed, imagined story line, the athlete can fully understand and anticipate the situation, building up the anxiety level. A game plan is then formulated to deal with this situation. It might begin with a stress management procedure (see following section) to reduce the anxiety level and calm down. Then the athlete rehearses going through the actions of the physical therapy regimen in a relaxed state.

Relaxation Strategies

It is essential for the injured athlete, facing the rigors of the rehabilitation process, to learn emotional self-control. Using a relaxation routine can help to reduce tension and enhance blood circulation.[3] Relaxation techniques can take several forms. There are relaxation tapes and soothing music. Some athletes use yoga and meditation. Relaxation massage can also help to reduce stress levels. Two specific techniques are briefly discussed here. Relaxation breathing techniques and progressive muscle relaxation fall under the category of muscle to mind strategies. Most athletes respond well to these methods.

Relaxation Techniques

- Relaxation tapes
- Soothing music
- Yoga
- Meditation
- Relaxation massage
- Relaxation breathing
- Progressive muscle relaxation

Clinical Guideline

With practice, relaxation breathing is one of the easiest ways to control the physiological response to anxiety. Techniques include learning how to take deep, full, slow breaths from the diaphragm. This will usually trigger a relaxation response. Having the athlete verbally "sigh" on exhalation helps to reduce tension. After holding a deep breath for 10 seconds, have the athlete exhale through the mouth with a spoken sigh. The athlete should focus on the quiet time between the exhale and the inhale. Another technique is rhythmic breathing. The athlete would inhale while counting to three or four, hold her breath for the same count, and exhale while doing a three or four count. A third technique combines imagery with breathing. Ask the athlete to pick her favorite pleasant, soothing color. First, she should inhale a deep slow breath through her nose. Then as she exhales through her mouth, she can imagine her breath flowing out the selected color.

Progressive muscle relaxation exercises involve contracting specific muscle groups, holding the contraction, and then easing off the tension in the muscle group. The athlete would use this technique from muscle group to muscle group throughout her body. With practice, she can learn to become aware of tension in her body and also voluntarily let go of the tension. The premise is that if her body is relaxed, her mind will not be anxious.

Concentration

One of the side effects of anxiety and stress is a disruption in concentration. The ability to eliminate distractions and focus one's attention can be taught. One method uses individual verbal and kinesthetic cues to bring back the concentration. These can be used to help the athlete focus her attention and turn away intrusive thoughts. It is best to learn to attend to the present moment, also called the "here and now."

Another refocusing method is to use a positive photo of the athlete in action performing her sport. Have her try to focus on the picture without letting a disrupting thought or feeling interfere. She should practice gently bringing back her attention when it is disrupted. Also, she could practice thinking of a single, positive thought related to the image in the photo. She should see how long she can do that without another thought interfering. These simple exercises take only a few minutes a day and can enhance concentration abilities.

Advanced Techniques

There are some other effective strategies that will require more advanced training. These include biofeedback, hypnosis, and Eye Movement Desensitization and Reprocessing, a relatively new treatment method for dealing with the psychological trauma of injury.[27]

Athletes usually have a history of dealing with pain and discomfort. There are also specific techniques that are successful for pain management. Research evidence shows that the athlete's tolerance for pain can be regulated by cognitive training.[28] These include various self-regulation strategies using external focus of attention; healthy, cheerful imagery; and coping rehearsals.[4,28] These pain control strategies should be used by a skilled, professional consultant.

Compliance Issues

Poor adherence to rehabilitation tends to be associated with psychological adjustment problems.[4] Compliance issues include keeping appointments and adhering to physical therapy regimens.

There is more to the recovery process than simply being there in body. There needs to be a positive attitude, an expectation of success, an intensity to the exercise regimen. The athlete can learn to take a more active role through psychological skills training such as goal-setting, imagery training, and mental rehearsal.

Dr. DiNubile has found that his female athlete patients have been much more compliant, in general, compared with his male patients. The key, he states, is to spend time with the athlete and let her know that you care about her sport participation; she will respond better by listening and taking personal responsibility. "Attitude affects recovery." This includes both the attitude of the physician and the athlete.

Sometimes, there may be a question of overcompliance.[3,4] Because of such factors as the pressure to return quickly from coaches, teammates, or family, the athlete may overdo the prescribed physical regimen. This could lead to setbacks, both physically and emotionally. Unfortunately, there are some coaches who view an injured athlete as worthless and communicate this thought to the team members. Athletes may try to do more than is necessary to try to expedite return to the field and to the favor of the coach.

Returning to the Playing Field

Traditionally, the sports medicine team has focused primarily on the physical rehabilitation of athletes. Therefore, the athlete was deemed ready to return to competition after meeting the prescribed physical guidelines.[3] Although it is apparent that some athletes adjust to the injury and recovery process, many do not. A total, whole-person healing may not have taken place. Sometimes the athlete is physically ready to return to competition but not emotionally prepared for the return to sport.[16]

The notion of returning to sport may evoke fears of reinjury, pain, and setbacks. There may also be a loss of confidence in ability.

Readiness to Return to Sport Concerns

- Will she be able to perform at her preinjury level?
- Will she be accepted back into the team?
- Has she lost her standing?
- Will she be treated differently?
- How is her fitness level?

Clinical Guideline

The athlete could be consumed by images of a disastrous comeback or even scenes of the original injury itself. This scenario has been exacerbated by the new shortened rehabilitation period caused by new medical techniques and insurance regulations.

It is important for the athlete to continue using the newly learned psychological skills on initial return to sports. Anxiety and tension can result in a loss of confidence, increased muscle tension, and a disruption in concentration. These states may result in reinjury or a compensating injury, loss of motivation, or depression.[3] It is advisable to screen for life stresses before reentry to the playing field and competition.

There is also important work, at this point, with the coach, teammates, parents, and significant others to prepare them and the athlete for reentry. This task includes establishing an atmosphere of optimism and eliminating any self-defeating attitudes.[3,6]

THE PSYCHOLOGIST IN THE SPORTS MEDICINE CLINIC

The research literature has documented the importance of psychological counseling in athletic injury rehabilitation.[3,4,6] The SPC can lay the groundwork for effective rehabilitation. The fundamental assumption is that a comprehensive mind-body approach will have the best results.

Having the SPC on site is beneficial to both the athlete and the sports medicine team, because it allows for a true multidisciplinary approach to rehabilitation. The SPC can provide both direct and indirect services to the athlete and to the treatment team. As a team member, the SPC can help to establish the trust for the rehabilitation team, facilitate pain management, enhance motivation, aid in compliance, and foster social support. The SPC can teach the injured athlete specific psychological rehabilitation strategies. The SPC can be a mediator between the coach, the rehabilitation team, and the injured athlete.

Sport psychology is becoming an integrated part of the injury recovery process. Collaborative efforts can be made for injury prevention, assessment, and rehabilitation.

The Sport Psychology Consultant on the Treatment Team

- Helps to establish trust for the rehabilitation team
- Facilitates pain management
- Enhances motivation
- Aids in compliance
- Fosters social support
- Teaches psychological rehabilitation skills
- Acts as a mediator between coach, clinic, and athlete

Clinical Guideline

CONCLUSION

The purpose of this chapter was to delineate the value of psychological assessment and treatment as part of the injury recovery process. It is clear from the research literature that the athlete's psychological state influences her reaction to injury. There is also significant evidence of the positive impact of psychological skills training on the rehabilitation of the athlete. The following suggestions are a summation of the information supplied here. The most important guideline is to view the athlete as an individual, with her own perceptions, fears, dreams, and goals.

Effective Strategies for a Healing Psychological Environment

- Establish trust.
- Look as the athlete as a whole person—not just an injury.
- Take her sport participation and injury seriously. Avoid thoughtless assumptions and gender stereotypes.
- Offer answers about the injury and rehabilitation process.
- Reinforce the importance of rehabilitation therapy by example and education.
- Allow the athlete to make decisions and help plan the recovery process.
- Acknowledge progress by sharing concrete evidence of progress by using a chart, log, or journal—based on the athlete's individual course of recovery.

- Plan for mood fluctuations throughout the rehabilitation process.
- Plan for setbacks.
- Don't assume that an athlete who has successfully completed physical rehabilitation is ready to return to sports.
- Seek professional psychological counseling for severe distress.
- Remain a positive model. Help the athlete to see this as an opportunity to find some positive meaning from injury and recovery.
- Listen, listen, listen.

Clinical Guideline

FUTURE RESEARCH

There is a scarcity of research literature regarding female athletes and the psychological dynamics of injury. Almost all the studies have been with male athletes. We do know that the athlete's perception influences the recovery process. Could there be a different impact when it is from the female perspective? There is a need to examine this area.

Recommendations for future research include:

- gender differences in psychosocial variables related to injury risk vulnerability
- gender differences and psychological adjustment to sport injury
- gender differences and ignoring pain and injury
- gender differences for coping strategies
- gender differences and compliance and adherence to rehabilitation
- gender differences and treatment by the sports medicine team
- self-worth and the injured female athlete
- the impact of cultural factors on psychological responses to injury

REFERENCES

1. Barnett NP, Wright P. Psychological considerations for women in sports. *Clin Sports Med.* 1994;13:297–313.
2. Williams JM, Andersen MB. Psychosocial antecedents of sport injury: Review and critique of the stress and injury model. *J Appl Sport Psy.* 1998:105–125.
3. Williams JM, Rotella RJ, Heyman SR. Stress, injury, and the psychological rehabilitation of athletes. In: Williams JM, ed. *Applied Sport Psychology.* 3rd ed. Mountain View, CA: Mayfield Publishing; 1998:409–428.
4. Heil J. *Psychology of Sport Injury.* Champaign, IL: Human Kinetics; 1993.
5. Petrie TA. Coping skills, competitive trait anxiety, and playing status: Moderating the effects of life stress-injury relationship. *J Sport Exerc Psy.* 1993;15:261–274.
6. Pepitas A, Danish SJ. Caring for injured athletes. In: Murphy SM, ed. *Sport Psychology Interventions.* Champaign, IL: Human Kinetics; 1995:255–281.
7. Wiese-Bjornstahl DM, Smith AM, Shaffer SM, Morrey MA. An integrated model of response to sport injury: Psychological and sociological dynamics. *J Appl Sport Psy.* 1998;10:46–69.
8. Brewer BW. Review and critique of models of psychological adjustment to athletic injury. *J Appl Sport Psy.* 1994;6:87–100.
9. Heil J, Henschen K. Assessment in sport and exercise psychology. In: Van Raalte JL, Brewer BW, eds. *Exploring Sport and Exercise Psychology.* Washington, DC: American Psychological Association; 1995:229–255.
10. Smith M, Scott SG, O'Fallon WM, Young ML. Emotional responses of athletes to injury. *Mayo Clin Proc.* 1990;65:38–50.
11. Saint-Phard D, Van Dorsten B, Marx RG, York KA. Self-perception in elite collegiate female gymnasts, cross-country runners, and track-and-field athletes. *Mayo Clin Proc.* 1999;74:770–774.
12. Brewer BW, Linder DE, Phelps CM. Situational correlates of emotional adjustment to athletic injury. *Clin J Sport Med.* 1995;5:241–245.
13. Crossman J. Psychological rehabilitation from sports injuries. *Sports Med.* 1997;23:333–339.
14. O'Leary A, Helgeson VS. Psychosocial factors and women's health: Integrating mind, heart and body. In: Gallant SJ, Keita GP, Royak-Schaler R, eds. *Health Care for Women: Psychological, Social, and Behavioral Influences.* Washington, DC: American Psychological Association; 1997:25–40.
15. Wasley D, Lox CL. Self-esteem and coping responses of athletes with acute versus chronic injuries. *Percept Motor Skills.* 1998;86:1402.
16. Morrey MA, Stuart MJ, Smith AM, Wiese-Bjornstahl DM. A longitudinal examination of athletes' emotional and cognitive responses to anterior cruciate ligament injury. *Clin J Sport Med.* 1999;9:630–669.
17. Brewer BW, Van Raalte JL, Linder DE. Role of the sport psychologist in treating injured athletes: A survey of sport medicine providers. *J Appl Sport Psy.* 1991;3:183–190.
18. Leddy MH, Lambert MJ, Ogles BM. Psychological consequences of athletic injury among high-level competitors. *Res Q Exerc Sport.* 1994;65:347–354.
19. McDonald SA, Hardy CJ. Affective response patterns of the injured athlete: An exploratory analysis. *Sport Psychologist.* 1990;4:261–274.
20. Smith AM, Scott SG, Wiese DM. The psychological effects of sport injuries. *Sports Med.* 1990;9:352–369.
21. Stanton AL. Psychology of women's health: Barriers and pathways to knowledge. In: Stanton AL, Gallant SJ, eds. *The Psychology of Women's Health: Progress and Challenges in Research and Application.* Washington, DC: American Psychological Association; 1995:3–21.
22. Roter DL, Hall JA. Gender differences in patient-physician communication. In: Gallant SJ, Keita GP, Royak-Schaler R, eds. *Health Care for Women: Psychological, Social, and Behavioral Influences.* Washington, DC: American Psychological Association; 1997:57–71.
23. Davis JO. Sports injuries and stress management: An opportunity for research. *Sport Psychologist.* 1991;5:175–182.

24. Ievleva L, Orlick T. Mental links to enhanced healing: An exploratory study. *Sport Psychologist*. 1991;5:25–40.

25. Smith AM. Psychological impact of injuries in athletes. *Sports Med*. 1996;22:391–405.

26. Heil J, Wakefield C, Reed C. Patient as athlete: A metaphor for injury rehabilitation. In: Hays KF, ed. *Integrating Exercise, Sports, Movement and Mind: Therapeutic Unity*. New York: Haworth Press; 1998:21–39.

27. Bauman NJ, Carr CM. A multi-modal approach to trauma recovery: A case history. In: Hays KF, ed. *Integrating Exercise, Sports, Movement and Mind: Therapeutic Unity*. New York: Haworth Press; 1998:145–160.

28. Pargman D. *Understanding Sport Behavior*. Upper Saddle River, NJ: Prentice–Hall; 1998.

CHAPTER 23

Ergogenic Aids

Mary Ann Everhart-McDonald

INTRODUCTION

Charlie Chaplin was quoted as saying: "Man's ingenuity has developed first and his soul afterwards. Thus, the progress of science is far ahead of man's ethical behavior."[1(p 1697)]

Winning at a Price

The desire to win has been pushed to far greater levels (beyond ethical boundaries) not only because of one seeking personal gratification but by governments seeking recognition[2] and by the monetary value of winning vs placing second. At the elite level little difference exists between first place (gold medal performance) and fourth place (little recognition). Refer to the Clinical Guidelines. At the 1997 International Amateur Athletic Federation's (IAAF) track and field World Championships, the 100-m women's finals recorded a 0.02 s difference between a world record, first place, and second place; a 0.22 s difference was recorded between first and fourth place. At the same world championships the high jump finals recorded a difference of only 0.03 m between first place and fourth place. At the 1999 Pan American games, in the 100-meter women's backstroke event there was only 0.77 s difference between first place and fourth place.

Athletes who use drugs have demonstrated increased risk-taking behaviors off the playing field.[5] Male athletes are more likely to demonstrate these increased risks than are the female athletes. Female athletes are less likely to take risks than the female nonathletes. Goldman reported a survey he had done confirming the results of a previous study by Dr.

Gabe Mirkin.[6] He asked 198 world class athletes "…if there was a pill that would let you win all the competitions over the next 5 years but it would kill you 5 years after you took it, would you take the drug?" More than 50% answered yes.

Use of Ergogenic Aids

Ergogenic aids are drugs and supplements thought to improve performance. These may include medications, herbs, food supplements, and procedures. Doping is banned by the National Collegiate Athletic Association (NCAA) and the International Olympic Committee (IOC), because it "contravenes the ethics of both sport and medical science. It threatens the integrity and dignity of Olympic sport, erodes public confidence in the Olympic Movement, and jeopardizes the health and well-being of athletes."[7(p 1)]

The drugs and supplements may be obtained from physicians, chemists, other athletes, and underground through the black market.[1,8–12]

Under the Dietary Supplement Health and Education Act passed by Congress in 1994, nutritional supplements are not regulated by the US Food and Drug Administration (FDA). No research or required test for substance purity is needed before the supplement is marketed. A small impurity in a food supplement may become a major health risk if taken in large quantities. All ingredients do *not* need to be listed on the food supplement label. In August 1999, elite track and field athletes tested positive for the banned anabolic-androgenic steroid, nandrolone.[13] It was believed the athletes were inadvertently taking this steroid in a food supplement.[14]

Ergogenic aids are no longer being used only by a few elite athletes.[11,15–17] Beginner, immature athletes are trying them.

Examples of the Miniscule Differences in Performances at the Elite Levels of Competition

100-m women's finals—1997 IAAF World Championships in Athletics[3]

Marion Jones (US)	10.83 s (wr)	1st
Zhanna Tarnopolskaya-Pintusevich (UKR)	10.85 s	2nd
Sevatheda Fynes (BAH)	11.03 s	3rd
Christine Arron (FRA)	11.05 s	4th

Women's High Jump—1997 IAAF World Championships in Athletics[3]

Hanne Haugland (NOR)	1.99 m	1st
Olga Kaliturina (RUS)	1.96 m	2nd
Inga Babakova (UKR)	1.96 m	2nd
Yuliya Lyakhova (RUS)	1.96 m	4th

Women's 100-m back stroke—1999 Pan American Games[4]

Kelly Stefanyshyn (CAN)	1:02.14	1st
Denali Knapp (US)	1:02.45	2nd
Beth Botsford (US)	1:02.48	3rd
Erin Gammel (CAN)	1:02.91	4th

Abbreviations: sec = second; wr = world record; US = United States of America; UKR = Ukraine; BAH = Bahamas; FRA = France; NOR = Norway; RUS = Russia; CAN = Canada; m = meter; min:s = minute:second.

Clinical Guideline

Use is reported to be greater in men than women.[4,9,10,18,19] The use of ergogenic aids has spread beyond the weightlifting and strength-related events.

Research does not always support the beneficial results reported by the athletes. This is partly related to the dose the athlete may take, which is 30 to 100 times greater than would be permitted by the FDA.[11,20] Far more research has been done with male athletes than female athletes. In some instances, the results can be inferred to the female athlete; however, as new research using female subjects is being completed, differences are being found.[16]

ANABOLIC-ANDROGENIC STEROIDS

Anabolic (tissue building)-androgenic (masculinizing) steroids (AAS) are derivatives of testosterone. There are *no* steroids that have a purely anabolic effect. An anabolic substance that promotes tissue growth is assumed to increase muscle mass and thus improve strength and power. AAS do counter the catabolic effect that naturally occurs with physically stressful activity. The AAS displace cortisol from the glucocorticosteroid receptors on muscle and other organ receptors.[11,18]

Biochemistry

The natural levels of testosterone present in women are significantly smaller than found in men (0.03 μg/dL and 0.65 μg/dL, respectively).[21] Approximately two-thirds of the testosterone in the plasma is bound to proteins such as sex hormone–binding globulin and albumin.[21,22] In women dehydroepiandrosterone sulfate is the androgen produced by the adrenal cortex; a small amount is synthesized in the ovaries. The dehydroepiandrosterone sulfate is converted in the peripheral tissues to more active steroids such as androstenedione and testosterone.[16] Evidence has shown that female and adolescent athletes have greater improvement in their performance but greater risk of the virilizing effects with lower doses of AAS than do male athletes.[2,18,23]

Oral testosterone is rapidly degraded by the liver. Many synthetic AAS have been designed to slow the hepatic metabolism, thus prolonging the effects of the drug.[22] Bjorkhem et al[24] administered a single dose of 10 mg methandienone (Dianabol) orally; it could be detected in the urine by gas chromatography-mass spectrometry up to 4 days after the dose. Others have reported it could be detected as long as 14 days after ingesting it.[25] Refer to the Clinical Guideline for a list of oral AAS frequently used and the doses reported in literature.[11,16,18,20,26,27]

The parenteral form of AAS has little effect on the hepatic metabolism. Oil-based injectables have a longer half-life than do the water-based ones. Bjorkhem et al[28] administered a single dose of 25 mg 19-norandrosterone (Deca-Durabolin) intramuscularly; it could be detected in the urine by gas chromatography-mass spectrometry up to 6 weeks after the injection. It must be remembered that the athlete rarely takes only one dose; the true excretion rate after prolonged use may be much longer than reported. Refer to the Clinical Guideline for a list of injectable AAS frequently used and the doses reported in literature.[16,26,27,29]

Frequently Used Oral AAS

Generic Name	Brand Name	Doses Reported	Maximum Normal Replacement Doses
Ethylestrenol	Maxibolin		
Fluoxymesterone	Halotestin		
Mesterolone	Proviron	50 mg/d	
Methandrostenolone	Dianabol	25–150 mg/d	5 mg/d
Methenolone acetate	Primobolan	100 mg/wk	
Methyltestosterone	Metadren		
Oxandrolone	Anavar	10–35 mg/d	10 mg/d
Oxymetholone	Anadrol-50		
Stanozolol	Winstrol	3–42 mg/d	6 mg/d

Abbreviations: mg/d = milligrams per day; mg/wk = milligrams per week.

Clinical Guideline

Frequently Used Parenteral AAS

Generic Name	Brand Name	Doses Reported	Normal Replacement Doses
Boldenone undecylenate	Equipoise (vet)		
Methandrostenolone injectable	Dianabol		
Methenolone enanthate	Primobolan	30 mg/2 d	
Nandrolone decanoate	Deca-Durabolin	100–200 mg/wk	50–100 mg every 3–4 wk
Stanozolol	Winstrol-V (vet)	50 mg/2 d	
Testosterone enanthate		100–800 mg/wk	50–400 mg every 2–4 wk

Clinical Guideline

Glossary of Terms

- Continuous dosing: Never taking a break from using the AAS.
- Cycling: Taking multiple doses of AAS over a specified period of time, stopping for a time and starting again.
- Drug holiday: The time when the AAS has been stopped before resuming the next cycle.
- Megadosing: Taking massive amounts of AAS.
- Plateauing: When a drug becomes ineffective at a certain level.
- Pyramiding: Gradually increasing the dose of AAS followed by gradual tapering of the dose after a maximum dose has been reached.
- Stacking: Using more than one AAS at a time; often combining oral and injectable forms.
- Tapering: Slowly decreasing the steroid intake.

Clinical Guideline

Terms found among users are listed and explained in the Clinical Guideline. Most AAS users will cycle the drugs; however, it has been found that as the duration of use increases so does the number of drugs per cycle.[30] Most users will cycle on the AAS from 4 to 8 weeks and then take a drug holiday for 2 weeks to as long as a year.[27,30]

Women are believed to use lower doses than men.[11] A review of 30 years of highly classified reports from the German Democratic Republic (GDR), which collapsed in 1990, has been done.[2] It reports the involvement of more than 2000 athletes and clearly presents doping programs for more than 400 athletes. The information includes doses taken, when the doses were taken, when drugs had to be stopped for competition, and side effects found. The Ministry for State Security reported higher doses were given to women and adolescent athletes (especially female swimmers less than 14 years old) than were being given to their male counterparts, because the positive results were much more dramatic. However, the problem of virilizing side effects was also documented in these reports.

Adolescent male athletes have been reported to use longer cycles and larger doses than are needed to obtain the desired physical effects.[17,31]

Athletes may stack the AAS for various reasons. Some believe that by using lower doses of multiple drugs they may avoid the plateauing effect. Others will vary the drugs being used to avoid detection with drug testing; they will discontinue the longer acting injectables as they switch to the oral AAS and later discontinue these for drugs not detected in the drug testing program such as growth hormone.

History

In 1939 the Bulletin of the Health Organization of the League of Nations indicated "that testosterone and its derivatives may enhance performance in sport."[11(p 381)] The first reported use of AAS was by the Russian male and female athletes in 1954.[32] After visiting the Soviet Union in 1954, Dr. Ziegler, a team physician for the US power lifters, began taking AAS himself and administering it to the team members.[11] In the early 1960s US, German, and Russian male strength athletes were using AAS; by the late 1960s the German female athletes were also using them.[2] By the 1970s the use of AAS had spread to the sprinters, middle distance runners, and swimmers.[2] The IOC banned the use of AAS in 1976.[33] By then the GDR was providing AAS "vitamins" to all its athletes except female gymnasts and those athletes in sailing events.[2] It was at the 1976 Olympics in Montreal that drug testing was able to identify some of the AAS being used. Of only 275 tests performed, 8 were positive.[32] In 1989, declines were reported in both male and female records for the "world best" performances; this was thought to be a result of the IOC ban, initiation of testing, and subsequent decreased use of AAS. With the presence of testing, for some (reported in the GDR reports) the challenge was how to avoid testing positive while still taking the banned substance as long as possible.[2]

In 1988 it became a felony in the United States to possess, with the intention to distribute, AAS without a prescription. In 1990, President Bush signed the Anabolic Steroids Control Act, which made AAS a Schedule III drug of the Controlled Substance Act.[11,15] Before 1990, reports of athletes obtaining AAS from physicians were as high as 20% to 35%; from the black market (including friends, coaches, gym operators), it was 60%.[1,8,9,30] Studies published after 1990 indicate a drop in the percent of athletes obtaining AAS from physicians to 10% to 15%.[11]

Medical Uses

In the early 1960s AAS (stanozolol) was used to counter the muscle and tissue atrophy of aging.[22] AAS has been used for constitutional delay of growth and for osteoporosis. Other reasons for AAS medical use include metastatic breast cancer with bone involvement, hypotestosteronemia, aplastic anemia, hereditary angioedema, endometriosis, and fibrocystic breast disease.[11,22,34] The medical indications for AAS are estimated to be less than 3 million prescriptions per year in the United States.[34]

The anabolic potency factor compared with testosterone in bioassay has been reported as follows: methyltestosterone, 1.15; mesterolone, 1.15; methandrostenolone, 1.7; stanozolol, 5.0; oxandrolone, 11.3; and nandrolone decanoate, 11.3.[35]

Prevalence

The exhaustive inquiry that had resulted after the positive drug test of Ben Johnson in 1989 was directed by Canadian commissioner, Honorable Mr. Justice Charles Leonard Dubin. The Dubin Inquiry examined the use of drugs and banned practices. The results "made clear that a drug-free athlete is usually a losing athlete."[1(p1697)] Many athletes, coaches, national sport organizations, and medical personnel will continue to debate this unproved statement.

It is difficult to document the true prevalence of use, but most estimates are thought to be low.[36] Athletes are hesitant to report the use of AAS for fear of jeopardizing their past accomplishments and for fear of causing legal problems by divulging the use of an illegal drug.

Various studies have reported the use in high school boys to be as low as 2.5% (evaluated the use only in the preceding 30 days) to 11% (included those who had tried or were using the drugs).[2,4] A survey of US households estimated the use of AAS to be more than 1 million people, with at least 300,000 Americans using the AAS in the past year.[37] On the basis of these numbers, the cost of use was estimated to be at least $500 million per year in the United States.[38] In 1993, research indicated the annual cost of AAS per person could range from $90.00 to $6780.00.[39]

Fewer studies have reported the use of AAS among female athletes; all indicated the use by female athletes was less than that of the male athletes. Several reports indicate approximately 20% of the use was by female athletes.[4,18,19] In the study by Lindstrom et al[38] only 10% of 33 female body builders were found to be using. Of those using, a higher rate of use was reported among female athletes participating on professional teams.[16] The National Survey estimated only 0.1% of the female population and 0.9% of the men had used AAS.[37]

Only anecdotal reports are available for estimates of use among the National Football League (50% was thought to be a conservative number).[40,41] Estimates of use were 80% to 90% of body builders and power lifters at a fitness club.[42]

Efficacy

Early studies that used low AAS doses in normal male subjects failed to show a significant improvement in performance or change in body composition.[25,35,43] Studies using male species (animal or man) with low hormone levels or females demonstrated an increase in muscle mass and a decrease in percent of body fat.[2,44] Debate continues as to whether AAS improve endurance. They have the potential to do so by increasing erythropoiesis, which in turn has been shown in blood doping situations to improve endurance.[45,46]

More recent studies in which athletes self-dose the AAS have demonstrated anabolic changes that include an increase in lean body mass with a decrease in percent of body fat and increase in mean muscle fiber area. Improvement in strength and power are documented.[11,43,47] Comparisons have been made between the athlete who does not use AAS but is involved in a heavy strength training program, use of AAS in the unconditioned individual, and the use in the athlete with and without concurrent intense strength training programs. Strength training in combination with AAS improved performance more than either AAS or strength training alone.[47] Little benefit was reported when taken by the unconditioned individual.[44] The GDR reported, after a critical period during which androgenic changes occurred in the female athletes, a "permanent" higher level of performance (strength) was reached and did not return to pre-AAS levels after the drug was withdrawn.[2] The anticatabolic effects have been shown to increase the athlete's tolerance to heavy exercise, increase the workout intensity of the athlete, decrease the recovery time needed between intense workouts, and increase the frequency of training sessions.[11]

Adverse Effects

Numerous potential and proven adverse side effects have been described that affect specific organ systems of the body. Some of these effects are considered to be permanent and could be life threatening.

Cardiovascular System

The cardiovascular system has been one of the earliest areas studied. An increased risk of atherosclerotic disease is correlated to the documented changes in cholesterol. An inverse relation exists between the high density lipoprotein cholesterol (HDL-C) and the risk of coronary artery disease (CAD). Men were found to have an increased risk of CAD with low values of HDL-C.[20,43,48] Cohen et al reported findings were similar in male and female users when comparing the cholesterol changes.[6,49] As the dose of AAS is increased, the values of HDL-C decrease.[48] Most studies have shown a significant decrease in the HDL-C values with AAS use of more than 2 weeks.[11,27,48,50,51] Hurley et al[43] compared the HDL-C values of the athletes who had not taken AAS for 10 weeks with values of the same athletes who had self-dosed the AAS for a minimum of 4 weeks; a 55% (±4%) decrease

in HDL-C was found. HDL-C depression resolved within 4 to 6 weeks after stopping AAS use.[26,43,48]

The degree to which the low density lipoprotein cholesterol (LDL-C) values increase appears to be variable. Hurley et al[43] reported a large 61% (±10%) increase in LDL-C values. Most studies report a mild elevation of LDL-C values.[11,43,51] Other studies (even those in which the athletes were self-administering the AAS) have shown no change in the LDL-C.[50,52] The changes in total cholesterol are not well documented. Some studies indicate a significant increase in the total cholesterol[11,43] and others have shown no change.[20,27,48–50]

Other side effects have not been well documented in research involving athletes. In the *Physician's Desk Reference* the risk of suppression of clotting factors II, V, VII, and X with a resultant increase in prothrombin time is mentioned.[53] A case report indicated a 34-year-old body builder suffered a left cerebrovascular accident; it left him with severe expressive and mild receptive deficits in addition to a mild right upper limb motor weakness. He had taken AAS for 4 years. On arteriography occlusion of a small suprasylvian branch of the middle cerebral artery was found.[54] An anecdotal report by 33-year-old Steve Courson, the former Tampa Bay Buccaneer offensive lineman, blamed his dilated cardiomyopathy on the heavy use of AAS, which had been prescribed by a team physician.[41] Ultrasonic video densitometric study of weight lifters' myocardium demonstrated an alteration of the myocardial texture but no change with the ventricle systolic or diastolic function.[55]

Hepatic System

The oral AAS with the 17-alpha alkyl derivatives of testosterone are thought to contribute to the adverse effects the AAS have on the liver. Few liver changes have been found with the use of parenteral AAS doses.[11,18] The length of AAS use is thought to be directly related to the risk of hepatic disease developing.[56]

Elevated liver function studies (SGOT, SGPT) are reported.[54] Most hepatic changes have been documented in individuals who have chronic disease, not in athletes. Thirty-three cases of hepatic tumors were documented; 14 patients were being treated for Fanconi's anemia, whereas 13 others were being treated with long-term AAS for other androgen-responsive illness.[56] Overly et al[56] reported the "first case" of hepatic carcinoma in a 26-year-old body builder who had taken a variety of AAS for 4 years to increase his muscle mass; he died 2 months after the diagnosis was made. He had no known risks factors other than the use of AAS. A rare liver disorder described in patients on long-term AAS is peliosis hepatic with subsequent rupture of the blood-filled sacs; this causes severe hemorrhage and liver failure.[11,25] Cholestatic jaundice has been reported in these same individuals.[11]

Endocrine

Testosterone is converted by the body to estradiol (a hormone more prevalent in women than in men). It is presumed that AAS also converts to estrogenic metabolites.[11,18,32] In the man this may cause irreversible gynecomastia.

Only a few studies in which the female athletes have self-administered the AAS are reported. Thirty-fold increases in serum testosterone levels have been documented; this is accompanied by a decrease in the sex hormone–binding globulin and a decrease in the thyroid-binding proteins.[50,57] The effect testosterone has on the menstrual cycle has been debated. A few studies have indicated there is no change in the menstrual cycle; however, in one such study the dose was 100 mg of testosterone implanted subcutaneously. These doses are much lower than those the female athletes are self-administering.[20,22,57] These researchers believed the menstrual cycle was dependent on progesterone and estradiol and not on the presence of testosterone. Malarkey et al[50] compared female weightlifters who were taking AAS to those who were not. Seven of nine women taking AAS had either amenorrhea or oligomenorrhea; all of the nonusers had normal menses. Spinder et al[58] studied women who became male transsexuals; the long-term dose of testosterone ranged from 6 to 36 months, with a dose of 250 mg/2 wk. No change was reported in the serum estrone and estradiol levels. Structural changes were documented in the ovaries; 69.2% of those studied met the criteria for the pathological diagnosis of polycystic ovaries. Sixty-nine percent had multiple cystic follicles develop; 80.8% had diffuse ovarian stromal hyperplasia.

The data regarding the effect on other hormones remain mixed. Some research indicates a decrease in the luteinizing hormone,[32,50,58] whereas other research shows no change.[20,50,57]

Teratogenic problems were of such concern to the GDR that most of the women being given AAS were also placed on birth control pills.[2] Before the twelfth week of gestation the male or female genitalia develop; if abnormal levels of testosterone are present, even in the female embryo, the male external genitalia and a masculine type of lower urinary tract anatomy will develop. In this same female embryo normal female gonads, fallopian tubes, uterus, cervix, and upper vagina may develop and function as expected.[21,59] After birth, when there is no further exposure to abnormal levels of testosterone, these infants show no further tendencies to virilization or abnormalities of growth or development.

It is the irreversible masculinizing effects that make the risks of taking AAS greater in the female athlete than in the male athlete.[11,50,60,61]

The distribution and increased amount of body hair are a permanent change; it involves growth over the pubis and along the linea alba to the umbilicus. Growth appears on the face and chest more often than on the back. Growth of hair decreases on the top of the head and recession of the scalp line occurs anterolaterally.

The deepening of the voice is a permanent change. Hypertrophy of the laryngeal mucosa and enlargement of the larynx occur.

Clitoral hypertrophy is a permanent change. Breast atrophy and increase in libido are reported to be reversible side effects.

The thickening of bones is a permanent effect. Body physique changes as the shoulders become broader and muscles enlarge.

The skin becomes thicker and more coarse. An increase in the quantities of melatonin given the skin a deeper hue. The increased secretion of the sebaceous glands may cause facial acne.

In the male, testicular atrophy and reversible decreased or abnormal spermatogenesis are reported. Also reported is an increase in the length and width of the penis.

Psychological Effects

Both anecdotal and research reports indicate use of AAS causes an increase in aggression and hostile behavior.[11,62] Pope et al,[63] using the medical diagnostic guidelines, DSM-III-R, studied 41 AAS users. They found 22% of the users had an affective syndrome disorder and 12% were considered to be psychotic. Depression, even suicidal ideation, followed by wide mood swings, has been reported.[11,41,42,62,64]

Several researchers suggested that AAS caused dependency.[42,64,65] With cessation of AAS use the athlete experienced withdrawal symptoms similar to that which would be found by one who was dependent on alcohol, cocaine, or opioids.

Musculoskeletal System

Anecdotal reports have indicated there is an increased risk of injury to the musculotendinous structures.[18] Foss et al[66] used animal studies; no evidence of tendon atrophy or significant change in tendon stiffness or strength qualities was found.

Infections

Users have a tendency to share contaminated needles previously used to inject AAS.[1,67,68] Acquired immunodeficiency syndrome was reportedly transmitted through a shared needle.[68] Abscess infections have been blamed on the nonsterile techniques the athletes use when sharing needles.[1]

Drug Test for AAS Use

The positive results from testing are believed to be far less than those who are actually using the drug.[36] Initially, testing was done only at competition; the athletes were able to use AAS while training without the risk of detection.

Unannounced testing was initiated in the early 1990s by the IAAF, the IOC, and other organizations. The laboratory compares testosterone (T) to epitestosterone (E) as a means of detecting the use of testosterone. The normal male T:E levels rarely exceed a 3:1 ratio. The level used to confirm a positive test is a 6:1 ratio.[69] If a result exceeds the 6:1 ratio, a mandatory investigation is conducted before the sample is declared a positive result. A review is made of previous tests, subsequent tests, and any results of endocrine investigations.

Using the T:E ratio method of identifying users is not foolproof. If the athlete has a naturally low T:E ratio, it is feasible for her to take just enough AAS to raise the ratio and still remain below the abnormal 6:1 ratio. Others have injected epitestosterone propionate to bring the ratio within normal range.[2]

CREATINE

The use of creatine as a food supplement has increased rapidly since early studies in 1990 began to show favorable ergogenic benefits as an energy substrate for muscle contraction. It is usually sold as creatine monohydrate and is readily available in health food stores. Creatine, unlike other ergogenic aids, has not been banned by the IOC or NCAA.

Biochemistry and Availability

Supplemental creatine was found to easily bind to phosphate, thus yielding phosphocreatine (PCr), a source of high-energy phosphate bonds. PCr was found to act as a substrate to donate phosphate for the formation of adenosine triphosphate (ATP). Without ATP, muscular contraction will not occur.[61] The storage capacity for PCr in the muscle fiber is probably limited by functional and storage reasons. Ninety-five percent of creatine is stored in skeletal muscle, especially type II fibers.[5] With high-intensity exercise, PCr stores are depleted after approximately 10 seconds; glycolysis then becomes the sole contributor of anaerobic ATP.[5]

The daily requirement is approximately 2 g.[70,71] Creatine may be found in steak, milk, and some fish. A small amount of creatine is produced in the liver, kidney, and pancreas.[5,72] Women are reported to have a higher total creatine content than men.[73] Creatine is degraded to creatinine and eliminated in the urine. Creatinine is not reabsorbed in the renal tubules.[61]

Studies have used loading doses that ranged from 5 g/day to 30 g/day for 5 days; some continued the study with a maintenance dose of 2 g/day for up to 58 days.[74–77] The greatest amount of increase in the intramuscular stores of creatine occurred during the first few days.[71,76] A more gradual increase in intramuscular stores of creatine was found when lower steady doses of supplement were used.[77]

Those individuals with a lower preloading level of creatine demonstrate the greater amount of uptake into the muscles.[71,76,78] Most research has involved only male athletes; however, Harris et al[76] reported little difference between male and female athletes.

Concomitant exercise and the intake of various foods influence creatine accumulation in skeletal muscle. Exercise with creatine supplementation demonstrates a pronounced enhancement of total creatine content in the muscle and performance more than either creatine or exercise alone.[76,79] Carbohydrates are hypothesized to increase the accumulation of skeletal muscle creatine by an insulin-mediated mechanism of action.[75] Vandenberghe et al[17] unexpectedly found the intake of caffeine with creatine supplementation counteracted the ergogenic actions of creatine loading. The mechanism of action is not known.

Benefits

The benefits of creatine supplementation are greatest in short duration (less than 30 seconds), high-intensity activities.[19,23,74,79,80] As much as a 13% improvement in the athlete's time to exhaustion during an intense, short duration run has been documented.[81] Harris et al[82] showed significant improvements in running times even in the longer distance runs of 1000 m. Most studies have documented the major benefits as an increase in muscle power and muscle strength.[23,33,83,84] Improvements in recovery time after creatine supplementation suggest the increase in total creatine concentration can increase PCr resynthesis shortly after an intense contraction, thus allowing faster recovery times.[78,85,86] Increased total body mass and an increase in fat-free mass have been reported.[19]

The medical use of creatine supplementation in individuals with various neuromuscular diseases has demonstrated an increased high-intensity strength performance and an increase in total lean body mass.[72]

No significant benefits have been found with endurance performance.[23] Thompson et al[70] studied 10 female swimmers using 2 g of creatine per day for 6 weeks. Unlike previous studies, the results showed no effect on muscle concentrations of creatine, no effect on the resynthesis of PCr, no effect on anaerobic muscle metabolism, and no effect on lean body mass.

Adverse Effects

Renal side effects from long-term use are being debated in the literature. Poortmans and Francaux[87] studied nine track athletes (eight men and one woman); two had used varying doses of creatine supplementation for 5 years. The mean duration of use by the group was 2.7 years. These authors found no differences when comparing these athletes with controls regarding the plasma creatine, creatinine, urea, or albumin levels. They concluded no renal metabolic changes had occurred in the group using "long-term" creatine. A case report indicated a 20-year-old man had interstitial nephritis develop after having used 20 g creatine per day for 4 weeks. He fully recovered with cessation of creatine intake.[88]

Because a limited amount of research is available regarding the side effects that may develop with prolonged use, it is recommended that the athlete take creatine supplements for no more than 3 consecutive months.[74] Creatine levels return to normal during the recommended month during which the athlete does not use the supplement.[77] Several authors recommend the resting albumin excretion rate be monitored as a means of identifying early renal dysfunction.[88,89]

It must be remembered that creatine is a food supplement that is not regulated by the FDA. When large doses are taken for an extended period of time, the risk of side effects from impurities (not identified in the product) is a potential hazard.

Performance Effects of Creatine Supplementation

- Increased time to exhaustion in sprint activities
- Increased muscle power
- Increased muscle strength
- Faster recovery times

Clinical Guideline

GROWTH HORMONE

Human growth hormone (GH) is a protein molecule produced and stored in the anterior pituitary gland.[11,61] It exerts its effects on all tissues of the body capable of growing. It is capable of increasing the size of cells and the number of cells.[18,61] GH increases amino acid transportation into tissues where it is synthesized to protein. It may increase lean body weight by mobilizing lipids from adipose tissue; the lipids are then used as energy sources.[18]

Biochemistry and Availability

The increase in the use of GH has developed for several reasons. Before 1985, the hormone was taken from cadavers and was not easily obtained; after 1985, it was synthetically engineered using recombinant DNA technology and became more readily available.[11,18,40] With the onset of testing for AAS, in 1984 athletes turned to the use of GH to maintain the benefits they had derived from the AAS after they were forced to stop the AAS to avoid detection at competitions.[11] Use is no longer limited to the elite level of athlete. Rickert

et al[90] found that 5% of male tenth graders had used GH and only 0.5% of the females (1 of 202) had used it. Most of the 426 students questioned were unaware of the potential side effects from the use of GH. Those who obtain GH on the black market are most likely to be using either the hormone from cadavers or some unknown compound being falsely distributed (ie, the marketing of "rhesus growth hormone" is thought to be highly unlikely because of the scarcity of the animal).[18]

The amount of GH secreted by an individual may vary. Higher levels of estrogen in females during the menstrual cycle generate higher levels of growth hormone production.[18] Psychological and physical stress increases the serum GH concentration.[18,91] Tenfold increases in GH levels were found 1 hour after recovery from sprint activity. A greater increase in GH levels was found among sprinters compared with endurance-trained athletes.[91] The level of physical activity described as a stimulus was 20 minutes of exercise at 75% of maximum oxygen uptake.[18] Exercise-induced muscle growth involves new ribonucleic acid (RNA) synthesis; GH supplemented growth results from an increase in the rate and translation of already existing RNA.[92]

Use

GH has been used medically to treat Turner's syndrome, GH-deficient children, and children with short stature.

Several studies have not shown improvements in muscle size or changes in protein synthesis rates in the muscles.[93,94] Anecdotal reports and other research support the hypothesis that with increased protein synthesis, more than protein breakdown, there is an increase in lean body weight with an increase in muscle mass.[18,93,95] Crist et al[95] indicated the changes reported were dose dependent. Reports indicate athletes are using much larger doses (some twentyfold greater) than those used for therapeutic reasons.[11]

Adverse Effects

Adverse side effects reported with long-term use include acromegaly, hypothyroidism, hypercholesterolemia, coronary artery disease, menstrual irregularities, impotence, myopathies, glucose intolerance–diabetes mellitus, Hodgkin's lymphoma, leukemia, and osteoporosis.[11,18,96,97] The risk of Creutzfeldt-Jakob disease persists with the use of GH obtained from cadavers.[98]

GH was added to the list of banned drugs by the IOC in 1988.[36] However, no test is available to differentiate the exogenous hormone from the normal endogenous hormone.

BLOOD DOPING

Blood doping refers to any technique that attempts to increase the red blood cell (RBC) count with the goal of increasing the oxygen-carrying capacity of the blood, thus improving exercise performance. Attempts to induce erythrocythemia have included the use of autologous and homologous transfusions, hypoxia that accompanies altitude training, and administration of erythropoietin (EPO). The first documented use of blood doping was in 1976 at the Olympic Games in Montreal.[11] In the 1984 Summer Games in Los Angeles, the US men's cycling team confessed to having received transfusions before competition.[99,100] Although blood doping was banned by the IOC in 1985, there has been no technique developed to identify those who are using this ergogenic aid.[36,101]

Transfusions

The technique of autologous transfusions has been well defined in the literature.[11,102] Refer to Figure 23–1 for the time course of hematology changes after the removal and reinfusion of blood. Approximately 900 mL of blood is withdrawn from the athlete, ideally 5 to 6 weeks before the planned reinfusion date. An immediate decrease of 11% was found in the hemoglobin (Hb) and hematocrit (Hct) of the donors.[102] Gradually over the next 6 weeks the body responds to the relative anemia by increasing the production of RBCs and the Hb and Hct return to normal. The means of storage of the donated blood is important. In the United States blood may be refrigerated at 4°C for a maximum of 21 days. During this time approximately 30% to 35% of the RBCs are lost to normal aging; the normal half-life of the RBC is 120 days. The RBCs are more fragile after refrigeration; because of this, additional RBCs are lost at the time of infusion. Blood may be frozen using a high

glycerol freeze technique at –80°C for up to 10 years. This technique interrupts the aging process of the cell. Only 10% to 15% of the RBCs are lost during storage. No further loss occurs at the time of reinfusion, because the RBCs are not considered to be more fragile than normal.[103] After the blood is reinfused, the Hb and Hct reached an 11% elevation after the first week; this was followed by a linear decline of Hb over the next 15 weeks until the normal levels were reached.[102]

The improvement in physical performance was found to be correlated with the increase in blood volume achieved up to approximately a Hb concentration level of 210 g/L.[46,104] Early studies that either did not withdraw sufficient amounts of blood or did not store the blood long enough for the body to replenish the loss failed to demonstrate improvement in performance.[105] Blood doping improves the performance of endurance events.[11,45,104,106] Blood doping was found to provide a thermoregulatory advantage that was not related to hydration status, especially in heat-acclimated athletes.[99] It reduced heat storage and increased sweating sensitivity.

A hypothesized medical concern is the danger of a "thicker" blood, especially the increased concentration of RBCs that may further result from dehydration. Concern is for cardiac changes that may develop from the increased stress on the heart or from the increased risk of thrombotic or embolic events. Increases in Hb concentration have not altered the stroke volume or the heart rate during maximal exercise.[46,102] Electrocardiograms after exercise have shown no abnormalities or suggestion of ischemia.[102]

The risks of disease or reactions associated with homologous transfusions are a concern. In the United States, the risk associated with receiving one unit of screened and

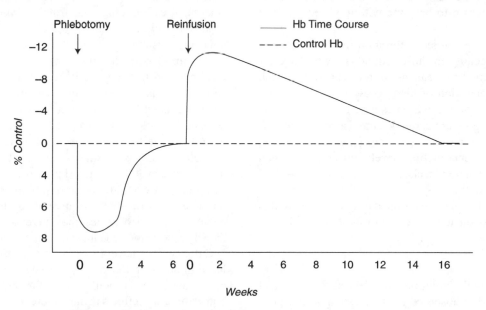

Figure 23–1 Time Course of Hematology Changes after the Removal and Reinfusion of ~900 mL of Autologous Freeze-Preserved Blood.

tested RBC is 1 in 200,000 for hepatitis B and between 1 and 3 in 10,000 for hepatitis C.[99] The risk of human immunodeficiency virus infection varies within the geographical regions of the United States. The risk of clerical error, bacterial infection, or serum reaction may cause serious side effects or death.

Altitude Training

Attempts to increase the RBCs through altitude training have been hindered by the "detraining" that occurs when the athlete is not able to perform to a maximal exercise capacity as she acclimates to the altitude. Altitude training can induce a 10% increase in the Hb. When the athlete returned to sea level, a 25% improvement in exercise endurance capacity was found.[102]

Erythropoietin

EPO is a glycoprotein hormone that regulates the production of RBCs in the bone marrow. It is produced by interstitial cells in the peritubular capillary bed of the adult kidneys and the perivenous hepatocytes in the liver.[11,107] Recombinant human EPO became available in 1985 after the gene that codes EPO was cloned.[11] With subcutaneous injection, EPO has a half-life of 20 hours but will increase the RBC production for a maximum of 2 weeks after that. EPO can be detected in the serum for 3 days after the injection and in the urine for 2 days.[99] EPO is used medically to treat uremic anemia, neoplastic disease, prematurity, and hemochromatosis.[108]

The ergogenic benefits of EPO are similar to those gained from transfusions.[99] The maximal aerobic power and physical performance were enhanced. The maximal aerobic power was reported to return to baseline within 3 weeks of the injection.[109]

The cause of the significant elevation in blood pressure documented, especially in those individuals who have received EPO for medical reasons, is not well understood. Reports of mild elevation of blood pressure have been reported in the healthy athlete. Studies have demonstrated the elevation in blood pressure paralleled the rise in Hct.[99,107,108] Research is implicating microcirculatory factors, including changes in plasma endothelin-1 levels, in factor VIII von Willebrand factor antigen levels, and in thromboxane A_2 and prostacyclin levels.[108]

EPO was placed on the IOC banned drug list in 1988. It is difficult to identify the users because of its short half-life.

CAFFEINE

Caffeine is a methylxanthine found in numerous plant species. It is quickly absorbed after ingestion with a peak blood value being reached within 30 minutes.[11,110] Reportedly, it has been used by athletes for many years; it is readily available and reports purport the benefits of this ergogenic aid.[111]

An improvement in endurance performance has been reported with the use of caffeine.[11,110,112,113] Costill et al[112,113] believed the onset of exhaustion could be delayed if muscle glycogen was spared. Caffeine enhances the rate of lipid catabolism during which the oxidation of fatty acids provides the initial energy source, thus sparing the glycogen. Varying degrees of improvement have been reported ranging from a 7.4% increase in work production with caffeine ingestion of 250 mg to a 19.5% improvement in endurance activities with ingestion of 330 mg. The latter study by Costill et al measured the performance of nine (two female) competitive cyclists; no differences were described between the sexes. Some research has failed to show an improvement in the time to exhaustion, even though an elevation in the fatty acid levels was reported. An earlier study by Perkins and Williams[114] studied 14 female cyclists who pedaled to exhaustion after ingesting 4 mg, 7 mg, and 10 mg caffeine per kilogram of body weight; no change in performance was documented.[110] Athletes have reported less difficult endurance performances after the ingestion of caffeine.[112] The mechanism for this is not well understood. Costill et al suggested an increase in neuronal excitability. They indicated that a reduction in the excitability threshold of the neurons may lower the threshold for muscle fiber recruitment and nerve transmission, thus making the activity seem easier. Other studies suggest caffeine may potentiate the role of hormones as neurotransmitters or perhaps increase the muscle contractility.[11]

Caffeine can be found in numerous food sources and medications (both over the counter and prescription). Refer to the Clinical Guideline for a list of caffeine sources, the amount of caffeine ingested from a given source, and the expected level of caffeine detected in the urine after 2 or 3 hours of ingestion.

Caffeine has been banned by the IOC; the maximum level allowed in the urine is 12 µg/mL.[115] Potentially far less caffeine is needed to act as an ergogenic benefit. The athletes studied by Costill et al[112] ingested 330 mg of caffeine 60 minutes before exercise; they demonstrated a 19.5% improved time to exhaustion. By referring to the Clinical Guideline, this would suggest the level of caffeine in the urine would be 4.95 µg/mL (far below the banned level of 12 µg/mL). It would be difficult to compete after ingesting multiple cups of coffee. A source of caffeine not previously mentioned is suppositories; they were used by US cyclers at the Olympic Summer Games in Los Angeles in 1984.[111]

Caffeine does have a variety of side effects in some athletes. In doses of 3 g to 10 g, it has caused seizures, tachycardia, and even ventricular dysrhythmias.[11] Less serious but bothersome side effects include increased anxiety, insomnia,

Caffeine Sources[110,114]

Source	Amount/Dose Ingested	Equivalent in Urine within 2–3 h
Decaffeinated coffee	2–5 mg	
Coffee	100 mg	1.50 µg/mL
Mountain Dew	54 mg	0.75 µg/mL
No Doz	100 mg	1.50 µg/mL
Anacin	32 mg	0.48 µg/mL
Cafergot	100 mg	1.50 µg/mL
Excedrin	65 mg	0.97 µg/mL
Fiorinal	50 mg	0.60 µg/mL
Midol	332 mg	0.48 µg/mL
Vivarin	200 mg	3.00 µg/mL

mg = milligrams; µg/mL = micrograms/milliliter.

Clinical Guideline

diarrhea, irritability, urine production, and withdrawal headaches.[110]

CONCLUSION—FUTURE DIRECTIONS

The cat (authority) and mouse (athlete using ergogenic aids) game will continue. As the pressures to win continue to escalate, the athlete and/or her "support" personnel will look for every means of gaining any possible advantage. Even though the drug testing equipment (high-resolution mass spectrometer) and tests become more elaborate, new sophisticated pharmacological methods continue to be created to enhance athletic performance.

Urine will continue to be the body fluid most likely tested for use of banned substances over the next several years. Some authorities still support the benefits of blood sampling; blood is needed to detect EPO and human GH or markers of their use. Others indicate that until guidelines have been determined to indicate abnormal levels of EPO, GH, and so on, little more would be determined from the blood than can now be obtained from the urine samples.

The International Skiing Federation used blood sampling as a part of doping control during a World Championship competition.[116] Ninety-nine athletes had blood samples drawn by the IAAF in 1993–1994.[116] One female athlete was found to have a grossly elevated testosterone level. Measurements of hemoglobin levels, EPO, GH, and insulin-like growth factor 1 did not suggest misuse in those athletes. However, some levels for testosterone and EPO were unexpectedly lower than the controls. Because of the sensitivity of blood testing, the importance of special circumstances (what time of day the sample is taken, the training environment of the athlete, the degree of strenuous activity that preceded the sample) needs to be taken into account.

Before blood sampling is used as the universal ans of detecting the use of banned substances, further research is needed to focus on developing more sensitive and specific tests to detect doping with endogenous substances. Also, tamperproof methods of collecting and processing blood samples would need to be established.

The purpose of drug testing is to maintain a fair and safe environment among all athletes. Drug testing programs must evaluate the athlete in competition and during the training period. Out-of-competition testing (short notice or no notice) is needed to address the use of "training" drugs such as anabolic steroids.

The IOC is reevaluating the drug test procedures and penalties. The United States Olympic Committee (USOC) has restructured the drug control program to "externalize" it immediately after the 2000 Summer Olympics. A Summit organized by USOC held in 1998 determined that drug testing of the elite athlete should be removed from direct control by the USOC because of a possible conflict of interest. The US AntiDoping Agency assumed the responsibility of testing athletes October 1, 2000. It is no longer under the management of the USOC. The NCAA continues to expand the testing program to athletes in sports other than track and field and football.

REFERENCES

1. Breo DL. Of MDs and muscles—lessons from two 'retired steroid doctors'. *JAMA*. 1990;263:1697–1705.

2. Franke WW, Berendonk B. Hormonal doping and androgenization of athletes: A secret program of the German Democratic Republic government. *Clin Chem*. 1997;43:1262–1279.

3. Results of 6th IAAF World Championships in Athletics Athena. 1997; www.iaaf.org/results/past/WCH97/data/W/HJ/Rf.html ww.iaaf.org/results/past/WCH97/data/W/100/Rf.html.

4. Results of 1999 Pan American Games, Winnipeg. 1999; www.swiminfo.com/results/published/267.asp.

5. Kokotailo PK, Henry BC, Koscik RE, Fleming MF, Landry GL. Substance use and other health risk behaviors in collegiate athletes. *Clin J Sport Med*. 1996;6:183–189.

6. Goldman R, Bush P, Klatz R. *Death in the Locker Room*. S. Bend, IN: Icarus Press; 1995.

7. USOC Drug Control Administration Division. United States Olympic Committee National Anti-Doping Program Policies and Procedures. Colorado Springs, CO.

8. Buckley WE, Yesalis CE, Friedl KE, Anderson WA, Streit AL, Wright JE. Estimated prevalence of anabolic steroid use among male high school seniors. *JAMA*. 1988;260:3441–3445.

9. Chng CL, Moore A. A study of steroid use among athletes: Knowledge, attitude and use. *Health Educ*. 1990;21:12–17.

10. DuRant RH, Rickert VI, Ashworth CS, Newman C, Slavens G. Use of multiple drugs among adolescents who use anabolic steroids. *N Engl J Med*. 1993;328:922–926.

11. Knopp WD, Thomas WW, Bach BR. Ergogenic drugs in sports. *Clin Sports Med*. 1997;16:375–392.

12. Scott DM, Wagner JC, Barlow TW. Anabolic steroid use among adolescents in Nebraska schools. *Am J Health-System Pharm*. 1996;53:2068–2072.

13. Associated Press. Top athletes questioning drug testing methods of IAAF. *Columbus Dispatch*. 8/20/99:9C.

14. Associated Press. Food supplements may be causing positive tests. *Columbus Dispatch*. 8/21/99.

15. Catlin D, Wright J, Pope H, Liggett M. Assessing the threat of anabolic steroids. *Phys Sportsmed*. 1993;21:37–44.

16. Strauss RH, Yesalis CE. Additional effects of anabolic steroids on women. In: Yesalis CE, ed. *Anabolic Steroids in Sports and Exercise*. Champaign, IL: Human Kinetics; 1993:35–48.

17. Vandenberghe K, Gillis N, Van Leemputte M, Van Hecke P, Vanstapel F, Hespel P. Caffeine counteracts the ergogenic action of muscle creatine loading. *J Appl Physiol*. 1996;80:452–457.

18. Haupt HA. Substance abuse by the athlete female. In: Pearl AJ, ed. *The Athletic Female*. Champaign, IL: Human Kinetics; 1993:125–140.

19. Kreider RB, Ferreira M, Wilson M, et al. Effects of creatine supplementation on body composition, strength, and sprint performance. *Med Sci Sports Exerc*. 1998;30:73–82.

20. Dewis P, Newman M, Ratcliffe WA, Anderson DC. Does testosterone affect the normal menstrual cycle? *Clin Endocrinol*. 1986;24:515–521.

21. Ganong WF. *Review of Medical Physiology*. Los Altos, CA: Lange Medical Publications; 1979.

22. Honour JW. Steroid abuse in female athletes. *Curr Opin Obstet Gynecol*. 1997;9:181–186.

23. Engelhardt M, Newmann G, Berbalk A, Reuter I. Creatine supplementation in endurance sports. *Med Sci Sports Exerc*. 1998;30:1123–1129.

24. Bjorkhem I, Lantto O, Lof A. Detection and quantitation of methandienone (Dianabol) in urine by isotope dilution—mass fragmentography. *J Steroid Biochem*. 1980;13:169–175.

25. Lamb DR. Anabolic steroids in athletics: How well do they work and how dangerous are they? *Am J Sports Med*. 1984;12:31–38.

26. Burkett LN, Falduto MT. Steroid use by athletes in a metropolitan area. *Phys Sportsmed*. 1984;12:69–74.

27. Peterson GE, Fahey TD. HDL-C in five elite athletes using anabolic-androgenic steroids. *Phys Sportsmed*. 1984;12:120–130.

28. Bjorkhem I, Ek H. Detection and quantitation of 19-norandrosterone in urine by isotope dilution-mass spectrometry. *J Steroid Biochem*. 1982;17:447–451.

29. Strauss RH, Liggett MT, Lanese RR. Anabolic steroid use and perceived effects in ten weight-trained women athletes. *JAMA*. 1985;253:2871–2873.

30. Frankle MA, Cicero GJ, Payne J. Use of androgenic anabolic steroids by athletes. *JAMA*. 1984;252:482.

31. Coward VS. If youngsters overdose with anabolic steroids what's the cost anatomically and otherwise? *JAMA*. 1989;261:1856–1857.

32. Million MB. Anabolic steroids in athletes. *Am Family Pract*. 1984;30:113–119.

33. Earnest CP, Snell PG, Rodriguez R, Almada AL, Mitchell TL. The effect of creatine monohydrate ingestion on anaerobic power indices, muscular strength and body composition. *Acta Physiol Scand*. 1995;53:207–209.

34. Council on Scientific Affairs. Medical and nonmedical uses of anabolic-androgenic steroids. *JAMA*. 1990;264:2923–2927.

35. Elashoff JD, Jacknow AD, Shain SG, Braunstein GD. Effects of anabolic-androgenic steroids on muscular strength. *Ann Intern Med*. 1991;115:387–393.

36. Catlin DH, Murray TH. Performance-enhancing drugs, fair competition, and Olympic sport. *JAMA*. 1996;276:231–237.

37. Yesalis CE, Kennedy NJ, Kopstein AN, Bahrke MS. Anabolic-androgenic steroid use in the United States. *JAMA*. 1993;270:1217–1221.

38. Lindstrom M, Nilsson AL, Katzman PL, Janzon L, Dymling JF. Use of anabolic-androgenic steroids among body builders—frequency and attitudes. *J Intern Med*. 1990;227:407–411.

39. Kouri EM, Pope HG, Katz DL. Use of anabolic-androgenic steroids: We are talking prevalence rates. *JAMA*. 1994;271:347.

40. Alzado. L. I'm sick and I'm scared. *Sports Illustrated*. 1991:21–26.

41. Hannon K. What price glory? *The Main Event*. 1988;Apr:13–14.

42. Hays LR, Littleton S, Stillner V. Anabolic steroid dependence. *Am J Psychiatry*. 1990;147:122.

43. Hurley BF, Seals DR, Hagberg JM, et al. High-density-lipoprotein cholesterol in bodybuilders v powerlifters. Negative effects of androgen use. *JAMA*. 1984;252:507–513.

44. Yesalis CE, Bahrke MS. Anabolic-androgenic steroids: Current issues. *Sports Med*. 1995;19:326–340.

45. Brien AJ, Simon TL. The effects of red blood cell infusion on 10-km race time. *JAMA*. 1987;257:2761–2765.

46. Ekblom B. Blood doping and erythropoietin: The effects of variation in hemoglobin concentration and other related factors on physical performance. *Am J Sports Med*. 1996;24(Suppl):S40–S42.

47. Alen M, Hakkinen K, Komi PV. Changes in neuromuscular performance and muscle fiber characteristics of elite power athletes self-

administering androgenic and anabolic steroids. *Acta Physiol Scand.* 1989;122:535–544.

48. Costill DL, Pearson DR, Fink WJ. Anabolic steroid use among athletes: Changes in HDL-C levels. *Phys Sportsmed.* 1984;12:113–117.

49. Moffatt RF, Wallace MB, Sady SP. Effects of anabolic steroids on lipoprotein profiles of female weight lifters. *Phys Sportsmed.* 1990;8:106–110.

50. Malarkey WB, Strauss RH, Leizman DJ, Liggett M, Demers LM. Endocrine effects in female weight lifters who self-administer testosterone and anabolic steroids. *Am J Obstet Gynecol.* 1991;165:1385–1390.

51. Webb OL, Laskarzewski PM, Gleuck CJ. Severe depression of high-density lipoprotein cholesterol levels in weight lifters and body builders by self-administered exogenous testosterone and anabolic-androgenic steroids. *Metabolism.* 1984;33:971–975.

52. Kantor MA, Bianchini A, Bernier D, Sady SP, Thompson PD. Androgens reduce HLD2-cholesterol and increase hepatic triglyceride lipase activity. *Med Sci Sports Exerc.* 1985;17:462–465.

53. *Physicians' Desk Reference.* Montvale, NJ: Medical Economics Company; 1999.

54. Frankle MA, Eichberg R, Zachariah SB. Anabolic-androgenic steroids and a stroke in an athlete: Case report. *Arch Phys Med Rehabil.* 1988;69:632–633.

55. DiBello V, Giorgi D, Bianchi M, et al. Effects of anabolic-androgenic steroids on weight-lifter's myocardium: An ultrasonic videodensitometric study. *Med Sci Sports Exerc.* 1999;31:514–521.

56. Overly WL, Dankoff JA, Wang BK, Singh UD. Androgens and hepatocellular carcinoma in an athlete. *Ann Intern Med.* 1984;100:158–159.

57. Dewis P, Newman M, Ratcliffe WA, Anderson DC. Does testosterone affect the normal menstrual cycle? *Clin Endocrinol.* 1986;24:515–521.

58. Spinder T, Spijkstra JJ, van den Tweel JG, et al. The effects of long term testosterone administration on pulsatile luteinizing hormone secretion and on ovarian histology in eugonadal female to male transsexual subjects. *J Clin Endocrinol Metab.* 1989;69:151–157.

59. Green TH. *Gynecology Essentials of Clinical Practice.* Boston: Little, Brown & Co; 1977.

60. AMA Council on Scientific Affairs. Drug abuse in athletes: Anabolic steroids and human growth hormone. *JAMA.* 1988;259:1703–1705.

61. Guyton AC. *Textbook of Medical Physiology.* Philadelphia: WB Saunders; 1976.

62. Pope HG, Katz DL. Psychiatric effects of anabolic steroids. *Psychiatric Ann.* 1992; 22:24–29.

63. Pope HG, Katz DL. Affective and psychotic symptoms associated with anabolic steroid use. *Am J Psychiatry.* 1988;145:487–490.

64. Kashkin KB, Kleber HD. Hooked on hormones? *JAMA.* 1989;262:3166–3170.

65. Rosse RB, Deutsch SI. Hooked on hormones? [letter] *JAMA.* 1990;263:2048–2049.

66. Foss ML, Goldin B, Plotkin M, Mackie MS. Effects of steroid drugs on the strength of cartilage and tendons. In: Craig T, ed. *The Medical Aspects of Sports: 16.* Chicago: AMA; 1974:25–30.

67. Rich JD, Dickinson BP, Flanigan TP, Valone SE. Abscess related to anabolic-androgenic steroid injection. *Med Sci Sports Exerc.* 1999;31:207–209.

68. Scott MJ, Scott MJ. HIV infection associated with injections of anabolic steroids. *JAMA.* 1989;262:207–208.

69. Wallach J. Athletes and steroid drugs. *JAMA.* 1984;252:565–566.

70. Thompson CH, Kemp GJ, Sanderson AL, et al. Effect of creatine on aerobic and anaerobic metabolism in skeletal muscle in swimmers. *Br J Sports Med.* 1996;30:222–225.

71. Ekblom B. Effects of creatine supplementation on performance. *Am J Sports Med.* 1996;24:S38–S39.

72. Tarnopolsky M, Martin J. Creatine monohydrate increases strength in patients with neuromuscular disease. *Neurology.* 1999;52:854–857.

73. Forsberg AM, Nilsson E, Werneman J, Bergstrom J, Hultman E. Muscle composition in relation to age and sex. *Clin Sci.* 1991;81:249–256.

74. Feldman E. Creatine: A dietary supplement and ergogenic aid. *Nutr Rev.* 1999;57:45–50.

75. Green AL, Hultman E, MacDonald IA, Sewell DA, Greenhaff PL. Carbohydrate ingestion augments skeletal muscle creatine accumulation during creatine supplementation in humans. *Am J Physiol.* 1996;271:E821–E826.

76. Harris RC, Soderlund K, Hultman E. Elevation of creatine in resting and exercised muscle of normal subjects by creatine supplementation. *Clin Sci.* 1992;83:367–374.

77. Hultman E, Soderlund K, Timmons JA, Cederblad G, Greenhaff PL. Muscle creatine loading in men. *J Appl Physiol.* 1996;81:232–237.

78. Greenhaff PL, Bodin K, Soderlund K, Hultman E. Effect of oral creatine supplementation on skeletal muscle phosphocreatine resynthesis. *Am J Physiol.* 1994;266:E725–E730.

79. Brannon TA, Adams GR, Conniff C, Baldwin KM. Effects of creatine loading and training on running performance and biochemical properties of rat skeletal muscle. *Med Sci Sports Exerc.* 1997;29:489–495.

80. Casey AD, Constantin-Teodosin S, Howell E, Hultman E, Greenhaff PL. Creatine ingestion favorably affects performance and muscle metabolism during maximal exercise in humans. *Am J Physiol.* 1996;271:E31–E37.

81. Bosco C, Tihanyi J, Pucspk J, Kovacs I, Gabossy A, Colli R. Effect of oral creatine supplementation on jumping and running performance. *Int J Sports Med.* 1997;18:369–372.

82. Harris RC, Viru M, Greenhaff PL, Hultman E. The effect of oral creatine supplementation on running performance during maximal short term exercise in man. *J Physiol.* 1993;467:74P.

83. Birch R, Noble D, Greenhaff PL. The influence of dietary creatine supplementation on performance during repeated bouts of maximal isokinetic cycling in man. *Eur J Appl Physiol.* 1994;69:268–270.

84. Greenhaff PL, Case A, Short AH, Harris R, Soderlund K, Hultman E. Influence of oral creatine supplementation on muscle torque during repeated bouts of maximal voluntary exercise in man. *Clin Sci.* 1993;84:565–571.

85. Greenhaff PL, Constantin-Teodosiu D, Case A, Hultman E. The effects of oral creatine supplementation on skeletal muscle ATP degradation during repeated bouts of maximal voluntary exercise in man. *J Physiol.* 1994;476:84P.

86. Cooke WH, Grandjean PW, Barnes WS. Effect of oral creatine supplementation on power output and fatigue during bicycle ergometry. *J Appl Physiol.* 1995;78:670–673.

87. Poortmans JR, Francaux M. Long-term oral creatine supplementation does not impair renal function in healthy athletes. *Med Sci Sports Exerc.* 1999;31:1108–1110.

88. Koshy KM, Griswold E. Interstitial nephritis in a patient taking creatine. *N Engl J Med.* 1999;340:814–815.

89. Greenhoff P. Renal dysfunction accompanying oral creatine supplements. *Lancet.* 1998;352:233.

90. Rickert V, Pawlak-Morello C, Sheppard V, Jay MS. Human growth hormone: A new substance of abuse among adolescents. *Clin Pediatr.* 1992;31:723–726.

91. Nevill ME, Holmyard DJ, Hall GM, et al. Growth hormone responses to treadmill sprinting in sprint- and endurance-trained athletes. *Eur J Appl Physiol Occup Physiol.* 1996;72:460–467.

92. Rogol AD. Growth hormone: Physiology, therapeutic use, and potential for abuse. *Exerc Sport Sci Rev.* 1989;17:353–377.

93. Yarasheski KE, Campbell JA, Smith K, Rennie MJ, Holloszy JO, Bier DM. Effect of growth hormone and resistance exercise on muscle growth in young men. *Am J Physiol.* 1992;262:E261–E267.

94. Yarasheski KE, Zachwieja JJ, Angelopoulos TJ, Bier DM. Short-term growth hormone treatment does not increase muscles protein synthesis in experienced weight lifters. *J Appl Physiol.* 1993;4:3073–3076.

95. Christ DM, Peake GT, Egan PA, Waters DL. Body composition response to exogenous GH during training in highly conditioned adults. *J Appl Physiol.* 1988;65:579–584.

96. Magnavita N. Hodgkin's lymphoma in a cyclist treated with growth hormone. *Am J Hematol.* 1996;52:65–66.

97. Magnavita N, Sica S, DiMario A, Leone G. Concurrent epiphyseal fracture and leukemia in a patient treated with growth hormone. *Am J Hematol.* 1996;51:95–96.

98. Dyer C. Growth hormone deaths blamed on MRC and DoH. *BMJ.* 1996;313:185.

99. American College of Sports Medicine. Position statement on the use of blood doping as an ergogenic aid. *Med Sci Sports Exerc.* 1996;28:i–viii.

100. Legwold G. Blood doping and the letter of the law. *Phys Sportsmed.* 1985;13:37–38.

101. Nash HL. New techniques may catch blood dopers. *Phys Sportsmed.* 1986;14:36–37.

102. Gledhill N. Blood doping and related issues: A brief review. *Med Sci Sports Exerc.* 1982;14:183–189.

103. Gledhill N. The ergogenic effect of blood doping. *Phys Sportsmed.* 1983;11:87–90.

104. Kanstrup I, Ekblom B. Blood volume and hemoglobin concentration as determinants of maximal aerobic power. *Med Sci Sports Exerc.* 1984; 6:256–262.

105. Williams MH, Lindhjem M, Schuster R. The effect of blood infusion upon endurance capacity and ratings of perceived exertion. *Med Sci Sport.* 1978;10:113–118.

106. Williams MH, Wisseldine S, Somma T, Schuster R. The effect of induced erythrocythemia upon 5-mile treadmill run time. *Med Sci Sport Exerc.* 1981;13:169–175.

107. Vaziri ND. Mechanism of erythropoietin-induced hypertension. *Am J Kidney Dis.* 1999;33:821–828.

108. Navarro JF, Mora C, Marcia ML. Elevation of blood pressure after erythropoietin therapy. *Am J Med.* 1996;101:329–330.

109. Ekblom B, Berglund B. Effect of erythropoietin administration on maximal aerobic power. *Scand J Med Sci Sports.* 1991; 88–93.

110. Slavin JL, Joensen DJ. Caffeine and sports performance. *Phys Sportsmed.* 1985;13:191–193.

111. Rogers CC. Cyclists try caffeine suppositories. *Phys Sportsmed.* 1985;13:39–40.

112. Costill DL, Dalsky GP, Fink WJ. Effects of caffeine ingestion on metabolism and exercise performance. *Med Sci Sports.* 1978;10:155–158.

113. Ivy JL, Costill DL, Fink WJ, Lower RW. Role of caffeine and glucose ingestion on metabolism during exercise. *Med Sci Sports.* 1979;11:6–11.

114. Perkins R, Williams M. Effects of caffeine upon maximal muscular endurance of females. *Med Sci Sports.* 1975;7:221–224.

115. Exum W, ed. *U.S. Olympic Committee Drug Education Handbook.* Colorado Springs, CO: USOC; 1996.

116. Birkeland KI, Ljungqvist A, Fagerhol M, et al. Blood sampling in doping control. *Int J Sports Med.* 1997;18:8–12.

CHAPTER 24

The Use of Recreational Drugs by Female Athletes

Amie S. Ward

INTRODUCTION

Drug abuse remains a significant health problem. An estimated 13 to 14 million Americans use illicit drugs, and 4.5% of American women currently use illegal drugs.[1] In the past decade, the media has brought the use of drugs of abuse by professional athletes to national attention, and large-scale efforts have been launched by such agencies as the International Olympic Committee (IOC), National Collegiate Athletic Association (NCAA), National Football League (NFL), National Basketball Association (NBA), and others to study the prevalence of drug use, institute relevant drug-testing policy, and generate aggressive educational programs. This chapter will focus on the use of "recreational" drugs by female athletes, with particular focus on prevalence of use as a function of drug class, medical and social consequences of such use with particular attention to female athletic conditioning and performance, and therapeutic approaches to the clinical management of the female substance abuser. Much of the information contained in this chapter is not specific to females, however, because many of the issues surrounding drug abuse are similar for both sexes and, until recently, very little research in the field of drug abuse has examined sex differences. Fortunately, in the last few years, the National Institute on Drug Abuse has rigorously promoted research designed to explain gender differences in drug abuse. For an update of ongoing research in this area, go to www.nida.nih.gov/STRC/Role6.html.

PREVALENCE

Why would a highly paid, world-renowned, well-respected sports figure risk career, family, and reputation to use an illicit substance? In fact, status may actually increase the likelihood of drug use among professional athletes. Celebrities such as nationally recognized athletes have less perceived risk of their drug use being discovered and even less perceived risk that it will be penalized. Recent surveys have indicated that the nonmedical use of drugs among athletes parallels drug use among nonathletes.[2,3] Furthermore, the prevalence of drug use among female athletes does not differ significantly from that of male athletes.[4]

The pressure for female athletes to succeed in competition is no less than for male athletes.[4] Increased participation in sports by women has fostered intensified competition, with a corresponding rise in the use of illicit drugs. The traditional performance enhancers, such as anabolic steroids, have been thoroughly discussed in Chapter 23. However, drugs that are typically abused by nonathletes for "recreational" purposes, such as amphetamines, cocaine, and ephedrine, can be perceived by athletes to have performance-enhancing and weight-reduction properties. The pressure to perform produces stress, which is compounded by the stress of training and the stress of time constraints. These stressors may be greater for female athletes, who often have to balance training and competition with family care responsibilities. As in the general population, female athletes often use drugs such as alcohol to relieve stress. In fact, national studies indicate that female athletes have higher rates of binge drinking than their nonathlete counterparts (50% vs 30%).[5,6]

Although recreational substance abuse by male athletes has been fairly widely studied, considerably less attention has been given to the use of drugs of abuse by female athletes. Several epidemiological studies have reported that the use of recreational drugs by female athletes has risen sharply since 1989. Alcohol is the most commonly used recreational substance, with approximately 49% of female athletes reporting occasional binge drinking, whereas 47% report consumption of more than four drinks per week. A recent survey administered to athletes at 125 universities indicated that 65% of female athletes reported having hangovers, 57% have had nausea or vomiting associated with drinking, 25% had impaired academic performance, 35% engaged in fights or arguments while intoxicated, 37% suffered memory loss after drinking, and 14% had legal troubles associated with drinking.[7]

The illicit use of amphetamines by female athletes is a serious concern, because these drugs are used for their perceived ergogenic properties and anorectic effects, as well as their general mood-enhancing properties. Amphetamines are dependence-producing and are associated with a pronounced abstinence syndrome, so it is quite likely that the athlete who initiates amphetamine use to enhance athletic performance on a regular basis will develop tolerance and dependence on the drug. Because amphetamine use for performance enhancement is extremely prevalent among athletes, it is difficult to determine the prevalence of recreational amphetamine use. In general, 42.9% of athletes report using amphetamines to improve athletic performance, and 20% report using amphetamines for extra energy.

The prevalence of cocaine/crack use among athletes has decreased over the past 10 years, despite the few widely publicized reports of cocaine-related arrests of several prominent professional male athletes. Data on cocaine use by female athletes are limited, but it is generally assumed that this population is not widely affected by cocaine abuse.

Marijuana use, which has shown an upward trend in the past 10 years in the general population, has likely followed the same trend among athletes. Whereas 23% of athletes reported using marijuana in 1983,[8] a more recent survey estimates that 29% of male college athletes and 25% of female college athletes currently smoke marijuana cigarettes compared with 41% and 34% of their respective nonathlete counterparts.

The use of smokeless tobacco by female athletes has also risen sharply in the past 10 years, despite a decrease among the general population. Although very few women reported use of smokeless tobacco in 1989, 11% of female athletes currently report regular use of smokeless tobacco.

There are no data to support the premise that depressant use is particularly problematic among female athletes. Barbiturates, sedatives, and pain medications are primarily used and abused by athletes as a result of injury, rather than recreationally or to enhance performance. Therefore, this class of drugs will not be discussed in this chapter.

Prevalence of Drug Use by Female Athletes

- The use of recreational drugs by athletes parallels drug use by nonathletes.
- Drug use by female athletes parallels drug use by male athletes.

- 49% of female athletes report binge drinking.
- 42.9% of athletes report using amphetamines for extra energy.
- 25% of female college athletes use marijuana.
- 11% of female athletes use smokeless tobacco.

Clinical Guideline

PHYSIOLOGICAL AND SOCIAL FACTORS

Considerable research has been directed toward delineating the effects of drugs of abuse on female physiology. Comparatively more research has been conducted on the effects of alcohol in women, but major research efforts to study the effects of the amphetamines, cocaine, and heroin have also recently been launched. There is virtually no research on the specific effects of drugs of abuse on the physiology of female athletes, but it is reasonable to assume that the effects of drugs on the conditioned female body are compounded by increased metabolic sensitivity and altered biological function that accompany high-intensity training.

The psychological and social factors affecting drug use by female athletes consist not only of those factors that affect the women in the general population but also by sets of issues that are unique to competitive athletes. These issues include, but are not limited to, competition-related pressures, weight management, self-esteem, and performance enhancement. This section will address the various drugs abused by female athletes, and the interaction of those drugs with female physiology and psychology.

Alcohol

Physiological Effects

Chronic alcohol intake affects every organ system in the human body. In the central nervous system, alcohol exerts its primary effects, such as intoxication and depressant effects, by means of its action as a γ-aminobutyric acid (GABA) agonist. GABA is an inhibitory amino acid that regulates a chloride ion channel; its primary activity is to increase the flow of chloride through the channel. Like alcohol, barbiturates and benzodiazepines are also agonistic to GABA. These neuromodulators facilitate the activity of GABA by means of their interaction with distinct peptide-binding sites in the chloride channel.

Functionally, the facilitation of GABA activity translates into a slowing of many central nervous system (CNS) functions, including planning and sequencing behavior into meaningful and goal-directed activity and impairing judgment. The acute consumption of alcohol is associated with these effects, as well as dose-related impairments in motor performance. Chronic effects of alcohol include gastritis, gastric ulcer, cirrhosis, peripheral neuropathy (caused primarily by alcohol-induced vitamin B deficiencies), amblyopia, anterior lobe cerebellar degenerative disease, Wernicke-Korsakoff syndrome, cardiomyopathy, thrombocytopenia, and anemia.

The effects of alcohol differ greatly for men vs women, owing partly to the higher average body water content in men (65% ± 2%) than in women (51% ± 2%).[9] Additional research has indicated that women have lower levels of alcohol dehydrogenase, an enzyme that metabolizes alcohol, and metabolize about one quarter as much alcohol as men.[10] This combination of factors produces an increased blood level of alcohol in women vs men, which means that women will have more intense reactions to a given dose of alcohol and will be less able to accurately predict the effects of that dose.

Physiological Effects of Alcohol

- Impaired judgment
- Impaired motor performance
- Gastritis
- Gastric ulcer
- Cirrhosis
- Peripheral neuropathy
- Amblyopia
- Anterior lobe cerebellar degeneration
- Wernicke-Korsakoff syndrome
- Cardiomyopathy
- Thrombocytopenia
- Anemia
- Impaired calcium absorption

Clinical Guideline

There is increasing evidence of a link between alcohol intake and the development of breast cancer,[11] and women who consume alcohol are at higher risk for the development of other alcohol-related disorders, such as fatty liver, hypertension, anemia, malnutrition, and gastrointestinal hemorrhage, than men.[12] The effects of alcohol on the female reproductive system are complex and not completely understood, but chronic heavy drinking is associated with inhibition of ovulation, infertility, and a wide variety of gynecological dysfunctions.[13]

Psychological Issues

The psychological factors associated with alcohol abuse in women are often different than those associated with alcohol abuse in men. For example, women seeking treatment for alcohol abuse report more depressive symptoms[14] and low self-esteem[15] than men, along with higher levels of guilt than men. Alcoholic women are more likely than alcoholic men to attribute the onset of their drinking to a stressful life event.[16]

Although the effects of alcohol on the physiological and psychological functioning of female athletes have not been systematically studied, it is reasonable to infer that the interaction between physiological and psychological factors with alcohol would be compounded in the female athlete. Because many biological systems are altered by athletic training, the effects of alcohol on these systems are enhanced. Of particular importance is that alcohol directly impairs calcium absorption and muscle coordination, which manifests as difficulty in training, decreased conditioning, and impaired performance.[3] Although research indicates that female athletes are generally aware of the effects of alcohol on their bodies and performance,[17] several studies have indicated that female athletes consume as much[18] or more[5] alcohol than their nonathlete counterparts. Although 85% of NCAA Division I female athletes report participation in alcohol education programs,[17] several studies have indicated no correlation between awareness of the effects of alcohol and the actual use of alcohol.[19] Female athletes become involved with alcohol for the same reasons as their nonathlete counterparts do but have additional issues that may lead to increased drinking:

1. Realization that athletic goals may not be attainable[19]
2. Competition stress[4,19]
3. Inability to relax after competition[20]
4. Training or career disruptions because of injury or replacement[20]
5. Escape from the sporting arena[21]
6. False sense of security that they will not be adversely affected by alcohol[22]

Alcohol abuse among athletes is additionally unique in its set of "enablers," individuals or institutions that protect the athlete from the need to confront his or her problem. One quarter of television commercials aired during network sports events advertise beer,[19] providing a link between drinking and the sports arena. Coaches and teammates often go to extra lengths to ensure that an athlete's alcohol problem is not brought to media attention. Although excessive alcohol use is banned by the Women's National Basketball Association (WNBA), it is only specifically banned by the NCAA for rifle sports and is subject to certain restrictions by the IOC. An interesting use of alcohol by a female athlete occurred in August 1997, when three-time Olympic gold medalist swimmer Michelle Smith was discovered adding a lethal concentration of Irish whiskey to her urine sample to mask the presence of other banned substances. Smith is the first world-class athlete suspended for manipulating a urine test.

Stimulants Banned by Various Sports Organizations

Drug	Organization
Amfepramone	IOC/USOC, USTA
Amfetaminil	IOC/USOC, USTA
Amineptine	IOC/USOC
Amiphenazole	NCAA, IOC/USOC, USTA
Amphetamine	NCAA, IOC/USOC, USTA, WNBA
Bemigride	NCAA, IOC/USOC, USTA
Benzphetamine	NCAA, IOC/USOC, USTA
Bromantan	NCAA, IOC/USOC, USTA
Caffeine (>12 μcg/mL)	NCAA (>15 mcg/mL), IOC/USOC, USTA
Cathine/norpseudoephedrine	IOC/UOC
Chlorphentermine	NCAA, IOC/USOC, USTA
Clobenzorex	IOC/USOC, USTA
Clorprenaline	IOC/USOC, USTA
Cocaine	NCAA, IOC/USOC, USTA, WNBA
Cropropamide	NCAA, IOC/USOC, USTA
Crothetamide	NCAA, IOC/USOC, USTA
Deoxyephedrine	IOC/USOC
Dexamphetamine	USTA
Diethylpropion	NCAA, IOC/USOC
Dimethylamphetamine	NCAA, IOC/USOC, USTA
Doxapram	NCAA
Ephedrine	NCAA, IOC/USOC, USTA*
Etaphedrine	IOC/USOC, USTA
Ethamivan	NCAA, IOC/USOC, USTA
Ethylamphetamine	NCAA, IOC/USOC, USTA
Fencamfamine	NCAA, IOC/USOC, USTA
Fenethyline	IOC/USOC, USTA
Fenproporex	IOC/USOC, USTA
Flurothyl	USTA
Furfenorex	IOC/USOC, USTA
Isoetharine	IOC/USOC
Isoproterenol	IOC/USOC
Leptazol	USTA
Levamphetamine	USTA
Ma huang	IOC/USOC
Meclofenoxate	NCAA, IOC/USOC, USTA
Mefenorex	IOC/USOC
Mesocarb	IOC/USOC, USTA
Metaproterenol	IOC/USOC
Methamphetamine	NCAA, IOC/USOC, USTA
Methoxyphenamine	IOC/USOC, USTA
Methylephedrine	IOC/USOC, USTA
Methylphenidate	NCAA, IOC/USOC, USTA
Morazone	IOC/USOC, USTA
Nikethamide	NCAA, IOC/USOC, USTA
Pemoline	NCAA, IOC/USOC, USTA
Pentylenetetrazol	NCAA, IOC/USOC, USTA
Phendimetrazine	NCAA, IOC/USOC, USTA
Phenmetrazine	NCAA, IOC/USOC, USTA
Phentermine	NCAA, IOC/USOC, USTA
Phenylpropanolamine	IOC/USOC, USTA*
Picrotoxine	NCAA, IOC/USOC
Pipradol	NCAA, IOC/USOC, USTA
Prolintane	NCAA, IOC/USOC, USTA

Propylhexadrine	IOC/USOC, USTA
Pseudoephedrine	IOC/USOC, USTA*
Pyrovalerone	IOC/USOC, USTA
Selegiline	IOC/USOC
Strychnine	NCAA, IOC/USOC, USTA

Abbreviations: NCAA = National Collegiate Athletic Association; IOC = International Olympic Committee; USOC = United States Olympic Committee; USTA = United States Tennis Association; WNBA = Women's National Basketball Association; μ/mL = micrograms per milliliter; * = Use monitored without penalty.

Clinical Guideline

Stimulants

Although alcohol is the most widely used recreational substance by athletes, as well as the general population, the use of stimulants by athletes is probably more problematic. Stimulants are used by female athletes not only for their direct stimulant effects but also for their anorectic and perceived ergogenic effects.

The use of stimulants has a very long history in sports. Athletes used stimulants as early as the third century BC in ancient Greece, according to the Greek physician Galen. The first documented case of stimulant use during sporting events was in 1865, when The Netherlands swimmers were caught using caffeine-containing drugs. In 1904, winning marathoner Thomas Hicks required several physicians to revive him after taking a brandy and strychnine combination during the race.[19] Amphetamines were found to be widely used by players in the NFL during the 1960s and 1970s.[23] Today, the use of amphetamines is strictly regulated by most sporting organizations.

Stimulants are indirect catecholamine agonists; their administration results in increased levels of CNS norepinephrine, dopamine, and in some cases, serotonin. The functional consequence of increased CNS catecholamine levels is behavioral activation. Acute behavioral effects of amphetamine administration include euphoria, increased energy, increased mental alertness, increased social activity, anorexia, and decreased fatigue. Although some reports have described mild psychomotor performance enhancement after amphetamine administration,[24,25] Laties and Weiss[26] report that amphetamine improves performance only under some conditions, such as fatigue. In terms of athletic performance, reports are mixed, with some researchers reporting very large performance improvements after amphetamine administration,[27] and others reporting no improvement.[28,29] A 1981 review of the literature reported that amphetamines do improve athletic performance by a margin of a few percent.[26] Although seemingly only a small advantage, even a 1% edge can be the difference between winning and losing.

Chronic administration of amphetamine produces tolerance to many of its effects. As the user escalates the dose to attain the initial desired effect of the drug, toxicities may occur. These include paranoid psychoses[30,31] and aggression,[32] as well as several pathophysiological changes. Centrally, monoaminergic systems are substantially altered, with dopamine, norepinephrine, and serotonin stores becoming depleted in several brain regions.[33-35] Repeated administration of amphetamine for as little as 3 months produces changes in cerebral vasculature, which include vascular filling or nonfilling, vessel fragmentation, and microhemorrhage.[36] The cardiovascular consequences of amphetamines are substantial and include increased blood pressure and tachycardia after acute administration and myocardial lesions after chronic administration. Thermoregulatory mechanisms are also altered after amphetamine administration. Peripheral hyperthermia and central hypothermia occur,[37,38] and hyperpyrexia is a major cause of death related to amphetamine abuse.[39] Chronic amphetamine use is associated with a pronounced withdrawal syndrome, which manifests as fatigue, decreased mental energy, limited interest in the environment, and anhedonia.[40]

For the athlete, the slight performance edge resulting from amphetamine administration may be accompanied by serious side effects: peripheral hyperthermia can lead to heat stroke in warm weather, elevated blood pressure and tachycardia, and the masking of fatigue, which can lead to injury, heat exhaustion, and cerebral collapse.

Although the performance effects of the amphetamines are the same for male and female athletes, the reasons that they are taken are slightly different between the sexes. Although both sexes use amphetamines to mask fatigue; promote self-confidence; and increase speed, power, and endurance,[41] female athletes also use the drugs for their anorectic properties to decrease body fat.[4] Anorexia and bulimia remain substantial problems among competitive female athletes[4] and are features of the much-researched "female athlete triad"[42]

Adverse Effects of Stimulants in Sports

- Peripheral hyperthermia >> Heat stroke
- Elevated blood pressure

- Tachycardia
- Masking of fatigue > > Injury, heat exhaustion, cerebral collapse

Clinical Guideline

The use of the stimulant ephedrine has recently gained attention because of its widespread and unregulated availability. Ephedrine is extracted from botanical ma huang[43] and is used by athletes for its thermogenic and stimulant effects.[44] Female athletes may be at particular risk for ephedrine abuse because of its lipolytic properties and its lack of masculinization properties. Gruber and Pope[45] conducted an investigation of drug use among female weightlifters, 56% of whom reported using ephedrine. These athletes reported using the drug in either its pure form or in readily available preparations such as "Ripped Fuel" or "Thermadrine." Reasons for ephedrine use included a desire to decrease body fat, increase energy, or avoid withdrawal. Several of the women expressed a belief that it was impossible to be competitive without using ephedrine, and all reported daily use of ephedrine for more than 1 year. All women reported using a dose above the recommended dose, and most reported the development of tolerance to the drug. Ephedrine use in this sample was associated with significant other pathological conditions, including amenorrhea (89%), muscle dysmorphia (97%), eating disorders (83%), other substance abuse (25%), childhood gender identity disorder (78%), and adult gender identity disorder (5%). Side effects of ephedrine are similar to those of the traditional amphetamines, and withdrawal symptoms include fatigue and weight gain.

Ephedrine Use Among Female Athletes

- Commonly used daily for more than 1 year
- Some believe it necessary for competition
- Often used above recommended dosage
- Tolerance develops rapidly
- Associated with amenorrhea, dysmorphia
- Associated with eating disorders, gender identity disorder

Clinical Guideline

Although cocaine use does not seem to be a major problem among female athletes, likely because of its street reputation as a dangerous drug, it deserves mention because it is a significant public health problem and because of recent media attention as a result of its use by professional male athletes. The effects of cocaine are similar to the effects of other stimulants, but the abuse liability of the drug is greater because of its rapid onset of action and short duration of action.[46] Athletes may use it to acutely enhance performance before competition[19] or recreationally between competitions.

Although data are limited on the specific effects of amphetamine on female physiology, research on the effects of cocaine on female physiology indicate that cocaine abuse is associated with alterations in menstrual cycle function, galactorrhea, amenorrhea, and infertility.[47] Significant to the athlete is that cocaine is associated with rhabdomyolysis, or muscle wasting.[48,49] Although the direct cause of cocaine-induced rhabdomyolysis is not known, Roth and colleagues[50] suggest that it may stem from arterial vasoconstriction or disruption of muscle metabolism, both of which are direct effects of cocaine.

Cocaine toxicity is also associated with sinusitis, nosebleed, nasal mucosa atrophy, nasal septum perforation, bowel ischemia, cellulitis, thallium poisoning, retinal artery occlusion, dermatological problems, and muscle and skin infections. Cocaine use has been associated with sudden death, as occurred in the two promising young athletes, Len Bias and Don Rogers. Bias, a 22-year-old University of Maryland All-American basketball player, was the first-round draft choice of the NBA champion Boston Celtics. Rogers was a 23-year-old Cleveland Browns star defensive back. Both athletes died from cardiac arrest after ingesting massive amounts of cocaine in June 1986, 1 week apart. Rogers died on the eve of his wedding day.

Marijuana

Marijuana, like alcohol, is not used by athletes to enhance athletic performance. However, media reports of athletes such as Celtics hoopster Robert Parish, tennis player Jennifer Capriati, and Pittsburgh Steeler Byron "Bam" Morris being arrested for possession of marijuana indicate that the drug is used by some athletes. Likely reasons for marijuana use by athletes are the same as those for alcohol use: to relieve stress and to relax and escape from the sporting arena.

Marijuana has been used for centuries for its intoxicating and euphoria-producing properties. Although the centrally active component of marijuana is delta-9 tetrahydrocannabinol (THC), marijuana contains more than 60 cannabinoids, many of which are biologically active. A receptor for THC in the human brain has only recently been discovered,[51] and even more recently, an endogenous compound for that receptor has been identified.[52] This compound has been named anandamide (*ananda* is the Sanskrit word for bliss). The acute effects of smoking marijuana are dose-dependent and include increased heart rate, euphoria, calmness, distortion of time estimation, perceptual changes, increased appetite, reddening of the conjunctiva, psychomotor performance deficits, and enhanced sensitivity to sound and touch.

The effects of chronic marijuana use are a subject of controversy. An early investigation of chronic users who smoked an average of seven marijuana cigarettes a day for an average of 8 years reported no serious physical or psychological consequences of chronic use.[53] More recent controlled studies have generally supported these findings,[54,55] but some adverse consequences of long-term use have been identified. Smoking marijuana narrows and inflames bronchial tubes and reduces lung capacity, which is significant for athletes. THC administration lowers sperm count and testosterone levels in men and produces altered hormonal levels and menstrual cycle perturbations in women.[56] Although marijuana use has historically and anecdotally been associated with an amotivational syndrome, experimental evidence has not supported that association.

Strong evidence exists for the development of tolerance and dependence on marijuana. Jones and colleagues[57] characterized a withdrawal syndrome in long-term, heavy users of marijuana that included restlessness and irritability; more recently, Haney and colleagues[58] described the development of tolerance to the euphoric effects of smaller doses of marijuana and a subsequent withdrawal syndrome that included irritability, sleep disturbances, and gastrointestinal complaints.

Recent legislation in several states has decriminalized the medical use of marijuana. Marijuana smoking is associated with decreased nausea induced by cancer chemotherapy, AIDS-related cachexia, and glaucoma-induced intraocular pressure increases. Despite its recent decriminalization, however, medical marijuana remains controversial, because Marinol, a synthetic form of THC, has been available by prescription for years.

Marijuana is banned by most sports organizations except the NBA and can be detected in urine for up to 30 days.

Adverse Effects of Marijuana

Acute effects:
    Increased heart rate
    Time estimation distortion
    Psychomotor performance deficits
Chronic effects:
    Narrowed and inflamed bronchial tubes
    Reduced lung capacity
    Altered menstrual cycle
    Tolerance and dependence

Clinical Guideline

Smokeless Tobacco

Smokeless tobacco has been a mainstay in baseball dugouts for decades. The use of smokeless tobacco in the form of snuff or chewing tobacco has increased steadily over recent years, especially among female athletes.[59]

Although smoke inhalation provides a more rapid uptake of nicotine into the bloodstream, similar peak blood nicotine levels are reached after administration of smokeless tobacco. Nicotine is readily absorbed and produces a wide variety of central and peripheral effects by means of its interaction with nicotinic cholinergic receptors. Acute cardiovascular effects of nicotine include increased blood pressure, increased heart rate, increased coronary blood flow, increased cardiac output, and cutaneous vasoconstriction.[60] Neuroendocrine effects include release of prolactin, growth hormone, vasopressin, ß-endorphins, cortisol, and adrenocorticotropic hormone.[61]

Athletes may use smokeless tobacco to increase vigilance and physical performance, but research suggests that performance enhancements after nicotine administration may be attributed to improvements in abstinence-induced performance decrements.[62] Further, Escher and colleagues[63] found that simple and complex reaction times were not improved after administration of smokeless tobacco to tobacco-using athletes and that several strength parameters were improved during abstinence from smokeless tobacco.

Another reason cited for nicotine use with particular relevance for female athletes is weight control. Weight changes associated with nicotine administration or cessation are transient, however, and the increases in metabolism resulting from nicotine administration do not necessarily translate to chronic decreased metabolism on cessation.[64] Athletes may also use smokeless tobacco to reduce stress. Because there is no experimental support for this particular coping strategy, however, it is likely that any nicotine-induced stress reduction is actually a relief from abstinence-induced anxiety.[65]

Like cigarettes, smokeless tobacco produces dependence[66,67] and has been associated with the development of oral cancer.[68] Withdrawal symptoms resulting from cessation of smokeless tobacco include irritability, anxiety, depression, impatience, fatigue, difficulty concentrating, headache, stomach distress, increased appetite, sleep disturbances, and constipation.

TREATMENT ISSUES

Most major sports organizations have implemented drug education and drug awareness programs for athletes. Efforts range from printed educational information to blood and urine toxicology screening. The IOC and United States Olympic Committee (USOC) have instituted widespread efforts to reach coaches and trainers, as well as athletes, and believe that drug testing is the most favorable way to deter drug use by athletes and promote fair competition. The USOC supports a Drug Control Hotline (1–800–233–0393) manned with knowledgeable counselors to discuss drug

Treatment Strategies for Alcohol Abuse

Treatment	Indication
Benzodiazepines	Restlessness
	Sleep disturbances
	Agitation
	Tremulousness
B vitamins	Prevention of Korsakoff's syndrome
Fluid administration	Dehydration caused by vomiting
Anticonvulsants	Seizures
Tranquilizers	Delirium tremens
Disulfiram	Relapse prevention
Alcoholics anonymous	Relapse prevention
Support network	Relapse prevention

Clinical Guideline

abuse issues with athletes. The NBA, WNBA, NCAA, and NFL have launched major efforts to educate players, detect drug use, and penalize athletes who use banned substances. The Hazelden Foundation, a well-known treatment center in Center City, Minnesota, oversees the NFL's drug awareness programs and offers drug treatment programs tailored to the special needs of athletes. The American Medical Association has a set of guidelines governing the medical care of athletes, which suggests rigid control over the prescription of stimulants, analgesics, androgens, and anabolic steroids to athletes. This section will discuss specific approaches to drug abuse treatment as a function of drug class. Although some treatment principles apply across drug classes, such as individual and group psychotherapy, behavior and cognitive therapies, and residential treatment programs, strategies have been found to be differentially effective for different classes of drugs.

Alcohol

The treatment of alcoholism and the management of alcohol withdrawal represent separate clinical issues. Alcohol treatment cannot begin until detoxification and withdrawal are complete. Alcohol withdrawal can be fatal, and the risk of death increases with the number of times the alcoholic withdraws from alcohol. Usually, however, the symptoms of alcohol are transient and short-lived. Treatment of alcohol withdrawal is symptomatic and prophylactic. Restlessness, sleep disturbances, agitation, and tremulousness should be treated with benzodiazepines as front-line treatment. Barbiturates, chloral hydrate, and phenothiazines can also be used. The B vitamins should be administered in large doses. Vomiting or diarrhea may produce dehydration that will require the parenteral administration of fluids. Otherwise, fluid administration is not necessary. During acute withdrawal, hyperventilation may produce respiratory alkalosis, which can lead to seizure activity if hypomagnesemia is present.[69] Anticonvulsants can be administered in this case. Delirium tremens may be present in severe withdrawal. If delirium develops, physical restraint may be necessary, and the administration of tranquilizers is warranted.

Sobriety and amelioration of the psychological conditions associated with alcoholism are the goals of treatment. As discussed previously, women who abuse alcohol may do so for a different set of reasons than men, and athletes may abuse alcohol for a different set of reasons than nonathletes. These issues should be addressed directly in therapy.

Most relapses occur within the first 6 months of abstinence,[70] so the first goal of treatment is to maintain total abstinence. Total abstinence is necessary for the therapist to accurately diagnose other psychopathology and for the patient to learn to cope with her issues without alcohol. Disulfiram (Antabuse) is useful in maintaining abstinence in some patients by inhibiting aldehyde dehydrogenase, the hepatic enzyme responsible for metabolism of alcohol. Inhibition of alcohol metabolism leads to an accumulation of acetaldehyde, which results in nausea and hypotension. Because it has a very long elimination half-life, disulfiram can be administered during office visits separated by 3 to 4 days.

A number of therapeutic strategies have been used for the treatment of alcoholism, and none has been found to be particularly superior to others. Most therapists encourage their patients to attend Alcoholic Anonymous meetings, although there are no data regarding the efficacy of this program in maintaining abstinence. Several studies, however, have indicated that the best predictor of treatment outcome for the female alcoholic is the presence or absence of social support,[71,72] which suggests that the involvement of teammates, coaches, trainers, and partners should be incorporated into the treatment program.

Several drugs have been investigated for the treatment of alcohol abuse, including serotonin reuptake inhibitors, lithium carbonate, the opioid antagonist naltrexone, and the excitatory amino acid antagonist acamprosate. Large-scale clinical trials with the latter two medications are currently under way.

Stimulants

Several athletes have received media attention for participation in treatment for stimulant (primarily cocaine) abuse, including Major League baseball players Dwight Gooden, Keith Hernandez, Darryl Strawberry, and Steve Howe, and All-Pro New York Giant Lawrence Taylor. Although relapse to cocaine abuse is common, as in the aforementioned cases, some treatment strategies have shown efficacy. There are virtually no data regarding the efficacy of treatment for amphetamine abuse. However, the burgeoning body of literature on cocaine abuse treatment provides some indication about what will be effective in treating the amphetamine abuser. Any treatment plan should incorporate a range of treatment strategies, including supportive counseling, drug education, peer support groups, and family or team meetings.

Several behavioral strategies have been used with some success for cocaine abuse. Because environmental stimuli acquire strong conditioned triggers for stimulant use, it is important to limit the patient's exposure to the settings and stimuli that have acquired such associations, especially during early abstinence from the substance. The weakening of these associations takes a very long time but can be accelerated in therapy through the implementation of a strategy called extinction.

The efficacy of extinction therapy depends on the stimuli used in the clinical setting and the generalizability of extinction training from the clinic to the athlete's natural setting. The technique involves exposing the athlete, by means of mental imagery, to a set of cues that trigger the desire to use stimulants and then teaching the athlete coping strategies to reject the desire to use in the presence of such cues.

Another technique that is likely to have efficacy in treating the stimulant-abusing athlete is contingency contracting. The therapist establishes a contract with the athlete stating that she will refrain from using stimulants. Urine is tested at regular intervals. If the athlete submits drug-free urine, she is "rewarded" with positive consequences; drug-positive urine tests result in aversive consequences. Consequences are established between the therapist and patient at the time of contracting. Positive consequences might include such reinforcers as money, vouchers for merchandise, or a preferred activity; negative consequences might include payment of money, loss of privileges, or engagement in an aversive activity.

Increasing the natural reinforcement density in the athlete's environment is another technique that may be used to treat stimulant abuse. This technique involves teaching the athlete to recognize and engage in other behaviors that are not compatible with stimulant abuse but that offer the athlete equal gratification.

Several pharmacotherapies have been tried for stimulant abuse, with little success. Dopaminergic agonists, such as bromocriptine, methylphenidate, and pergolide, have shown a modicum of promise in reducing some of the anergia and dysphoria accompanying cocaine abstinence,[73] but dopamine antagonists and serotonergic agents have not proven successful. Several antidepressants have shown promise in stimulant users with a comorbid depression. The monoamine oxidase inhibitor selegiline and the GABA agonists baclofen and gabapentin are currently being investigated for cocaine abuse.

Treatment Strategies for Stimulant Abuse

Treatment	Indication
Extinction	Cue-induced craving
Contingency contracting	Abstinence maintenance
Increasing reinforcement density	Reinforcement replacement
Dopamine agonists	Withdrawal symptoms

Clinical Guideline

Marijuana

There is no research on the efficacy of treatment for marijuana. However, the recent characterization of a marijuana withdrawal syndrome suggests that treating the symptoms of marijuana may be one avenue for therapy. In addition, the author has demonstrated that marijuana smoking can be reduced with alternative reinforcers.[74] Because the number of persons seeking treatment for marijuana abuse has recently increased, several studies have been initiated to investigate possible pharmacotherapies for marijuana abuse. The novel antidepressants bupropion and nefazodone, are currently under investigation.

Smokeless Tobacco

Treatment of nicotine dependence has become big business. Although current efforts are directed at smoking cessation, these strategies can also be used in the treatment of smokeless tobacco dependence. Nicotine replacement systems, in the form of nicotine gum, transdermal nicotine delivery patches, and nasal spray, have been approved in the United States for several years, and the novel antidepressant bupropion (Zyban) was recently approved by the Food and Drug Administration for smoking cessation. These treatments reduce the severity of withdrawal but should be accompanied by techniques to help the athlete cope with urges to use tobacco. Other strategies may be useful: close inspection of a Major League baseball dugout after a game would likely reveal an accumulation of sunflower seed shells!

CONCLUSION

Recreational drug use by athletes is a cause for serious concern. The reasons for initiation and maintenance of drug use by the general population are compounded by the complex set of issues of the female athlete. Body image issues and the desire to lose or maintain weight are factors that are unique to women in general and put them at risk for drug use. The female athlete carries with her all of those issues and more: the desire for a competitive edge, the stressors that accompany intensive training and competition, and the "macho" stereotype that presents role conflicts in sports. The interplay of these factors renders the female athlete particularly vulnerable to drug abuse.

Drug use by athletes is particularly problematic from a sociocultural standpoint. Americans love sports, and athletes are perceived as superheroes to many sports fans. Athletes set standards of behavior for the youth of our country, so that drug-using athletes send messages that drug use is acceptable, if not encouraged, and that athletes are immune to the consequences of drug abuse. Although all major sport-

ing organizations have set policies against drug abuse and penalties for violation of those policies, the monetary and social issues in the sports industry set the stage for drug abuse. Although drug treatment, stringent testing, and strict penalties for drug use should be necessary restraints to drug use, prevention efforts will undoubtedly be the most successful deterrent to drug use by young athletes. The recent initiation of research into sex differences in drug abuse will hopefully allow for more specifically tailored treatment and prevention strategies for the female athlete.

REFERENCES

1. Drug Abuse and Addiction Report. *25 Years of Discovery to Advance the Health of the Public.* NIDA—the 6th Triennial Report to Congress. Washington, DC: National Institutes of Health; 1999.

2. Toohey JV. Nonmedical drug use among intercollegiate athletes at five American universities. *Bull Narc.* 1978;30:61–64.

3. Bell JA, Dodge TC. Athletes' use and abuse of drugs. *Phys Sports Med.* 1987;15:99–108.

4. Duda M. Female athletes: Targets for drug abuse. *Phys Sports Med.* 1986;14:142–146.

5. The Higher Education Center for Alcohol and Other Drug Prevention. *College Athletes and Alcohol and Other Drug Use.* Infofacts Resources, 1997.

6. Wechsler H, Davenport A, Dowdall G, Grossman S, Zanakos S. Binge drinking, tobacco, and illicit drug use and involvement in college athletics. *J Am Coll Health.* 1997;45:195–200.

7. Johnson R. Available on-line: www2.ari.net/rjohnson/articles/DRINKERS/CNS.html.

8. Clement DB. Drug use survey: Results and conclusions. *Phys Sports Med.* 1983;11:64–67.

9. Van Theil DH, Tarter RE, Rosenblum E. Alcohol, its metabolism and gonadal effects: Does sex make a difference? *Adv Alcohol Sub Abuse.* 1988;131–169.

10. Frezza M, DiPadova C, Pozzato G, Terpin M, Baroona E, Lieber CS. High blood alcohol levels in women: The role of decreased gastric alcohol dehydrogenase activity and first-pass metabolism. *N Engl J Med.* 1990;322:95–99.

11. Longnecker MP, Berlin JA, Orza MJ, Chalmers TC. A meta-analysis of alcohol consumption in relation to breast cancer in women. *JAMA.* 1988;260:652–656.

12. US Dept of the Treasury and US Dept of Health and Human Services. *Report to the President and the Congress on Health Hazards Associated with Alcohol and Methods to Inform the General Public of These Hazards.* Washington, DC: US Dept of the Treasury; 1980.

13. Mello NK. Some behavioral and biological aspects of alcohol problems in women. In: Kalant OJ, ed. *Alcohol and Drug Problems in Women.* New York: Plenum Press; 1980.

14. Corrigan EM. *Alcoholic Women in Treatment.* New York: Oxford University Press; 1980.

15. Beckman LJ. Self-esteem of women alcoholics. *J Stud Alcohol.* 1978;39:491–498.

16. Griffin ML, Weiss RL, Mirin SM. A comparison of male and female cocaine abusers. *Arch Gen Psych.* 1989;46:122–126.

17. Martin M. The use of alcohol among NCAA Division I female college basketball, softball, and volleyball athletes. *J Ath Train.* 1998;33:163–167.

18. Carr CN, Kennedy SR, Dimick KM. Alcohol use among high school athletes. *Prev Res.* 1996;3:1–3.

19. Special Report. Drug use and abuse in sports: Denial fuels the problem. *Phys Sport Med.* 1982;10:114–123.

20. Heyman S. Psychological factors in athletes' substance use. *Prev Res.* 1996;3:3–5.

21. Tricke R. Preventing substance use in young athletes. *Prev Res.* 1996;3:6–9.

22. Ungerleider S. Sports, drugs, and other societal reflections. *Prev Res.* 1996;3:10–11.

23. Mandell AJ. The Sunday syndrome: A unique pattern of amphetamine abuse indigenous to American professional football. *Clin Toxicol.* 1979;15:225–232.

24. Hamilton MJ, Smith PR, Peck AW. Effects of bupropion, nomifensine and dexamphetamine on performance, subjective feelings, autonomic variables and electroencephalogram in healthy volunteers. *Br J Clin Pharm.* 1983;15:367–374.

25. Peck AW, Bye CE, Clubley M, Henson K, Riddington C. Comparison of bupropion hydrochloride with dexamphetamine and amitriptyline in healthy subjects. *Br J Clin Pharmacol.* 1979;7:469–478.

26. Laties VG, Weiss B. The amphetamine margin in sports. *Fed Proc.* 1981;40:2689–2692.

27. Smith GM, Beecher HK. Amphetamine sulfate and athletic performance. *JAMA.* 1959;170:542–557.

28. Karpovich PV. Effect of amphetamine sulfate on athletic performance. *JAMA.* 1959;170:558–561.

29. DeMeersman R, Getty D, Schaefer DC. Sympathomimetics and exercise enhancement: All in the mind? *Pharm Biochem Behav.* 1987;28:361–365.

30. Ellinwood EH Jr. Amphetamine psychosis. I. Description of the individuals and process. *J Nerv Ment Dis.* 1967;144:273.

31. Snyder SH. Catecholamines in the brain as mediators of amphetamine psychosis. *Arch Gen Psych.* 1972;27:169.

32. Ellinwood EH Jr. Amphetamine psychosis: Individuals, settings, and sequences. In: Ellinwood EH, Cohen S, eds. *Current Concepts in Amphetamine Abuse.* Rockville, MD: National Institute of Mental Health; 1972:143–157.

33. Ricuarte GA, Seiden LS, Schuster CR. Further evidence that amphetamines produce long-lasting dopamine neurochemical deficits by destroying dopamine nerve fibers. *Brain Res.* 1984;303:359–364.

34. Schuster CR, Lewis M, Seiden LS. Fenfluramine. Neurotoxicity. *Psychopharm Bull.* 1986;22:148–151.

35. Seiden LS, Fischman MW, Schuster CR. Changes in brain catecholamines induced by long-term methamphetamine administration in rhesus monkeys. In: Ellinwood EH, Kilbey M, eds. *Cocaine and Other Stimulants.* New York: Plenum Press; 1977:179–185.

36. Rumbaugh CL. Small vessel cerebral vascular changes following chronic amphetamine intoxication. In: Ellinwood EH, Kilbey M, eds. *Cocaine and Other Stimulants.* New York: Plenum Press; 1977:241–251.

37. Gessa GL, Clay GA, Brodie BB. Evidence that hyperthermia produced by d-amphetamine is caused by peripheral action of the drug. *Life Sci.* 1969;8:135–141.

38. Jellinek P. Dual effect of dexamphetamine on body temperature in the rat. *Eur J Pharmacol.* 1971;15:389–392.

39. Kalant H, Kalant O. Death in amphetamine users: Causes and rates. In: Smith DE, ed. *Amphetamine Use, Misuse, and Abuse.* Boston: GK Hall & Co, 1979:169–188.

40. Gawin FH, Ellinwood EH. Cocaine and other stimulants. *N Engl J Med.* 1988;318:1173.

41. Catlin DH, Hatton CK. Use and abuse of anabolic steroids and other drugs for athletic enhancement. *Adv Intern Med.* 1991;36:399–424.

42. Skolnick A. "Female athlete triad" risk for women. *JAMA.* 1993;270:921–923.

43. Caldwell J. The metabolism of amphetamines and related stimulants in animals and man. In: Caldwell J, ed. *Amphetamines and Related Stimulants: Chemical, Biological Clinical and Social Aspects.* Boca Raton, FL: CRC Press; 1980.

44. Grunding P, Bachman M. *World Anabolic Review.* Houston, TX: MB Muscle Books; 1996.

45. Gruber AJ, Pope HG. Ephedrine abuse among 36 female weightlifters. *Am J Addictions.* 1998;7:256–261.

46. Hatsukami DK, Fischman MW. Crack cocaine and cocaine hydrochloride: Are the differences myth or reality? *JAMA.* 1996;76:1580–1588.

47. Phillips J, Wynne RD. *Cocaine: The Mystique and the Reality.* New York: Avon Books; 1980.

48. Merigian KS, Roberts JR. Cocaine intoxication: Hyperpyrexia, rhabdomyolysis, and acute renal failure. *J Clin Toxicol.* 1987,25.135–148.

49. Krohn KD, Slowman-Kovacs S, Leapman SB. Cocaine and rhabdomyolysis. *Ann Intern Med.* 1988;208:639–640.

50. Roth D, Alarcon FJ, Fernandez JA, Preston RA, Bourgoignie JJ. Acute rhabdomyolysis associated with cocaine intoxication. *N Engl J Med.* 1988;319:673–677.

51. Matsuda LA, Lolait SJ, Brownstein MJ, Young AC, Bonner TI. Structure of a cannabinoid receptor and functional cloned cDNA. *Nature.* 1990;346:561–564.

52. Devane WA. Isolation and structure of a brain constituent that binds to the cannabinoid receptor. *Science.* 1992;258:1946–1949.

53. Mayor's Committee on Marijuana. *The Marijuana Problem in the City of New York.* Lancaster, PA: Jacques Catell Press; 1944.

54. Stefanis C, Dornbush R, Fiuk M. *Hashish: Studies of Long-term Use.* New York: Raven Press; 1977.

55. Beaubrun MH, Knight F. Psychiatric assessment of 30 chronic users of cannabis use and 30 matched controls. *Am J Psychol.* 1973;130:309.

56. Grinspoon L, Bakalar JB. Marijuana. In: Lowinson JH, Ruiz P, Millman RB, Langrod JG, eds. *Substance Abuse: A Comprehensive Textbook.* Baltimore, MD: Williams & Wilkins; 1997:199–206.

57. Jones RT, Benowitz N, Bachman J. Clinical studies of cannabis tolerance and dependence. *Ann NY Acad Sci.* 1976;282:221–239.

58. Haney M, Ward AS, Comer SD, Foltin RW, Fischman MW. Abstinence symptoms following smoked marijuana in humans. *Psychopharmacology.* 1998;141:395–401.

59. Anderson WA, Albrecht RR, McKeag DB, Hough DO, McGraw CA. A national survey of alcohol and drug use by college athletes. *Phys Sports Med.* 1991;19:91–110.

60. Benowitz NL. Clinical pharmacology of nicotine. *Ann Rev Med.* 1986;37:21–32.

61. Seyler LE, Pomerleau OF, Fertig JB, Hunt D, Parker K. Pituitary hormone response to cigarette smoking. *Pharmacol Biochem Behav.* 1986;24:159–162.

62. Heishman SJ, Taylor RC, Henningfield JE. Nicotine and smoking: A review of effects on human performance. *Exp Clin Psychopharm.* 1994;2:345–395.

63. Escher SA, Tucker AM, Lundin TM, Grabiner MD. Smokeless tobacco, reaction time, and strength in athletes. *Med Sci Sports Exerc.* 1998;1548–1551.

64. Schwid SR, Hirvonen MD, Keesey RE. Nicotine effects on body weight: A regulatory perspective. *Am J Clin Nutr.* 1992;55:878–884.

65. Parrot AC. Stress modulation over the day in cigarette smokers. *Addiction.* 1995;90:233–244.

66. Hatsukami DK, Gust SW, Keenan RM. Physiologic and subjective changes from smokeless tobacco withdrawal. *Clin Pharm Ther.* 1987;41:103–107.

67. Hatsukami DK, Anton D, Keenan R, Callies A. Smokeless tobacco abstinence effects and nicotine gum dose. *Psychopharmacology.* 1992;106:60–66.

68. US Department of Health and Human Services. *The Health Consequences of Using Smokeless Tobacco: A Report of the Advisory Committee to the Surgeon General.* Washington, DC: US Department of Health and Human Services, Public Health Service; 1986.

69. Mendelson JH. Biologic concomitants of alcoholism. *N Engl J Med.* 1970;283:24–32.

70. Casteneda R, Cushman P. Alcohol withdrawal: A review of clinical management. *J Clin Psychol.* 1989;50:278–284.

71. MacDonald JG. Predictors of treatment outcome for alcoholic women. *Int J Addictions.* 1987;22:235–248.

72. Havassy BE, Hall SM, Tschann JM. Social support and the relapse to alcohol, tobacco, and opiates: Preliminary findings. *NIDA Research Monograph.* 1987;76:207–213.

73. Dackis CA, Gold MS. Pharmacological approaches to cocaine addiction. *J Subst Abuse Treat.* 1985;2:139–145.

74. Ward AS, Comer SD, Haney M, Foltin RW, Fischman MW. Effects of a monetary alternative on marijuana self-administration. *Behav Pharmacol.* 1997;8:275–286.

Sports-Specific Injuries

Nadya Swedan

INTRODUCTION

The nature, prevalence, risks, and rates of injury occurrence are related to many factors. Most clinicians would agree that type of sporting activity is one of the most important variables. Certain injuries are common to particular sports—terms such as swimmer's shoulder, tennis and golfer's elbow, turf toe, and march fracture are truly valid in the athletic arena. The nature of the sport suggests the nature of the injury. Level of contact, equipment, protective gear, shoes, weather, and playing surfaces are extrinsic factors affecting injury rates. Intrinsic factors include flexibility, proprioception, skill level, conditioning, training, strength, joint alignment, range of motion, previous injuries, and gender.

Injuries occur more frequently in games than in practice, reflecting the increased effort and decreased precautions of competition. Injuries also occur more frequently in the second half of games[1] or later in the time span of activity with respect to recreational sports. Minor injuries often do not receive medical attention; injuries requiring medical management and time off from play comprise approximately one-third in education settings.[2(p 400)] Contact sports increase the risk of all types of injuries; those other than musculoskeletal include abdominal, eye, dental, head trauma, and nerve injuries, both central and peripheral. Burners or stingers can occasionally be secondary to brachial plexus, cervical nerve root, and cervical spinal cord injury.[3] Position on a team predicts risks and injury patterns.[4] Activities requiring explosive bursts of speed, cutting and turning maneuvers, and jumping and landing increase risk of injury to the lower extremities.

Sports injuries are usually "acute macrotrauma" or "repetitive microtrauma."[5(p 541)] Whether caused by an acute injury or insidious as a result of overuse, the mechanism of injury has been the subject of many studies. As expected, a survey of recreational athletes in Australia found player collision, overextension, and falling particularly during running, catching, jumping, and riding to precede most injuries.[6] However, subacute injuries must also be considered, as untreated mild complaints can lead to weakness that may precede more severe injuries. A recent study of physical education students suggested that many athletes forget and underreport musculoskeletal injuries.[7]

GENDER

As literature begins to address gender-related sports injuries, it is fortunate that trends reveal that girls and women report and seek medical care for injuries more commonly than men.[8] As more girls and women become active in sports, gender is becoming identified with certain sports injuries, although epidemiological studies suggest injury rates to be more a factor of sport than gender.[9,10] Much research has focused on knee injuries in female athletes, particularly anterior cruciate ligament (ACL) injuries, because overall rates are higher than in men and, more often, noncontact.[10–14] Injury factors specific to female athletes that have been identified in research include playing surface (particularly natural vs. artificial turf), shoe type, including cleat number and size,[15] knee joint laxity and proprioception,[16,17] skill level,[18] anatomical alignment and posture,[19] muscle firing patterns,[20] and hormonal cycles in relation to ligament laxity.[21] Higher rates of injuries have also been attributed to less preplay conditioning, training, and less optimal coaching, playing surfaces, and equipment for female athletes.

The most common reported overall sports injuries are ankle sprains; knee and hand injuries are also common. Research suggests that across genders, knee pain and/or injuries occur more frequently in women participating in all athletic activities, including basketball[12] and soccer,[11] skiing,[22] tennis,[23] and military duties.[24] Although lower extremity injuries make up most sports-related injuries,[6(p 391)] hand and wrist injuries have been described as contributing to 25% of sports injuries, with the right hand injured three times more often than the left.[25(p 191)] In a study done on school-age children, there was a statistically significant higher proportion of hand injuries in girls.[26(p 283)] In another study on school-age children,[27] there was a significant increased amount of patellofemoral pain syndrome and recurrent and acute patellar dislocation in girls vs boys.

SPORTS-SPECIFIC INJURIES

Aerobics

An extremely popular predominately female athletic activity, aerobic classes now include dance classes, step, mini-trampoline, tae-bo, aero-boxing, power yoga, and classes with weights. Injuries vary on the basis of activity, intensity, and frequency of classes. Improper posture, alignment, and high-velocity movements can cause disc pathology, shoulder impingement, and overuse syndromes. Improperly gripped and weighted equipment can lead to rotator cuff tendinitis, instability, and wrist tendinitis. Morton's neuromas, plantar fasciitis, stress fractures, jumper's knee, and iliotibial band syndrome are common. Ankle and knee sprains occur frequently from improper landing. Abdominal exercises with extreme rotation and unsupported flexion and extension and improper squats are a common cause of spine injury at all levels. Because aerobic classes are often attended for weight and body shape maintenance, eating disorders are frequent.

Bowling

One of the first organized sports for women, bowling was highly attended as an industrial league sport[28] and remains popular as both recreational activity and sport today. Injuries include lumbar sprains and disc pathology, knee sprains, patellofemoral symptoms, wrist tendinitis, lateral and medial epicondylitis, and finger sprains and tendon injuries.

Basketball

Beginning as an industry-sponsored sport, basketball is now a popular women's sport with participation at all school levels and professionally. Because of this popularity, inju-

ries in basketball have been well studied. Contact injuries, sprains and strains, and knee injuries, particularly ACL tears, have been well documented. ACL injuries in female athletes have been researched as occurring approximately three times more frequently[12,14] than in male athletes, with greater likelihood of surgery. Ankle injuries are most frequent and can be recurrent and chronic. Achilles tendinitis and plantar fasciitis also occur. Stress fractures of the tibia, navicular, and metatarsals should be considered. In addition to ACL, collateral ligament, and meniscal injuries, jumper's knee (Sinding-Larsen-Johanson disease) occurs along with patellar tendinitis and pes anserine bursitis. In young athletes, Osgood Schlatter's disease and osteochondritis desiccans should be considered. Eye injuries are frequent, including eyelid injury, periorbital contusions, corneal abrasions, and orbital fractures.[29] Dental injuries, concussions, and traumatic brain injuries can also occur. (One study reports mild TBI rates in high school students as 1.04 per 100, slightly higher than that in boys.[30]) Upper extremity overuse injuries from shooting include rotator cuff tendinitis, medial epicondylitis, wrist sprains, dorsal proximal interphalangeal dislocations, volar dislocations, jersey finger (flexor digitorum profundus avulsion), and mallet finger.[31]

Cheerleading

Often overlooked in the sports medicine field, cheerleading is an athletic activity with serious risks. Falls can cause fractures and trauma. Cheerleading has claimed the highest percentage of direct fatalities and catastrophic injuries in US female student athletes.[32] Jumping and landing leads to ankle and knee injuries. Falls can cause fractures and trauma. Overuse injuries include those to the upper extremities with rotator cuff tendinitis, impingement, and shoulder and wrist instabilities.[33] Wrist and lumbar sprain occur from repetitive motions, lifts, and improper technique. Stress fractures should be considered.[34] Eating disorders are common among cheerleaders.[35]

Climbing

As indoor and outdoor climbing gain popularity, women are proving their negotiating skills as some consider themselves better climbers than men. Upper extremity injuries are related to handholds. Elbow sources of pain include medial epicondylitis, anterior capsular injury, brachialis tendinitis, and brachialis tears ("climber's elbow").[36(p 197)] Wrist extensor and finger flexor tendinitis can occur. Finger injuries, including spiral fractures, dislocations, and ruptures of the flexor digitorum sublimis; annular pulley tears, specifically A2 pulley tears, have been described in extreme climbers.[36(p 200)] Flexion contractures and joint effusions can occur as a result of chronic injury. Nerve compressions include cubital and radial tunnel syndrome and carpal tunnel syndrome.[37]

Cycling

Although most children in the United States learn equal bicycling skills, cycling as a sport has only recently been popular among women. Introduced to the Olympics just recently in 1984, competitive cycling demands a rigorous training schedule. Seating and cleating malalignment can cause patellofemoral pain, posterior knee pain resulting from biceps femoris insertional tendinitis, patellar tendinitis, iliotibial band syndrome, pes anserine bursitis, and medial plica, along with Achilles tendinitis. Pelvic malalignment through the sacroiliac joints has also been described.[38(pp 424-425)] Trauma from road crashes leads to clavicular fractures, shoulder dislocations, scaphoid fractures, Colles fractures, radial head fractures,[39] and road rash. Candidiasis and skin irritation can occur with long workouts. Neuropathies include ulnar nerve in Guyon's canal and cubital tunnel. Tarsal tunnel syndrome and Morton's neuroma can occur as a result of shoe pressures. Interdigital neuromas and pudendal neuropathies can also occur.[40(p 561)]

Dance

Training for dance often begins at a young age. Injuries vary between types of dance; however, hip flexor tendinitis, patellofemoral complaints, pelvic epiphysial avulsion fractures, and spondylolysis, including facet pain, are concerns in both adult and younger dancers.[41(pp 395-396)] En pointe (on toes) usually begins at age 12, introducing a host of ankle, foot, and toe problems. Turnout (external hip rotation) can cause hip flexor and sartorius tendinitis and pyriformis syndrome. Knees are subject to rotation, squatting, jumping, and landing, resulting in patellar tendinitis and Achilles tendinitis with occasional rupture, as well as stress fractures in the leg and metatarsals.[42] Foot and ankle injuries include flexor hallucis tendinitis, anterior and posterior impingement, Morton's neuroma, cuboid syndrome, sesamoiditis, and spiral fracture of the fifth metatarsal head ("dancer's fracture").[43]

Diving

A rigorous and demanding sport requiring spine and extremity flexibility, strength, and control, dives from 10-m platforms cause more injuries than springboard because of the high velocity on water entry. Cervical sprains and injuries can occur, including brachial plexus injuries. Injuries to the lumbar spine include spondylolysis, spondylolisthesis, and lumbar facet arthropathy.[44] Multidirectional shoulder laxity can lead to instability, tendinitis, bursitis, and rotator cuff tears. The impact on water entry commonly causes distal upper extremity injuries, including medial collateral ligament, triceps strains and tears, ulnar neuritis, dorsal impaction syndromes, lunate subluxation, dorsal ganglion cysts, and ulnar collateral ligament injuries. Head contusions, scalp lacerations, and phalangeal injuries occur from striking the board. Jumping results in ankle and leg injuries, including patellar tendinitis and pain syndromes; tibial and metatarsal stress fractures can also occur. Medical issues include perforation of tympanic membrane, retinal detachment, and ocular contusions, as well as otitis externa. Landing flat on the water can result in hemoptysis and pulmonary contusions.[44] Vertigo can be a chronic and problematic complication. As an aesthetic, disciplined sport, eating disrorers must also be considered.

Equestrian Events

Young riders are mostly girls; women have higher reported rates of injuries but lower rates of morbidity than male riders.[45] Overuse injuries include adductor and hamstring sprains and contractures, ischial bursitis, patellofemoral symptoms, and Achilles tendinitis. Myositis ossificans of the adductor muscles should be considered.[46 (p 562)] Lumbar and pelvic pain syndromes, including degenerative and discogenic pain, are common. Medical concerns include environmental allergies, asthma, and skin irritation, including blistering of hands, chapping of thighs, intertrigo, and contact dermatitis. Falls lead to head injuries, spine fractures, and upper extremity fractures, most commonly to the clavicle, humerus, elbow, and wrist and hand.[45]

Fencing

Because activities are done primarily on one side of the body, overuse injuries on that side are more common. Ankle sprains and foot injuries are quite common; knee ligament sprains and meniscal tears also occur. Iliotibial band syndrome, plantar fasciitis, and leg overuse injuries occur. Wrist and hand tendinitis can also occur. Lumbar sprains, along with other causes of back pain, are described. Contusions and lacerations can occur from the weapon.[47]

Field Hockey

A sport quite popular among scholastic and collegiate young women, field hockey can result in various sports-related injuires; most to the lower extremities, as well as the upper extremities, face, and head. Like most field sports, ankle sprains are most frequent. Back pain is quite common secondary to constant flexion while maneuvering a stick, and rotation required during play; disc herniation can occur. Knee injuries include meniscal, collateral ligament, patellofemoral, and ACL. Dorsal hand and finger injuries occur, including dorsal ganglions and DeQuervain's tenosynovitis, and lateral epicondylitis. Falls result in clavicle fractures or shoulder injuries. Because of the contact nature of the sport, as well as the use of sticks and balls, contusions, lacerations, and concussions can occur. Ocular injuries also may occur.[48]

Golf

Golf is a sport that continues to increase in popularity among girls and women; improper conditioning and technique can lead to overuse injuries, including AC synovitis, shoulder impingement and instability, and rotator cuff tendinitis. Lateral epicondylitis (tennis elbow) usually occurs in the leading arm and medial epicondylitis (golfer's elbow) in the trailing arm.[49(p 571)] Ulnar wrist pain should be evaluated for hook of hamate fractures. DeQuervain's tenosynovitis, extensor carpi ulnaris tendinitis, stenosing tenosynovitis (trigger finger), and wrist ganglia can occur. Rib stress fractures have also been described. Low back pain is frequent due to lumbar sprain, disc pathology, and osteoporotic and trauma-induced lumbar and low thoracic vertebral compression fractures.[50]

Gymnastics

Girls begin training at ages as early as 4 to 5; hyperextension of all joints can lead to chronic instability and injury as gymnasts push the limits of strength, balance, and flexibility. This is a whole-body demanding sport requiring early discipline and control. Repetitive spine movements in many planes result in spondylolysis, spondylolisthesis, and discogenic sources of back pain. Wrist pain is also quite frequent. Stress fractures of the distal radial physis are frequent: younger gymnasts can have widening of the distal radial growth plate, which may develop into a shortened radius after skeletal maturity.[51(p 30)] Triangular fibrocartilage tears, ganglion cysts, and extensor tendinitis are also prevalent.[52] Elbow dislocations, shoulder instabilities, impingement, and tendinitis can occur. Ankle and knee injuries are frequent as well. In adolescence, pelvic apophyseal avulsion fractures can occur prior to growth plate closure.[53(p 575)] Body image disorders and components of the female athlete triad are common to gymnasts of all age levels.[54]

Ice Hockey

Since the US women's Olympic win in 1996, women's ice hockey has been a growing force. Injuries include lacerations and contusions, especially to the face, eyes, and hands. Concussions and cervical injuries can also occur. AC separations are seen in older players, clavicular fractures in younger players.[55(p 575)] Other upper extremity injuries include rotator cuff, shoulder dislocations, sternoclavicular, first metacarpal fractures, and scaphoid fractures along with jersey and mallet fingers. Hamstring, groin, and adductor sprains and contusions are quite common. Osteitis pubis

can occur. Knee injuries are most frequent, often because of contact, particularly medial collateral ligament (MCL) and medial meniscus injuries. ACL tears can also occur. Ankle sprains, bursae, and foot injuries, including navicular fractures, can be common. Rib injuries and abdominal trauma including the spleen and kidney are also described.[55]

Military Training

The higher incidence of overall injuries in women midshipmen actually decreases over time served in the military.[56] March fractures (stress fractures of the metatarsals) are common. With the obstacle course presenting the site of highest knee injuries, military training is associated with a higher ACL injury risk in women than men. Overall risk of serious injuries is equal to men.[56]

Rowing

Rowing requires repetitive high-resistance movements that can lead to overuse injuries. Thoracic and lumbar pain is frequent because of the forces transmitted through flexion and extension as the shell (boat) is propelled through the water. Rib stress fractures,[57] disc pathology, and spondylolysis should be considered, both from overuse and from "catching a crab" in which the oar gets pulled under the boat. Sciatica can also be present as a result of seat fit. Ischial tuberosity bursitis can also occur.[58] Patellofemoral and iliotibial band syndromes can occur as a result of hill and squat training along with loaded flexion.[59 (p 377)] Forearm and wrist tendinitis, DeQuervain's tenosynovitis, and extensor tendinitis are common because of "feathering" (rotating) the oar. "Interstitial syndrome" has been described as a result of compression of the extensor carpi radialis longus and brevis as a frequent cause of wrist pain.[51] Palm and finger blistering is frequent and can lead to infection, which may spread to teammates by sharing oars.[60]

Rugby

Rugby is an aggressive contact field sport in which little to no protective gear is worn. Women's rugby teams are more prevalent in Europe, Australia, and New Zealand but increasing in the United States. Overall injury rates are lower in women than men.[61] Shoulder dislocations, AC sprains, and instabilities occur along with facial and eye injuries. Clavicle and finger fractures with occasional rib fractures occur as well. Like all field sports, ankle sprains are the most frequent injuries. Knee injury rates have been reported to be higher than women's soccer, and MCL vs ACL injuries can be related to position played.[4] Quad and hamstring strains, hip pointers, and quadriceps contusions can lead to myositis ossificans.[62]

Running

Appealing to all levels of athletes, women now compete in events of all distance. The popularity of marathons and endurance events in older women has resulted in a higher frequency of overuse injuries, the most common of which include iliotibial band syndrome, plantar fasciitis, metatarsalgia; Achilles and posterior tibial tendinitis; and "shinsplints" often secondary to improper conditioning, stretching, footwear, running surface, and alignment. Sprinters frequently have hamstring sprains.[63(p 613)] Knee pain is common and associated with patellofemoral symptoms, plica, quadriceps and patellar tendinitis, and meniscal degeneration. Gluteal and greater trochanteric bursitis, sacroiliitis, and iliotibial band syndrome can result from running on banked or uneven surfaces. Osteitis pubis can also be a cause of pelvic pain. "Shinsplints" can be secondary to periostitis, compartment syndrome, tibial stress fractures, or tendinitis. Additional sites of stress fractures include femoral neck, pubis, fibula, and metatarsals.[64(p 412)] Hallux valgus and rigidus also occur. Morton's neuromas, tarsal tunnel, and bunions and blisters can also occur frequently in women because of restriction of shoe size. Eating disorders associated with stress fractures and amenorrhea—the female athlete triad—have a higher incidence in runners who desire to maintain an ultralight frame. In endurance events, postural hypotension can cause exercise-associated collapse upon completion of the event; hyponatremia and heatstroke are more serious causes of collapse, which can take the athlete out of the event.[65]

Scuba Diving

It has been speculated that women are more susceptible to decompression sickness, but this is still under debate.[66(pp 355–356)] Pregnancy is a contraindication to scuba diving. Injuries are not frequently reported but are often secondary to equipment, marine life, and terrain. Hypothermia is a concern.

Skating

Despite the prevalence and popularity of women skaters, specific injuries to skaters have not been well studied. Women frequently participate in figure, ice dancing, pair, speed, and in-line skating. Collisions, falls, and jumping and landing can result in fractures of the ankle, tibia, distal radius, femur, and patella, along with wrist sprains, AC separations, ulnar collateral ligament injuries, meniscal tears, and knee and wrist ligament tears. Feet and ankles are susceptible to malleolar bursitis, Haglund's deformities, bunions, Achilles tendinitis, and lacerations, resulting in superficial peroneal injuries.[67] Tibial and metatarsal stress fractures, compartment syndromes, hip adductor, flexor, and hamstring injuries can occur. Pair skaters are susceptible to wrist ganglions from lifts. Figure skaters can also be at risk for spondylolysis and listhesis; back pain in all skaters is frequent and can also be due to lumbar sprain and disc pathology. Younger skaters can be at risk for tibial tubercle apophysitis and physeal fractures of the knee.[67(p 598)] Judged on aesthetics and requiring lithe, overly viewed physiques, figure skaters are at high risks for eating disorders and the female athlete triad.[68]

Skiing

A woman's Olympic event since 1924,[69] skiing is notorious for knee injuries. Types of skiing vary in use of equipment and injury with incidences greatest in alpine (downhill) and telemark and less in cross-country. Releasable bindings are invaluable in preventing knee injuries; boot type can also play a role.[22] As in most sports, ACL injuries are known to occur with greater frequency in women. MCL, meniscal, and patellar dislocations also occur. Female skiers have also been documented to have greater incidences of anemia and iron deficiency.[69(p 351)] Older skiers can be susceptible to hip and femur fractures. Upper extremity injuries secondary to falling include "skier's thumb" (ulnar collateral ligament tear), AC joint separations, rotator cuff tears, and shoulder dislocations.[70] Fractures include those of the humerus, olecranon, and scaphoid. Collisions with other skiers, objects, and ski and lift equipment can result in oral and facial injuries.[71] Environmental hazards include terrain, trees, tree wells, and ice; deep heavy snow can increase knee injury risks also. Head injuries can result in death, and the use of helmets is widely recommended in downhill skiing.

Snowboarding

Increasing in popularity among all winter athletes, snowboarding is a sport associated with young, daring personalities. Ease of control of one piece of equipment allows for flips and jumps in half-pipes along with intense downhill speed. A recent study reports snowboarding as associated with a greater likelihood of overall injury than skiing.[72] Skiers with knee injuries have also turned to snowboarding, because the closed-chain mechanism of the snowboard is relatively knee sparing. Most common injuries are to the wrist and forearms, including scaphoid fractures.[70] Shoulder dislocations can also occur. In one study 6.8% of all injuries in snowboarders were distal radius fractures.[73] Chest injuries and rib fractures are also reported.[74] Helmets should be encouraged to prevent head injuries because of the likelihood of backward falls. Snowboarders' ankle has been described as a fracture of the lateral process of the talus.[75]

Soccer

Soccer is known as the most popular sport in the world, and has had a dramatic increase in female participation recently.[76] Injuries include both contact and noncontact, and can be variable based on surface of play (indoor vs outdoor), position, and level of competition. While studies suggest a higher incidence of overall injuries in girls vs boys,[1(p 77), 77(p 480)] generally, rates of injuries in women vs men are similar,[78(p 602)] with the exception of an increased rate of noncontact ACL injuries. Meniscal injuries, collateral ligament sprains, and patellar syndromes, including tendinitis, also occur. Thigh and calf contusions are common and must be followed to rule out myositis ossificans. Stress fractures, tibial periostitis, and stress syndromes, along with compartment symdromes, can also be present. Ankle sprains, Achilles tears and sprains, and turf toe are common. "Footballer's ankle," or anterior ankle impingement syndrome, is associated with tibiotalar osteophytes.[79(p 605)] Heel pain in young girls can be evidence of Sever's disease (calcaneal apophysitis).[53(p S74)] Adductor, hip flexor, and iliotibial band tendinitis and strains can occur from kicking. Foot injuries include midfoot sprains, metatarsal stress fractures and sesamoid injuries along with hallux rigidus and reverse turf toe ("soccer toe.") Head and neck injuries can result from "heading" the ball, or impact with the field, other players, or the goalpost. Fractures are more common in the upper extremities due to falls or collisions; goalkeepers suffer more upper extremity injuries.[77(p 482)] Dental and facial trauma can also occur.

Softball, Baseball, and Fast-Pitch Softball

These sports have been popular with girls and women for the past century. Hyperextension injuries and sprains of the fingers and wrists are common along with navicular and hook of hamate fractures, scapholunate instability, and triangular fibrocartilage and extensor carpi ulnaris sprains. The "foot first" sliding techniques result in ankle sprains and fractures and knee injuries, in particular collateral ligament injuries. Collision injuries also occur. Sprinting can lead to hamstring and quadriceps sprains and strains. Pitching injuries include multidirectional, anterior, and posterior instability, which can lead to or be associated with superior labrum anterior posterior (SLAP) lesions and glenoid labrum tears.[80] Other reported injuries include suprascapular neuropathy, stress fractures of the ribs and humerus, and stress-induced epiphysiolysis at the proximal humeral physis.[80(p 541)] Pitchers' techniques and injuries have been widely studied; the underhand pitch of fast-pitch softball is not known to cause less incidence of injuries.[81(p 460)] Bicipital and rotator cuff tendinitis, medial epicondylitis, and ulnar stress fractures along with tears of the ulnar collateral ligament

can occur. Radial neuropathy has also been described.[82] Osteochondritis dissecans of the capitellum can also occur with extreme overuse. In young pitchers, medial apophyseal injury can occur. This, along with other overuse injuries of the medial epicondyle, is referred to as "little leaguer's elbow."[53(S73)]

Swimming

Swimming is a highly popular and publicized sport among girls and women, and training often begins at a young age. "Swimmers shoulder" is the most frequently occurring overuse injury with components of impingement, tendinitis, bursitis, and instability. This is a result of the overhead reach of the freestyle and butterfly strokes and the high yardage demanded of most swimmers (some swim up to and more than 10,000 yards per day; approximately 3000–4000 strokes per arm per day). Breaststrokers can develop patello-femoral and medial patterns of knee pain, including chronic MCL strain due to repetitive open chain valgus and rotation stress. Lumbar extension in the butterfly and breaststroke kick can lead to increased incidence of spondylolysis.[83(p 367),84] A frequent medical problem is external otitis, "swimmer's ear." Despite the common belief that swimming is beneficial for exercise-induced asthma, the chemicals used in pool maintenance can be a bronchial irritant. The heavy training schedule and focus on body shape contribute to eating disorders and amenorrhea. Injuries secondary to cross-training may occur almost with equal frequency as those caused by overuse injuries in swimming.[85]

Tennis

Because tennis is popular as a professional and recreational sport, overuse injuries are common,[23] including "tennis elbow" (lateral epicondylitis, secondary to overload of weak extensors, improper raquet grip size, and poor technique), medial epicondylitis, rotator cuff tendinitis, and stress fractures. Ulnar collateral ligament sprain and median and ulnar nerve entrapments can also occur. Ulnar stress fractures have also been documented. Hook of hamate fractures can occur along with tenosynovitis of the wrist and fingers, especially DeQuervain's tenosynovitis.[86] Thoracic and abdominal muscle sprains and tears can also occur. Back pain can be secondary to lumbar sprain, sacroiliitis, spondylolysis, and disc pathology. "Tennis leg," partial rupture of the medial head of the gastrocnemius,[87] can occur, along with patellar tendinitis, and Achilles tendinitis and rupture. Ankle sprains are common, along with overuse injuries of feet, including plantar fasciitis, turf toe, and "tennis toe" (subungual hematoma). Shoulder impingement and rotator cuff tendinitis are also common from serving, volleying, and overheads.[88]

Triathlon

Races combining swimming, biking, and running require many hours of training and result in overuse injuries associated with each sport, along with the traumatic injuries due to biking collisions. Triathletes' average age is in the mid 30s,[89] and numbers of women participants are growing. In addition to the previously described specific sport injuries, open water swimming and cycling can cause cervicothoracic strain.[40] Eating disorders can be common, along with dehydration, anemia, and hyponatremia, resulting from the endurance nature of training and events.

Volleyball

Volleyball is a popular sport among female athletes at all levels. The jumping, overhead motions, and contact nature of the team sport leads to a variety of injuries. Like most team sports, the most common injuries are inversion ankle sprains.[90] Finger injuries are also quite common because players strike the ball with open hands. Ulnar collateral ligament injuries (gamekeeper's thumb), "jammed fingers," and mallet fingers must be evaluated for avulsion fractures. Wrist sprains, scaphoid fractures, and pisiform fatigue fractures also may occur. Shoulder overuse syndromes, including rotator cuff tendinitis, impingement, and AC sprains and chronic impingement, can even lead to suprascapular neuropathy.[91] Lumbar spine injuries include spondylolysis as extension occurs in play. Lumbar sprain is also common. Knee injuries have also been fairly well studied and include ACL tears, patellar tendinitis (jumper's knee), and patellofemoral pain. Tibial stress fractures should be considered as a cause of leg pain.

Waterskiing

A recreationally popular sport, waterskiing requires great strength, balance, and control over high speeds. Injuries that can occur from impact with the water (or objects) include shoulder dislocations, rib fractures, contusions, and head trauma. Hamstring and quadriceps strains, MCL strains, and meniscal tears along with ACL injuries occur. Posterior cruciate ligament tears can occur as a result of rotational injuries. Jumps can result in bruised heels, ankle fractures and sprains, and disc herniations. Cervical, thoracic, and lumbar sprains are common. Forearm, particularly flexor and pronator, tendinitis is a common overuse injury along with subacromial bursitis. Wrist and hand injuries can occur; blistering and skin infections along with tympanic membrane ruptures can occur also. Vaginal douches are possible during falls and may lead to abscess, lacerations, or miscarriage.[92]

Weightlifting

Introduced as an Olympic event for women in 2000, weightlifting is also recreationally popular. Injuries are a result of excess weight, overtraining, and poor technique. These include cervical and lumbar sprains and disc herniations, shoulder sprains and tendinitis, including AC joint sprains, rotator cuff sprains, pectoralis rupture and instability, lateral epicondylitis, flexor carpi radialis and DeQuervain's tendinitis, knee sprains, including patellofemoral and meniscal pain, and patellar tendinitis.[93] The tendency for these athletes to use supplements and performance enhancers should be considered. Bodybuilders have a high incidence of eating disorders and amenorrhea.

INJURY PREVENTION

Knowledge of incidence and mechanism of sports injuries facilitates injury prevention. Identifying and studying causes of injury can be complicated by the combination of factors that result in each injury; therefore isolating and controlling a single risk of injury is unrealistic. Defining an injury has also been variable—a universal rating system for significance and severity of injury could make studies more interreliable. The prevalence of nontreated minor injuries that may lead to severe injuries is uncertain; this is an important area of consideration when addressing injury prevention.

Injury prevention techniques, such as jumping and landing training,[94] and sliding, falling, and rolling techniques to reduce risk of injury should be included in practice, training, and rehabilitation. Programs incorporating such neuromuscular training have been shown to reduce knee injury incidence in high school soccer and basketball players.[95] Similarly, training workshops to teach techniques to avoid injury in skiing have been found to reduce knee injuries.[96] Implementing safety regulations and modifying equipment, clothing, and rules in sports have also been proven to reduce injuries.[32] Examples include secure goalposts, breakaway bases, streamlined clothing, and releasable telemark and trick ski bindings. Fingernail extensions and jewelry should be discouraged, because these can increase finger and skin injuries. Education of athletes, parents, and coaches; continuity of medical care; preseason conditioning; and appropriate sports injury management and rehabilitation will reduce injury incidence. As girls' and women's sports become more organized and recognized, preventative strategies more regularly applied, and treatment and rehabilitation strategies more clearly defined, numbers of sports injuries and medical complications at all levels of activity will decline.

REFERENCES

1. Nelson C. Taking a critical look at youth soccer injuries. *Sports Med Digest.* 1999;21:76–84.

2. Ehrendorfer S. Survey of sport injuries in physical education students participating in 13 sports. *Wien Klin Wochenschr.* 1998:110:397–400.

3. Perlmutter GS, Leffert RD, Zarins B. Direct injury to the axillary nerve in athletes playing contact sports. *Am J Sports Med.* 1997;25:65–68.

4. Levy AS, Wetzler MJ, Lewars M, Lauglin W. Knee injuries in women collegiate rugby players. *Am J Sports Med.* 1997;25:360–362.

5. Fronek J. Baseball and softball. In: Safran MR, McKeag DB, Van Camp SP, eds. *Manual of Sports Medicine.* Philadelphia: Lippincott-Raven; 1998:541–543.

6. Jago D, Finch C. Sporting and recreational injuries in a general practice setting. *Aust Family Phys.* 1998;27:389–395.

7. Twellaar M, Verstappen FTJ, Huson A. Is prevention of sports injuries a realistic goal? A four-year prospective investigation of sports injuries among physical education students. *Am J Sports Med.* 1996;24:528–534.

8. Almeida SA, Trone DW, Leone DM, et al. Gender differences in musculoskeletal injury rates: A function of symptom reporting? *Med Sci Sports Exerc.* 1999;31:1807–1812.

9. Clarke KS, Buckley WE. Women's injuries in collegiate sports. *Am J Sports Med.* 1980;8:187–191.

10. Arendt EA, Agel J, Dick R. Anterior cruciate ligament injury patterns among collegiate men and women. *J Athletic Training.* 1999;34:86–92.

11. Arendt E, Dick R. Knee injury patterns among men and women in collegiate basketball and soccer. NCAA Data and Review of Literature. *Am J Sports Med.* 1995;23:694–701.

12. Messina DF, Farney WC, DeLee JC. The incidence of injury in Texas high school basketball: A prospective study among male and female athletes. *Am J Sports Med.* 1999;27:294–299.

13. Baker MM. Anterior cruciate ligament injuries in the female athlete. *J Women's Health.* 1998;7:343–349.

14. Ireland ML. Anterior cruciate ligament injury in female athletes: Epidemiology. *J Athletic Training.* 1999;34:150–154.

15. Tancred B. Footwear: The hidden component in sporting injuries? A commentary. *Am J Phys Med Rehabil.* 1996;75:66–67.

16. Rozzi SL, Lephart SM, Gear WS, Fu FH. Knee joint laxity and neuromuscular characteristics of male and female soccer and basketball players. *Am J Sports Med.* 1999;27:312–319.

17. Decoster LC, Bernier JN, Lindsay RH, Vailas JC. Generalized joint hypermobility and its relationship to injury patterns among NCAA lacrosse players. *J Athletic Training.* 1999;34:99–105.

18. Harmon KG, Dick R. The relationship of skill level to anterior cruciate ligament injury. *Clin J Sport Med.* 1998;8:260–265.

19. Loudon JK, Jenkins W, Loudon KL. The relationship between static posture and ACL injury in female athletes. *JOSPT.* 1996;24:91–96.

20. Huston LJ, Wojtys EM. Neuromuscular performance characteristics in elite female athletes. *Am J Sports Med.* 1996;24:427–434.

21. Wojtys EM, Huston LJ, Lindenfeld TN, Hewett TE. Association between the menstrual cycle and anterior cruciate ligament injuries in female athletes. *Am J Sports Med.* 1998;26:614–619.

22. Tuggy ML, Ong R. Injury risk factors among telemark skiers. *Am J Sports Med.* 2000;28:83–89.

23. Bylak J, Hutchinson MR. Common sports injuries in young tennis players. *Sports Med.* 1998;26:119–132.

24. Gwinn DE, Wilckens JH, McDevitt ER, et al. The relative incidence of anterior cruciate ligament injury in men and women at the United States Naval Academy. *Am J Sports Med.* 2000;28:98–102.

25. Barton N. Sports injuries of the hand and wrist. *Br J Sports Med.* 1997;31:191–196.

26. Sorensen L, Larsen SE, Rock ND. The epidemiology of sports injuries in school-aged children. *Scand J Med Sci Sports.* 1996;6:281–286.

27. DeHaven KE, Lintner DM. Athletic injuries: Comparison by age, sport and gender. *Am J Sports Med.* 1986;14:218–224.

28. Emery L. From Lowell Mills to the Halls of Fame: Industrial league sport for women. In: Costa DM, Guthrie, SR. *Women and Sport: Interdisciplinary Perspectives.* Champaign, IL: Human Kinetics; 1994:107–121.

29. Caborn DNM, Coen MJ. Basketball. In: Safran MR, McKeag DB, Van Camp SP, eds. *Manual of Sports Medicine.* Philadelphia: Lippincott-Raven; 1998:544–545.

30. Powell JW, Barber-Foss KD. Traumatic brain injury in high school athletes. *JAMA.* 1999;282:958–963.

31. Krivickas LS. Basketball. In: Agostini R, Titus S, eds. *Medical and Orthopedic Issues of Active and Athletic Women.* Philadelphia: Hanley & Belfus; 1994:465–477.

32. Cantu RC, Mueller FO. Fatalities and catastrophic injuries in high school and college sports, 1982–1997. *Physician Sportsmed.* 1999;27:35–48.

33. Hutchinson MR. Cheerleading injuries: Patterns, prevention, case reports. *Physician Sportsmed.* 1997;9:83–96.

34. Meade KM. Something to cheer about: Preventing and treating cheerleading injuries. *Adv Directors Rehabil.* 1998;2:24–25.

35. Gottlieb A. Cheerleaders are athletes too. *Pediatr Nurs.* 1994;20:630–633.

36. Holtzhausen LM, Noakes TD. Elbow, forearm, wrist, and hand injuries among sport rock climbers. *Clin J Sports Med.* 1996;6:196–203.

37. Bach A. Mountaineering and climbing. In: Safran MR, McKeag DB, Van Camp SP, eds. *Manual of Sports Medicine.* Philadelphia: Lippincott-Raven; 1998:583–585.

38. Hopkins SR. Bicycling. In: Agostini R, Titus S, eds. *Medical and Orthopedic Issues of Active and Athletic Women.* Philadelphia: Hanley & Belfus; 1994:419–429.

39. Hunter RE. Cycling: Road, velodrome and mountain biking. In: Safran MR, McKeag DB, Van Camp SP, eds. *Manual of Sports Medicine.* Philadelphia: Lippincott-Raven; 1998:551–552.

40. Scott WA. Endurance events: Marathon, ultramarathon, triathlon. In: Safran MR, McKeag DB, Van Camp SP, eds. *Manual of Sports Medicine.* Philadelphia: Lippincott-Raven; 1998:558–561.

41. Schafle MD. The child dancer. In: Agostini R, Titus S, eds. *Medical and Orthopedic Issues of Active and Athletic Women.* Philadelphia: Hanley & Belfus; 1994:395–397.

42. Schafle MD. Dance. In: Safran MR, McKeag DB, Van Camp SP, eds. *Manual of Sports Medicine.* Philadelphia: Lippincott-Raven; 1998:553–555.

43. Garrick JD. Dance. In: Agostini R, Titus S, eds. *Medical and Orthopedic Issues of Active and Athletic Women.* Philadelphia: Hanley & Belfus; 1994:398–405.

44. Rubin BD. Diving: Platform and springboard. In: Safran MR, McKeag DB, Van Camp SP, eds. *Manual of Sports Medicine.* Philadelphia: Lippincott-Raven; 1998:556–557.

45. Finnegan MA. Equestrian events. In: Agostini R, Titus S, eds. *Medical and Orthopedic Issues of Active and Athletic Women*. Philadelphia: Hanley & Belfus; 1994:439–444.

46. Korompilias AV, Seaber AV. Equestrian activities. In: Safran MR, McKeag DB, Van Camp SP, eds. *Manual of Sports Medicine*. Philadelphia: Lippincott-Raven; 1998:562–563.

47. Jaffe R, Knowles JM. Fencing. In: Safran MR, McKeag DB, Van Camp SP, eds. *Manual of Sports Medicine*. Philadelphia: Lippincott-Raven; 1998:564–565.

48. Laurencin CT, Gorun WJ III. Field hockey. In: Safran MR, McKeag DB, Van Camp SP, eds. *Manual of Sports Medicine*. Philadelphia: Lippincott-Raven; 1998:566–567.

49. Mallon WJ. Golf. In: Safran MR, McKeag DB, Van Camp SP, eds. *Manual of Sports Medicine*. Philadelphia: Lippincott-Raven; 1998:571–572.

50. Metz JP. Managing golf injuries. *Physician Sportsmed*. 1999;7:41–56.

51. Teitz CC. Upper extremity injuries in female athletes. *Women's Health: Orthop Ed*. 1999;2:27–31.

52. Mandelbaum BR, Nattiv A. Gymnastics. In: Safran M, McKeag DB, Van Camp SP, eds. *Manual of Sports Medicine*. Philadelphia: Lippincott-Raven; 1998:573–574.

53. Smith J, Wilder RP. Musculoskeletal rehabilitation and sports medicine. 4. Miscellaneous sports medicine topics. *Arch Phys Med Rehabil*. 1999;80:S68–89.

54. Nattiv A, Stryer BK, Mandelbaum BR. Gymnastics. In: Agostini R, Titus S, eds. *Medical and Orthopedic Issues of Active and Athletic Women*. Philadelphia: Hanley & Belfus; 1994:378–387.

55. Bartolozzi AR III, Palmeri M, DeLuca PF. Ice hockey. In: Safran MR, McKeag DB, Van Camp SP, eds. *Manual of Sports Medicine*. Philadelphia: Lippincott-Raven; 1998:575–577.

56. Cox JS, Lenz HW. Women midshipmen in sports. *Am J Sports Med*. 1984;12:241–243.

57. Sinha AK, Kaeding CC, Wadley GM. Upper extremity stress fractures in athletes: Clinical features of 44 cases. *Clin J Sports Med*. 1999;9:199–202.

58. Jenkinson DM. Rafting/rowing/kayaking/canoeing. In: Safran MR, McKeag DB, Van Camp SP, eds. *Manual of Sports Medicine*. Philadelphia: Lippincott-Raven; 1998:592–594.

59. Musnick DJ. Rowing. In: Agostini R, Titus S, eds. *Medical and Orthopedic Issues of Active and Athletic Women*. Philadelphia: Hanley & Belfus; 1994:373–377.

60. Karlson KA. Rowing injuries: Identifying and treating musculoskeletal and nonmusculoskeletal conditions. *Physician Sportsmed*. 2000;28:40–50.

61. Carson JD, Roberts MA, White AL. The epidemiology of women's rugby injuries. *Clin J Sport Med*. 1999;9:75–78.

62. Brukner P. Rugby. In: Safran MR, McKeag DB, Van Camp SP, eds. *Manual of Sports Medicine*. Philadelphia: Lippincott-Raven; 1998:595–596.

63. Shaw DR. Track and field. In: Safran MR, McKeag DB, Van Camp SP, eds. *Manual of Sports Medicine*. Philadelphia: Lippincott-Raven; 1998:613–614.

64. Colliton JW. Running. In: Agostini R, Titus S, eds. *Medical and Orthopedic Issues of Active and Athletic Women*. Philadelphia: Hanley & Belfus; 1994:406–418.

65. Noakes TD. Hyponatremia in distance athletes. Putting the IV on the "Dehydration Myth." *Physician Sportsmed*. 2000;28:71–76.

66. Beerman G. Scuba diving and the marine environment. In: Agostini R, Titus S, eds. *Medical and Orthopedic Issues of Active and Athletic Women*. Philadelphia: Hanley & Belfus; 1994:355–362.

67. Smith W. Speed skating, in-line skating, figure skating. In: Safran MR, McKeag DB, Van Camp SP, eds. *Manual of Sports Medicine*. Philadelphia: Lippincott-Raven; 1998:597–599.

68. Smith AD. Figure skating. In: Agostini R, Titus S, eds. *Medical and Orthopedic Issues of Active and Athletic Women*. Philadelphia: Hanley & Belfus; 1994:388–394.

69. Gibbs P. Skiing. In: Agostini R, Titus S, eds. *Medical and Orthopedic Issues of Active and Athletic Women*. Philadelphia: Hanley & Belfus; 1994:347–354.

70. Steadman JR, Dean MT. Alpine skiing. In: Safran MR, McKeag DB, Van Camp SP, eds. *Manual of Sports Medicine*. Philadelphia: Lippincott-Raven; 1998:600–601.

71. Gassner R et al. Incidence of oral and maxillofacial skiing injuries due to different injury mechanisms. *J Oral Maxillofac Surg*. 1999;57:1068–1073.

72. Nakaguchi H, Fujimaki T, Ueki K, et al. Snowboarding head injury: Prospective study in Chino, Nagano, for two seasons from 1995 to 1997. *J Trauma: Inj Infect Crit Care*.1999;46:1066–1069.

73. Sasaki K, Michiaki T, Kiyohige Y, et al. Snowboarder's wrist: Its severity compared with alpine skiing. *J Trauma: Inj Infect Crit Care*. 1999;57:1068–1073.

74. Machida T, Hanazaki K, Ishizaka K, et al. Snowboarding injuries of the chest: Comparison with skiing injuries. *J Trauma: Inj Infect Crit Care*. 1999;46:1062–1065.

75. Cronin WM, McKeon JP. Wild jumps and bumps: Snowboarders' ankle is more than a casual sprain. *Adv Directors Rehabil*. 2000;2:27–28.

76. Delfico AJ, Garrett WE. Mechanisms of injury of the anterior cruciate ligament in soccer players. *Clin Sports Med*. 1998;17:779–785.

77. Putukian M. Soccer. In: Agostini R, Titus S, eds. *Medical and Orthopedic Issues of Active and Athletic Women*. Philadelphia: Hanley & Belfus; 1994:478–488.

78. Ticker JB. Soccer: Futsal and indoor. In: Safran MR, McKeag DB, Van Camp SP, eds. *Manual of Sports Medicine*. Philadelphia: Lippincott-Raven; 1998:602–603.

79. Johnson DL, Neef RL. Soccer: Outdoor. In: Safran MR, McKeag DB, Van Camp SP, eds. *Manual of Sports Medicine*. Philadelphia: Lippincott-Raven; 1998:604–605.

80. Fronek J. Baseball and softball. In: Safran MR, McKeag DB, Van Camp SP, eds. *Manual of Sports Medicine*. Philadelphia: Lippincott-Raven; 1998:541–543.

81. Hebert PA. Softball. In: Agostini R, Titus S, eds. *Medical and Orthopedic Issues of Active and Athletic Women*. Philadelphia: Hanley & Belfus; 1994:459–464.

82. Werner SL. Down the middle. *Adv Directors Rehabil*. 1997;8:29–30.

83. Kenal K. Swimming and water polo. In: Agostini R, Titus S, eds. *Medical and Orthopedic Issues of Active and Athletic Women*. Philadelphia: Hanley & Belfus; 1994:363–372.

84. Richardson AB. Swimming. In: Safran MR, McKeag DB, Van Camp SP, eds. *Manual of Sports Medicine*. Philadelphia: Lippincott-Raven; 1998:609–610.

85. McFarland EG, Wasik M. Injuries in female collegiate swimmers due to swimming and cross training. *Clin J Sports Med*. 1996;6:178–182.

86. Rettig AC. Wrist problem in the tennis player. *Med Sci Sports Exerc*. 1994;26:1207–1212.

87. Safran MR, Stone DA. Tennis and other racket sports. In: Safran MR, McKeag DB, Van Camp SP, eds. *Manual of Sports Medicine*. Philadelphia: Lippincott-Raven; 1998:611–612.

88. Fieseler CM. Tennis. In: Agostini R, Titus S, eds. *Medical and Orthopedic Issues of Active and Athletic Women*. Philadelphia: Hanley & Belfus; 1994:445–454.

89. Kenal K. Triathlon. In: Agostini R, Titus S, eds. *Medical and Orthopedic Issues of Active and Athletic Women.* Philadelphia: Hanley & Belfus; 1994:430–433.

90. Hirshman HP. Volleyball. In: Safran MR, McKeag DB, Van Camp SP, eds. *Manual of Sports Medicine.* Philadelphia: Lippincott-Raven; 1998:615.

91. Davidson CJ, Harty DJ. Volleyball. In: Agostini R, Titus S, eds. *Medical and Orthopedic Issues of Active and Athletic Women.* Philadelphia: Hanley & Belfus; 1994:489–502.

92. Caldwell GL. Waterskiing: Standard and wakeboarding. In: Safran MR, McKeag DB, Van Camp SP, eds. *Manual of Sports Medicine.* Philadelphia: Lippincott-Raven; 1998:618–619.

93. Luetzow WF, Hackley D. Power lifting, weight lifting, and body building. In: Safran MR, McKeag DB, Van Camp SP, eds. *Manual of Sports Medicine.* Philadelphia: Lippincott-Raven; 1998:586–588.

94. Hewett TE, Stroupe AL, Nance TA, Noyes FR. Plyometric training in female athletes: Decreased impact forces and increased hamstring torques. *Am J Sports Med.* 1996;24:765–773.

95. Hewett TE, Lindenfeld TN, Riccobene JV, et al. The effect of neuromuscular training on the incidence of knee injury in female athletes: A prospective study. *Am J Sports Med.* 1999;27:699–705.

96. Ettinger CF et al. A method to help reduce the risk of serious knee sprains incurred in alpine skiing. *Am J Sports Med.* 1995;25:531–537.

Social Influences—The Experience of the Female Athlete

Linnea S. Hauge

"She didn't know it couldn't be done, so she went ahead and did it."

—*Bridget O'Donnell*

cited in *"BITS & PIECES"* e-mail service
from Daily Inbox.com and *BITS & PIECES* magazine

The female sport experience is as individual as its participants. Are there social influences that impact *all* female sport experiences? Champions of social causes might posit that social structures such as media or government have had an impact on all female sport experiences. However, the successes of female athletes who are unaware of these social structures may suggest otherwise. Certainly, a woman's sport experience is an individual experience that is likely affected by myriad of social influences.

SPORTS PARTICIPATION: THE INFLUENCE OF GENDER ROLES

The phrase "throw like a girl" and the intended implication that girls are not skilled sport participants by nature of their gender exemplify how gender roles have influenced who does and does not participate in sport. Girls and women have made significant advances in participation opportunities, with one in three college women currently participating in competitive sport.[1] Despite these advances and the publicized successes of many female athletes, many still face societal barriers to participation. These barriers are most often intangible in that female athletes are often confronted with stereotypes about the physical and emotional nature of athletic performance. For example, commonly accepted sport language often implies that a weaker sex exists ("girls' push-ups") or that female athletes are second-class athletes (ie, Lady Tigers).[2] Female athletes often face marginalization of their sport experiences, in which others do not see the value of their choice to participate. A woman's motivation to participate in sport, whether it is to achieve success, compete with others, enjoy social benefits of a sports team, or gain fitness, should be recognized as important, and a healthy sport experience should be encouraged. An athlete's perception of the value of her sport experience is important in identifying health and fitness goals, whether it be from a performance, maintenance, or recovery perspective. Furthermore, the lay press has made and continues to make recent significant contributions to health care by reporting the value of physical activity in disease prevention, especially for women.

For the sports medicine professional who provides care to female athletes, it is important to develop an understanding of the patient's sport experience and its contribution to her whole person. Of course, personal sport involvement is one way to begin to understand a patient's sport experience. Having personal experience in sport is likely to increase one's empathy toward a patient, as well as assist in establishing patient trust. However, a lack of athletic experience does not preclude a sports medicine professional from empathizing with patients, gaining patients' trust, or providing excellent care.

THE MEDIA'S INFLUENCE ON WOMEN'S SPORT AND FITNESS

Brandy Chastain and Mia Hamm, Venus and Sarena Williams, Rebecca Lobo and Sheryl Swoopes: these women, by their astounding athletic accomplishments in major sports events, have been the foci of media spotlights. Their names and faces have become recognizable. They have surpassed the single sports sound bite and achieved even greater recognition by means of marketing affiliations with major corporations. They are, albeit the beginning of the twenty-first century, anomalies. Few female athletes have achieved their level of recognition for their sporting achievements. It is a recent, and still unusual, phenomenon that female sports results appear on the front page of the sports section and that female athletes in team sports are paid to market products for major corporations. Historically, media attention has been paid to female athletes in lean sports where aesthetics, especially feminine attributes, are valued and rewarded as part of a competition (i.e., gymnastics, ice skating). Furthermore, the marketing of female athletes tends to focus on their physical attractiveness and personal lives rather than their athletic accomplishments.[2]

LEGISLATING PARTICIPATION: THE ADVENT AND ENFORCEMENT OF TITLE IX

Quite possibly one of the greatest influences on women's sport participation in the last century has been the advent of Title IX of the Education Amendments of 1972.[3] It states:

> No person in the United States shall, on the basis of sex, be excluded from participation in, be denied the benefits of, or be subjected to discrimination under any education program or activity receiving Federal financial assistance....[3]

Its immediate impact was relatively ineffective, largely because of judicial interpretation and application of other legislation that weakened Title IX. However, widespread changes and enforcement began to take place with the passage of the Civil Rights Restoration Act of 1988, and the U.S. Court of Appeals decision in *Cohen v Brown University* in 1993. Furthermore, educational institutions recognized the financial liabilities associated with noncompliance with the 1991 Supreme Court decision in *Franklin v Gwinnett*, which awarded a large sum of money for damages to a female student who had been sexually harassed by a teacher in her school.[4] Twenty years after its legislative debut, Title IX began to effect educational changes that have had, quite possibly, their greatest impact on scholastic sport opportunities for girls and women. More specifically, the application of Title IX has increased opportunities for female sport participation, financial and educational support for female athletes, and availability of expert training and coaching in public school and collegiate settings.[4]

Although there have been several positive changes in scholastic sport, the advent and enforcement of Title IX have also created a fair amount of ill will within some physical education and athletic departments, especially in the collegiate ranks. Administrative decisions aimed at Title IX compliance have often included a more equitable division of athletic budgets, resulting in spending increases in women's athletics and spending decreases in men's athletics. The female athletes who have benefited most from Title IX have

also suffered, often having to endure unreceptive and even hostile climates within their own athletic departments.

Despite one's philosophical or political bent on Title IX and its impact on school sport, the point of this discussion is that health care providers recognize the possible strife that their athletic patients bring along with their physical health concerns. The climate among male and female athletes, coaches, and administrators at some institutions remains chilly,[1] and the Title IX debate across the United States has become more heated only in the last decade. These dynamics lend further credibility to the proposition that "sport is a microcosm of life," and as such, all athletic participants learn and practice valuable life skills through joyous *and* difficult experiences.

A Title IX Primer

1. Title IX applies to educational institutions receiving direct or indirect federal funding. It does not apply to private settings such as health and fitness clubs.
2. Title IX mandates *equitable* educational opportunities for males and females, and programs can choose to comply in one of three ways:
   a. Substantial proportionality where athletic opportunities for females should be substantially proportionate to the school's enrollment of females, or
   b. Demonstration of a history and continuous practice of expanding options for the underrepresented group, or
   c. To ensure that the interests of women are met.[5]

THE ECONOMICS OF WOMEN'S SPORTS

One of the results of the enforcement of Title IX has been, and continues to be, the increased financial support for female scholastic athletes. As NCAA Division I female participant numbers continue to rise (5% between 1996–1997 and 1997–1998), so does funding of their athletic scholarships (14% increase between 1996–1997 and 1997–1998).[6] Female athletes comprised 40% of Division I athletes in 1997–1998 and received a comparable percentage of athletics-scholarship budgets, 32% of recruiting budgets, and 36% of total team operating budgets.[6] Women's teams have strides to make in terms of receiving an equitable portion of coaching budgets—that same year, coaches of women's teams earned 28% of total salary budgets.[6] Some women's teams have made incredible strides, however. For example the University of Tennessee women's basketball team made a profit of almost $500,000 last year, and their average fan support of 16,559 is greater than the fan support of 13 National Basketball Association (NBA) teams.[6] Moreover, last summer's Women's NBA crowds averaged more than

10,000 per game and continue to grow in popularity along with the Women's National Collegiate Athletic Association tournament crowd.[6]

The phenomenon of increasing participation opportunities for female scholastic athletes has begun to be realized in the realm of professional athletics, where women's participation opportunities are improving. The success of the U.S. Women's Soccer Team and the arrival of professional basketball leagues for women are two examples of new opportunities that are providing collegiate female athletes with access to sport careers. These opportunities are exciting for players and spectators, and are expected to continue growing.

A HEALTHY ENVIRONMENT FOR PERFORMANCE

An effective coach or trainer designs experiences and provides encouragement that maintains a mastery-oriented approach to training and competition. A mastery-oriented approach encourages an athlete to set performance goals that focus on achievements and gains within the athlete's control. Maintaining and improving on personal bests encompass a mastery-oriented approach to training. This same approach can be applied to the process of maintaining or recovering an athlete's physical health. Furthermore, an ego-oriented approach in which the athlete compares herself to other competitors and their successes can be detrimental to motivation, especially during periods of injury or overtraining.

An important part of the mastery-oriented approach is goal setting. Process-oriented goals within an athlete's control and evaluation of these goals are key to improving performance and maintaining or recovering physical health. Outcome goals, such as "place in the top three finishers in the race," may not be helpful. An athlete does not typically control others' performances, and therefore these goals base their success on an uncontrollable entity. Process goals should include realistic short-term goals (weekly through monthly) and long-term goals (monthly through yearly). These goals can be most effective if they are identified and written by the athlete in positive, specific terms. The goals should be measurable (ie, it is clear when they are accomplished). Finally, the performer should reevaluate the goals periodically to assess progress.

For the recreational athlete interested in the health benefits of physical activity, fitness goals may be incorporated into their goal setting. It is advisable to focus on maintaining or improving the five components of health fitness (eg, cardiovascular endurance, muscular endurance, muscular strength, flexibility, and body composition). Certified fitness specialists will have the equipment, knowledge, and skill needed to measure a woman's physical fitness. Exercise and sport science departments at your local university are often an affordable and reliable resource for providing these services.

Adhering to a program of physical activity is sometimes a challenge to the recreational athlete. Furthermore, maintaining the motivation to maintain a rigorous training schedule is a common problem in the ranks of amateur and professional athletes. There are several strategies that athletes can use to improve adherence to exercise and training regimens, including:

1. Select training facilities that are convenient to work or home
2. Exercise at appropriate intensity levels
3. Keep a log of exercise and training activities
4. Make written plans to incorporate exercise or training into your day
5. Use mental imagery during training sessions to focus on external factors, such as surrounding scenery
6. Create visible reminders such as notes or signs that emphasize the value of and past successes associated with exercise and/or training
7. Set process-oriented training goals, evaluate, and enjoy healthy rewards for your accomplishments
8. Recruit a friend or family member to participate in exercise or training sessions
9. Vary your workout activities
10. Plan for and take appropriate rest and recovery periods
11. Choose and participate in activities that you enjoy![7]

What can you do to contribute to a female athlete's continued and healthy participation during periods of injury? Try to avoid marginalization of a person's sport experiences by identifying and recognizing *her* perceived value of that sport experience. Unfortunately, the value of a woman's sport experience is often challenged when an injury occurs. The loss of an athlete's opportunity to participate will likely be significant, despite her level of performance or success. An athlete's feelings of loss about her identity as an athlete, the loss of training time, and physical and mental preparation often accompany injuries. Sincere understanding and encouragement are the requisite part of patient/doctor communication during these difficult periods.

PROVIDING EXCELLENT CARE TO THE FEMALE ATHLETE

Treating the whole athlete is critical to developing and maintaining an athlete's health. This process can be enhanced when a sports medicine professional takes time during a history and physical to identify the nature of a woman's sport experience, especially:

1. The duration, frequency, and intensity of the athlete's training regimen
2. Competition schedule
3. The number of years as a participant in her sport(s)
4. Family and social support perceived by the athlete
5. Training goals and objectives
6. Reason and motivation for participation in her sport(s)
7. Plan for continued participation in sport and/or fitness activities
8. The role that sport participation plays in her life in terms of time and value
9. Sport-related health indicators such as nutrition practices and knowledge
10. Athlete's satisfaction with personal fitness measures, including body composition, muscular endurance, muscular strength, cardiovascular endurance, and flexibility

Furthermore, be willing to recognize and bracket your own biases and beliefs that you may have about female athletes and the sports in which they compete. Knowing your own limitations will be important to establishing rapport and creating an environment that is conducive to questions and patient input.

CONCLUSION

Recognizing the structures and nuances of the social world in which female athletes participate is an important step in understanding the experiences of female athletes. Given the nature of sport and the growing impact that female athletes are having on sport, the need for competent, knowledgeable caretakers will also increase. Those who are sincerely interested in understanding the psychosocial factors associated with female sports participation will benefit most from the opportunities to support, treat, and heal female athletes.

REFERENCES

1. Heywood L. Despite the positive rhetoric about women's sports, female athletes face a culture of sexual harassment. *Chronicle of Higher Education*. January 8, 1999.
2. Cohen GL. Media portrayal of the female athlete. In: Cohen GL, ed. *Women in Sport: Issues and Controversies*. Newbury Park, CA: Sage; 1993:171–184.
3. Title IX of the Education Amendments of 1972 (20 U.S.C. Sec. 1681).
4. Lindgren JR, Taub N. *The Law of Sex Discrimination*. 2nd ed. Minneapolis, MN: West; 1993.
5. Healy PH. A lightning rod on civil rights. *Chronicle of Higher Education*. September 17, 1999.
6. Suggs W. More women participate in collegiate athletics. *Chronicle of Higher Education*. May 21, 1999.
7. Weinberg RS, Gould D. *Foundations of Sport and Exercise Psychology*. 2nd ed. Champaign, IL: Human Kinetics; 1999.

Sources

FOREWORD

Donna Lopiano

Pages xvii–xix Data from presentation by Dr. Donna Lopiano, Executive Director, Women's Sports Foundation, New York, at the *1999 National Institute of Health Workshop*, Marriott Hunt Valley Inn, Hunt Valley, MD, June 11, 1999.

FOREWORD

Camille Duvall

Figure F–1 Courtesy of Camille Duvall, 2000, New York, New York.

Figure F–2 Courtesy of Camille Duvall, 2000, New York, New York.

INTRODUCTION

Figure I–1 Courtesy of the United States Olympic Committee, 2000, Colorado Springs, Colorado.

Figure I–2 Courtesy of the United States Olympic Committee, 2000, Colorado Springs, Colorado.

Figure I–3 Courtesy of the United States Olympic Committee, 2000, Colorado Springs, Colorado.

Figure I–4 Courtesy of the United States Olympic Committee, 2000, Colorado Springs, Colorado.

The Present (p. xxxvi) Data from Women's Sports Foundation, *National Girls and Women in Sports Day Promotional Materials*, East Meadow, New York, 1999.

PROLOGUE

Figure P–1 Courtesy of Kofi Sekyi Amah, 2000, New York, New York.

Figure P–2 Courtesy of Kofi Sekyi Amah, 2000, New York, New York.

Figure P–3 Courtesy of Kofi Sekyi Amah, 2000, New York, New York

Figure P–4 Courtesy of Kofi Sekyi Amah, 2000, New York, New York.

Figure P–5 Courtesy of Kofi Sekyi Amah, 2000, New York, New York.

Table P–1 Reprinted from B.W. Kibler, Determining the Extent of the Functional Deficit, in *Functional Rehabilitation of Sports and Musculoskeletal Injuries*, W.B. Kibler et al., eds., pp. 16–19, (c) 1998, Aspen Publishers, Inc.

Table P–2 Data from T. Field, Massage Therapy in W.B. Joans and J.S. Levin, *Essentials of Complimentary and Alternative Medicine*, pp. 383–391, (c) 1999, Lippincott Williams & Wilkins and J.C. Tan, Physical Modalities, *Practical Manual of Physical Medicine and Rehabilitation*, pp. 133–155, (c) 1998, Mosby.

Table P–3 Data from J.A. Green and R. Shellenberger, Biofeedback Therapy in W.B. Joans and J.S. Levin, *Essentials of Complimentary and Alternative Medicine*, (c) 1999, pp. 410–425, Lippincott Williams & Wilkins and J.C. Tan, Physical Modalities, *Practical Manual of Physical Medicine and Rehabilitation*, (c) 1998, pp. 133–155, Mosby.

CHAPTER 2

Figure 2–1 Courtesy of Mayo Clinic, 1996, Rochester, Minnesota.

Figure 2–2 Courtesy of Mayo Clinic, 2000, Rochester, Minnesota.

Figure 2–3 Courtesy of Mayo Clinic, 2000, Rochester, Minnesota.

Figure 2–4 Courtesy of Mayo Clinic, 2000, Rochester, Minnesota.

Figure 2–5 Courtesy of Mayo Clinic, 2000, Rochester, Minnesota.

Figure 2–6 Courtesy of the American Academy of Orthopaedic Surgeons, 2000, Rosemont, Illinois.

Figure 2–7 Courtesy of Mayo Clinic, 2000, Rochester, Minnesota.

Figure 2–8 Courtesy of Mayo Clinic, 2000, Rochester, Minnesota.

Figure 2–9 Courtesy of Mayo Clinic, 2000, Rochester, Minnesota.

Figure 2–10 Courtesy of Mayo Clinic, 2000, Rochester, Minnesota.

Figure 2–11 Courtesy of Mayo Clinic, 2000, Rochester, Minnesota.

Figure 2–12 Courtesy of Mayo Clinic, 2000, Rochester, Minnesota.

Figure 2–15 Courtesy of Geoffrey Crowley, 2000, Toowong Rehabilitation Centre Pty, Ltd., Toowong, Australia.

Figure 2–16 Courtesy of Geoffrey Crowley, 2000, Toowong Rehabilitation Centre Pty, Ltd., Toowong, Australia.

CHAPTER 3

Figure 3–2 Courtesy of Evanston Hospital, 2000, Evanston, Illinois.

Figure 3–3 Courtesy of Evanston Hospital, 2000, Evanston, Illinois.

Figure 3–4 Courtesy of Evanston Hospital, 2000, Evanston, Illinois.

Figure 3–5 Courtesy of Evanston Hospital, 2000, Evanston, Illinois.

Figure 3–6 Courtesy of Kofi Sekyi Amah, 2000, New York, New York.

Table 3–1 Courtesy of J. Alleva, 2000, Evanston, Illinois.

CHAPTER 4

Exhibit 4–1 Data from Syllabus-exercise Prescription as an Adjunct to Manual Medicine in M.R. Bookout, P.E. Greenman, eds., *Continuing Medical Education Course*, Michigan State University: College of Osteopathic Medicine, September 30–October 2, 1994.

Exhibit 4–2 Reprinted with permission from J. Travell and D. Simons, Myofascial Pain and Dysfunction: *The Trigger Point Manual*, Vol. 2, The Lower Extremities, (c) 1992, Lippincott Williams & Wilkins.

Exhibit 4–3 Reprinted with permission from J. Laycock, Incontinence. Pelvic Floor Re-education. Nursing: *The Journal of Clinical Practice, Education and Management*, now *British Journal of Nursing*, (c) 1991, Vol. 4, No. 39, 15–7 and courtesy of P.E. Chiarelli, 2000, University of New Castle, Callaghan Campus, NSW, Australia.

Exhibit 4–4 Reprinted with permission from W.B. Kibler et al., Principles of Rehabilitation after Chronic Tendon Injuries, *Clinics & Sports Medicine*, (c) 1992, No. 11, pp. 668–669, W.B. Saunders Company.

Exhibit 4–5 Reprinted with permission from W.B. Kibler et al., Principles of Rehabilitation after Chronic Tendon Injuries, *Clinics & Sports Medicine*, (c) 1992, No. 11, pp. 668–669, W.B. Saunders Company.

Exhibit 4–6 Reprinted with permission from W.B. Kibler et al., Principles of Rehabilitation after Chronic Tendon Injuries, *Clinics & Sports Medicine*, (c) 1992, No. 11, pp. 668–669, W.B. Saunders Company.

Figure 4–1 Reprinted with permission from A. Vleeming et al., eds., The Self Blocking Mechanism of the Sacroiliac Joints and Its Implications for Sitting, Standing, and Walking, *Handout for Integrative Function of the Lumbar Spine and Sacroiliac Joint Course* in San Diego, California, November 9–11, p. 154,1995.

Figure 4–2 P. Greenman, *The Principles of Manual Medicine*, 2nd Ed., Figure 17.2, (c) 1996, p. 307, Lippincott Williams & Wilkins.

Figure 4–3 Reprinted with permission from A. Vleeming et al., eds., The Self Blocking Mechanism of the Sacroiliac Joints and Its Implications for Sitting, Standing, and Walking, *Handout for Integrative Function of the Lumbar Spine and Sacroiliac Joint Course* in San Diego, California, November 9–11, p. 478,1995.

Figure 4–4 P. Greenman, *The Principles of Manual Medicine, 2nd Ed.*, Figure 20.15B, (c) 1996, p. 462, Lippincott Williams & Wilkins.

Figure 4–5 Reprinted with permission from R. Don Tigny, Function of the Lumbosacroiliac Complex as a Self Compensating Force Couple with a Variable, Force-Dependent Transverse Axis: A Theoretical Analysis, from *2nd Disciplinary World Congress on Low Back Pain, The Integrated Function of the Lumbar Spine and Sacroiliac Joints*, San Diego, November, 1995, p. 507.

Figure 4–6 Reprinted with permission from J. Travell and D. Simons, *Myofascial Pain and Dysfunction: The Trigger Point Manual*, Vol. 2, The Lower Extremities, (c) 1992, Lippincott Williams & Wilkins.

Figure 4–7 Courtesy of Heidi Prather, D.O., Washington University Hospital, 2000, St. Louis, Missouri.

Figure 4–8 Reprinted with permission from J. Portersfield, Conditions of Weightbearing Asymmetrical Overload Syndrome (AOS), handout, *3rd Interdisciplinary World Congress on Low Back Pain and Pelvic Pain*, p. 253, Vienna, Austria, November 1998,

CHAPTER 5

Clinical Guideline, Classification of Jumper's Knee According to Symptoms (p. 60) Reprinted with permission from M.E. Blazina and R.K. Kerlan et al., Jumper's Knee, *Orthopaedic Clinics of North America*, Vol. 4, No. 3, (c) 1973, pp. 665–678, W.B. Saunders Company.

Clinical Guideline, Considerations in Evaluating Acute Lateral Patella Dislocations (p. 64) J.L. Halbrecht and D.W. Jackson, Acute Dislocation of the Patella, J.M. Fox and W. Del Pizzo, eds. *The Patellofemoral Joint*, (c) 1993, pp. 123–134. Reproduced with permission of The McGraw–Hill Companies.

Clinical Guideline, Rehabilitation Goals (p. 64) L.Y. Griffin, Rehabilitation of the Knee Extensor Mechanism, J.M. Fox and W. Del Pizzo, eds., *The Patellofemoral Joint*, (c) 1993, pp. 279–290. Reproduced with permission of The McGraw-Hill Companies.

Clinical Guideline, Jump-Training Program (p. 81) Reprinted with permission from T.E. Hewett et al., Plyometric Training in Female Athletes, *American Journal of Sports Medicine*, Vol. 24, pp. 765–773, (c) 1996, The American Orthopaedic Society for Sports Medicine.

Clinical Guideline, Glossary of Jump-Training Exercises (p. 82) Reprinted with permission from T.E. Hewett et al., Plyometric Training in Female Athletes, *American Journal of Sports Medicine*, Vol. 24, pp. 765–773, (c) 1996, The American Orthopaedic Society for Sports Medicine.

Clinical Guideline, Stretching and Weight-Training Program (p. 82) Reprinted with permission from T.E. Hewett et al., Plyometric Training in Female Athletes, *American Journal of Sports Medicine*, Vol. 24, pp. 765–773, (c) 1996, The American Orthopaedic Society for Sports Medicine.

Clinical Guideline, Rehabilitation for Acute Traumatic Dislocation of the Patella (p. 85) L.Y. Griffin, Rehabilitation of the Knee Extensor Mechanism, *The Patellofemoral Joint*, J.M. Fox and W. Del Pizzo, eds. pp. 279–290. Reproduced with permission of The McGraw-Hill Companies.

Clinical Guideline, Rehabilitation for Patellofemoral Stress Syndrome (p. 86) L.Y. Griffin, Rehabilitation of the Knee Extensor Mechanism, *The Patellofemoral Joint*, J.M. Fox and W. Del Pizzo, eds. pp. 279–290. Reproduced with permission of The McGraw-Hill Companies.

Clinical Guideline, Accelerated Rehabilitation for ACL Petellar Tendon Graft (PTG) Reconstruction (Isolated), (p. 86) Reprinted with permission from K. Wilk, et al., Rehabilitation after Anterior Cruciate Ligament Reconstruction in the Female Athlete, *Journal of Athletic Training*, Vol. 34, No. 2, pp. 177–193, (c) 1999, Figure 3, National Athletic Trainers' Association.

Clinical Guideline, Female ACL Rehabilitation: Special Considerations and Specific Exercise Drills (p. 89) Reprinted with permission from K. Wilk, et al., Rehabilitation after Anterior Cruciate Ligament Reconstruction in the Female Athlete, *Journal of Athletic Training*, Vol. 34, No. 2, pp. 177–193, (c) 1999, Figure 4, National Athletic Trainers' Association.

Figure 5–1 Reprinted with permission from S. Dye et al., Conscious Neurosensory Mapping of the Internal Structures of the Human Knee Without Intraarticular Anesthesia, *American Journal of Sports Medicine*, Vol. 26, pp. 773–777, (c) 1998, The American Orthopaedic Society for Sports Medicine.

Figure 5–2 Reprinted with permission from J.A. Goss and R.F. Adams, Location Injection of Corticosteroids in Rheumatic Diseases, Journal of Musculoskeletal Medicine, Vol. 10, (c) 1993, pp. 83–92, *Journal of Musculoskeletal Medicine*.

Figure 5–3 Reprinted by permission from J.V. Ciullo, 1993, "Lower Extremity Injuries" in *The Athletic Female*, edited by A.J. Pearl (Champaign, IL: Human Kinetics), 270.

Figure 5–4 F.H. Fu and M.J. Seel et al., Patellofemoral Biomechanics in *The Patellofemoral Joint*, J.M. Fox and W. Del Pizzo, eds., pp. 49–62. Reproduced with permission of The McGraw-Hill Companies.

Figure 5–5 Reprinted with permission of M.H. Bourne, et al., Anterior Knee Pain, *Mayo Clinic Proceedings*, Vol. 63, No. 5, pp. 482–491, (c) 1988, Mayo Clinic Proceedings.

Figure 5–6 R.D. Ferkel, Lateral Retinacular Release, J.M. Fox and W. Del Pizzo, eds., *The Patellofemoral Joint*, (c) 1993, pp. 309–323. Reproduced with permission of The McGraw-Hill Companies.

Figure 5–7 Reprinted with permission of M.H. Bourne, et al., Anterior Knee Pain, *Mayo Clinic Proceedings*, Vol. 63, No. 5, pp. 482–491, (c) 1988, Mayo Clinic Proceedings.

Figure 5–8 Reprinted from Sports Medicine 1990; 10(2):132–138 with permission. (c) Adis International, Inc.

Figure 5–9 D. Patel and C.T. Laurencin et al., Synovial Folds plicae, in *The Patellofemoral Joint*, J.M. Fox and W. Del Pizzo, eds., pp. 193–198. Reproduced with permission of The McGraw–Hill Companies.

Figure 5–10 Reprinted by permission from J.V. Ciullo, 1993, "Lower Extremity Injuries" in *The Athletic Female*, edited by A.J. Pearl (Champaign, IL: Human Kinetics), 278.

Figure 5–11 Courtesy of Cincinnati Sportsmedicine and Orthopaedic Center, 2000, Cincinnati, Ohio.

Figure 5–12 Courtesy of Cincinnati Sportsmedicine and Orthopaedic Center, 2000, Cincinnati, Ohio.

Figure 5–13 Courtesy of Cincinnati Sportsmedicine and Orthopaedic Center, 2000, Cincinnati, Ohio.

Figure 5–14 Courtesy of Cincinnati Sportsmedicine and Orthopaedic Center, 2000, Cincinnati, Ohio.

Figure 5–15 Courtesy of Cincinnati Sportsmedicine and Orthopaedic Center, 2000, Cincinnati, Ohio.

Figure 5–16 J.L. Halbrecht and D.W. Jackson, Acute Dislocation of the Patella, J.M. Fox and W. Del Pizzo, eds. *The Patellofemoral Joint*, (c) 1993, pp. 123–134. Reproduced with permission of The McGraw-Hill Companies.

Figure 5–17 R.D. Ferkel, Lateral Retinacular Release, J.M. Fox and W. Del Pizzo, eds., *The Patellofemoral Joint*, (c) 1993, pp. 309–323. Reproduced with permission from The McGraw-Hill Companies.

Figure 5–18 J.G. Aronen et al.: Practical, Conservative Management of Iliotibial Band Syndrome, *The Physician and Sportsmedicine*, Vol. 21, No. 6, Fig. 1 only, p. 60, (c) 1993. Reproduced with permission of The McGraw-Hill Companies.

Figure 5–19 Reprinted with permission from E.A. Arendt, J. Agel et al., Anterior Cruciate Ligament Injury Patterns among Collegiate Men and Women, *Journal of Athletic Training*, Vol. 34, No. 2, (c) 1999, pp. 86–92, Hughston Sports Medicine Foundation, Inc.

Figure 5–20 Reprinted with permission from Principles of Diagnosis and Treatment, *The Crucial Ligaments*, J.A. Feagin, ed., (c) 1988, Churchill Livingstone/W.B. Saunders Company.

Figure 5–21 Courtesy of Cincinnati Sportsmedicine and Orthopaedic Center, 2000, Cincinnati, Ohio.

Figure 5–23 Courtesy of Cincinnati Sportsmedicine and Orthopaedic Center, 2000, Cincinnati, Ohio.

Figure 5–24 Courtesy of Cincinnati Sportsmedicine and Orthopaedic Center, 2000, Cincinnati, Ohio.

Figure 5–25 Courtesy of Cincinnati Sportsmedicine and Orthopaedic Center, 2000, Cincinnati, Ohio.

Figure 5–26 Courtesy of Cincinnati Sportsmedicine and Orthopaedic Center, 2000, Cincinnati, Ohio.

Figure 5–27 Courtesy of Cincinnati Sportsmedicine and Orthopaedic Center, 2000, Cincinnati, Ohio.

Figure 5–28 Courtesy of Cincinnati Sportsmedicine and Orthopaedic Center, 2000, Cincinnati, Ohio.

Figure 5–29 Courtesy of Cincinnati Sportsmedicine and Orthopaedic Center, 2000, Cincinnati, Ohio.

Figure 5–30 Courtesy of Cincinnati Sportsmedicine and Orthopaedic Center, 2000, Cincinnati, Ohio.

Figure 5–31 Courtesy of Cincinnati Sportsmedicine and Orthopaedic Center, 2000, Cincinnati, Ohio.

Figure 5–32 Courtesy of Cincinnati Sportsmedicine and Orthopaedic Center, 2000, Cincinnati, Ohio.

Figure 5–33 Reprinted with permission from D.M. Daniel et al., Use of the Quadriceps Active Test to Diagnose Posterior Cruciate-ligament Disruption and Measure Posterior Laxity of the Knee, *Journal of Bone & Joint Surgery*, Vol. 70A, No. 3, pp. 386–391, (c) 1988, Journal of Bone and Joint Surgery.

Figure 5–34 Reprinted with permission of C.D. Harner and J. Hoher, Evaluation and Treatment of Posterior Cruciate Ligament Injuries, *American Journal of Sports Medicine*, Vol. 26, pp. 471–482, (c) 1998, The American Orthopaedic Society for Sports Medicine.

Figure 5–35 Reprinted with permission from P.A. Indelicato, Injury to the Medial Capsuloligamentous Complex, *The Crucial Ligaments*, J.A. Feagin, ed., pp. 197–206, (c) 1988, Churchill Livingstone/W.B. Saunders Company.

Figure 5–36 Reprinted with permission from R. Warren et al., Anatomy of the Knee in J.A. Nicholas and E.B. Hershman, eds., *The Lower Extremity and Spine in Sports Medicine*, (c) 1986, pp. 657–694, CV Mosby.

Figure 5–39 Courtesy of Cincinnati Sportsmedicine and Orthopaedic Center, 2000, Cincinnati, Ohio.

Figure 5–40 Courtesy of Cincinnati Sportsmedicine and Orthopaedic Center, 2000, Cincinnati, Ohio.

Figure 5–41 Courtesy of Cincinnati Sportsmedicine and Orthopaedic Center, 2000, Cincinnati, Ohio.

Figure 5–42 M.L. Ireland, Anterior Cruciate Ligament Injury in Female Athletes: Epidemiology, *Journal of Athletic Training*, Vol. 34, No. 2, pp. 150–154, (c) 1999, National Athletic Trainers' Association.

CHAPTER 6

Figure 6–1 Courtesy of Nadya Swedan, M.D., (c) 2000, New York, New York.

Figure 6–2 Courtesy of Nadya Swedan, M.D., (c) 2000, New York, New York.

Figure 6–6 Courtesy of Nadya Swedan, M.D., 2000, New York, New York.

Figure 6–7 Courtesy of Kofi Sekyi Amah, 2000, New York, New York.

CHAPTER 7

Figure 7–1 Adapted with permission from C.C. Norkin and P.K. Levangie, *Joint Structure and Function*, p. 451, (c) 1992, FA Davis Company.

Figure 7–2 Courtesy Richard Jackson, PT, OCS, 2000.

Figure 7–3 Courtesy Richard Jackson, PT, OCS, 2000.

Figure 7–4 Adapted with permission from C.C. Norkin and P.K. Levangie, *Joint Structure and Function*, p. 451, (c) 1992, FA Davis Company.

Figure 7–5 Adapted with permission from C.C. Norkin and P.K. Levangie, *Joint Structure and Function*, p. 451, (c) 1992, FA Davis Company.

CHAPTER 8

Appendix 8–A Courtesy of Carol Mushett, 2000, Atlanta, Georgia.
Figure 8–1 Courtesy of Harper Run Communications, 2000, Battle Creek, Michigan.

CHAPTER 9

Figure 9–1 Courtesy of Castlemead Publications, 1999, Hertfordshire, United Kingdom.
Figure 9–2 Courtesy of Castlemead Publications, 1999, Hertfordshire, United Kingdom.
Figure 9–3 Reprinted with permission from S.M. Tanner, The Tanner Stages, *Clinics and Sports Medicine*, Vol. 13, No. 2, pp. 337–353, (c) 1994, W.B. Saunders Company.
Figure 9–A1 Courtesy of Judy Anne Donahue, ATC, 2000, Rockville Centre, New York.
Figure 9–A2 Courtesy of Judy Anne Donahue, ATC, 2000, Rockville Centre, New York.
Figure 9–A3 Courtesy of Judy Anne Donahue, ATC, 2000, Rockville Centre, New York.
Figure 9–A4 Courtesy of Judy Anne Donahue, ATC, 2000, Rockville Centre, New York.
Figure 9–A5 Courtesy of Judy Anne Donahue, ATC, 2000, Rockville Centre, New York.
Figure 9–A6 Courtesy of Judy Anne Donahue, ATC, 2000, Rockville Centre, New York.
Figure 9–A7 Courtesy of Judy Anne Donahue, ATC, 2000, Rockville Centre, New York.
Figure 9–A8 Courtesy of Judy Anne Donahue, ATC, 2000, Rockville Centre, New York.
Figure 9–A9 Courtesy of Judy Anne Donahue, ATC, 2000, Rockville Centre, New York.
Figure 9–A10 Courtesy of Judy Anne Donahue, ATC, 2000, Rockville Centre, New York.
Figure 9–A11 Courtesy of Judy Anne Donahue, ATC, 2000, Rockville Centre, New York.
Figure 9–A12 Courtesy of Judy Anne Donahue, ATC, 2000, Rockville Centre, New York.
Figure 9–A13 Courtesy of Judy Anne Donahue, ATC, 2000, Rockville Centre, New York.

CHAPTER 10

Figure 10–1 D.C. Cumming et al.: Defects in Pulsatile LH Release in Normally Menstruating Runner, *Journal of Clinical Endocrinology and Metabolism*, No. 60, pp. 810–812, 1985; (c) The Endocrine Society.
Figure 10–2 A.B. Loucks et al., Alterations in the Hypothalamic-Pituitary-Adrenal Axes in Athletic Women, *Journal of Clinical Endocrinology and Metabolism*, No. 68, pp. 402–411, 1989; (c) The Endocrine Society.
Figure 10–3 A.B. Loucks et al., Alterations in the Hypothalamic-Pituitary-Adrenal Axes in Athletic Women, *Journal of Clinical Endocrinology and Metabolism*, No. 68, pp. 402–411, 1989; (c) The Endocrine Society.
Figure 10–4 D.C. Cumming et al.: Defects in Pulsatile LH Release in Normally Menstruating Runner, *Journal of Clinical Endocrinology and Metabolism*, No. 60, pp. 810–812, 1985; (c) The Endocrine Society.

CHAPTER 11

Clinical Guideline, Daily Nutritional Needs of Pregnancy (p. 177) Data *from Recommended Dietary Allowances, 10th Ed.*, The Food and Nutrition Board, National Research Council, National Academy Press, (c) 1989, J. Hautvast, Adequate Nutrition in Pregnancy Does Matter, (c) 1997, and M. Brown, Nutrition in Female Athletes.
Figure 11–1 Reprinted by permission of FA Davis Company, Cailliet R.: *Low Back Pain Syndrome*, Ed. 5. FA Davis, Philadelphia, 1962,1968, 1981, 1988, 1995.
Figure 11–2 Courtesy of Kofi Sekyi Amah, 2000, New York, New York.
Figure 11–3 Courtesy of Kofi Sekyi Amah, 2000, New York, New York.
Figure 11–4 Courtesy of OPTP, 2000, Minneapolis, Minnesota.
Figure 11–5 Courtesy of N. Swedan, M.D., 2000, New York, New York.
Figure 11–6 Courtesy of N. Swedan, M.D., 2000, New York, New York.

CHAPTER 12

Figure 12–1 Courtesy of OPTP, 2000, Minneapolis, Minnesota.
Figure 12–2 Courtesy of Judy Anne Donahue, ATC, 2000, Rockville Centre, New York.
Figure 12–A1 Courtesy of Judy Anne Donahue, ATC, 2000, Rockville Centre, New York.
Figure 12–A2 Courtesy of Judy Anne Donahue, ATC, 2000, Rockville Centre, New York.
Figure 12–A3 Courtesy of Judy Anne Donahue, ATC, 2000, Rockville Centre, New York.
Figure 12–A4 Courtesy of Judy Anne Donahue, ATC, 2000, Rockville Centre, New York.
Figure 12–A5 Courtesy of Judy Anne Donahue, ATC, 2000, Rockville Centre, New York.
Figure 12–A6 Courtesy of Judy Anne Donahue, ATC, 2000, Rockville Centre, New York.
Figure 12–A7 Courtesy of Judy Anne Donahue, ATC, 2000, Rockville Centre, New York.

Figure 12–A8 Courtesy of Judy Anne Donahue, ATC, 2000, Rockville Centre, New York.

Figure 12–A9 Courtesy of Judy Anne Donahue, ATC, 2000, Rockville Centre, New York.

Figure 12–A10 Courtesy of Judy Anne Donahue, ATC, 2000, Rockville Centre, New York.

Figure 12–B1 Courtesy of Judy Anne Donahue, ATC, 2000, Rockville Centre, New York.

Figure 12–B2 Courtesy of Judy Anne Donahue, ATC, 2000, Rockville Centre, New York.

Figure 12–B3 Courtesy of Judy Anne Donahue, ATC, 2000, Rockville Centre, New York.

Figure 12–B4 Courtesy of Judy Anne Donahue, ATC, 2000, Rockville Centre, New York.

Figure 12–B5 Courtesy of Judy Anne Donahue, ATC, 2000, Rockville Centre, New York.

Figure 12–B6 Courtesy of Judy Anne Donahue, ATC, 2000, Rockville Centre, New York.

Figure 12–B7 Courtesy of Judy Anne Donahue, ATC, 2000, Rockville Centre, New York.

Figure 12–B8 Courtesy of Judy Anne Donahue, ATC, 2000, Rockville Centre, New York.

Figure 12–B9 Courtesy of Judy Anne Donahue, ATC, 2000, Rockville Centre, New York.

Figure 12–B10 Courtesy of Judy Anne Donahue, ATC, 2000, Rockville Centre, New York.

CHAPTER 14

Figure 14–1 Courtesy of Jeff Caven Photography, 1999, Taos, New Mexico.

CHAPTER 16

Figure 16–1 Courtesy of N. Swedan, M.D., 2000, New York, New York.

Figure 16–2 Courtesy of N. Swedan, M.D., 2000, New York, New York.

CHAPTER 17

Figure 17–2 Reprinted by permission of the American Cancer Society, Inc.

Figure 17–3 Courtesy of Sandra K. Hoffman, M.D. 2000, Kalamazoo, Michigan.

Figure 17–4 Courtesy of Kofi Sekyi Amah, 2000, New York, New York and Asics Corporation, 2000, Kobe, Japan.

Figure 17–5 Courtesy of Kofi Sekyi Amah, 2000, New York, New York and Asics Corporation, 2000, Kobe, Japan.

Figure 17–6 Courtesy of Kofi Sekyi Amah, 2000, New York, New York and Asics Corporation, 2000, Kobe, Japan.

Figure 17–7 Courtesy of Sandra J. Hoffman, M.D., 2000, Kalamazoo, Michigan.

CHAPTER 18

Clinical Guideline, Optimal Calcium Intake (p. 277) Adapted from NIH Consensus Conference. Optimal Calcium Intake. NIH Consensus Development Panel on Optimal Calcium Intake. Journal of the American Medical Association, 272, pp. 1942–1948, 1994.

Figure 18–1 By permission of Mayo Foundation.

Figure 18–2 Reprinted with permission from C. Johnston et al., Calcium Supplementation and Increase in Bone Mineral Density in Children, The *New England Journal of Medicine*, Vol. 327, pp. 82–87. Copyright (c) 1992 Massachusetts Medical Society. All rights reserved.

Figure 18–3 Reprinted from Anonymous, Effects of Hormone Therapy on Bone Mineral Density: Results from the Postmenopausal Estrogen/Progestin Interventions (PEPI) Trial. The Writing Group for the PEPI, *Journal of the American Medical Association*, Vol. 276, 1996, pp. 1389–1396.

Figure 18–4 Reproduced from Journal of *Bone and Mineral Research*, 1999, 14S1, S158 with permission of the American Society for Bone & Mineral Research.

Figure 18–5 Reproduced from Journal of *Bone and Mineral Research*, 1992, 7: 761–769, with permission of the American Society for Bone & Mineral Research.

Figure 18–6 Reproduced from Journal of *Bone and Mineral Research* 1997;12:255–260 with permission of the American Society for Bone and Mineral Research.

Figure 18–7 Reproduced from Journal *of Bone and Mineral Research*, 1995; 10: 1788–1795 with permission of the American Society for Bone & Mineral Research.

Figure 18–8 Reproduced from Journal of *Bone and Mineral Research* 1995; 10: 1015–1024 with permission of the American Society for Bone & Mineral Research.

Figure 18–9 Reprinted with permission from M.L. Rencken and C.H. Chesnut, Bone Density at Multiple Skeletal Sites in Amenorrheic Athletes, *Journal of the American Medical Association*, Vol. 276, pp. 238–240. Copyrighted 1996, American Medical Association.

Figure 18–10 Courtesy of Mayo Clinic and Foundation, 2000, Rochester, Minnesota.

Figure 18–11 Courtesy of Mayo Clinic and Foundation, 2000, Rochester, Minnesota.

Figure 18–12 Courtesy of Mayo Clinic and Foundation, 2000, Rochester, Minnesota.

Figure 18–13 Courtesy of Mayo Clinic and Foundation, 2000, Rochester, Minnesota.

CHAPTER 19

Clinical Guideline, Diagnostic Criteria for Anorexia Nervosa (p. 299) Reprinted with permission from the *Diagnostic and Statistical Manual of Mental Disorders*, Fourth

Edition. Copyright 1994 American Psychiatric Association.

Clinical Guideline, Diagnostic Criteria for Bulimia Nervosa (p. 299) Reprinted with permission from the Diagnostic and Statistical Manual of Mental Disorders, Fourth Edition. Copyright 1994 American Psychiatric Association.

Clinical Guideline, Age of Menarche in Populations of Athletes (p. 302) Reprinted by permission from M.J. De Souza, J.C. Arce, D.A. Metzger, 1994, Endocrine basis of exercise-induced amenorrhea. In *Women and Sports: Interdisciplinary Perspectives*, edited by D.M. Costa and S.R. Guthrie.

Figure 19–1 Reprinted from *Clinical Endocrinology: An Illustrated Text*, 2nd Ed., G.M. Besser, p. 12.12, 1987, by permission of the publisher, Mosby.

Figure 19–2 Copyright 1999. Icon Learning Systems, LLC, a subsidiary of Havas MediMedia USA Inc. with permission from ICON Learning Systems, LLC, illustrated by Frank H. Netter, MD. All rights reserved.

CHAPTER 20

Appendix 20–A Reprinted with permission from American Academy of Pediatrics Committee on Sports Medicine and Fitness: Medical Conditions Affecting Sports Participation. *Pediatrics*. 1994;94(5);757–760.

Clinical Guideline, Sports Concussion Guidelines (p. 325) Adapted with permission from J.P. Kelly and J.H. Rosenberg, Diagnosis and Management of Concussion in Sports, *Neurology*, Vol. 48, (c) 1997, pp. 575–580, Lippincott Williams & Wilkins.

Exhibit 20–1 Reprinted with permission from J.E. Peltz et al., Summary Report of History Questionnaire, Stanford University, PPE *Medicine & Science in Sports & Exercise*, (c) 1999, Vol. 31, No. 2, p. 1730, Lippincott Williams & Wilkins.

Exhibit 20–4 Reprinted with permission from American Academy of Pediatrics Committee on Sports Medicine and Fitness: Medical Conditions Affecting Sports Participation. *Pediatrics*. 1994;94(5);757–760.

Exhibit 20–5 Reprinted with permission from G.P. Gidwani and E.S. Rome, Eating Disorders, *Clinical Obstetrics and Gynecology*, (c) 1997, Vol. 40, pp. 604, Table 2, Lippincott Williams & Wilkins.

CHAPTER 22

Anecdotal Testimony (p. 348) Courtesy of N. DiNubile, M.D., 1999, Philadelphia, Pennsylvania.

Anecdotal Testimony (p. 348) Courtesy of Carole Oglesby, 1999, Philadelphia, Pennsylvania.

Clinical Guideline, Topics of Injury Education (p. 349) Reprinted by permission from J. Heil, 1993, *Psychology of Sport Injury*, (Champaign, IL:Human Kinetics), 141.

CHAPTER 23

Figure 23–1 Reprinted with permission from N. Gledhill, Blood Doping and Related Issues: A Brief Review, *Medical Science Sports Exercise*, Vol. 14, p. 185, (c) 1982, Lippincott Williams & Wilkins.

Index